Diving Medicine

W0050835

Olaf Rusoke-Dierich

Diving Medicine

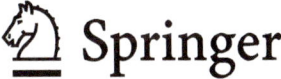 Springer

Olaf Rusoke-Dierich
Townsville, Queensland, Australia

Translated from the original German edition 'Tauchmedizin' by Olaf Rusoke-Dierich
© Springer-Verlag GmbH Deutschland 2017; ISBN 978-3-662-49853-8

ISBN 978-3-030-08865-1   ISBN 978-3-319-73836-9   (eBook)
https://doi.org/10.1007/978-3-319-73836-9

© Springer International Publishing AG, part of Springer Nature 2018
Softcover re-print of the Hardcover 1st edition 2018
This work is subject to copyright. All rights are reserved by the Publisher, whether the whole or part of the material is concerned, specifically the rights of translation, reprinting, reuse of illustrations, recitation, broadcasting, reproduction on microfilms or in any other physical way, and transmission or information storage and retrieval, electronic adaptation, computer software, or by similar or dissimilar methodology now known or hereafter developed.
The use of general descriptive names, registered names, trademarks, service marks, etc. in this publication does not imply, even in the absence of a specific statement, that such names are exempt from the relevant protective laws and regulations and therefore free for general use.
The publisher, the authors and the editors are safe to assume that the advice and information in this book are believed to be true and accurate at the date of publication. Neither the publisher nor the authors or the editors give a warranty, express or implied, with respect to the material contained herein or for any errors or omissions that may have been made. The publisher remains neutral with regard to jurisdictional claims in published maps and institutional affiliations.

Printed on acid-free paper

This Springer imprint is published by the registered company Springer International Publishing AG part of Springer Nature
The registered company address is: Gewerbestrasse 11, 6330 Cham, Switzerland

Preface

When I wrote the chapters of diving medicine as a medical student in 1994–1996, I tried to make it both easy to understand and medically profound. At that time I was a divemaster, and as I loved both scuba diving and free diving, I frequently went to the Red Sea for diving. After publishing the chapters for physiology and diving medicine, I wrote other chapters about diving history, physics and diving equipment. Being a young doctor and father at the same time, I was too busy to finish them off. Later I worked in hyperbaric chambers in Bremen and Hamburg, and then I moved to Australia and worked for years in different emergency departments. During that time, I also finished off my dissertation in medicine. Since 2007, I worked as a GP and completed my specialisation in this field. Recently, I re-discovered my book and updated it to the newest standard. I tried to make this a comprehensible, precise and compendious book. I am looking forward to feedback about the contents of this book to email: divemedforum@yahoo.com. With hopefully much constructive response, this book might be in its potentially future editions grow. As I imagined everything I read, I edited lots of pictures and graphs to illustrate the information. I was fascinated by complex theories of decompression, like the nucleation theory, and also tried to summarise the essence of core contents.

Olaf Rusoke-Dierich
Townsville, QLD, Australia

Acknowledgements

Many thanks to my wife, Judith, for her motivation and support.

Many thanks to my father Wolfgang Dierich. He himself has published several books. One of it was "Das große Handbuch der Flieger" (Manual for Pilots). He was an inspiration and encouraged me to follow his steps.

Many thanks to Dr. med. Peusch-Dreyer, Dr. med. Gensler and Dr. med. Lutz. They gave me the opportunity to practice hyperbaric medicine.

Many thanks to Hubertus Bartmann. He gave me the opportunity to publish my first chapter about diving physiology and medicine in his Diving Manual, Ecomed Publishing.

Many thanks in particular to Dr. Bruce Wienke. With his help and review, I was able to produce the ▶ Chaps. 9 "Decompression Theory". He supplied me with extremely helpful information and inspired my fascination with bubbles and physics. I hope this will help me to contribute in this field in the future.

Also thanks to my friend, Dr. Ken Stark, who constantly encouraged me to make a "different" book and made sure that I set my priorities and focused on my book. He was always pleased to see me having switched on my computer, iPhone and iPad and ready to go.

Many thanks to Springer Publishing and its entire team for helping me to produce this book. I received lots of professional and friendly support from them in this project.

Many thanks to the inventor of the Internet. Though the information is readily available on the Internet, it must be reviewed critically.

And finally, many thanks to the reader.

Contents

III   Diving Physiology and Anatomy

IV   Diving Medicine

Abbreviations

ABT	Actual Bottom Time	ECG	Electrocardiography
ACD	Air Consumption Depth	ECHM	European Committee for Hyperbaric Medicine
ADH	Antidiuretic Hormone		
AED	Automatic External Defibrilator	EDTC	European Diving Technology Committee
AGE	Arterial Gas Embolism		
AIDA	Association International pour le Développement de l'Apnée	EEG	Electroencephalography
		EHS	Exertional Heat Stroke
ANP	Atrial Natriuretic Peptide	END	Equivalent Narcotic Depth
ANS	Autonomic Nervous System	ENT	Ear, Nose and Throat
ARDS	Adult Respiratory Distress Syndrome	EOS	Equation of State
ASTM	Asymmetric Tissue Model	ESD	European Scientific Diver
AV	Atrioventricular		
		FEV_1	Forced Expiratory Volume
BCD	Buoyancy Control Device	FSW	Feet of Sea Water
BHR	Bronchial Hyperreactivity	FVC	Forced Vital Capacity
BMI	Body Mass Index		
BNP	Brain Natriuretic Peptide	GIBT	Gastrointestinal Barotrauma
BT	Barotrauma		
BTPS	Body Temperature and Pressure, Saturated	H_2	Hydrogen
		HBO	Hyperbaric Oxygenation
BW	Body Weight	He	Helium
		HPNS	High-Pressure Nervous Syndrome
Ca	Calcium	HSA	Handicapped Scuba Association
$CaCO_3$	Calcium Carbonate		
CAGE	Cerebral Arterial Gas Embolism	IAHD	International Association of Handi-capped Divers
CMAS	Confédération Mondiale des Activités Subaquatiques		
		IAND	International Association of Nitrox Divers
CNS	Central Nervous System		
CO_2	Carbon Dioxide	IANTD	International Association of Nitrox and Technical Divers
COPD	Chronic Obstructive Pulmonary Disease		
		ICAM	Intracellular Adhesion Molecule
CPR	Cardiopulmonary Resuscitation	IDA	International Divers Association
CT	Computer Tomography	IEBT	Inner Ear Barotrauma
CVGE	Cerebral Venous Gas Embolism	IEDCS	Inner Ear Decompression Sickness
		LEM	Linear-Exponential Model
DAN	Divers Alert Network		
DBT	Dental Barotrauma	MET	Metabolic Equivalent of Task
DCI	Decompression Illness	MOD	Maximum Operation Depth
DCS	Decompression Sickness	MRI	Magnetic Resonance Imaging
DM	Diffusion Model	MSW	Meter of Sea Water
DON	Dysbaric Osteonecrosis	MTM	Multitissue Model
EAD	Equivalent Air Depth	N_2	Nitrogen
EAN	Enriched Air Nitrox	NBO	Normobaric Oxygen Therapy

NEHS	Nonexertional Heat Stroke	RDP	Recreational Dive Planner
Nitrox	Nitrogen Oxygen Gas Mixture	RGBM	Reduced Gradient Bubble Model
NO	Nitrous Oxide	RNT	Residual Nitrogen Time
NOS	Nitrous Oxide Synthase	ROS	Reactive Oxygen Species
np	Negative Pressure	RV	Residual Volume
NSBT	Nasal Sinus Barotrauma		
		SAC	Surface Air Consumption Rate
O_2	Oxygen	SBT	Skin Barotrauma
OBT	Ocular Barotrauma	SCUBA	Self-Contained Underwater Breathing Apparatus
OTU	Oxygen Tolerance Unit		
		SPGM	Split Phase Gradient Model
PADI	Professional Association of Diving Instructors	SSI	Scuba Schools International
		STPD	Standard Temperature, Pressure and Dry
PBT	Pulmonary Barotrauma		
pCO_2	Carbon Dioxide Partial Pressure	TBT	Total Bottom Time
PEEP	Positive End-Expiratory Pressure	TBT	Tympanic Membrane Barotrauma
PEF	Peak Expiratory Flow	TK	Total Lung Capacity
PFO	Patent Foramen Ovale	TM	Thermodynamic Model
pH	Acid-Base Unit	TT	Tank Time
pN_2	Nitrogen Partial Pressure		
PNS	Peripheral Nervous System	UPTD	Unit Pulmonary Toxic Dose
pO_2	Oxygen Partial Pressure	UV	Ultraviolet Radiation
pp	Positive Pressure		
P_{ss}	Supersaturation Gradient	VC	Vital Capacity
P_{us}	Undersaturation Gradient	VGE	Venous Gas Embolism
		VPM	Variable Permeability Model

Introduction

Contents

Diving History

© Springer International Publishing AG, part of Springer Nature 2018
O. Rusoke-Dierich, *Diving Medicine*, https://doi.org/10.1007/978-3-319-73836-9_1

1

Diving is not a particular invention of modern society. Seas have vast quantities of food and treasures. Therefore, diving was already used since ancient times to recover shells, pearls, sponges or dye. To explore the underwater world, mankind developed more or less usable tools to do so. Only recently diving was made accessible for everyone. Unfortunately, this isn't to the benefit of all. This still relatively pristine sensitive habitat is disturbed by diving tourism. On the other side, more and more people, who discovered the miracles under water, campaign for the preservation of the marine environment.

1.1 Diving in Ancient Times

Diving in ancient times primarily served the gathering of food, tools and jewellery. For example the purple colour of specific snails, which had to be brought up from under water, was more expensive than gold at certain times. It was a very popular dye for colouring textiles. It was only available to the rich. The coloured fabrics signalled power and wealth. Raw materials like corals, pearls and mother of pearl were used to decorate artisan objects as well as jewellery or used as currency. Early findings from archaeology in the rubble of Bismaya (Babylon) from 4500 BC prove that pearls were already available as this time. In ancient Egypt (approx. 3000 BC) mother of pearl, pearls, sponges, purple dye and coral were common trading objects. These items were partly imported from the West Coast of India. All this suggests that already at this time diving was used to recover these assets.

The first written reports about diving originated from ancient Greece. *Aristotle* described the work of sponge divers in the third century before Christ. One must assume that the divers have reached depths of about 30 m at the time and stayed there for 2–3 min. Some of the sponge divers used diving bells, which extended their diving time by supplying additional air. Certainly, there must have been many diving accidents, because little was known about diving physics at this time. Aristotle mentioned even the first decompression disorders, particularly of skeletal changes.

There are several documents from the Greek historiography, such as *Heodot* and *Thucydides*, which showed the use of divers for warlike purposes. Divers equipped with reed pipes, which were used as snorkels, approached ships of enemies and ripped out their anchor ropes. These ships then drifted off and ran aground or against cliffs. Also clay pots or leather bags as breathing devices were described. However, whether they really were used is doubtful, because weights to counteract buoyancy would have been necessary and air supply would have been only very limited. It seems more likely that the description of these devices were rather created for dramaturgical effects.

Alexander the Great (335 BC) was watching elephants, wading through deep water by breathing with their trunks. This triggered his interest for exploring the underwater world. Diving bells made of wood were constructed for military purposes. This "cymbas amphidromes" resembled 2-m wooden barrels, which were sealed with tar and held together with bronze bands. The opening was facing downwards to get in and out. Inside was a bench to sit on. Alexander together with his companion Nearchus dived down in one of these barrels. Weighted with copper bars and stones, they sank. After reaching the surface, Alexander was doing well, but his companion, however, was unconscious. The two of them must had have struggled underwater, because they had to breath in and out into the barrel, which certainly caused carbon dioxide levels to increase dramatically. Since not oxygen but carbon dioxide triggers respiratory response, their shortness of breath must have been quite considerable.

There were other reports of diving about military divers from ancient Rome. *Pliny the Elder* denounced that people put themselves in danger not only in harvesting food but also in collecting raw material for luxury items. In ancient China diving must have been a common practice too, because mother of pearl, coral, sponges and pearl were used frequently (◼ Fig. 1.1).

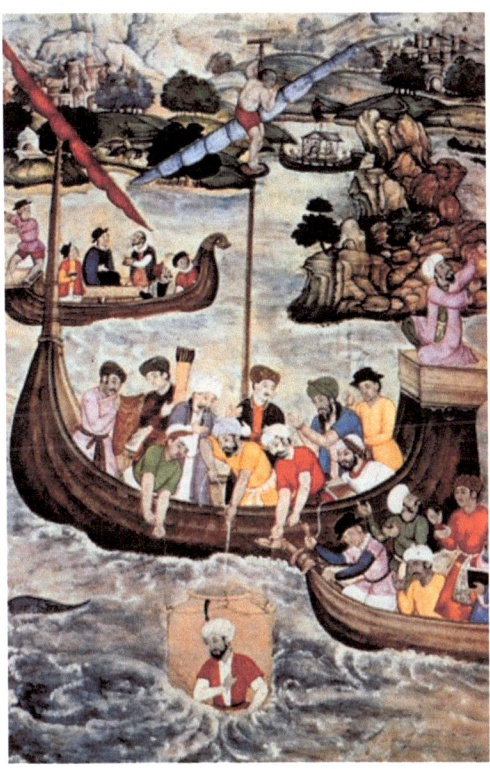

□ **Fig. 1.1** Alexander the Great. (Wikipedia)

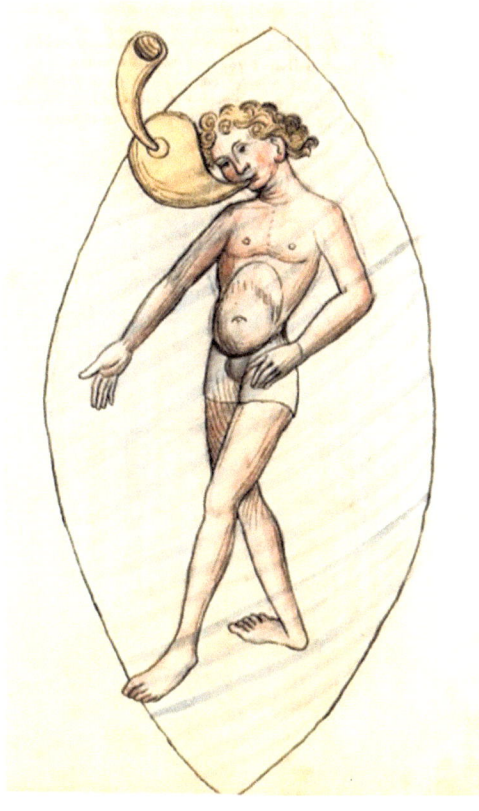

□ **Fig. 1.2** Diver with snorkel (Wikipedia)

1.2 Diving in the Middle Ages

In the middle ages, several considerations were undertaken to use diving equipment for military purposes or for recovering treasures. *Konrad Kyeser* 1405 described a diving suit in his book *Bellifortis*. The diving suit was made of leather. The diving helmet consisted either of a metal helmet or a leather hood (□ Fig. 1.2). The windows were made of curved glass. The air was provided via a long tube from the surface. The consideration and reports about such suits can be found frequently in different time periods in history. It is hard to believe that these equipments were used, as long snorkels like that are not suitable for diving. The lung would not have the strength to expand against the high ambient pressure. Thus, breathing would be impossible. *Roberto Valturio* had similar considerations about such suits. In 1472 he described how to construct a submarine, which was supposed to be suitable for crossing rivers. This submarine was designed however only in theory and was never built.

Even *Leonardo da Vinci* (1452–1519) drew up plans for wetsuits and submarines in his *Codex Atlanticus*. Also with these, it is questionable whether these designs were suitable for diving. He didn't want to disclose them to mankind, "due to the malicious nature of people who would murder from the bottom of the sea by breaking up ships, sinking them together with all people". Even if his inventions were not practical, he almost had a prophetic outlook into the future. In 1531, *Guglielmo de Lorena* built a diving bell, with a window. This diving bell reached to the waist and thus allowed working with hands under water. This type could be immersed up to maximum 20 m for a short time. This bell was used to recover Roman ships in the lakes south of Rome.

1

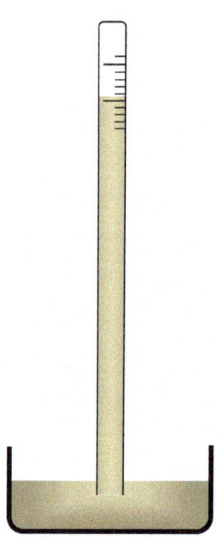

■ **Fig. 1.3**   Mercury column of Torricelli

1.3   The Century of the Physicists

The seventeenth century was determined by discoveries about physical fundamentals. Basics of today's physics were established. Newton, Pascal, Fahrenheit, Torricelli and Halley are just a few of the great thinkers of this century, which still have their recognition in the field of physics today.

The Italian mathematician *Evangelista Torricelli* (1608–1647) developed the mercury barometer and thus created a tool to measure variations in ambient pressure. He placed a single-sided closed glass tube in a bowl of mercury. Only the open side of the 1-m-long glass tube, which was facing down, was connected with the mercury in the bowl. At normal atmospheric pressure, the mercury levels rose to 76 cm. In his honour, the earlier classification for pressure was "torr" (■ Fig. 1.3).

1 mm in the column of mercury (Hg) equals 1 torr.

$$1\,\text{Torr} = 1\,\text{mmHg} = 133,322\,\text{Pa}$$

$$100\,\text{kPa} = 75,006\,\text{Torr}$$

Blaise Pascal (1623–1662) son of a French financial official developed his mathematical-physical talent early in life. At the age of 16, he wrote his first paper on conic sections and was influential in developing fundamentals in geometry. At the age of 20, he developed a calculator. At the age of 23, he began to study science. Specifically the behaviour of liquids and gases in relation to pressure caught his interest. He focused in conditions of pressure changes above and under water. Pascal developed later a formula that describes pressure. This formula is used today and describes the SI unit for pressure. One pascal is the pressure which occurs when a certain force (1 Newton) is exerted on one square meter.

$$1\,\text{Pa} = 1\,\text{N}\,(\text{Newton}) \bullet \text{m}^2$$

Sir *Isaac Newton* (1642–1727) is probably one of the most famous physicists. In his book *Philosophiae Naturalis Principia Mathematica*, which was published in 1687, he describes a variety of physical laws, which effectively dominate science till now.

Robert Boyle (1627–1691), son of the Earl of Cork, was born in Ireland. In his childhood and teenage years, he attended various schools in Switzerland, France and Italy. At the age of 19, he withdrew from his just-inherited estate near London and utilised his fortune for research. Like other famous scientists of that time, he moved then to Oxford. In 1660 he discovered the relationship between pressure and volume of gases. His first work in the field of physics is *New Experiments Physico-Mechanical, Touching the Spring of the Air and its Effects, Made, for the most part, in a New Pneumatical Engine*. Boyle experimented tirelessly. He noticed 1 day shortly after exposing a snake to decompression a peculiar glimmering in its eyes, which he recognised as gas bubbles. Probably this is the first decompression sickness that was scientifically documented: "what the air's presence contributes to life, the little bubbles generated upon the absence of the air in the blood, juices, and soft parts of the body...; ...disturb or hinder the due circulation of the blood,...what I once observed in a viper, ...that it had manifestly a conspicuous bubble moving to and from in the waterish humour of one of its eyes". In addition to these studies, he focused on the salinity of ocean water. The silver nitrate test developed by him is used even today to determine the chloride content of seawater. The law about pressure and volume described simultaneously by him and the French *Abbe Edme Mariotte* (1620–1684) is one of the most important physical laws in diving.

> Boyle's and Mariotte's Law
> P·V = constant

Alfonso Borelli (1608–1689) invented a diving apparatus to work under water for a prolonged time. This apparatus had already a separate air inlet and outlet to breath. It was a suit with a helmet made of leather. This suit was fitted with a sort of fins that the divers "could move like a frog". The air was absorbed through a hole in the helmet and release to a second flow outwards. However, this diving apparatus didn't seem to be too practical: "...a significant effect of the compressed air were observed o those going down with the diving bell into the sea, by the same in the beginning before they even reached it , the air and blood was prompted out of the mouth, ears and nose".

Gabriel Daniel Fahrenheit (1686 1736) a glassblower from Germany developed the first mercury thermometer in 1715. The temperature scale is common in England and the United States nowadays. Fahrenheit has chosen the temperature interval between a cold mixture of ice, liquid and solid ammonium chloride (−17.8 °C) and the blood temperature of a healthy human being. These intervals were divided into 96 equal parts. Nowadays the interval reaches from the boiling point (212 °F) of water to the ice point (32 °F). The modern interval is divided into 180 parts. The unit is called Fahrenheit degrees (°F).

Anders Celsius (1701–1744), a Swedish astronomer, developed another type of classification for temperature. This classification in

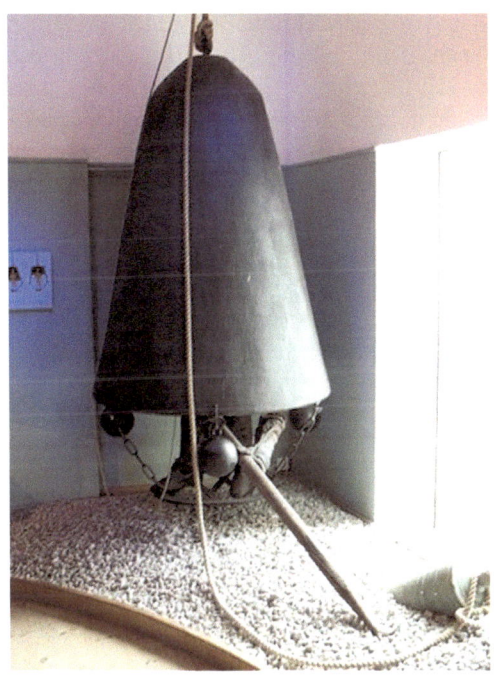

☑ **Fig. 1.4** Diving bell. (Wikipedia)

degrees Celsius (°C) is common in many parts of the world for measuring temperature.

The physicist *Edmund Halley* (1656–1742) is often associated with the comet named after him, which appears about every 74 years on our firmament. But Edmund Halley reported successful attempts leaving a diving bell with a diving suit, which was connected to the diving bell via a hose. Later, he came up with the idea to supply the diving bells with fresh air from barrels. At depths less than 10 m, the bell was directly supplied with air from the surface. With leather hoses air has been pumped directly into the diving bell. Used air was released to the outside through a second hose or through a valve (☑ Fig. 1.4).

1.4 The Age of Reason

This time epoch was thriven by an urge for research and discovery in science. Also in regard to diving, already well-known techniques were

1

modified and became more functional. Diving suits, quite similar to later helmet diving suits, were developed and successfully used. Additionally, knowledge expanded in physics and became more detailed. Interrelations of natural processes appeared increasingly understood.

Jacob Leupold described in 1715 in his scripts ("Theatrum Pontificale") diving and diving bells. The diving devices had copper helmets with windows. As it is evident from these reports that divers could remain underwater for more than an hour. One connection hose supplied fresh air, the second disposed the used air, and the third was for communication. The diving depth was limited as air pumps at the surface were not powerful enough to ensure sufficient air supply at greater depths.

John Lethbridge designed a diving apparatus in 1749, which made him a wealthy man. As he suffered from poverty, he was researching ways to retrieve sunken treasures in the River Thames. His diving apparatus consisted of a 2-m oak barrel, which had a window embedded at its head-facing end. It had holes for the arms, which were stocked with leather cuffs. This made it possible to manually work under water. Basically it was a mini-submarine. However, the dive time and depth were limited. The air could be renewed only on the surface. Therefore, he reported that he had to resurface every 30 min. The length of the dive time he mentioned seems quite long in regard to high concentrations of carbon dioxide inside the barrel during such a dive. The maximum diving depth must have been about 21–22 m, as in contrast to the rest of the body the arms were affected by the high ambient pressure. This would result in compression of the arms, and their perfusion would be reduced or suspended below such depth (◻ Fig. 1.5).

In 1772 *Ferminet* built a diving suit with air supply. The air supply was delivered by a weighted container under water. From this container a spring motor supplied the diving suit with air. The used air was fed back into the container. Thus, only a short period for diving would have been possible. A further development of Ferminet was that the air container

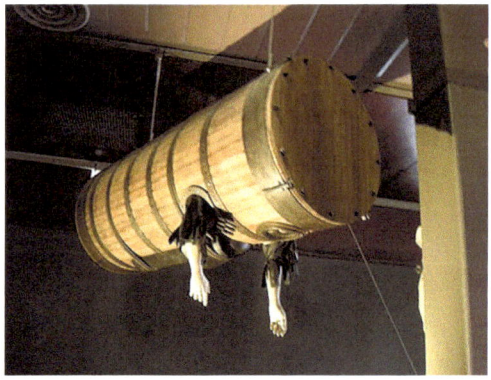

◻ **Fig. 1.5**   Diving apparatus of Lethbridge. (Wikipedia)

was located on the diver's back, which made him more independent in his movements.

In 1774 simultaneously *Joseph Priestley* in England and *Carl Wilhelm Scheele* in Sweden discovered oxygen. In the same year, the use of pure oxygen was recommended in diving bells.

John Dalton (1776–1844) described a physical law that explains partial pressures of individual gases in a gas mixture. The total pressure is the sum of the partial pressure of various gases.

$$p_A + p_B + p_C + \ldots = p_{total}$$

Joseph Henry (1797–1878) was a watchmaker and silversmith in America. Later he became professor in mathematics and natural science. He described in his law the correlation between the dissolved gas and ambient pressure. Till now, this law has great relevance in diving physics.

1.5 Diving During the Times of Industrialization

A real boom in technical achievements arose in the century of industrialization. These achievements included also the field of diving. Already existing devices were improved and made more efficient, and new equipment was added. This allowed people to reach out to the new habitat under water. This progress mainly was thriven by retrieval of new resources and scientific purposes. New technology for underwater work has been developed. These achievements were very helpful in particular for archaeologists and biologists. In 1788 specific diving bells for underwater work were designed by Englishman *Smeaton*, who built the first caisson construction site. The original idea of diving bells developed by Halley was picked up again and equipped with better air supply. The bellow was replaced by a piston pump. Such diving bells helped in the renovation of the foundations of a bridge in Northumberland. These diving bells had even a separate pressure chamber at the surface. The first helmet diving equipment came to use in the early 1800s.

Peter Kreeft from Pomerania constructed relatively handy diving equipments. They consisted of small copper helmets, with windows and two terminals for air supply and voice connection. The helmet was open at the bottom. From the surface, air was pumped into the helmet and thus displaced the water. It was a kind of miniature diving bell. Below the helmet, the diving suit was attached. This garment was cut like a sweater. The diving suit was tightened with a belt at the waistline. A safety line was attached to the belt, which led to the surface. The hose for the air supply consisted of leather which was sealed with wax and resin. This kind of diving helmet was improved by *Augustus Siebe* (1788–1872), as they repeatedly were flooded as they were very sensitive to changes in position. Augustus Siebe went as a young man from England and opened his workshop, in which ground-breaking inventions in diving technology had been developed. The hydraulic pump, a welder, an arc lamp, a helmet diving system and submersible pumps (lever and crank pumps) were produced in this workshop. Lots of these inventions and their development were omnipresent in the early years of diving. Helmet divers were supplied with air pumps from the surface. Improvements in performance of pumps made it possible to reach greater depths. A waterproof jacket was riveted onto Siebe's helmet. This jacket was made of linen, which was sealed with rubber. Weights were added to the belt to reduce buoyancy. In 1837, Siebe developed a complete helmet diving suit. The soles of the suit contained lead to secure a firm footing at the ground whilst diving. In 1851 a new crank pump was presented by Siebe. This pump had the advantage over previously used hand pumps that the airflow was continuous and slow. In conventional pumps, violent pressure oscillations in the helmet due to irregular pumping occurred, which resulted frequently in barotraumas of the sinuses and ears. At this time divers were frequently used during retrieval operations. There was a high incidence of diving accidents. Over and over it happens that connection hoses busted, which caused sudden pressure drops and so-called divers squeeze with associated skin or lung damage. Smaller accidents might have caused only skin damage, minor circulatory problems and shortness of breath. But often, such an accident was fatal due to a massive lung oedema and cardiopulmonary arrest. Also an initially unexplained diver's disease after diving was described for caisson workers. They named this disease "caisson disease," until such incidents were classified as decompression-related sickness (◘ Fig. 1.6).

W.H. James developed autonomous diving equipment in 1825. A metal tank containing air, holding approx. 30 bars, could be carried independently by divers. If necessary, air could be directly let into the helmet via a lever. Thus, there was always fresh air supplied to the helmet. Divers could exhale over breathing tubes that led through a check valve to the outside.

At the beginning of the nineteenth century, only speculations about the depth of the oceans existed. Long before, Magellan tried to measure the depth in 1521. He had a line of 745 meters weighted with a cannonball, which he tried to sink on one of his trips over the Atlantic Ocean. This cannonball wasn't hitting the ground, which implied that the sea was immensely deep, beyond human imagination. Some of the scientists took over the ancient image of the seas and designated it as bottomless ("abyssos"). *Pierre Laplace* (1749–1827) estimated later the maximum ocean depth to be 12 miles.

1

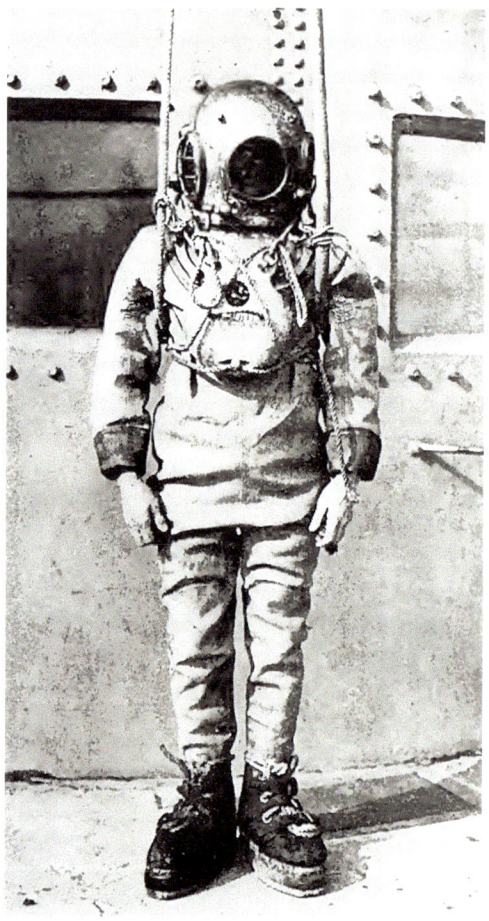

🔳 **Fig. 1.6**   Diving suit of Augustus Siebe. (Form book of Haldane)

Finally, in the mid-eighteenth century, the depth of the ocean could be determined for the first time. Thanks to the just-developed echo sounder, the deepest point of the world's oceans, the Mariana Trench, could be measured. Shortly afterwards, the first telegraph line was laid from Europe to America.

Rouquayrol and *Denayrouze* invented the modern diving suit. In common diving suits at this time, air were supplied from the surface, and adequate air supply underwater was difficult to maintain at changing ambient pressures. Air supply to divers was frequently associated with ear and sinus barotrauma, as often pressure fluctuations occurred with associated short-term pressure increase within diving suits. Moreover, it was quite dangerous when one of

the hoses broke or the diver quickly descended. Henceforth, these difficulties were supposed to be eliminated with the new type of diving equipment. The first autonomous regulator for underwater was developed by Benoit Rouquayrol (1826–1875) and Auguste Denayrouze (1837–1883). Originally, the regulator by Rouquayrol was developed only for miners. This breathing apparatus could be used in flooded tunnels. This inspired the Navy Lieutenant Denayrouze on the idea to develop such a device also for diving. In 1860 the "regulator for the handling of compressed gases" ("aérophore") was registered as a patent. A full face mask, a nose clip and an underwater kerosene lamp with separate air supply from the surface were included in that diving equipment. In 1862, the full face mask has been replaced with a partial mask made of rubber, a nose clip and a mouthpiece made of rubber. This breathing apparatus had a one-stage diaphragm-controlled regulator. Some similarities are even found in today's devices. There were two ways to use it. Air could be pumped from the surface into a metal container that was on the back of the diver. Pressure fluctuations, which were caused by pumping, were buffered in these compressed air tanks. But the 50 kilogram air tank could be also filled up to a pressure of 40 bars and operated without supply from the surface. Therefore, diving independently from the surface for a limited time was possible. This diving apparatus was forgotten and only a century later again "reinvented" and improved. The sophisticated version is our today's scuba diving (🔳 Fig. 1.7).

Paul Bert's (1830–1886) medical interests focused on the impact of pressure on humans. His interest grew through numerous record attempts in ballooning. He attributed the phenomenon of altitude sickness on low oxygen partial pressure in accordance with Dalton's Law. Then, he focussed on hyperbaric conditions. In numerous animal experiments, he linked seizures in animals during recompression to arterial gas embolism. For the first time, he proved that gas embolism after hyperbaric exposure is caused by nitrogen. He was the first who described in detail the pathophysiology and aetiology of decompression sickness. He

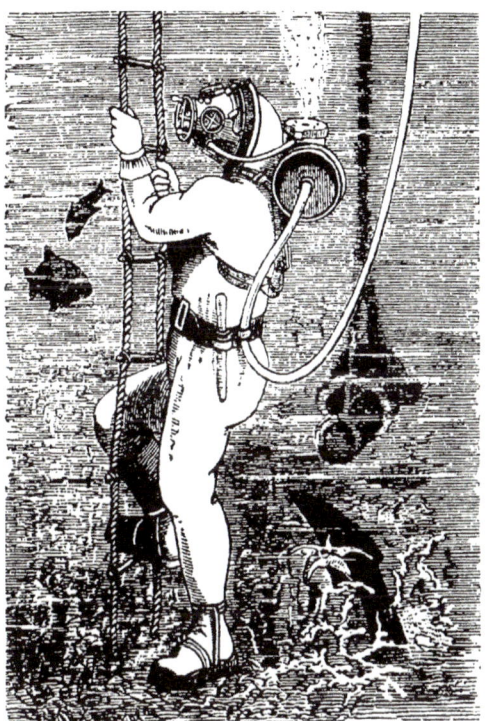

◘ **Fig. 1.7** Diving suit of Denayrouze. (Wikipedia)

connected ascent rates with the occurrence of DCS and established the uniform decompression with ascent rates of 1.5 m per minute. His diving tables had no decompression stops.

Towards the end of the nineteenth century, in 1889, *Dräger* developed fittings and carbon dioxide systems for beer dispensing equipment. This was followed by compressed air tanks, which could be filled up to 150 bars. Later on they were leading in hyperbaric technology.

In 1893, the first underwater camera was built by *Louis Boutan*. It produced excellent pictures and was used up to 50 m under water.

1.6 Diving in the Twentieth Century

In the twentieth century, diving technology progressed rapidly. Technical, physical and medical knowledge have been expanded and supplemented. *John Scott Haldane* (1860–1936) presented in his book *Respiration* the basics of stepped decompression. His theory was validated in his studies in hyperbaric chambers. However, it was only possible to verify the theory of decompression with experiment up to six bars at this time. He coined the term of the "eternal bottom time" from 0 to 10 m water depth. His principles of calculations of saturation and desaturation are more or less incorporated in the present dive tables and computers. His dive tables were not continuous like the one of Paul Bert, but stepwise with decompression stops. These decompression stops were held in certain depths. Because of the usual unit in feet (ft) in the Anglo-American regions, levels at 3, 6, 9, 12 or 15 m were used. Initially, Haldane didn't involve different body compartments for his calculation of nitrogen saturation. Despite complying with his tables, deadly diving accidents still occurred.

At the beginning of the century, the first oxygen diving equipment has been developed. Oxygen could be supplied into the helmet by manual operation. The oxygen came from a separate tank, which could be filled up to 100 bars. The excess amount of carbon dioxide was washed out of the exhaled air by caustic soda, and pure oxygen was again led into the helmet. *Hermann Stelzner*, the chief engineer of Dräger, developed his autonomous oxygen circulation device in 1907. This invention was later refined and designed for use on submarines. These oxygen devices were approved for depths up to 30 m. In the course of time, the units were getting smaller and more usable.

"Dry" test dives in hyperbaric chambers were carried out by *Stelzner* and *Gottsleben* in an equivalent depth of 80 m for 80 min in 1914. Stelzner described that the ambient air at 80 m depth was "pure oxygen". When he smoked his cigarette in the hyperbaric chamber, he noticed a bright glare. The cigarette was quickly finished off. This was the result of the nine times higher partial pressure of oxygen at this depth compared to normal ambient pressure. He must have been lucky that the pressure chamber didn't go up in flames, as at this ambient pressure, high oxygen contents create a highly inflammable environment. The decompression took 150 min and was calculated after the Haldane tables. Initially the

1

decompression was trouble-free and resulted only in mild joint pain. From 3 m water depth onwards, both participants collapsed with severe joint pains. They returned back to 5 m depth where the pain resolved and remained there for 100 min. Then they surfaced slowly within 80 min.

It turned out that the Haldane tables were not suitable for any depth. New tables have been developed. These tables had long decompression breaks and shorter bottom times as today's tables. However, the maximum ascent rate at that time was 20 m per minute instead of the current 10 m per minute. With this new dive tables, a diver of the newly formed US Navy diver's corps reached a submarine lying at a depth of 91 m in 1915. Since hyperbaric workers repeatedly suffered from DCI, Dräger developed a pressure suit for the treatment of "compressed air illness" in 1915. In that suit, pressure could be increased to 5 m water depth. Injured divers remained in this suit until the symptoms disappeared. An improvement was the development of the diver's bags, which could reach a pressure of 15 m water depth. This pressure could be also achieved by giving pure oxygen, which reduced the treatment time.

In 1919 the American physicist *Elihu Thomson* suggested to use a mixture of helium and oxygen, to avoid inert gas narcosis. He postulated that the diving depth could be increased by 50% with that kind of air mixture. As we know now, far greater depths can be achieved with such air mixture. In 1923 many animal experiments were conducted by *Meyer* and *Hoff*, to explore the impact of the inert gas narcosis. Again, the issue of inert gas narcosis remained the subject of numerous investigations and hypotheses. To date, no conclusive proof in explanations about the development of the inert gas narcosis can be given.

The French Navy officer *Yves le Prieur* and the designer *Fernez* in 1926 developed a light and independent diving apparatus, the Fernez-le Prieur diving apparatus. Unfortunately, the advantages of the diving apparatus, which previously was invented by Rouquayrol and Denayrouze with automatic release of air to breathe and pressure adjustments, were not integrated. The Fernez-le Prieur diving apparatus had no respiration-dependent air supply, but a constant flow of air designed as an open system.

In 1930 the American Explorer *William Beebe* made in collaboration with *Otis Burton* deep dive tests with hundreds of meters depth. A 2.5-m bathysphere reached 300 m. Due to the increased ambient pressure, the electric cable was pressed into the diving chamber, and the operation had to be abandoned. Another unmanned diving attempt was made at 600 m. In 1932, a manned bathysphere reached 500 m. In 1934, the bathysphere reached 908 m, which corresponded to the maximum length of the power cord.

In 1938 *Max Nohl* dived for the first time with a Heliox mixture (80% helium/20% oxygen) and reached 127 m in the Lake Michigan. In the same year, *Philippe Tailliez* developed a diving mask, which enclosed the nose and eyes. Thus, with that kind of mask, it was possible to dive deeper, without carrying the risk of ocular barotraumas. In 1939, *Behnke* and *Yarbough* discovered the correlation between fat solubility of substances and their narcotic effects. Behnke and *Shaw* introduced hyperbaric oxygen as a standard recompression therapy in 1937. *Hans Hass* began to excite the public for the underwater world with his travelogues and movies in the mid-twentieth century.

The development of a new regulator was ground-breaking for the development of diving in 1943. *Jacques Yves Cousteau* visited the engineer *Emile Gagnan* to develop a safe and complete diving apparatus. Gagnan used the technique of wood gasification for vehicles. The prototype worked out only unsatisfactory. In the horizontal position, it was easy to breathe. But the diver couldn't breathe at all head down and in an upright position, and the regulator blew off. The problem with this regulator was that the membrane of the regulator and the exhalation valve weren't at the same level (◘ Fig. 1.8).

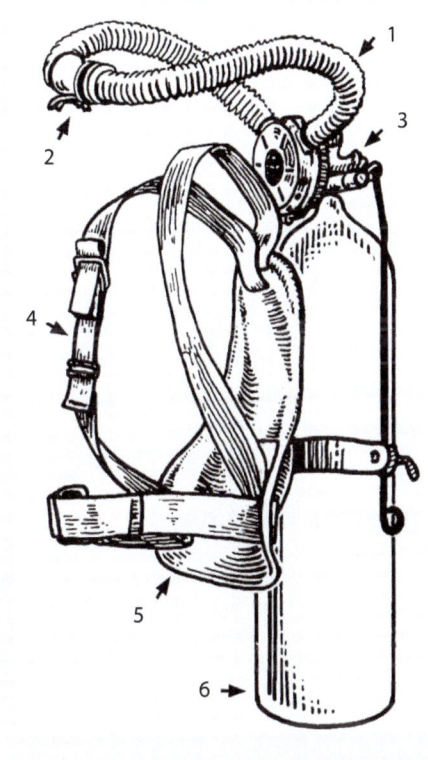

● **Fig. 1.8** SCUBA-Aqualung by Pearson Scott Foresman. (Wikipedia)

Rouquayrol and Denayrouze were facing this problem 100 years previously and solved it. Cousteau and Gagnan solved this problem "again" and reported the functional aqualung as a patent. This diving apparatus contained 3 compressed air tanks with 150 bar each, a high-pressure regulator in the size of an alarm clock on the tank outlet, which reduced the pressure to 8 bar, and a low-pressure regulator which adapted the pressure to the environment via a control membrane, allowing to breathe easily. Almost at the same time in 1944, Dr. Christian James Lambertsen filed a patent of diving equipment for the US Navy, which he described later as "SCUBA" (self-contained underwater breathing apparatus).

In 1943 the commander of the French Navy *Louis de Corlieu* reinvented the fins. Fins were already described by Leonardo da Vinci and Alfonso Borelli.

The exploration of the seas continued. Already extinct animals, such as the "archaic snail", were discovered. In 1960, *Jacques Piccard* reached the Mariana Trench 10,916 m deep with the Bathyscaphe "Trieste". Even in this depth, they found animals. *Bühlmann* and *Keller* built an underwater research centre in the Lake Zurich. There they retrieved important medical diving data. New, sophisticated models of decompression were originated. Physiological interrelationships in diving were connected and described. In the 1970s numerous underwater stations were built, mainly by the former Soviet Union. People lived in these stations for several days. Simultaneously, many deep diving with mixed gases were carried out. For the very first time, the "helium tremor" was described, which later on was named high-pressure nervous syndrome (HPNS).

The Swiss professor *Albert Bühlmann* developed in the early 1960s his diving tables, which are based on Haldane. It contained 16 different compartments ranging from 2.65 to 635 min. The calculations were dependent on supersaturation and ambient pressure. His compartment half-lives were running in a linear fashion. His proposed formulas allowed calculations for altitude diving. Later in the 1980s, these tables were modified and used for Swiss recreational divers. Dr. *Max Hahn* modified these tables for the use in Germany. At the same time like Bühlmann, *Hempleman* developed the diffusions model (DM), which is a dissolved-phase model. Dr. *Robert Workman*, a doctor of the US Navy, brought up the "M-values". The M-values are explaining how much supersaturation is tolerated by each compartment. Workman adopted the theory of supersaturation based on Haldane and modified it according to his research. The calculations of Haldane are somewhat inaccurate in deep and long dives. Workman corrected the ratio for the tolerated supersaturation over the ambient pressure of Haldane from 2:1 to 1.58:1. He also noticed that the fast compartments tolerate a bigger supersaturation-ratio compared to the slow

1

ones. Additionally, the ratio decreases with increasing depth. .

The newest models for bubble formation are described by *D.E. Young (VPM)* and *B.R. Wienke (RGBM)*. They explained the existence of microbubbles, which are responsible for bubble formation. Compared to the VPM, which is tested in gel and represents an in vitro model, the RGBM includes more components and represents more an in vivo model. All calculations are based on bubble physics. This is a completely new approach in the explanation of the development of bubbles. It allows more dynamic calculations of bubble formation. The results are incorporated in algorithms of some diving computers. This development gave new inside in the development of DCI and represents the most modern approach in diving physics.

Recently, free diving became more and more popular. It became more and more attractive because of the availability of improved diving equipment. Scuba and free diving developed rapidly. Again and again, new deep diving records for free diving were achieved. In the 1950s and 1960s, it seemed mathematically impossible to dive beyond the 50-m mark. There was a long-standing head-to-head race between Jacques Mayol and Enzo. First, they broke through the unimaginable 50-m mark

and shortly after through the 100-m mark. Again and again, the "absolute" deep diving limit was breached and corrected to greater depth. In hunting for new records, fatal accidents occurred over and over again. In 2007, Herbert Nitsch set the world record in Spetses, Greece, when he reached a depth 214 m!

Diving increasingly evolved into a recreational sport. More people were interested in scuba diving, and diving equipment became better and more convenient. The development of various materials increased comfort and durability of the equipment. Lots of organisations about diving and diving schools started operating. Now there is a worldwide network of divers.

Suggested Reading

Acott C. A brief history of diving and decompression illness. S Pac Underw Med Soc J. 1999;29(2):98–109.

Edmonds C, Lowry C, Pennefather J. Diving and subaquatic medicine, fourth edition, Chapter 1 History of diving. CRC Press, Boca Raton, 2002:1–10.

Gierschner N. Meine illustrierte Chronologie und Bibliografie der Tauchgeschichte. Berlin: Tauch-Info-Büro; 2007.

Jung M. Das Handbuch zur Tauchgeschichte. Stuttgart: Naglschmid; 1999.

Männche KH. Geschichte des Tauchens. Eigendruck/ Bremen: Taucheinsatzzug der DLRG Bremen-Nord; 1993.

Basic Diving Equipment

© Springer International Publishing AG, part of Springer Nature 2018
O. Rusoke-Dierich, *Diving Medicine*, https://doi.org/10.1007/978-3-319-73836-9_2

2

The ABC equipment includes diving mask, snorkel and fins. There are different kinds of diving *masks* available. All popular diving masks for sport divers cover the eyes and nose. The lip is nowadays commonly made out of silicone. Usually masks have one glass for each eye. The glass should have the description "Tempered Glass" or "Safety Glass". These glasses can be exchanged with prescription glasses, if needed. The visual acuity thus can be corrected. But this can be also achieved with wearing contact lenses. However, only soft contact lenses should be used as nitrogen bubbles might form under hard contact lenses on decompression (■ Figs. 2.1, 2.2, and 2.3).

Apnoea diving masks have a slightly smaller mask volume. As the nose is included in the mask space, equalisation is possible by blowing air through the nose into the mask space. There are also full face masks, which are used mainly by professional divers. The whole area of a full face mask is filled with air and connected to the air supply. The regulator is built into the mask itself. This allows the diver to speak and communicate with others via radio intercom. In general, glasses of diving masks have the tendency to fog under water. This can be prevented by usage of silicone sprays. A similar effect can be achieved by simply applying saliva onto the dry glass followed by washing it off with plain water. Masks should sit comfortable and tightly, so that no water can enter. When putting the mask on, it should be avoided to get hair under the lip of the mask, since this could lead to water entering into the mask space. Same applies to beards. The mask strap should be adjusted neither too tight nor too loose. If it is too loose, the mask easily can slip and produce water inlet. If the mask is too tight, it could not only cause pressure sores but also enable water to enter into the mask.

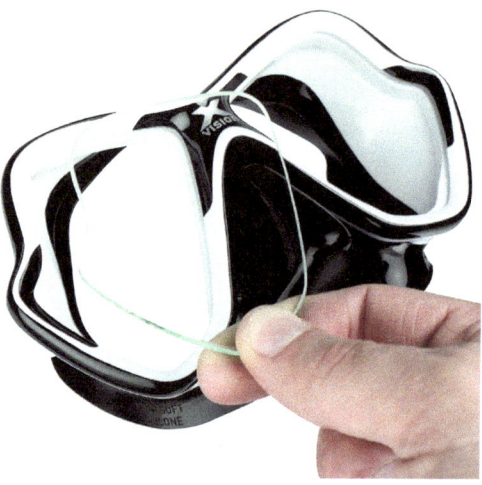

■ **Fig. 2.2** Exchangeable lenses. (Mares)

■ **Fig. 2.1** Complete scuba equipment. (With kind permission of Mares/Photo: A. Balbi)

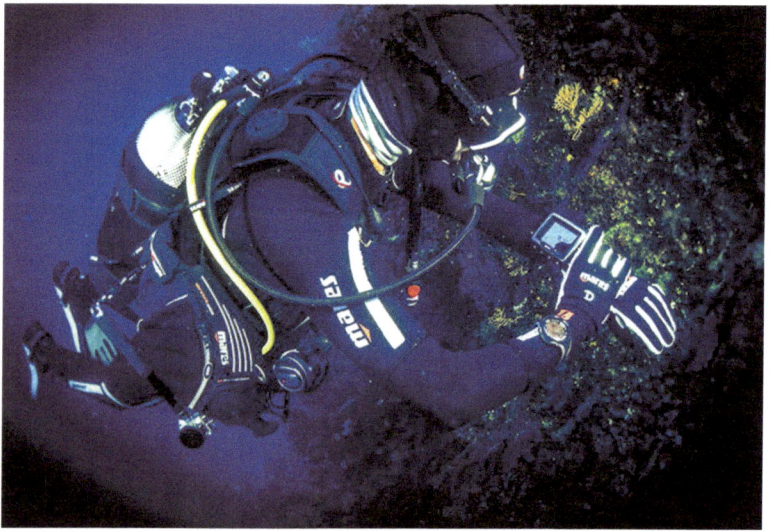

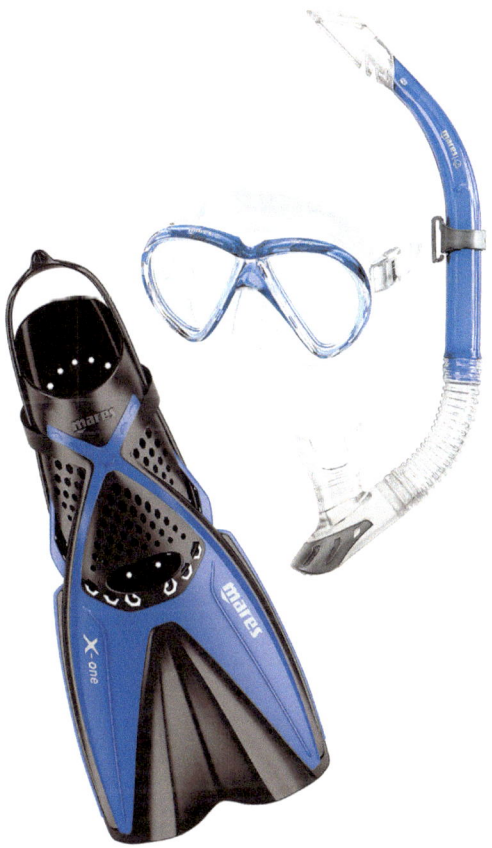

◘ **Fig. 2.3**   Basic diving equipment. (Mares)

Snorkels are usually 35 cm long for adults and 30 cm for children. This prevents negative barotrauma of the lung, as well as accumulation of increased CO_2 caused by the increased functional dead space. With increasing length of the snorkel, the risk for the above increases. The internal diameter of the snorkel for adults is 18–25 mm and 12–25 mm for children. The upper end should be marked with a bright colour that it is visible to boats on the surface. When the snorkel meets this standard, it bears the mark of "GS" (tested safety) (◘ Fig. 2.3).

Fins increase the thrust when swimming in water. They can be closed or open at the heels. Closed fins are used without boots. If they have open heels, they can be used with boots. Fins also differ in their elasticity. The harder the fins are, the more strenuous is their use. The advantage of harder fins is that they are faster and

more targeted in manoeuvring. The softer fins are, the less effort has to be made. Apnoea fins are soft and long. Freediving is less dependent on speed or manoeuvring. Apnoea fins are more effective with wide and slow strokes and have a good efficiency with relative low energy consumption. Mono-fins have a good efficiency too. High speed can be achieved with little effort. Swimming with mono-fins requires entire body movement and not just of the legs. As the strain is not only distributed only to the legs, the workload is more evenly distributed, resulting in a lower exhaustion rate and a broader distribution of lactate in the body. However, their use takes some time to learn, and manoeuvrability is limited (◘ Fig. 2.4).

Diving suits prevent the body from cooling. Two types of diving suits need to be distinguished, dry and wet diving suits. Dry suits completely protect the body from any water contact. The suit is waterproof, and water entry is prevented by tight fittings on arms, legs and neck. Under dry suits warm clothing, usually made of wool, is required. Fabrics with more air padding have better insulating effects. Because there is no water contact with the skin, less body heat is emitted to its surrounding. Thus dry suits have larger insulating effects compared to wetsuits and therefore are used for diving in cold environments. As openings of dry suits are very tight, vacuum within the suit can occur during diving. Therefore, dry suits have to be inflated to compensate the pressure loss during the descent. The effect is conversely on ascending. Gas can expand, therefore reinforcing the uplifting force. Hence, air must be released from the suit. Due to filling and emptying, dry suit diving is more demanding and requires special skills and training. As dry suits have less buoyancy than wetsuits, fewer weights are needed. Wetsuits are made of neoprene. They are not completely sealed. A thin layer of water remains between the skin and neoprene. The water under the neoprene absorbs heat from the skin and warms up. The neoprene should sit tight, to allow only minimal exchange of water to prevent the loss of warmed water and the entering

2

◘ **Fig. 2.4**   a + b
apnoea fins. (With kind
permission of Mares/
Photo: A. Balbi)

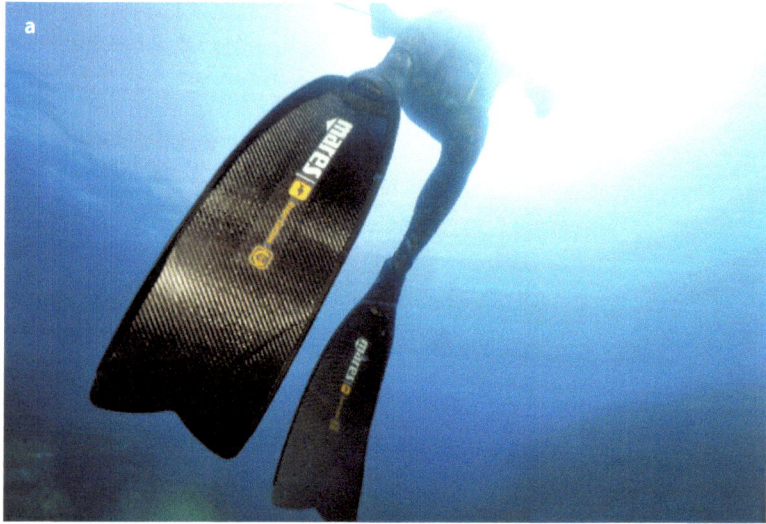

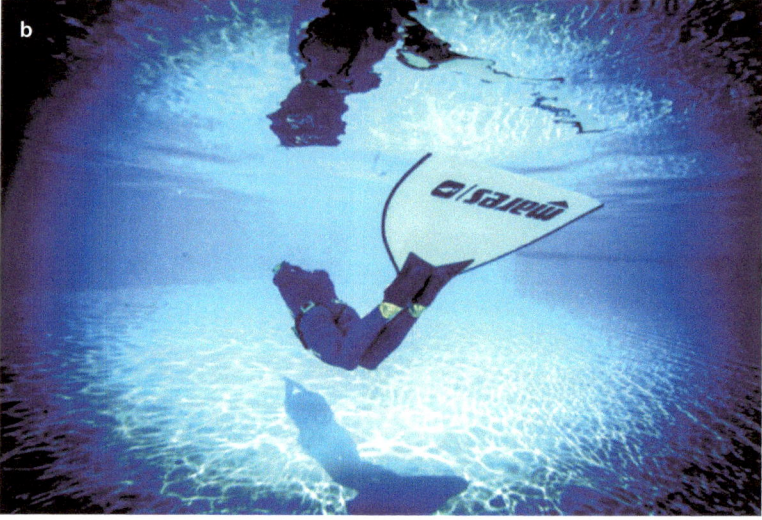

of cold water. This reduces heat loss by convection. The neoprene itself is insulating due to its air bubbles (◘ Figs. 2.5 and 2.6).

The thicker neoprene is the better is its insulation. However, insulation decreases during diving as air bubbles inside the neoprene shrink according to the ambient pressure. This causes a reduction in thickness of the neoprene. In dry suits, pressure changes don't really matter as pressure inside the suit adjusts continuously and insulation isn't affected. In general, to prevent heat loss, it is important to wear a hood. Because scalp vessels don't adjust adequately to cold outside temperatures with vasoconstriction, much of the body heat is lost via the scalp.

To counteract buoyancy of the neoprene, *weights* are needed. Neoprene provides uplift and tank downforce. To achieve neutral buoyancy, uplift forces need to be equal to downforces. This is achieved with weights. These are usually made of lead. All these weights are usually worn on a belt around the waist. Some can be integrated in the BCD. They come in a solid form or as small beads contained in bags. Weights in bags are softer and reduce pressure points along the belt area. Weights are available in various sizes and can be adjusted as required.

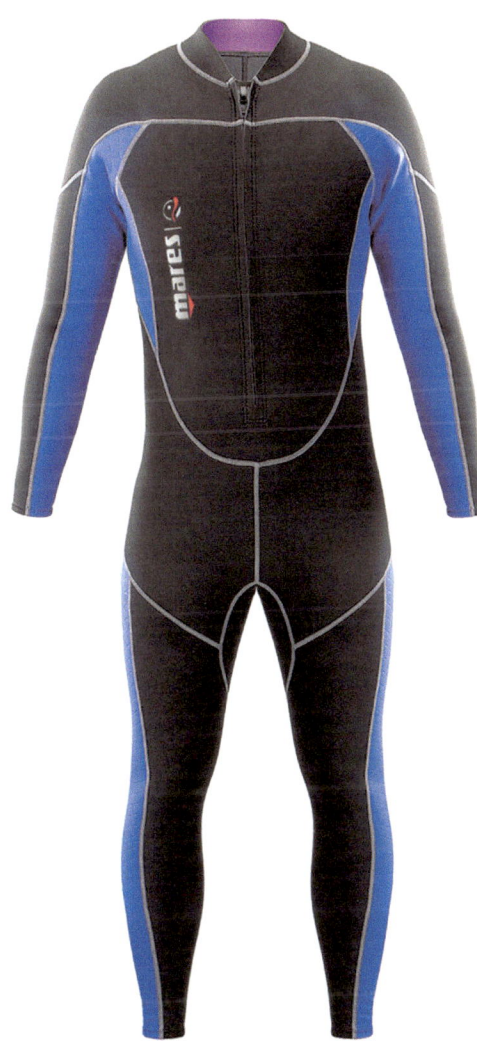

Fig. 2.5 Wetsuit. (Mares)

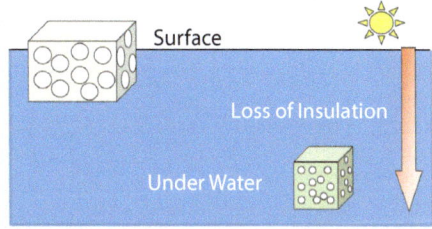

Fig. 2.6 Loss of insulation under water depending on the diving depth

The thicker the neoprene, the more weights are needed. In addition to the thickness of the diving suit, the weight of the gas tank needs to be taken in consideration in the adjustment of the weights as well, as steal tanks are heavier than aluminium tanks and both come in different sizes. It is important to choose the right amount of weights. If there is too much weight, levelling out buoyancy under water might be difficult. This causes higher air consumption due to greater physical effort. If weights are too light, the diver is at risk of unwanted rapid ascends towards the surface, particularly being close to the surface. The optimal weight can be checked at surface before the dive. When the diver in full equipment just floats at the surface with normal breathing and sinks on full exhalation, the correct weights are chosen. If the diver doesn't sink on full exhalation, more weights are needed. If the diver sinks while breathing normally, weights have to be reduced.

Scuba Diving

© Springer International Publishing AG, part of Springer Nature 2018
O. Rusoke-Dierich, *Diving Medicine*, https://doi.org/10.1007/978-3-319-73836-9_3

In scuba diving, air is obtained from tanks for breathing. For recreational diving, scuba tanks are usually filled with normal compressed air up to 200 bar. Via different stages, the pressure is reduced to a level so that the diver can breathe normally. Tanks are made either of steel or aluminium. However, aluminium scuba tanks are only allowed in certain countries. Aluminium scuba tanks are lighter than the one made of steel. Both can be filled up to 200 bar. Scuba tanks shouldn't be emptied completely for safety and maintenance reasons. They always should have more than 50 bar left at the end of each dive. If tanks are completely emptied, moist air might enter and cause the inside to rust. Rust particles in return might block of the sinter filter and block off air supply. Additionally, pressure display on poorly maintained pressure gauges might not reflect the real pressure in scuba tanks. That bears the risk of running out of air under water even when the pressure gauge displays that some air is still left. Besides, residual, "spare", air should always be kept in case of emergency situations, which could arise at anytime. Scuba tanks have to be serviced in regular intervals. Tanks made of steel have to undergo a visual test usually every 2.5 years and a hydrostatic test every 5 years. These dates vary in different countries. Aluminium bottles have to be serviced every 6 years. Information about the permitted filling pressure, the last maintenance and the gas mixture can be seen on the stamp marking on the scuba tank's top, close to the outlet. Tanks can capture something between 3 and 18 l. The most common type of scuba tanks for sport divers has around 10–11 l (◘ Fig. 3.1).

The pressure of scuba tanks with 200 bar has to be reduced to be used for breathing. This is achieved by the first and second stage. The first stage reduces high pressure to intermediate

◘ **Fig. 3.1** Example of stamp markings of a scuba tank

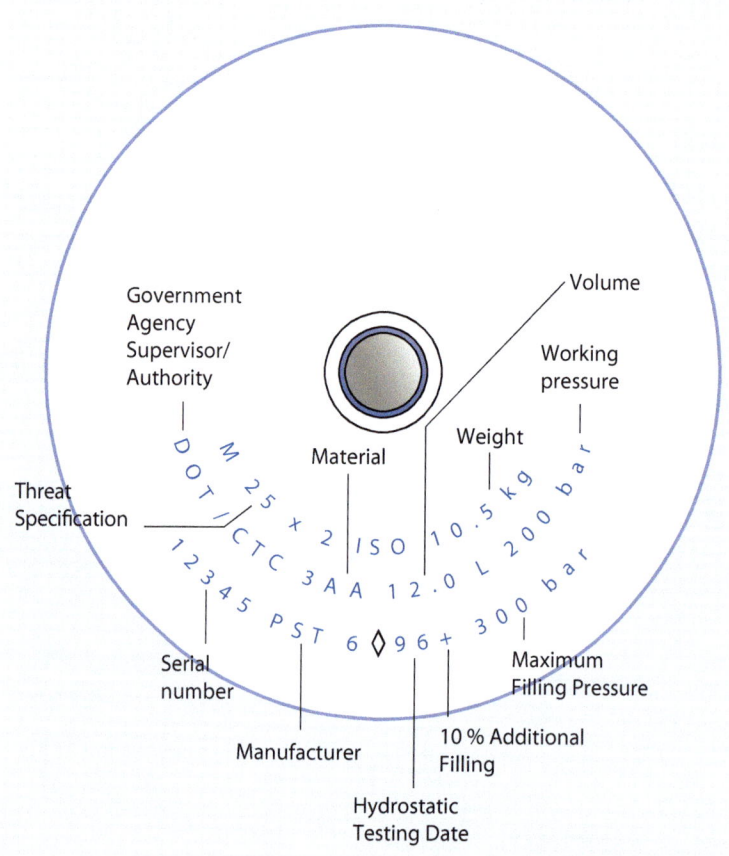

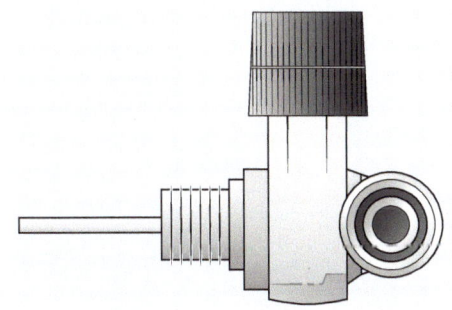

Fig. 3.2 Tank valve. (Wikipedia)

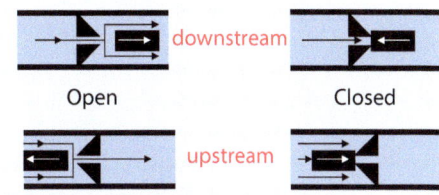

Fig. 3.3 Upstream and downstream valve

pressure, and the second stage adjusts the intermediate pressure to the actual breathing demand. A cylinder valve with a knob (K-valve type) is located at the top end of the gas tank. For safety reasons J-valves, with a switch instead of a knob, are not used anymore. By turning the valve, the scuba tank opens or closes. Closing valves only requires a gentle touch. If it is closed to tight, the valve might get damaged and seals wear out quickly. After completely opening of valves, the knob needs to be turned back slightly by half a turn. This avoids damages to the valve by accidental blows or thermal tensions. The tank valve or pillar valve has either a DIN or a yoke (A-clamp) connection with an O-ring. If the cylinder valve has a yoke connection, DIN-adapters might have to be used to connect the first stage. The tank valve has a sinter filter on the inside to trap small particles (■ Fig. 3.2).

The first stage reduces the tank pressure to 4–10 bar intermediate pressure. The pressure inside the first stage is independent to diving depth and therefore remains unchanged. Three outlets are departing from the first stage. The hose on the left side is for the BCD. On the right side, there are outlets for regulator, pressure gauge or dive console and octopus (second, alternative regulator).

Generally, there are two types of valves in regulators, a "downstream" or an "upstream" valve. The downstream valve opens with pressure, the upstream valve against pressure. First stages of most diaphragm pressure regulators have upstream valves. First stages of most piston regulators have downstream valves (■ Fig. 3.3).

First and second stages are either diaphragm or piston regulators. The first stage receives air from the tank with its high pressure in the first chamber. In the second chamber, the pressure is reduced to intermediate pressure. Another chamber is filled with water, which is connected to the outside with its ambient pressure. The water chamber in the first stage of the *diaphragm first stage* is separated to the second air-filled chamber with a membrane. The advantage of this is that only few parts of the regulator are exposed to water and the inner mechanism is environmentally sealed. Hence, these regulators are less likely to be damaged by salt water or freezing. In the second air-filled chamber, a spring counteracts the high pressure of the first chamber. On inhalation the diaphragm lifts and air flows from the first to the second air chamber. After the inhalation, the diaphragm returns to its neutral position, and the valve lifter closes, which interrupts the air flow between the air chambers. If the tank pressure drops, the pressure in the air chamber still remains the same. This helps to open the valve till the desired pressure is restored in the second air chamber, which then closes the valve again (■ Fig. 3.4).

Piston regulators are more delicate than diaphragm regulators. Piston regulators have pistons as a part of the pressure regulator. The middle section of this piston is connected to the outside and thus to the ambient pressure. This water-filled chamber has a spring, which counteracts the high pressure of the tank in the first air chamber. The opening to the high pressure of the piston sits on a valve seat and is closed. On inhalation the piston gets pulled down, and air flows till the intermediate pressure is high

Fig. 3.4 **a** Balanced diaphragm first stage; **b** unbalanced diaphragm first stage

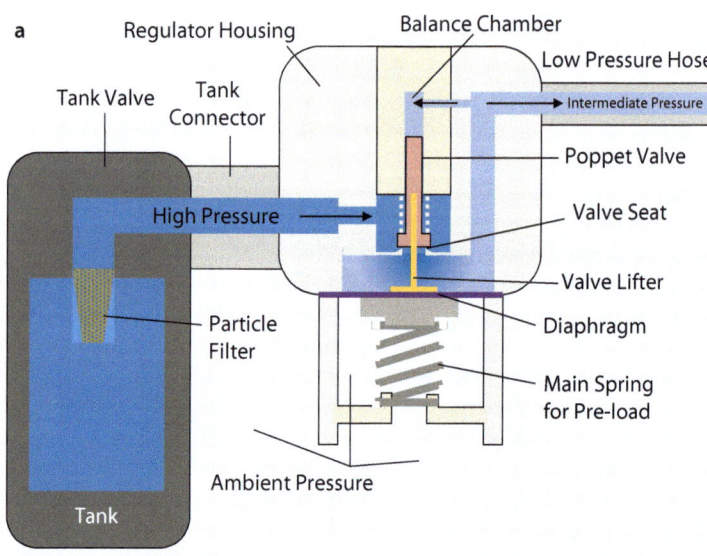

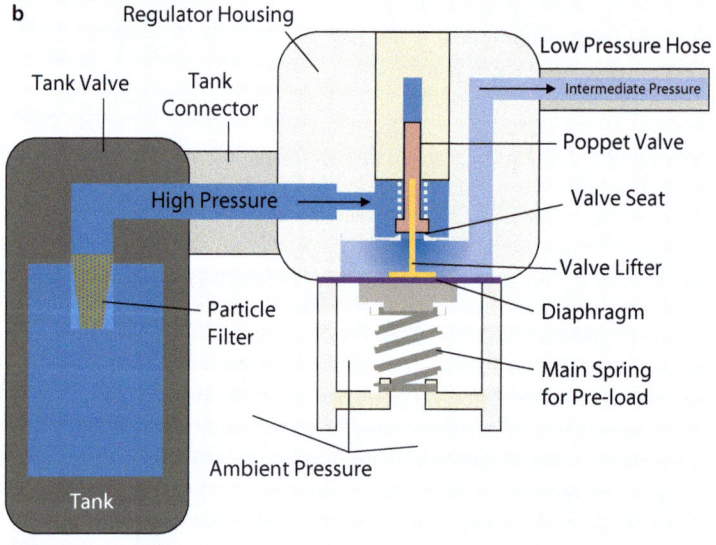

enough to push the piston back into its neutral position to interrupt airflow. The piston itself is sealed with O-rings from the second air chamber. The inside of the piston is in conjunction with the second air chamber and thus has the same pressure. In piston regulators, at decreasing tank pressure, the intermediate pressure drops as well. The thin passage of the piston is quite vulnerable due to its small diameter (**Fig. 3.5**).

There are compensated and uncompensated ("balanced" or "unbalanced") first stages. In compensated first stages, the intermediate pressure is constant, and the valve has a feedback loop to the second chamber. They are more independent to the tank pressure and diving depth than uncompensated first stages. The medium pressure of uncompensated first stages depends on the tank pressure. In general, uncompensated first stages are more

□ **Fig. 3.5** Balanced
piston first stage

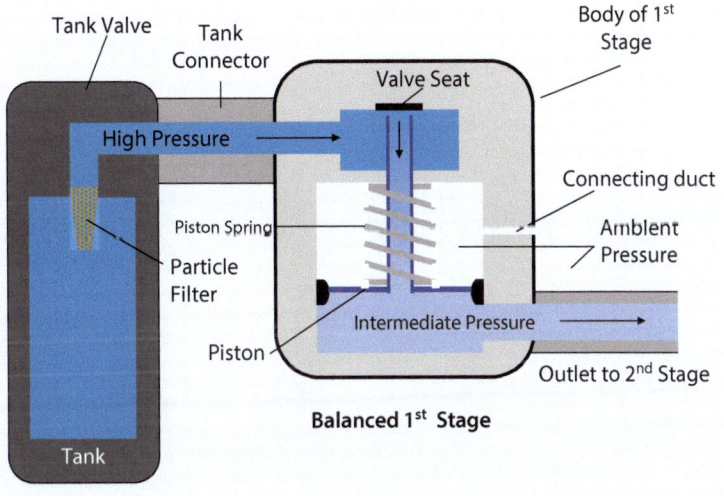

□ **Fig. 3.5** Balanced
piston first stage

robust and cheaper in maintenance due to their simple design. The air of uncompensated piston first stages enters directly from the first high-pressure chamber to the second intermediate pressure chamber, behind the piston.

At water temperatures below 10 °C, freezing of the first stage might occur. The temperature of inland lakes below 3 m is usually 5–10 °C. Different factors play a role in the freezing of the first stage:

— Air moisture
— Pressure reduction
— Cold environment

According to the law of Gay-Lussac and the Joules-Thompson effect temperatures drop when pressure is reduced. Pressure of scuba tanks is reduced in the first stage from up to 200 bar to approx. 4–10 bar. It may happen that even at normal temperatures in some places of the first stage, the ambient temperature drops to minus 20–30 °C for a very brief time. In combination with cold environment, this effect is accumulative and might cause freezing. Moisture in the air of scuba tanks may cause freezing of the first stage too. Compressed air is supposed to be "dry". However, there might be moisture in compressed air caused by poorly maintained compressors or by incorrect handling during the filling process of scuba tanks. It

can be discriminated between inner and outer freezing. Outer freezing occurs when cold water surrounds delicate parts of the spring. Freezing of these parts can block the piston. Due to the "fail safe" construction of regulators, air continually blows off when the first stage is frozen. The diver is still able to breathe, but the scuba tank pressure decreases rapidly, and the diver is running out of air quickly. Especially first stages of piston-controlled high-pressure regulators are affected by that. Causes for inner freezing are freezing of the valve or the sinter filter by moist compressed air. This could be caused during regular maintenance or by blowing off the second stage, where water may enter in the first stage itself. Inner freezing causes a sudden interruption of air supply. This type of freezing happens equally in membrane- and piston-controlled first stages.

Compressed air reaches the second stage through the intermediate pressure hose. In the *second stage,* pressure is further reduced and adjusted to the breathing demand. The air chamber in the second stage gets its air supply from the first stage. The air supply is regulated via a downstream valve. A spring closes the valve. The air flow on exhalation is interrupted by a valve and thus prevents water penetration on inhalation into the second stage of the regulator. The air chamber is separated from

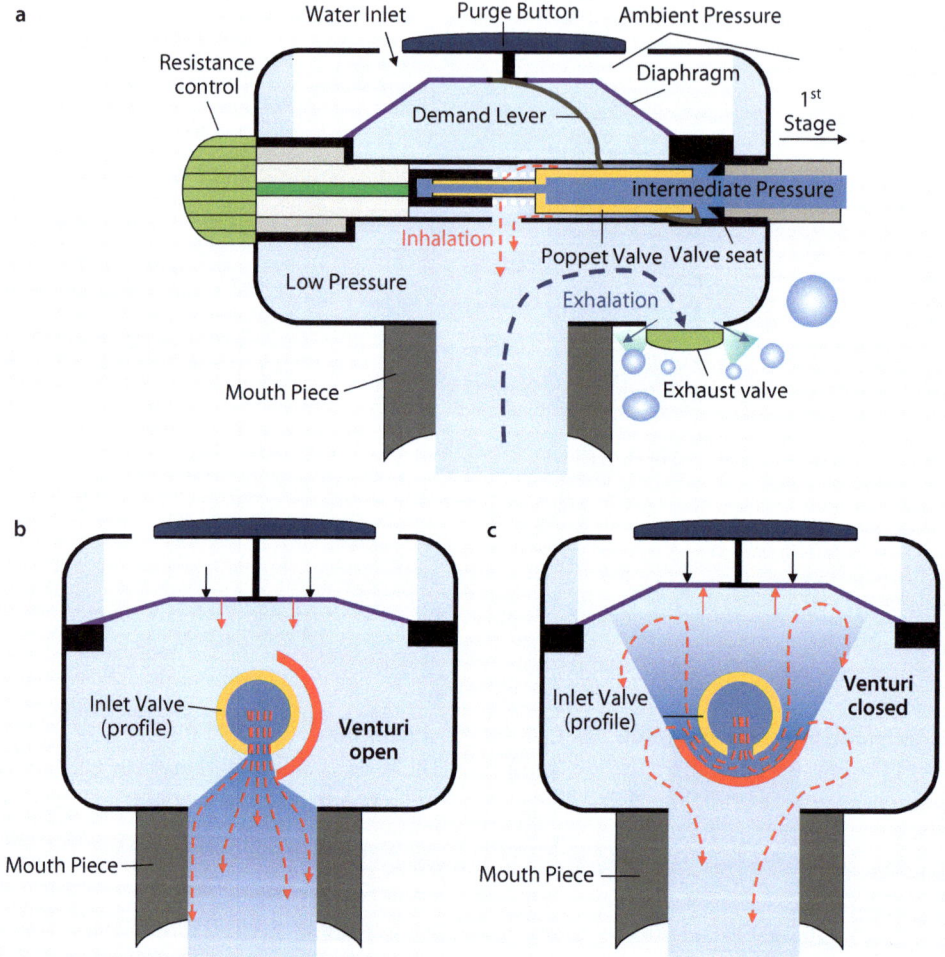

■ **Fig. 3.6**   **a** Compensated second stage; **b** Venturi open; **c** Venturi closed

the surrounding water by a membrane. On inhalation the membrane gets pulled in. The membrane itself is connected to the downstream valve with a lever. This lever tightens the spring and therefore opens the downstream valve when the diaphragm gets pulled in. Hence, air flow can adapt to various breathing demands. Air flow and supply can be additionally adjusted in different ways. A simple lever just before the mouthpiece of the regulator can increase or decrease flow resistance. Another effective mechanism to alter air flow is achieved by VIVA (venturi-initiated vacuum effect).

Hereby, air passes from the hose either directly or with some turbulence caused by VIVA into the air chamber of the second stage. This either increases or, if closed, decreases airflow. Reduced airflow in rough conditions like waves prevents the regulator from blowing out. If opened, VIVA enhances airflow and assists on inhalation, which makes airflow easier and more sensitive to inhalation (■ Fig. 3.6).

The *BCD* (= buoyancy control device) has different functions. The main feature is buoyancy control underwater. Wetsuits create an upforce while the scuba tank and the lead belt

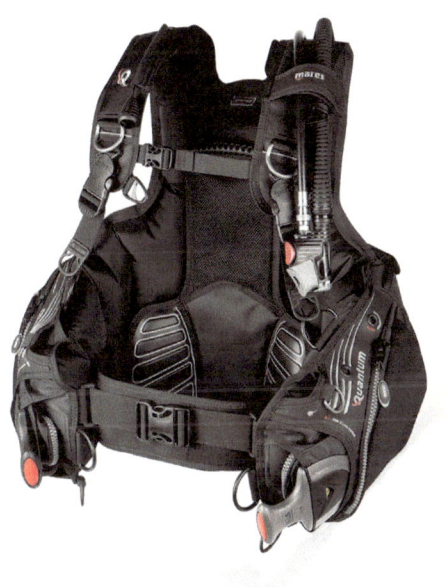

Fig. 3.7 BCD. (Mares)

a mouthpiece of the inflator hose. The BCD has various drain valves in different positions. The main drain valve is on the left upper side where the inflator hose enters the vest. By pulling on the hose, this valve opens. But air only can escape, if the diver is in more or less in an upright position. The valve on the lower back of the BCD, usually positioned on the right side, can be release, if the diver is upside down. BCDs have mountings, where the scuba tank can be attached. Usually BCDs have several pockets and clips for attaching diving equipment or for storage (■ Fig. 3.7).

a downforce. During diving the buoyancy of neoprene is continuously changing due to changing depth and hence has to be balanced. BCDs are connected to the first stage with a medium pressure hose and can be inflated by simply pressing a button. The hose is usually attached to the inflator hose of the BCD on the left side. It can be also inflated by the mouth via

Suggested Reading

Brum J (2012). Breath in, breath out. www.alertdiver.com/Breath_In_Breath_Out. Accessed 24 Mar 2014.

Farley MB. Scuba equipment care and maintenance. St Helena: Marcor Publishing; 1996.

Graver D. Scuba diving. 4th ed. Champaign: Human Kinetics; 2009.

Kromp T, Mielke O. Tauchen – Handbuch modernes Tauchen: Teil 1: Open Water Diver (OWD). Stuttgart: Franckh-Kosmos; 2014.

Kromp T, Roggenbach HJ, Peter BP. Praxis des Tauchens. 3 Auflage ed. Bielefeld: Delius Klasing Verlag; 2008.

Oldenhuizing J. Diving equipment functioning & care. Scuba Publications, Cannes la Boca, France, 2004.

Scheyer W. "Lungenautomat". Technik und Funktion der Atemregler. Stuttgart: Verlag Stephanie Naglschmid; 1991.

Dive Tables and Dive Computers

© Springer International Publishing AG, part of Springer Nature 2018
O. Rusoke-Dierich, *Diving Medicine*, https://doi.org/10.1007/978-3-319-73836-9_4

Dive tables and dive computers provide guidelines for safe diving. Diving depth and profile, as well as surface interval times, are incorporated in their algorithms. Common dive tables usually apply only for recreational diving, not for decompression diving. For diving in altitude special diving tables are required. The purpose of diving tables is to avoid decompression accidents and ensure safe diving. Nitrox diving tables incorporate the risk of oxygen toxicity, and diving time as well as depth is adjusted accordingly (◘ Fig. 4.1).

Basic dive training provides a good understanding of dive tables, of dive profile planning, as well as of dive safety. However, dive computers replaced dive tables. They are easy to use, more accurate and flexible in regard to dive profiles than dive tables. Dive tables are only suitable for non-deco dives. Dive computers can include deco stops. Regardless of using tables or computers, the deepest point of diving should be always at the beginning, followed by a steady ascend from then on. The time spent at the deepest point is called "actual bottom time" (ABT). By understanding ABT, beginners get a good feeling of diving limitations. All tables have a column of diving depth with ABT. Based on depth, ABT and repetitive dives pressure groups (A–Z) are determined (1.) at the end of each dive. According to the duration of the surface interval and the previous pressure group, a new pressure group is determined in a new column (2. + 3.). On the backside of the table, the columns indicate according to the group how much time needs to be added (RNT, residual nitrogen time) to the ABT to the next dive, which is then the "total bottom time" (TBT) (white 4.). The new ABT at a specific depth has a maximum limit (blue 4.), which should not be exceeded. The following dive then can be calculated accordingly. By setting the diving depth, the adjusted ABT can be used in the new group (1.). This process can be repeated. (Following fragments from the PADI dive table recreational dive planner, RDP, were adopted.) Other dive tables are similar but may have a different design and differ slightly in their values. Each recreational

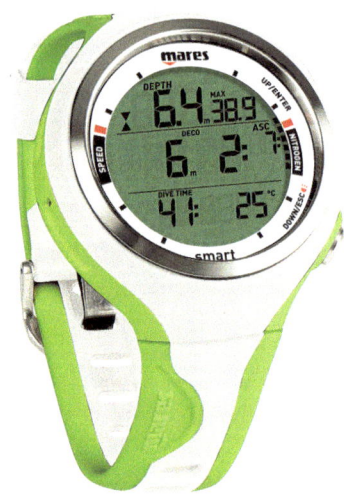

◘ **Fig. 4.1**   Diving computer. (Mares)

dive planner of different providers requires specific training. They may also contain further information, like general information, but also flying after diving, etc. (◘ Fig. 4.2).

Dive tables and dive computers may include parameters of dive profiles illustrated in the following picture. According to different providers, these parameters may vary (◘ Figs. 4.3 and 4.4).

Dive computers replaced diving tables as they are more accurate, safer, integrate dive profiles, more flexible and therefore more user-friendly. Various dive computers are based on different calculation models. For example, Mares and Suunto use the RGBM, UWATEC uses Haldane and Bühlmann ZHL-12 or ZHL-16 and Seiko use Randy Bohrer, to name a few of them. Dive computers are of course pressure-proof. They measure ambient pressure, time and temperature. Some of them display tank pressure and the Earth's magnetic field (compass). The tank pressure can be measured either by direct connection to the tank or wirelessly via a high-pressure sensor integrated in the first stage. In some computers, individual user data could be entered and various gas mixtures calculated. Some models have a function to dynamically calculate dive profiles. The remaining diving time, dive time itself, safety or deco stops, water temperature and ascent and descent speed and

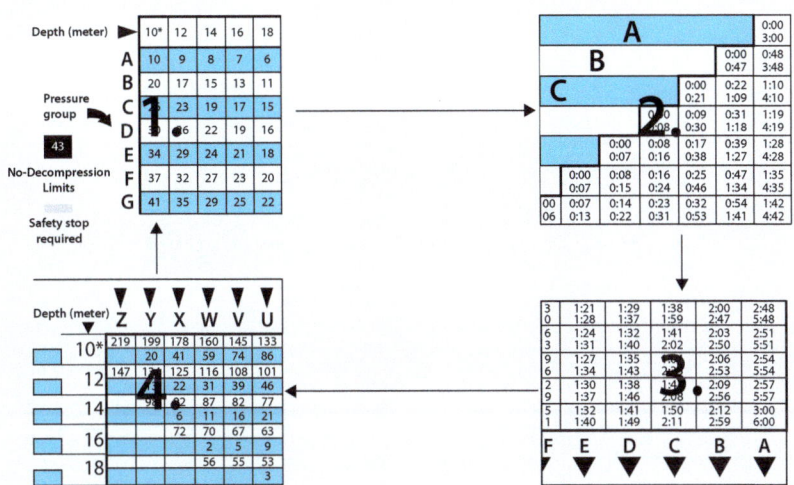

Fig. 4.2 Extract of a PADI recreational dive planner

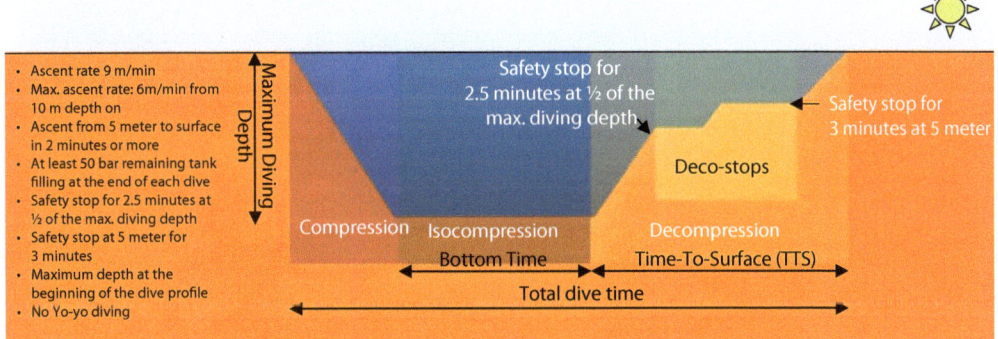

Fig. 4.3 Parameter of diving profiles

Parameters listed at left of Fig. 4.3:
- Ascent rate 9 m/min
- Max. ascent rate: 6m/min from 10 m depth on
- Ascent from 5 meter to surface in 2 minutes or more
- At least 50 bar remaining tank filling at the end of each dive
- Safety stop for 2.5 minutes at ½ of the max. diving depth
- Safety stop at 5 meter for 3 minutes
- Maximum depth at the beginning of the dive profile
- No Yo-yo diving

time where flying is not recommended can be displayed. Failure to comply with ascent rates or safety stops results in acoustical and optical warning signals. Dive computers can be set differently in various ways. This allows individual adaptation to diving environments and individual parameters of the diver. Dive computers have also a logbook function. Thus previous dives can be reviewed. Previous dives and their profile as well as data can be displayed on computer. Commonly, specific computer programs are required for doing this. This might be a useful tool for medical staff in reconstruction of diving accidents (◻ Figs. 4.1, 4.4 and 4.5).

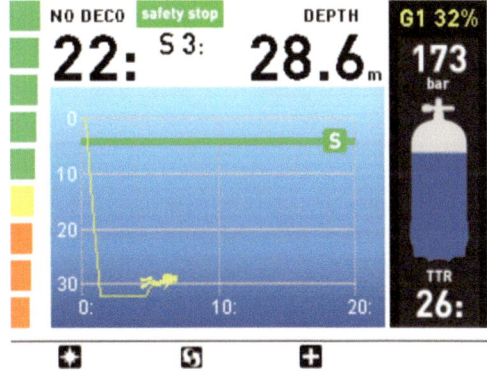

Fig. 4.4 Display of a diving computer. (Mares)

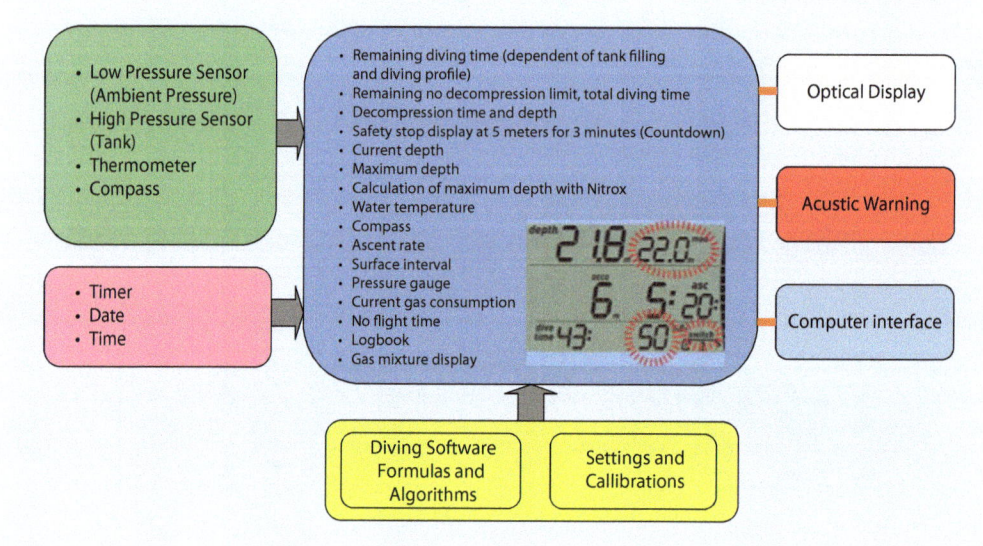

■ **Fig. 4.5**   Structure and function of dive computers. (With kind permission of Mares)

Tech Diving

Reference – 38

© Springer International Publishing AG, part of Springer Nature 2018
O. Rusoke-Dierich, *Diving Medicine*, https://doi.org/10.1007/978-3-319-73836-9_5

5

Tech diving exposes divers to environments beyond normal recreational diving. For tech diving usually specific equipment is required. Tech diving includes (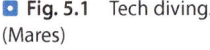 Fig. 5.1):

— Diving >40 m
— Decompression diving
— Mixed gases (trimix, heliox and hydrox)
— Diving in confined spaces (wreck diving, cave diving and ice diving)
— Changing of gas mixtures in different diving depth
— Rebreather diving

Tech diving is mainly a domain of professional divers. It requires special training to deal with technically complex equipment, to learn different guidelines, to use different gas mixtures and to apply decompression stops. Nitrox diving belongs actually not to tech diving, but it should be mentioned in this chapter, because it uses mixed gases in recreational diving. Nitrox is a gas mixture that differs from the normal breathing air. A greater percentage of oxygen is added to the gas mixture to reduce nitrogen. This allows increased bottom time and decreases risk of decompression accidents. The proportion of oxygen ranges from 22% to 40%. But for scuba diving, typically either 32% or 36% (EAN 32 and EAN 36) is used. EAN stands for "enriched air nitrox", and the number displays the fraction of oxygen in the gas mixture. Diving tanks for nitrox have to be specially marked. In nitrox mixtures nitrogen content is reduced. This means that less nitrogen is absorbed at a specific depth. This reduces the real depth to a sallower equivalent depth (EAD = equivalent air depth). For example nitrox 36% reduced the real depth of 27 to 20 m calculated depth. This means that during the dive at 27 m as much nitrogen is absorbed as in a dive with normal breathing gas at 20 m (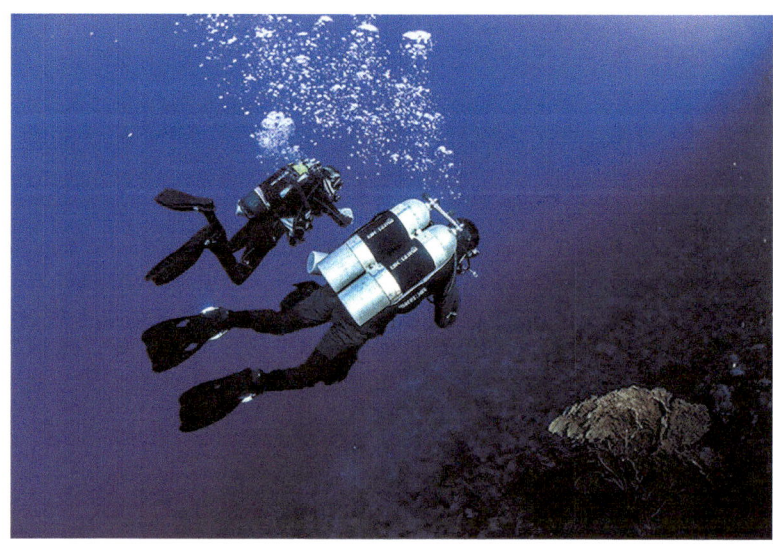 Fig. 5.2).

$$EAD\,(equivalent\,air\,depth)$$

$$EAD = \left(\frac{(1-F_mO_2)(d+x)}{(1-F_aO_2)}\right) - x$$

F_mO_2 = fraction of oxygen in mixed gases; F_aO_2 = fraction of oxygen in normal breathing

Enriched Air Nitrox

Fig. 5.2 Nitrox label. (Wikipedia)

Fig. 5.1 Tech diving. (Mares)

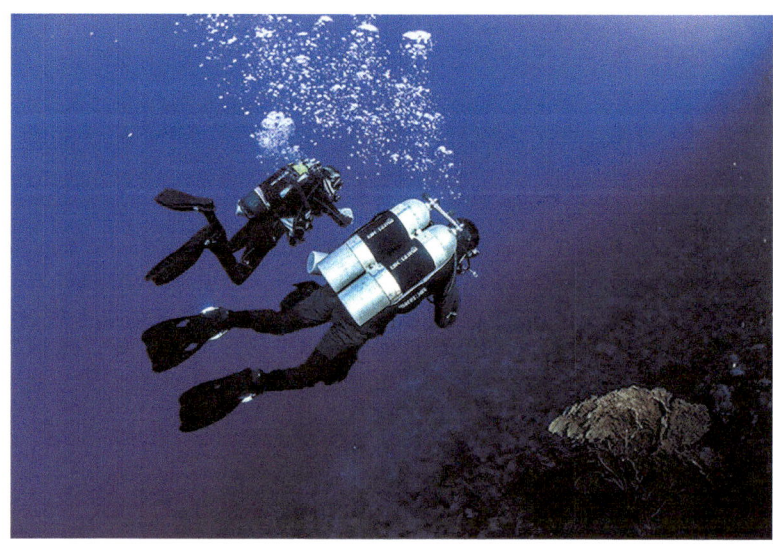

air; d = depth; x = value as function of f_{amb} multiplied with either 10 (m) and 33 (ft) in sea water or 10.3 (m) and 34 (ft) in fresh water, f_{amb} = ambient pressure fraction of sea level ambient pressure = ambient pressure at surface [bar].

The higher the proportion of oxygen, the higher the risk of oxygen poisoning. Therefore, it is necessary to calculate the maximum operating depth depending on the oxygen content of the mixed gas to avoid oxygen poisoning. The upper limit for the partial pressure of oxygen is 1.6 bar which sets maximum diving depth to 39 m with nitrox 32% and 33 m with nitrox 36% in recreational diving. For extreme diving, altitude diving, cold water diving, etc., the upper limit for the partial pressure of oxygen is 1.4 bar. At depths beyond this limit, the risk of acute oxygen poisoning and epileptic seizure increases rapidly.

MOD (maximum operation depth)

$$MOD = \left[\left(\frac{p_m O_2}{FO_2} \right) - 1 \right] \cdot x$$

FO_2 = fraction of oxygen in mixed gases; $p_m O_2$ = maximum partial pressure of oxygen; d = depth; x = value as function of f_{amb} multiplied with either 10 (m) and 33 (ft) in sea water or 10.3 (m) and 34 (ft) in fresh water, f_{amb} = ambient pressure fraction of sea level ambient pressure = ambient pressure at surface [bar].

Gas mixtures containing helium (He) are used for commercial diving at greater depth. Helium has for deep dives more favourable properties than nitrogen (N_2). Firstly, helium is lighter than nitrogen. According to Graham's law, lighter gases diffuse faster than heavier ones. Therefore, helium diffuses quicker between compartments than nitrogen. The lighter a gas, the quicker the diffusion and therefore its in- and outgassing. That means it gets quicker in and out of the body. Helium is less soluble and therefore rather remains in faster compartments like in blood. In contrast, heavier gases like nitrogen are more soluble in water and fat and hence more

relevant for in- and outgassing of slower compartments. Helium is faster in in- and outgassing and less soluble in water and fat than nitrogen. Due to these properties, nitrogen is better for short, shallow dives and helium better for longer exposure at greater depth. Additionally, gases with higher molecular weight produce bigger bubbles than smaller ones. Hence, nitrogen bubbles are bigger compared to helium bubbles, even with the same amount of gas. Switching breathing gases at unchanged depth can result in a sudden change of bubble size. This is caused by isobaric counter diffusion (ICD) [1]. It was first described by Graves, Lambersen, Idicula and Quinn in 1973. The definition of ICD is that different gases diffuse in opposite directions at constant ambient pressure. It can be distinguished between superficial ICD and deep tissue ICD. Superficial ICD occurs in diving suites containing different gases than the breathing gas, mainly resulting in skin manifestations. Deep tissue ICD is caused by switching from one breathing gas to another, often resulting in inner ear DCS manifestations. That is possible as diffusion of gases is driven by partial pressure of each individual gas and not by the total sum of gas. Gas bubbles have certain compositions of different gases. If gas mixtures are changing, gas compositions in tissue are changing too. As there are different gases in gas bubbles, gas transfer between tissues and bubble occurs to balance out these differences, even if there is no change of ambient pressure.

A switch from nitrox mixture to helium mixture could provoke bigger bubbles with a risk of DCI after switching, as this can increase the total tissue gas loading. The tissues have already a high gas loading with nitrogen. If the gas is switched to helium, there is an additional loading with helium in the blood and tissue. As helium diffuses faster into blood and tissues than nitrogen diffuses out, the total gas load increases. That always causes problems. Hence, normal air or any nitrox mixture never should be switched to heliox or trimix mixtures (■ Fig. 5.3).

5

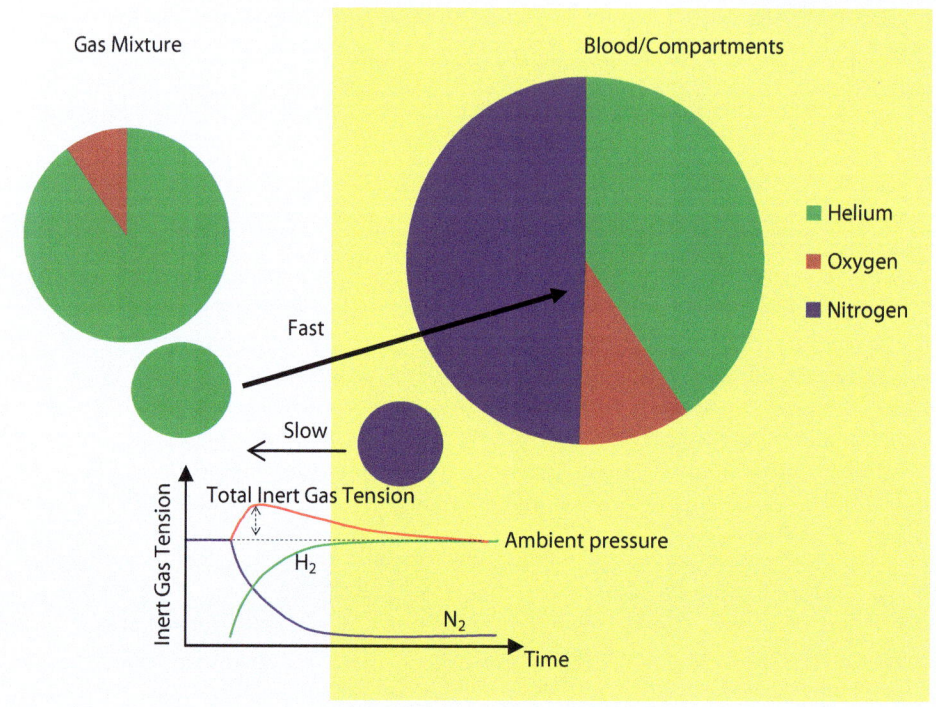

☐ **Fig. 5.3**   Changes in gas tension when switching from nitrox to heliox mixture

Switching from heliox/trimix to normal breathing gas decreases tissue gas loading. Helium diffuses out on a faster rate than nitrogen diffuses in. This results in a faster helium elimination compared to the nitrogen uptake. Hence, total gas loading is decreasing. However, it may lead to a nitrogen influx into the bubble, as the gas bubbles mainly contain helium and only little nitrogen. This might lead to a temporary increase of the size of the bubble due to nitrogen and might cause acute, mainly vestibular, symptoms just after changing the gas mixture. This is not an uncommon phenomenon in commercial divers (☐ Fig. 5.4).

To avoid problems with gas switching, gas mixtures should be changed gradually according to the depth. Helium is replaced by oxygen in heliox and by oxygen and nitrogen in trimix. In general, it might be better to switch to pure oxygen from 9 m than to normal air, to increase gas elimination and avoid ICD.

Mixed gas diving with trimix, heliox or hydrox reduces the risk of inert gas narcosis. Helium and hydrogen have a lower narcotic potency such as nitrogen. Therefore greater depths can be reached with these gas mixtures. The equivalent narcotic depth (END = equivalent narcotic depth) is calculated when helium with its fraction is used in certain depth. The formula for that is:

$$END(\text{equivalent narcotic depth})$$

$$END = (d+x) \bullet (1 - F_{He}) - x$$

F_{He} = fraction of helium in mixed gases; d = depth; x = value as function of f_{amb} multiplied with either 10 (m) and 33 (ft) in sea water or 10.3 (m) and 34 (ft) in fresh water, f_{amb} = ambient pressure fraction of sea level ambient pressure = ambient pressure at surface [bar].

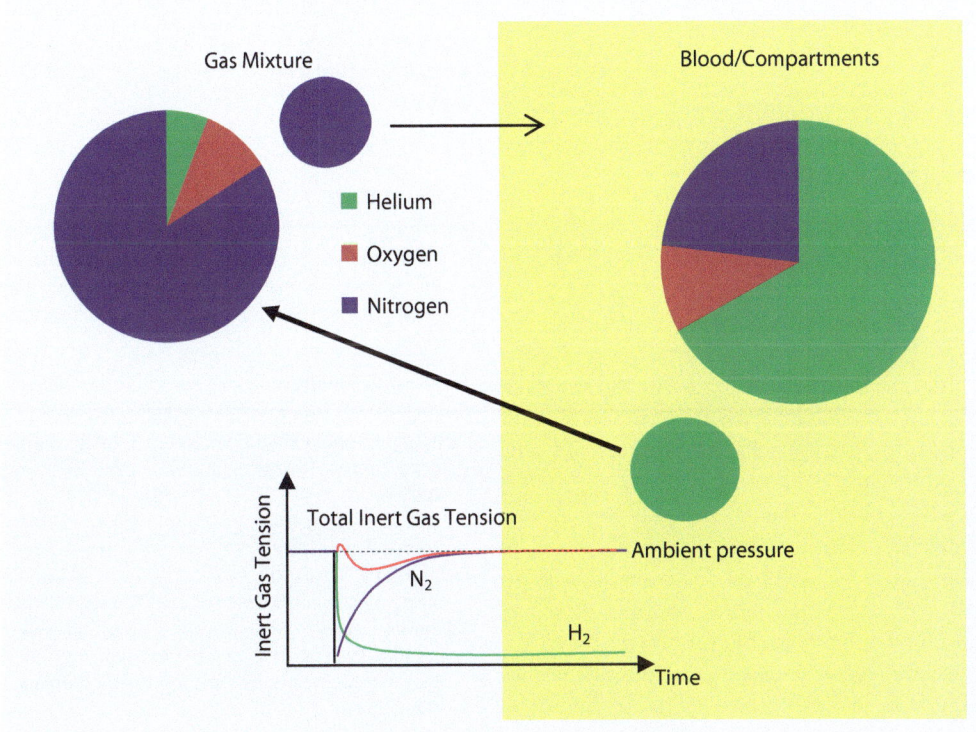

◘ Fig. 5.4   Changes in gas tension when switching from heliox to nitrox mixtures

Rebreathers are closed diving systems. The excess CO_2 is filtered with a carbon filter. This has the advantage that the dive can be extended and no bubbles are produced to obstruct the view. Incorrect devices might either eliminate completely CO_2 and therefore the physiological respiratory trigger or cause CO_2 poisoning by excess of unfiltered CO_2.

The following other formulas might be helpful for tech diving:

Individual air consumption rates

$$SAC = \frac{\Delta P \cdot x}{t(d+x)}$$

SAC = surface air consumption rate [bar or PSI/minute]; ΔP = used pressure of the scuba tank (bar or PSI); t = time; d = depth; x = value as function of f_{amb} multiplied with either 10 (m) and 33 (ft) in sea water or 10.3 (m) and 34 (ft) in fresh water, f_{amb} = ambient pressure fraction of sea level ambient pressure = ambient pressure at surface [atm].

Air consumption at specific depth

$$ACD = \frac{SAC}{x} \cdot d$$

ACD = air consumption depth; SAC = surface air consumption rate; d = Tauchtiefe; x = value as function of f_{amb} multiplied with either 10 (m) and 33 (ft) in sea water or 10.3 (m) and 34 (ft) in fresh water, f_{amb} = ambient pressure fraction of sea level ambient pressure = ambient pressure at surface [bar].

Diving time $(TT = tank\ time)$ depending on the tank filling in a specific depth

$$TT = \frac{\text{Tank pressure}}{ACD}$$

Formula (Bühlmann) for non decompression limit (NDL) in correlation of tissue nitrogen absorption and elimination:

$$NDL = -t_{1/2} \times \log 2 \left[\frac{PIN_2 - P_{t.tol}N_2(t_e)}{PIN_2 - P_t N_2(t_o)} \right]$$

$t_{1/2}$ = Half-life of the individual tissue; PIN_2 = Initial partial pressure of N_2 in the gas mix; $P_{t.tol}N_2(t_e)$ = Partial pressure of tissue N_2 after exposure; $P_t N_2(t_o)$ = Partial pressure of tissue N_2 at the start of the exposure.

The bottom time corresponds to the time, in which a risk-free surfacing from a certain depth without safety or decompression stops can be conducted. This formula however is no guarantee to be prevented from the development of a decompression sickness as several factors play a role for its development, which are not included in this formula. Perfusion, respiratory function, training, body structure and conditioning are additional factors.

Reference

1. Lambertsen JL, Bornmann RC. Isobaric inert gas counter-diffusion. Bethesda: Undersea and Hyperbaric Medical Society Publication 54WS(IC)1-11-82; 1979.

Suggested Reading

Fahlman A. On the physiology of hydrogen diving and its implication for hydrogen biochemical decompression. Carlton University, Ottawa, Ontario Canada, 2000.

Gentile G.: The technical diving handbook, G. Gentile Productions, 1998.

Richardson D. Taking 'tec' to 'rec': the future of technical diving. S Pac Underw Med Soc J. 2003; 33(4):202–205.

Taylor GH. Counter-diffusion: using isobaric mix switching to reduce decompression time. NOAA Undersea Research Center, University of North Carolina at Wilmington.

Diving Physics

Physics is an important part in understanding diving medicine. Some physical laws apply differently under water. They might have great impact on diving and dive safety. It mainly affects gases, as they are subject to physical changes under pressure. By recalling the behaviour of gases under changing pressures, application of diving guidelines suddenly make sense and mechanisms, aetiology as well as pathogenesis of diving accidents become understandable.

Contents

Composition of the Normal Air

© Springer International Publishing AG, part of Springer Nature 2018
O. Rusoke-Dierich, *Diving Medicine*, https://doi.org/10.1007/978-3-319-73836-9_6

Normal air is a combination of various gases (◘ Fig. 6.1, ◘ Table 6.1). Plants need carbon dioxide for their metabolism. The end product of plant metabolism is oxygen. Oxygen in return is required by animals and human beings for their metabolism. The end product of their metabolism again is carbon dioxide. Thus a stable cycle of gas absorption and emission emerged in the course of evolution. But air is also composed of other gases, which are not utilised in metabolism. Nitrogen is the main component. The remaining gases are noble gases (argon, neon, krypton, xenon) as well as hydrogen and helium. Nitrogen, noble gases, helium and hydrogen are only slightly reactive and are also referred to as inert gases. These gases don't participate in metabolic processes due to their chemical properties.

◘ **Table 6.1**   Composition of the normal air

Gas	Fraction (F)	Mol
Oxygen	0.20948	31.999
Carbon dioxide	0.00031	44.010
Nitrogen	0.78084	28.013
Argon	0.00934	39.948
Neon	0.00002	20.183
Helium	0.000005	4.0026
Hydrogen	0.0000005	2.0159
Other	0.0000045	
Total	1	28.964

◘ **Fig. 6.1**   Composition of the normal air

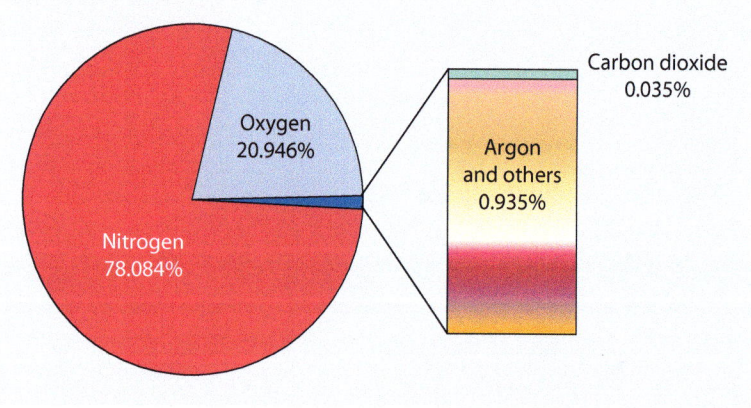

Pressure

© Springer International Publishing AG, part of Springer Nature 2018
O. Rusoke-Dierich, *Diving Medicine*, https://doi.org/10.1007/978-3-319-73836-9_7

Pressure is defined as force per unit area:

$$P = \frac{F}{A}$$

p = pressure; F = force; A = area

Pressure increases with increasing force over the same area. In a closed cavity filled with gas, pressure disperses evenly on the walls with the force directed perpendicular to the wall. With negative pressure suction is directed to the centre. Today's standard unit for pressure is Pascal. However, in diving the old description [bar], or in Anglo-American regions [PSI], is still used:

$$1\,bar = 100\,kPa = 10\,N/cm^2$$

Pressure increases with increasing depth. Underwater a water column is positioned above the diver and creates pressure. For example, in 20 m depth a 20-m water column exerts pressure on the body due to its mass. As sea water has a higher density than freshwater, the same volume of sea water produces a bigger mass and therefore more pressure. Hence, divers at 30 m depth in salt water would have equivalent pressure as at approximately 31 m depth in freshwater (Fig. 7.1).

The pressure of the water column affects only gas-filled cavities in the body (Boyle-Mariotte's law). The solid parts of the body won't be affected, as these parts aren't compressed significantly. Fluids aren't compressible unlike gases. Solid body parts react almost like above surface to pressure. However, during immersion in water, the effects of gravity on the body are almost eliminated. As a result, blood that normally is retained in the legs is redistributed throughout the entire body. As underwater, the atmosphere above water is subject to pressure changes. It is commonly referred to as atmospheric pressure (atm) pressure. The current pressure at specific depth or altitude is referred as ambient pressure. Above the mean sea level, an approximately 400 km thick layer makes the Earth's atmosphere. Of course, gas has less mass than water. Hence, pressure changes above sea level require greater distances. On the mean sea level (MSL), atmospheric pressure is approximately 1 bar. The exact value is 1.035 bar = 1 atm = 103.5 kPa = 760 mmHg. At 10 km altitude the ambient pressure is 0.264 bar. For comparison, pressure differences between 10 km altitude and sea level correspond to pressure changes from surface to 8 m depth. Additionally, weather influences atmospheric pressure with high- and low-pressure areas (Fig. 7.2).

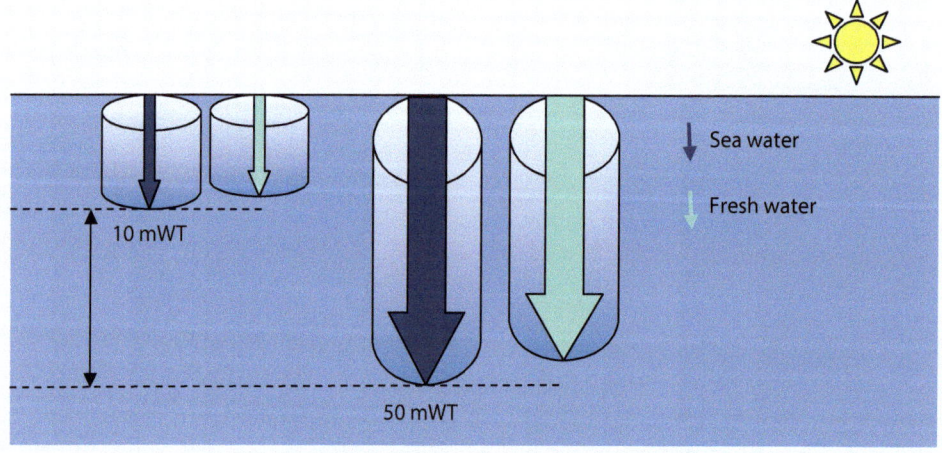

 Fig. 7.1   Water column: Pressure equivalent for sea water and fresh water

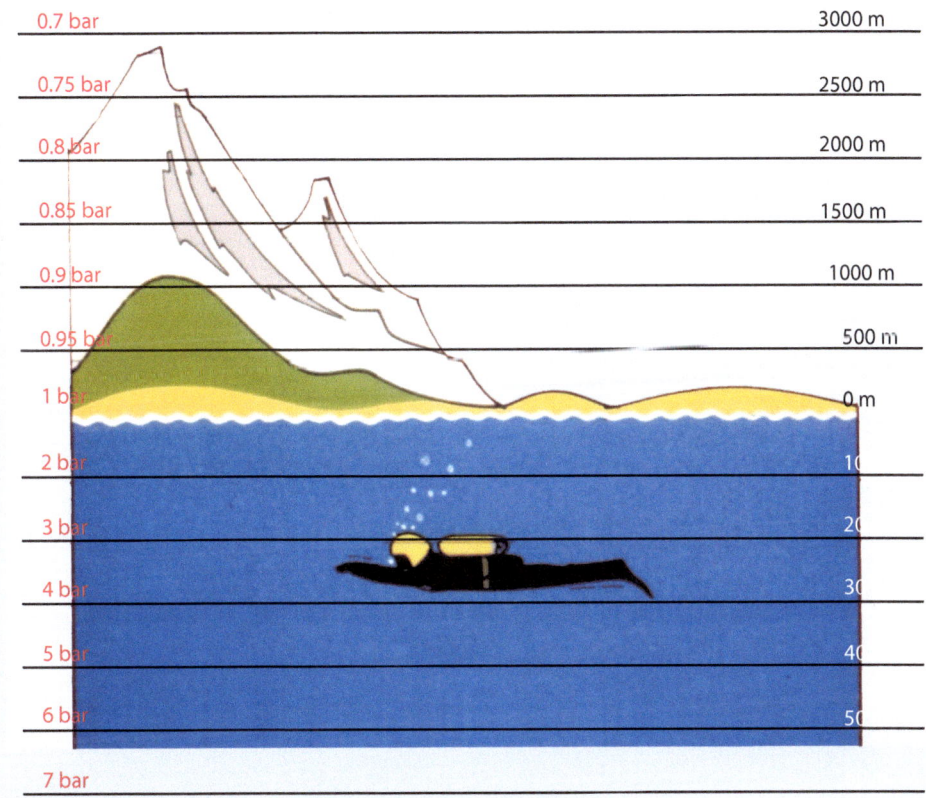

◾ **Fig. 7.2** Ambient pressure above and below mean sea level. (Ecomed)

Physical Behaviour of Gas

© Springer International Publishing AG, part of Springer Nature 2018
O. Rusoke-Dierich, *Diving Medicine*, https://doi.org/10.1007/978-3-319-73836-9_8

The physical properties of gases are characterised by their loose molecular structure. Thus, gas is more susceptible to external factors compared to liquids or solid materials. Gas has higher entropy than solids. This makes gases more vulnerable to pressure and temperature changes. The entropy of gases changes with temperature and pressure. These characteristics have been known for centuries and described by physicists.

8.1 Dalton's Law

Dalton's law describes partial pressures of gases in a gas mixture. It describes the fraction but also the sum of individual gases. The partial pressure of a gas corresponds to the percentage or fraction (f) of the individual gas in a gas mixture:

$$P_i = f_i \cdot P$$

And the absolute or total pressure is always the sum of individual partial pressures of the component gas mixture (◘ Fig. 8.1):

$$P = P_{i1} + P_{i2} + P_{i3} + \ldots P_{in}$$

P_i = partial pressure of an individual gas; f_i = percentage or fraction of a gas in a gas mixture; P = absolute ambient pressure

Normal air is a gas mixture, which is composed of different gases. The composition of the gases under atmospheric conditions at sea level has an absolute pressure of approx. 1 bar. Thus the partial pressure of oxygen is 0.21 bar, nitrogen 0.78 bar and 0.01 bar for the remaining gases. If ambient pressure changes, absolute pressure but also partial pressures of individual gases will change accordingly. For example, partial pressure of gases is twofold by doubling the absolute pressure to 2 bar (equivalent to 10-m depth).

◘ **Fig. 8.1**   Dalton's law

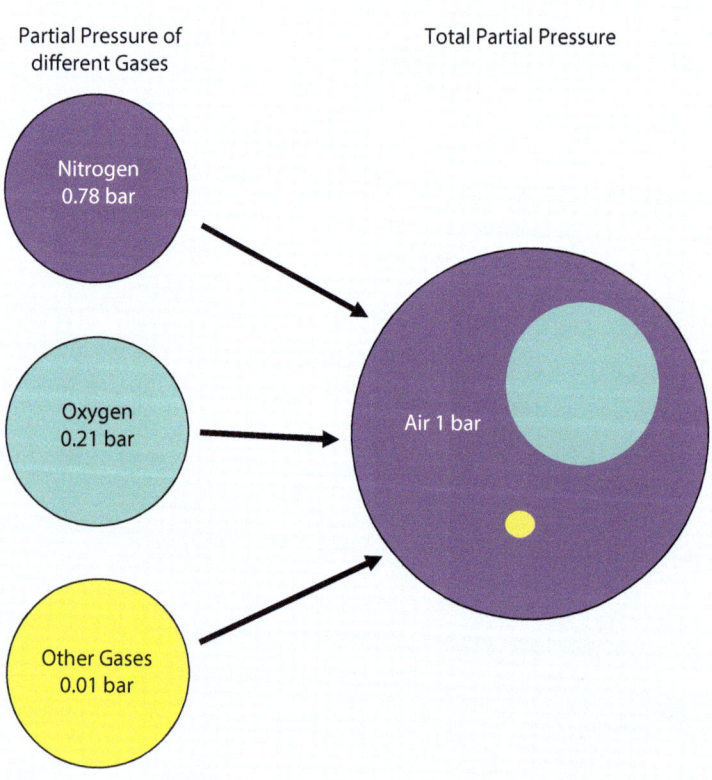

Partial Pressure of different Gases

Total Partial Pressure

Nitrogen 0.78 bar

Oxygen 0.21 bar

Other Gases 0.01 bar

Air 1 bar

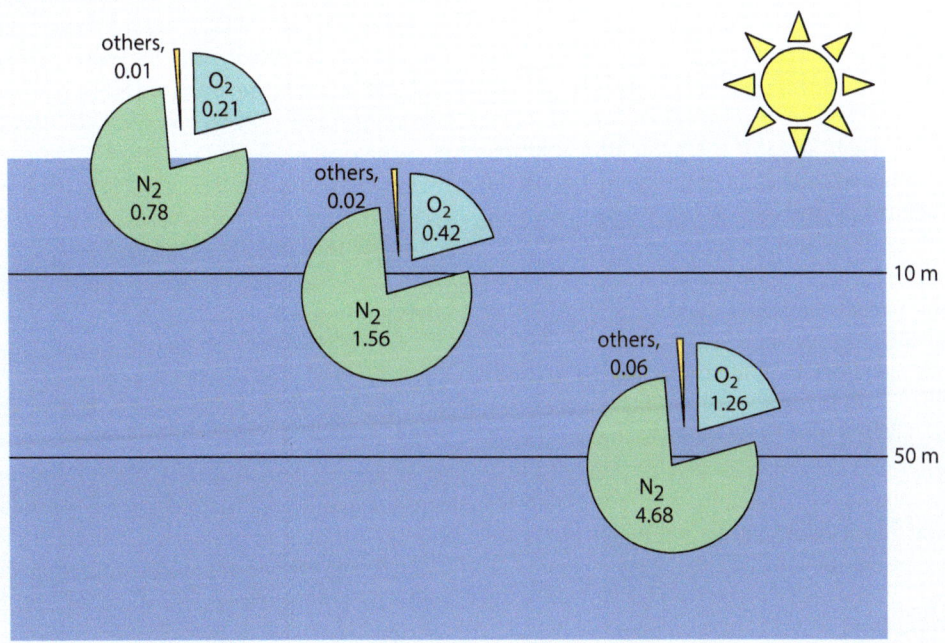

◘ **Fig. 8.2** Partial pressure of individual gases at different ambient pressures in %

Oxygen has 0.42 bar, nitrogen 1.56 bar and the remaining gases 0.02 bar (◘ Fig. 8.2).

and carbon dioxide intoxication or the development of DCS.

Example

A diver at 50-m water depth breathes normal air. The total pressure at 50 m is 6 bar. At this depth there is a sixfold higher ambient pressure compared to the surface. The air is compressed and thus denser. The same gas volume as on the surface contains "more" gas. As the molecules move closer at increased pressure, more gas molecules can be packed in the same gas volume. However, the percentage in the composition of the individual gases doesn't change. To yield the total pressure of 6 bar, the partial pressures of all individual gases increase accordingly (1.26 bar O_2 + 4.68 bar N_2 0.06 bar rest = 6 bar). The body becomes eventually saturated with these gases and their different partial pressures. This can cause problems during diving as well as ascent and after diving, e.g. inert gas narcosis, oxygen

8.2 Henry's Law

The amount of gas that can be absorbed at the same temperature in liquids is proportional to the solubility coefficient of the particular gas and to their partial pressure. The gas then diffuses into liquid and physically dissolves:

$$p_x = c_x \cdot k_H$$

c_x = concentration of the gas x in a solution; k_H = Henry's law constant of the gas x (varies with solvent and temperature; p_x = partial pressure of the gas x

The Henry's law constant k_H can be correlated with the Bunsen coefficient α:

$$k_H = \alpha_x \frac{1}{RT^{STP}}$$

then

$$p_x = \alpha_x \frac{1}{RT^{STP}}$$

c_x = concentration of the gas x in a solution; α_x = Bunsen coefficient of the gas x; p_x = partial pressure of the gas x; R = gas constant; T^{STP} = 273.15 K

During descending, ambient pressure and thus partial pressures and concentrations of breathing gases increase. Gases with higher concentrations in blood then diffuse into body tissues with lower concentrations or vice versa. This law is important to get to understand saturation and desaturation mechanisms of nitrogen in the body. The upload of nitrogen in the body and its elimination is a major factor for the development of DCI.

Example

Individual gases in the diver's tissues at the surface are in physical solution and correspond to the partial pressures of the gases in the environment. On descending the ambient pressure increases. The tissues of the diver have lower partial pressures compared to the inspiratory air. Therefore, the breathing gases diffuse from the lungs into the body until the body is saturated and has the same partial pressures as the breathing air. Because the lung has only a certain respiratory capacity and tissues take dif-

ferently long to completely saturate, this process may take a while. During the ascent this process is exactly reversed. The gases of the body diffuse into the lungs to get eliminated. The lungs however have only a limited capacity. Additionally, different tissue half-lives of gas saturation or desaturation result in a delay to release these gases. If decompression times are exceeded, the capacity of bloods keeping the gases saturated can be exceeded, and inert gas starts forming bubbles (◻ Fig. 8.3).

8.3 Boyle or Boyle-Mariotte's Law

Boyle (1662) and Mariotte (1676) independently established this gas law. It postulates that the product of pressure and volume of an individual gas is constant in a confined space at constant temperature. The mass of the gas remains however unchanged. In contrast to liquids, gas is to a greater degree compressible. The reason for this is the bigger distance of gas molecules and the weaker forces between them compared to solid materials. There are no strong molecular bonds; hence the molecules move more freely (higher entropy). If the pressure drops, molecules depart from each other and thus the total volume increases:

$$P \cdot V = \text{constant}$$

P = pressure; V = volume

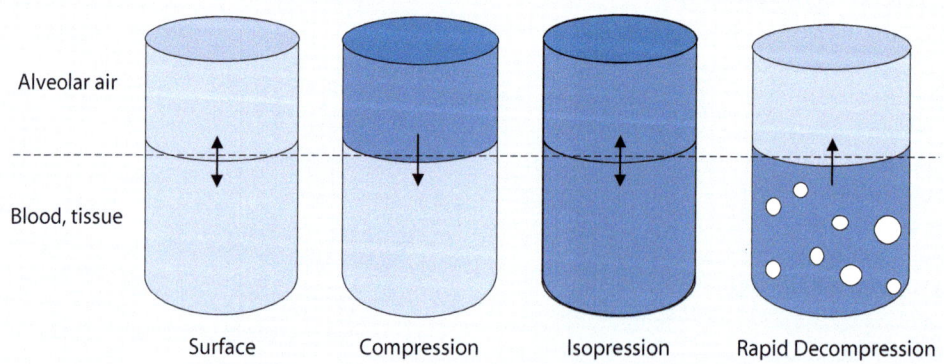

◻ **Fig. 8.3** Saturation depending to the partial pressures of the surroundings while descending and ascending according to Henry's law

Fig 8.4 Boyle-Mariotte's law gas volume dependent on ambient pressure

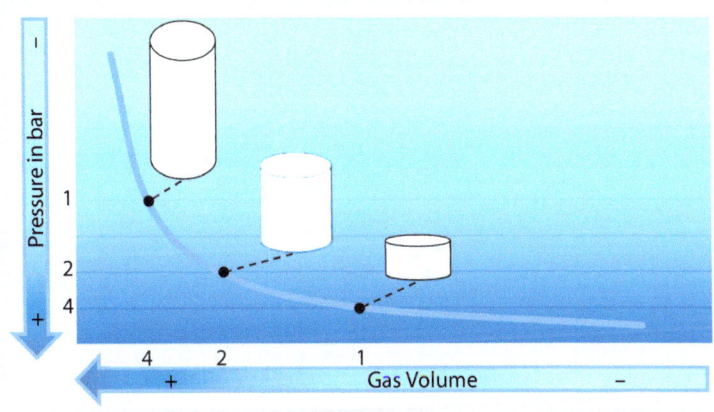

By changing either pressure or volume, one of these factors behaves inversely proportional to the other influencing factor:

$$P \sim \frac{1}{V} \; or \; V \sim \frac{1}{P}$$

That means volume decreases at increasing pressure and volume increases with decreasing pressure. And if the pressure increases, the volume decreases and vice versa (Fig. 8.4).

Formula for Volume and Pressure Changes :

$$\frac{P_1}{P_2} = \frac{V_2}{V_1}$$

P_1 = initial pressure; P_2 = actual ambient pressure; V_1 = initial volume; V_2 = actual volume

This formula explains the mechanism of barotraumas where the change of pressure causes changes in the gas volume and therefore damage to the body.

Example

During descending the diver feels pressure in his ears. The pressure is a direct result of decreasing gas volume in the middle ear. The middle ear is a closed body cavity and thus is sensitive to pressure changes. An increase in pressure causes a reduction in gas volume in the middle ear. The result is that the eardrum curves inward and starts hurting due to the tension. A remedy for this is equalising, which restores the gas volume in the middle ear. On the other hand, decompression causes an increase of gas volume. If a scuba diver holds his breath during ascent, the increased gas volume can't escape. Therefore, pressure within the lungs increases, the lung extends and it may result in a ruptured lung with its severe consequences.

8.4 Fick's Law of Diffusion

Diffusion requires two compartments, with varying substance concentrations. The boundary of these compartments is known as the exchange surface (Fig. 8.5).

The diffusion of substances during a specific time is proportional to the diffusion coefficient, the exchange surface and the concentration difference of these substances. The diffusion rate not only depends on the partial pressure of the individual gas but also on the exchange surface and the properties of the diffusing substance:

$$J_{diff} = F \cdot D \cdot \frac{\Delta C}{\Delta X} [\text{mol} / \text{s}]$$

J_{diff} = diffusion flux; ΔQ = amount of the diffusing substance; Δx = diffusion course; D = diffusion coefficient; F = exchange surface; ΔC = concentration difference

◻ Fig. 8.5 Diffusion

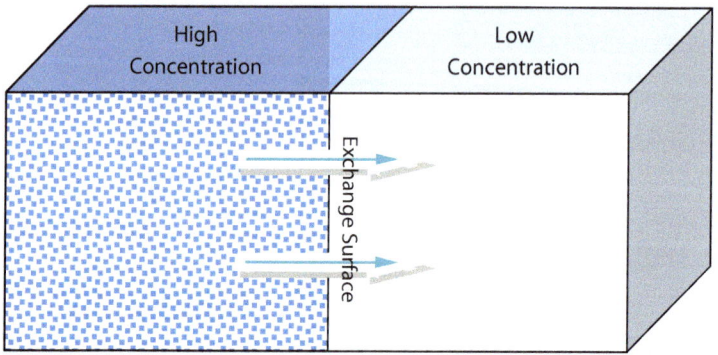

Because cells have a lipid membrane, the oil-water partition coefficient k must be included in the equation. The new equation is

$$J_{diff} = \kappa F \cdot D \cdot \frac{\Delta C}{\Delta X} \left[mol / s \right]$$

For gases the formula can be further modified. The concentration difference ΔC of the substances will be replaced with the partial pressure difference ΔP multiplied with the solubility coefficients α of the various gases (Henry's Law). The solubility coefficient α, the diffusion coefficient D and the oil-water partition coefficient k are then grouped together to the Krogh's diffusion coefficient K ($\alpha \cdot D \cdot k = K$). Converted for gases the new formula of the 1st Fick's law of diffusion is now

$$V_{diff} = F \cdot K \frac{\Delta P}{\Delta x} \left[m^3 / s \right]$$

V_{diff} = diffusing volume; Δx = diffusion distance; K = Krogh's diffusion coefficient; F = exchange surface; ΔP = partial pressure difference

As shown in this formula exchange surface, partial pressure difference and solubility coefficient are important parameters in gas diffusion. During diving differences of partial pressures between inspiratory and expiratory air and body tissue are created. Partial pressures of tissues and blood at higher ambient pressure balance gradually out. The most important gas in

this process during diving is nitrogen. Initially strongly perfused tissues become saturated. The increased perfusion is usually related to a high number of blood vessels. Because all these vessels have also a large exchange surface, nitrogen diffuses faster and easier into these tissues. The diffusion is slower in less perfused tissues. Additionally, each tissue has a different composition and each gas has different solubilities. Both affect diffusion in and out of tissues. Because of all this, it takes different time to saturate all tissues. As a result, there are different no-decompression limits for each compartment to avoid the point of critical supersaturation. Under extreme environmental conditions, tissues might be saturated even faster, despite adhering to dive tables. Theoretically on decompression the desaturation process of all tissues is expected to be exactly reversed. Instead of being saturated, tissues are desaturated. However, practically that isn't really the case as desaturation takes longer than saturation. Blood circulation in addition to the fat content of tissues influences greatly the saturation or desaturation nitrogen half-lives of tissues. The delayed desaturation is among other things responsible for late DCI, which may occur even hours or days after diving.

Fick and Wienke (1989) proposed a new diffusion rate equation in regard to bubble physics:

$$\frac{\partial c_t}{\partial t} = \nabla \left(D \cdot \nabla c_t \right) + \bar{Q} \left(c_a - c_v \right) - Z_{met} - Z_b$$

D = diffusion rate; c_t = gas concentration tissue; c_a = arterial gas concentration; c_v = venous gas concentration; $\bar{Q}$ = blood perfusion rate; Z_{met} = metabolic gas consumption rate; Z_b = bubble growth gas consumption

Example

A diver goes diving in the 16 °C cold Pacific Ocean. Within 5 days two dives daily were conducted. Since he has only his 5-mm wetsuit without hood, he freezes during the entire dives. He also has to fight with strong currents. Because the last dive was more than 20-m deep and it was not a decompression dive, they didn't even make a safety stop. 2 hours later he showed the first symptoms of a decompression accident. Due to the cold-water temperature and the high physical exertion, the metabolism and the blood flow to the muscles were increased. In addition to cardiovascular activity, also respiration was increased. Therefore, tissues became faster saturated with nitrogen as under normal conditions. During the ascend nitrogen could be not eliminated enough. Therefore, the nitrogen concentration in the diver's body was so high that bubbles were formed, which resulted then in his decompression accident.

8.5 Charles's Law

Charles's law proposes that gas volume is proportional to temperature:

$$\frac{V}{T} = \text{constant}$$

V = volume; T = temperature
    That means, if the temperature is increasing, the gas volume increases too:

$$\frac{V_1}{T_1} = \frac{V_2}{T_2}$$

V = volume; T = temperature; 1 = initial; 2 = consecutive

Example

Charles's law explains why after diving a hot shower should be avoided, as already existing gas bubbles may increase their volume with increased temperature and trigger a DCI. Additionally, nitrogen solubility decreases with increasing temperatures, leading to an increase release of free nitrogen into vessels and tissue.

8.6 Gay-Lussac's Law

This law describes the dependence of pressure and gas volume from temperature:

$$\frac{P}{T} = \text{constant}$$

P = pressure; T = temperature
    That means, if the temperature is increasing, the pressure increases too (◘ Fig. 8.6):

$$\frac{P_1}{T_1} = \frac{P_2}{T_2}$$

P = pressure; T = temperature; 1 = initial, 2 = consecutive

8.7 Combined Gas Law

The combined gas law is an amalgamation of Charles's law, Gay-Lussac's law and Boyle's law. It describes the interaction of volume, temperature and pressure. With increasing temperature gas molecules move away from each other and entropy increases. The gas expands with pressure remaining constant. If the gas can't expand and the volume remains constant, the pressure increases. Conversely, if temperature increases, the pressure is increased at constant volume:

$$\frac{P \cdot V}{T_{abs}} = \text{constant}$$

P = pressure; V = volume; T_{abs} = absolute temperature

■ **Fig. 8.6** Pressure changes at different temperatures according to Gay-Lussac's and Charles's law

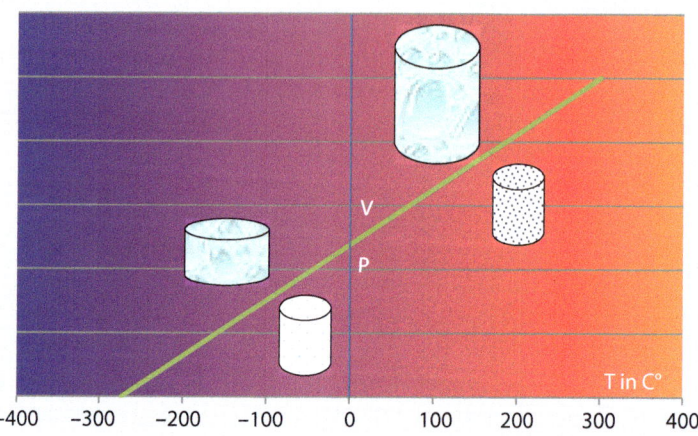

8

With modification of one of these factors, this formula is

$$\frac{P_1 \cdot V_1}{T_1} = \frac{P_2 \cdot V_2}{T_2}$$

P_1 = initial pressure; V_1 = initial volume; T_1 = initial temperature; P_2 = end pressure; V_2 = end volume; T_2 = end temperature

Example

Icing of the regulator may occur during diving. Beginning at about 5–10-m depth in freshwater lakes, there is a so-called thermocline with a constant temperature of 4 °C. Icing of the regulator results from a decline in pressure from the scuba tank (approx. 200 bar) to the 1st stage of the regulator (approx. 10–14 bar) together with cold environmental temperatures. Only small amounts of residual humidity can cause freezing of the 1st stage of the regulator and hence interfere with the air supply. Another temperature-related issue might cause trouble during or after diving. The combined gas law also explains warming of scuba tanks during their filling. Air is compressed during that process into the constant volume of a scuba tank with increasing pressure. The volume remains the same, but the pressure increases in only a short time. After the filling the scuba tanks lose some pressure

by cooling down, so they have to be topped up again.

8.8 Ideal Gas Law

The ideal gas law was postulated by Emile Clapeyron in 1834. It is a combination of Boyle's law, Charles's law and Avogadro's law. It describes the behaviour of hypothetical ideal gas under different conditions:

$$P \cdot V = n \cdot R \cdot T = N \cdot k \cdot T$$

R = universal gas constant = 8.13145 J/molK = 62.364 mmHg/molK = 8.3144621 bar/molK; T = temperature; N = number of molecules; n = number of moles; k = Boltzmann constant = 1.38066×10^{-23} J/K; $k = R/N_A$; A = Avogadro's number = 60.221×10^{23} /mol

The ideal gas law is only accurate under low pressures and high temperatures. A compressibility factor (Z) corrects it to the true gas law:

$$P \times V = Z \times n \times R \times T$$

If concentration needs to be included, the equation has to be rearranged with

$$C = \frac{n}{V}$$

$$P = C \times R \times T$$

8.9 Graham's Law of Effusion and Diffusion

Thomas Graham (1805–1869) described the effusion and diffusion of gases. Effusion is the process of molecules' travel through a small pinhole from a place of higher concentration to low concentration. Diffusion is a shift from an area of higher concentration to and area of lower concentration. The rates of diffusion and effusion both depend on the velocities of the gas molecules and are linked to the molecular weight. The rate of effusion or diffusion at constant temperature and pressure is indirectly proportional to the square root of the molecular weight:

$$R \propto \frac{1}{\sqrt{m}}$$

R = rate of diffusion or effusion; m = molecular weight

Because gases with a lower molecular weight are less cumbersome, they diffuse faster than the ones with higher molecular weights and vice versa. In diving that relates to the usage of different gas mixtures. For example, the diffusion rate of He compared to N_2 is 2.6 times higher. This means it in- and out-gases quicker which makes it more favourable for deep dives to avoid DCI. Additionally, due to its lower molecular weight, He has a lower density, which is beneficial for deep diving in regard to respiration and ventilation.

Suggested Reading

Anderson M. The physics of scuba diving. Nottingham: Nottingham University Press; 2011.

Dierich W. Das Grosse Fliegerhandbuch. 1 Auflage ed. Stuttgart: Motorbuchverlag; 1990.

Schmidt RF, Lang F, Heckmann M. Physiologie des Menschen. 31 Auflage ed. Berlin: Springer; 2010.

Taylor L. Diving physics. In: Bove AA, Davis JC, editors. Diving medicine. 4th ed. Philadelphia: Saunders; 2004. p. 11–35.

West JB. Respiratory physiology. 5th ed: Williams & Wilkins; 1995.

Decompression Theory

© Springer International Publishing AG, part of Springer Nature 2018
O. Rusoke-Dierich, *Diving Medicine*, https://doi.org/10.1007/978-3-319-73836-9_9

9.1 Classical Decompression Theory

The French physician *Paul Bert* (1833–1886) recognized the problem of accidents during and after decompression and therefore recommended a slow ascent. *John Scott Haldane* developed dive tables for the US Navy in 1908. Fundamentals of his research are incorporated in today's dive tables. His calculations included exponential saturation and desaturation, five different body compartments, gradual decompression in 3-m intervals and the concept of maximum supersaturation with the so-called Haldane factor [6]. He postulated that the partial pressure of inert gases in all tissues should not exceed twofold (2:1) of the ambient pressure during the ascent to avoid decompression accidents. In other words, a direct reduction to an ambient pressure from a twofold overpressure is regarded not to cause any DCS symptoms. For example, a direct ascent from 10 m after a saturation dive without deco stop is supposed to be safe. However, Workman corrected the value later to 1.58:1, considering only partial pressures of inert gases, primarily nitrogen. Haldane assumed that the main factor of a decompression accident during rapid ascents is caused by fast compartments. He postulated that slow compartments are responsible for decompression accidents during slow ascents and decompression stops. He established the basic principle of compartment saturation and desaturation based on tissue perfusion. He set the ascent rate initially to 18 m/min than later to 9 m/min.

■ **Haldane Equation**

$$p_{t_{(amb)}} = p_{t_{(t_0)}} + \left(p_{alv_{(amb)}} - p_{t_{(t_0)}} \right)(1 - e^{-k*\Delta t})$$

The Haldane equation is a good way to calculate loading and off-loading at steady pressure. It is based on half-lives and saturation times, reflecting general principles of pharmacodynamics. The initial tissue partial pressure $p_{t_{(t_0)}}$ reflects the starting point and the ambient

alveolar partial pressure $p_{alv_{(amb)}}$ the end point. The initial tissue partial pressure $p_{t_{(t_0)}}$ is added as the calculation doesn't start at 0 but at the given tissue pressure. The constant (k) is related to halftime $(T_{1/2})$ calculations with

$$k = \frac{\ln 2}{T_{1/2}}$$

Loading and off-loading is a continuous process. On inspiration there is a loading of gas into the arterial system expected, if p_{alv} is higher than p_{art}. During descending there is always a loading. On ascending the alveolar and arterial partial pressure is almost equal, so no or minimal ingassing is possible, depending on the ascent rate. Vice versa on expiration, there is an off-loading, if p_{ven} is higher than p_{alv}. On descending there is never an off-loading as the alveolar partial pressure is always greater than the venous one. On ascending there is not always an off-loading. Loading and off-loading is depending on the partial pressure difference between alveolar gas mix and blood. Gas exchange, between blood and tissue, is more complex and varies between compartments. Slow compartments, for example, still can load even with decreasing ambient pressure, if the alveolar partial pressure is higher than their tissue partial pressure. The pressure gradient determines the initial rate of loading and off-loading. The initial rate follows a more or less steep curve. The flatter the curve is the lesser the rate changes. During pressure reduction loading of $p_{t_{(amb)}}$ of slow compartments can slow down as the gradient between ambient and initial tissue partial pressure is reduced.

For linear changing pressure, Schreiner later modified the Haldane equation to enable computer calculations.

■ **Schreiner Equation**

$$p_{t_{(t)}} = p_{alv_{(0)}} + R\left(t + -\frac{R}{k} \right)$$
$$- \left(p_{alv_{(0)}} - p_{t_{(t)}} - \frac{R}{k} \right) e^{-k \times t}$$

9.2 Modern Decompression Theory

Different models followed the Haldane model, which were not only based on the tissue perfusion. Other models included, for example, diffusion-limiting models for gas transport in and out of tissues. Models, like the one of Hempleman, were more conservative. Albert A. Bühlmann, Max Hahn and Edward D. Thalmann reformed the dive tables in the 1980s. They were precise and detailed. The calculation of Bühlmann included 16 compartments (ZH16) [5] with half-lives of 4 min up to 635 min (◻ Table 9.1). The US Navy E-L algorithm from 2008 combines an exponential and linear saturation and desaturation models. The saturation time

has been extended and as a result the tables became safer.

Extended knowledge and inclusion of more factors have emerged in diving theory since mid last century. An important step was the development of M-values [bar] with "M" standing for "maximum". Robert D. Workman brought up this concept in the 1960s. Bühlmann added more details to it later on. It describes that each compartment has its own maximum saturation capacity. The M-value describes the maximum inert gas saturation in certain compartments, without incurring symptoms of DCS. It is believed that tissues can hold an excess amount of gas. Therefore, the supersaturation allows higher values than the expected saturation at ambient pressure. This represents a tolerated gradient between

◻ **Table 9.1** Bühlmann ZH16

Compartment	Halftime N₂ in minutes	Saturation time in hours and minutes	b	a (ZH16A – theoretical)	a (ZH16B – table)	a (ZH16C – computer)
1	4	0:24	0.5050	1.2599	1.2599	1.2599
2	8	0:48	0.6514	1.0000	1.0000	1.0000
3	12.5	1:15	0.7222	0.8618	0.8618	0.8618
4	18.5	1:51	0.7825	0.7562	0.7562	0.7562
5	27	2:42	0.8126	0.6667	0.6667	0.6200
6	38.3	3:50	0.8434	0.5933	0.5600	0.5043
7	54.3	5:26	0.8693	0.5282	0.4947	0.4410
8	77	7:42	0.8910	0.4701	0.4500	0.4000
9	109	10:54	0.9092	0.4187	0.4187	0.3750
10	146	14:36	0.9222	0.3789	0.3789	0.3500
11	187	18:42	0.9319	0.3497	0.3497	0.3295
12	239	23:54	0.9403	0.3223	0.3223	0.3065
13	305	30:30	0.9477	0.2971	0.2850	0.2835
14	390	39:00	0.9544	0.2737	0.2737	0.2610
15	498	49:48	0.9602	0.2523	0.2523	0.2480
16	635	63:30	0.9653	0.2327	0.2327	0.2327

inert gas pressure and ambient pressure. Other names for supersaturation are limits for tolerated overpressure, supersaturation limit or critical tension. The Workman M-value line begins at sea level, where Bühlmann's M-value line starts at 0 bar absolute. Therefore, Bühlmann's M-value line can be used for altitude diving too. However, Bühlmann's M-values are slightly incorrect at the section of low ambient pressure as they violate the second law of thermodynamics. The M-value curve should be exponential at decreasing pressure and shouldn't be used in a linear way as it is used in his calculations (🔲 Fig. 9.1).

In general, fast compartments absorb more nitrogen in correlation to the depth than slower ones during a normal dive. However, if diving time is long enough, eventually all compartments are filled up. This is called saturation dive (🔲 Table 9.2).

With

$$\Delta M = \frac{1}{b}$$

and

$$M_0 = a$$

and a minimum permissible (tolerated) ambient pressure

$$P_{\min} = (p - a)b$$

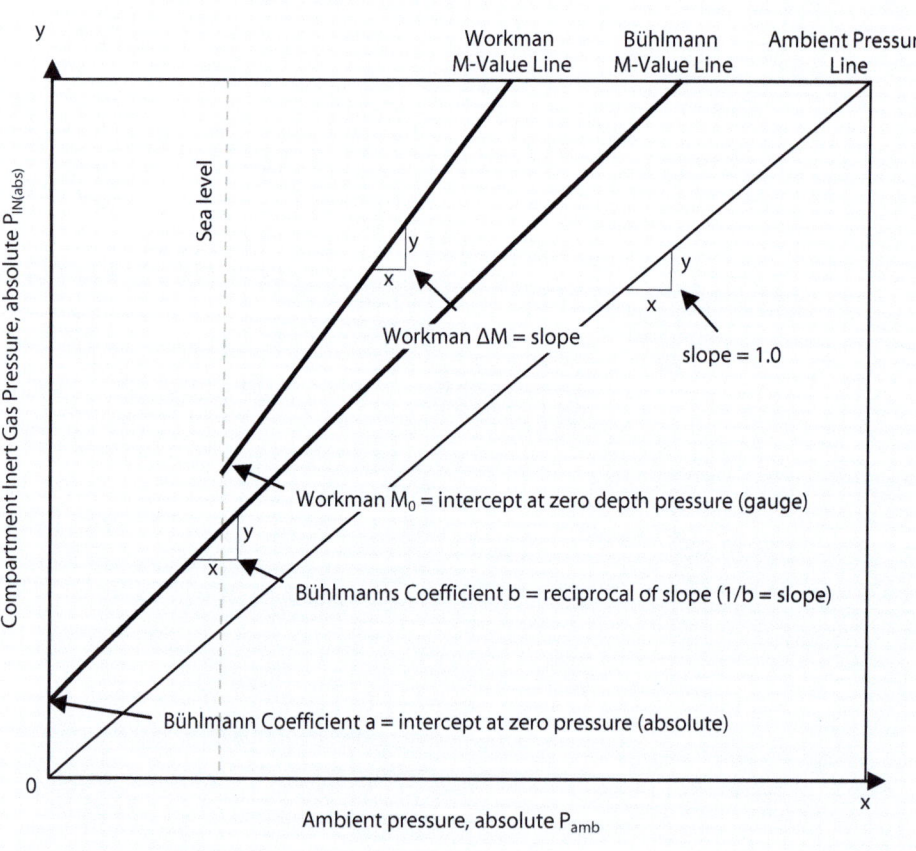

🔲 **Fig. 9.1**   Workman and Bühlmann's M-value lines. (Erik Baker [2])

□ **Table 9.2** Equations for the maximal saturation capacity

Workman	Bühlmann
$M = M_0 + \Delta M d$	$P_{t.\,tol}\text{i.g.} = (P_{amb}/b) + a$

$P_{t.tol}$ i.g. tolerated absolute inert gas pressure in the hypothetical compartment, P_{amb} absolute ambient pressure, a critical intercept/point of intersection at 0 bar ambient pressure, b critical slope/reciprocal value of the M-value line gradient

Values (M_0) closer to the surface are relevant for nonstop diving and values at depth, ΔM, rather for decompression diving. The USN sets the M_0 (= $152.7\tau^{-1/4}$ fsw = $46.5\tau^{-1/4}$ msw) and the ΔM ($3.25\tau^{-1/4}$ fsw = $0.99\tau^{-1/4}$ msw). This can be contrasted with the original Haldane constant critical tension M:

$$M = 1.58P$$

with the corresponding critical gradient

$$G = \frac{M}{0.79} - P$$

P = ambient pressure; G = critical gradient or the critical ratio

$$R = \frac{M}{P}$$

R = critical ratio

For diving in altitude, a correlation to the ambient pressure must be made:

$$d = P_a - P_z$$

P_a = absolute pressure; P_z = surface pressure

$$P_z = x \exp(-0.0381z) = x\alpha^{-1}$$

$$x = 33\,(\text{ft}),\, x = 10\,(\text{m})$$

$$\alpha = \exp(0.0381z);\text{ with } z \text{ in multiples}$$
$$\text{of } 1000\,\text{ft}\,(304.8\,\text{m}).$$

At altitude, no testing has been performed for critical tensions. Critical tensions below 10 msw (33 fsw) fall more rapidly than in the linear case. An exponentially decreasing extrapolation scheme, called similarity, is used for its calculation:

$$\frac{M(d)}{d + x\alpha^{-1}} = \frac{M(\delta)}{\delta + x}$$

$x = 33$ (ft) or 10 (m)

It can be assumed that there is a linear relationship between a safe pressure reduction and the degree of saturation. An empirically determined formula includes the current ambient pressure (P_1); a low pressure (P_2), to which can be ascended safely; and the constants a and b (these constants apply to the following formula and different from the one above). The values of the constants a and b vary depending on different authors ($a = 1.518$–1.401; $b = 0.42$–0.57):

$$P_1 = aP_2 + b$$

An approaching or exceeding of M-values increases the risk of DCI. However, M-values are only a guideline, not absolute values. Decompression accidents can also occur below M-values. M-values aren't reflecting the tolerable saturation gradients or the tolerable number of gas bubbles. A certain number of gas bubbles are considered safe (N_{safe}). The more excess gas bubbles are present, by approaching the M-value line, the more likely is a decompression accident to occur. To calculate the excess gas bubbles, the safe number of gas bubbles has to be subtracted from the total number of gas bubbles (N_{actual}):

$$\text{Excess gas bubbles} = N_{actual} - N_{safe}$$

The closer the dive profile is to the ambient pressure line, the safer the dive could be considered. The closer dive profile and inert gas saturation come to the M-value, the greater is the probability of a DCI. Between the ambient pressure line and the M-value line, a "conservatism factor" can be placed. This factor is outlined in percentage. The smaller it is, the more conservative and therefore safer the dive profile is. A dive table or computer is as safe as its conservatism factor and vice versa. The ambient pressure line is 0% and the M-value line 100%. In general, a conservatism factor of 50% is recommended. Other methods apply the gradient factor (GF) by Erik Baker [2]. There is a high and low GF with values ranging from% 0 to 100% or 0.0 to 1.0. The farther the value of the gradient is away from the M-value line, the more secure is the dive profile. The GF-line doesn't have to run parallel to the ambient pressure line, because the high and the low GF might have different values. The GF will be calculated as follows:

$$GF = \frac{\text{Tissue Tension} - \text{Ambient Pressure}}{M_{\text{Value}} - \text{Ambient Pressure}}$$

It reflects simply a decimal fraction or percentage of the M-value gradient. It is specified as a ratio, where the low GF appears on the top and the high GF at the bottom of the ratio, e.g. GF 30/80% or GF 70/20%. The ratio determines how the dive profile is set. For example, a GF 30/80% has its deco stops rather in greater depth. In a GF 70/20%, the deco stops would rather be at shallow depth and less frequent in greater depth. The determination of the GF influences therefore the dive profile (Fig. 9.2).

However, the GF is not validated by any data like the RF (reduction factor) of the early RGBM works. The RF is correlated to data with the M-values and imbedded in various diving computers and diving tables. The M-value in correlation to RF (ξ) is

$$M_\xi = \xi G + P$$

Combined with the formula of Bühlmann or Workman

$$G = M - P$$

The new formula for the critical gradient (G) with the RF is

$$M_\xi = \xi (M - P) + P$$

A certain inert gas supersaturation is tolerated during diving. The distance between the inert gas pressure gradient and the supersaturation gradient represents a safety gap, in which an acceptable number of gas bubbles are assumed, without causing any symptoms of a DCI. Repeated pushing of the limits of dive tables or computers narrows the safety gap and hence increases the risk of DCI. Deco and safety stops reduce the number of gas bubbles and avoid inert gas saturation close to the M-value line or above (Figs. 9.3 and 9.4).

$$\text{Supersaturation Gradient}\,(\text{Bühlmann})$$

$$P_{SS} = M - d = M_0 + d(\Delta M - 1)$$

M = maximal saturation capacity; M_0 = initial saturation capacity of the tissue; ΔM = difference of the saturation capacities ($M - M_0$); d = depth; P_{SS} = supersaturation gradient (difference of dissolved gas in tissue and ambient pressure)

The inert gas pressure gradient is the driving force in gas transfer between the lungs, blood and tissues. The gas transfer in blood and tissue is assumed to be exponential. By the given pressure difference and exposure time, the gas transfer can be calculated:

$$P_{(t_e)} = P_{(t_0)} + \left(P_{\text{alv}} - P_{(T_0)}\right)\left(1 - e^{-k \cdot t}\right)$$

$P_{(t_e)}$ = inert gas partial pressure at the end of exposure; $P_{(t_0)}$ = inert gas partial pressure at the beginning of exposure; P_{alv} = alveolar inert gas partial pressure; t = exposure time; k = perfusion constantwith

$$k = \frac{\ln 2}{T_{1/2}}$$

$T_{1/2}$ = halftime; k = perfusion constant

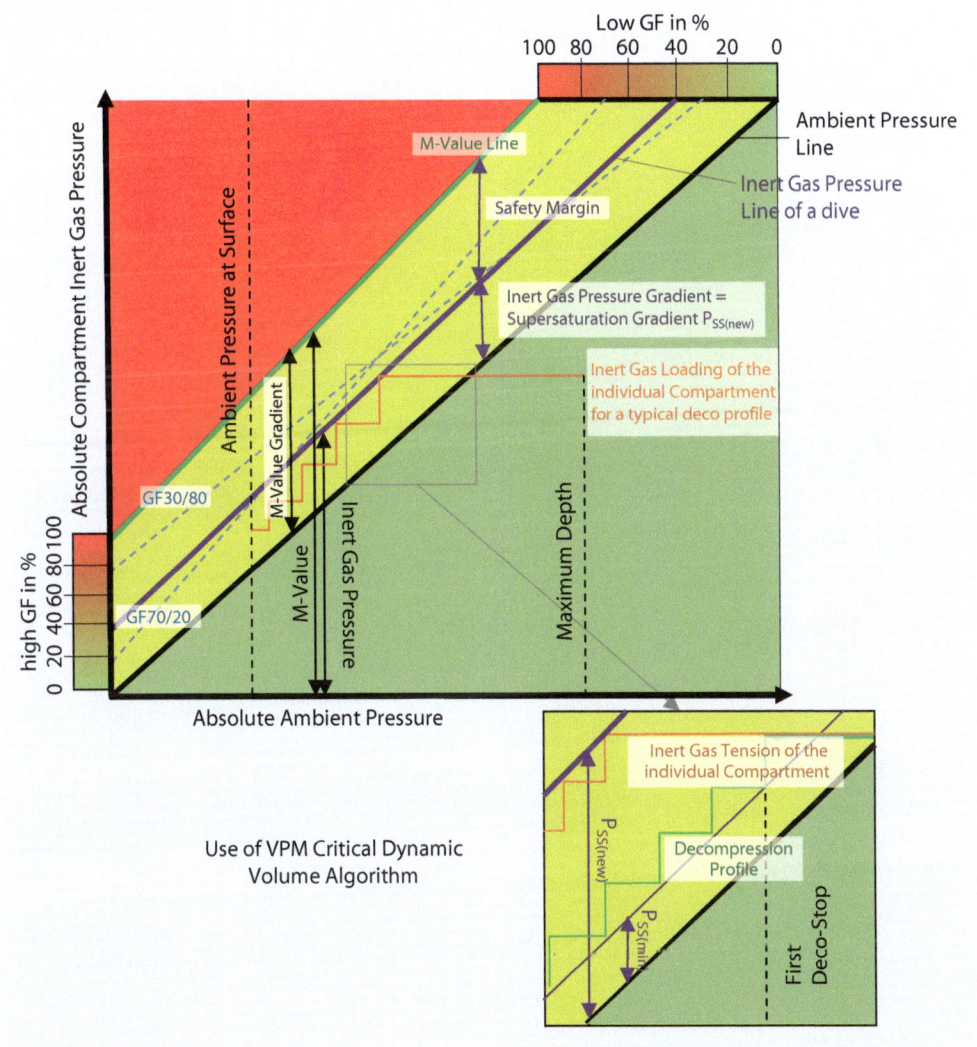

Fig. 9.2 Schematic illustration of the different gradients in correlation to the inert gas pressure and ambient pressure. (Erik Baker [2])

■ **Decompression Models for the Computer Algorithms** [14]

The most commonly used model is the *multitissue model (MTM)*, which is based on the Haldane model. Haldane created the critical ratio model with its pressure ratio of 2 to 1 for decompression. This means that there should be no bubble formation, if the inert gas partial pressure of compartments doesn't exceed the ambient pressure by 2:1 due to the ascent rate. That means that unlimited diving with no decompression stops is possible with a twofold pressure reduction, e.g. from 10 msw to the surface or from 30 msw to 10 msw. His calculations were used in the first half of the last century. In the late twentieth century, his model

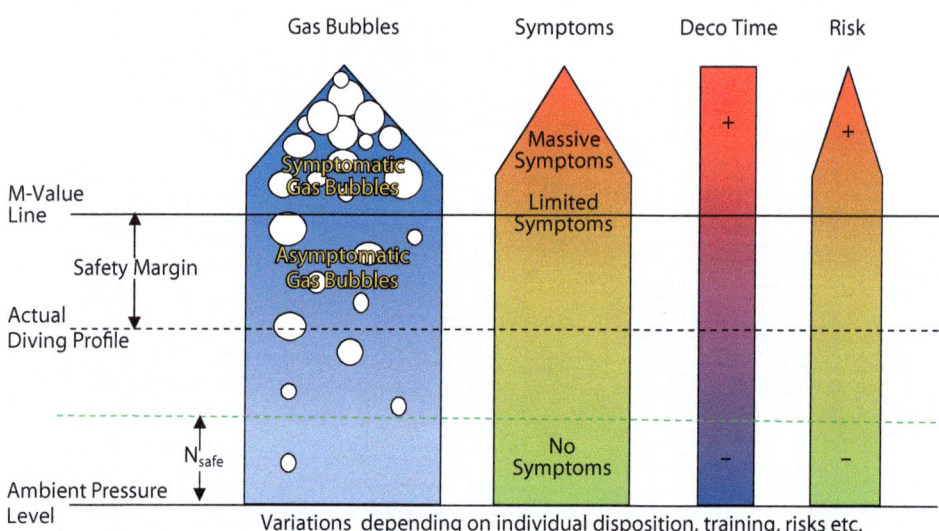

◘ Fig. 9.3   Effects of the diving profile in correlation to the *M*-value. (Erik Baker [2])

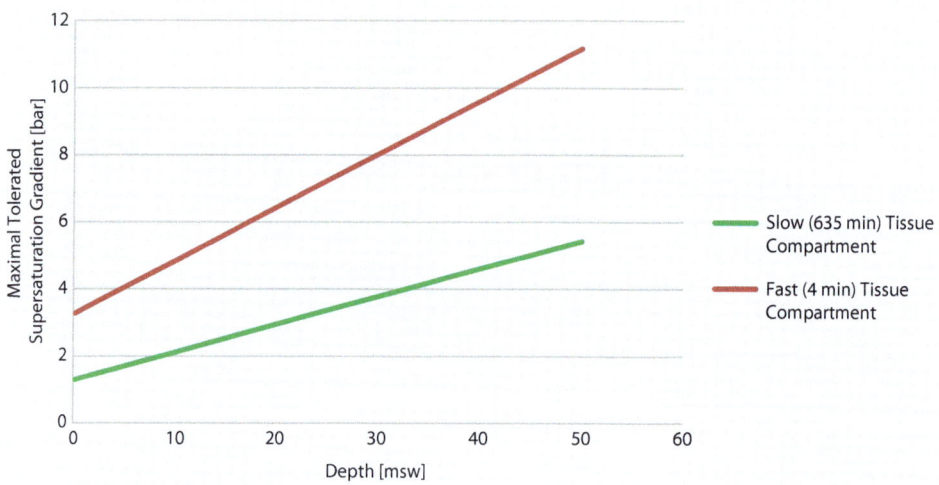

◘ Fig. 9.4   Maximal supersaturation of slow and fast tissue compartments in correlation to the depth

was adjusted by including the *M*-values from Workman. Haldane's model was too conservative for fast compartments and not conservative enough for slow compartments. Hence, it was later adjusted by Workman to 1.58:1. Workman only included nitrogen in this ratio with its fraction of 0.78 as this is the causative gas for DCI. Bühlmann reduced that ratio to 1.53: 1, as he was taking 1.53 bar as the inspiratory nitrogen partial pressure in the alveoli (BTPS) at 2 bar, not the nitrogen partial pressure in standard conditions (STPD). In other words a supersaturation of 0.53 bar is assumed to be tolerated. These values can be only used for saturation dives, where all compartments are fully saturated. This requires exposure times of approx 600 min. Studies from the US Navy and Bühlmann compared exposure times and tolerated inert gas partial pressures. It showed depending on compartments and exposure time that different nitrogen exposures are tolerated. For example, a dive to 40 m for 20 min and a decompression time of 2–3 min was tolerated without DCI. Bühlmann concluded that the pN_2 for a tissue with a $T_{1/2}$ of 20 min at this exposure was 1.93 bar, which leaves 0.93 bar of tolerated overpressure for this tissue and exposure time. His calculations assumed that independent from exposure time at 1 bar, the tolerated overpressure for nitrogen for all compartments was 1.26–1.3 bar, which corresponds to a diving depth of about 3 m (Fig. 9.5).

Bühlmann extended the calculations by introducing more compartments. Bühlmann also included calculations allowing for altitude diving. He expressed a linear relationship between maximum inert gas pressure in the compartments and ambient pressure. But this linear relationship violates the second law of thermodynamics, as the falloff is exponentially with decreasing pressure from the measured value at arbitrary altitude. The MTM is used for dive tables as well as dive computers and from various navies around the world. It is supported by studies with US Navy divers. However, it seems that computers using the MTM with different models (USN and ZHL16) have a weaker correlation compared to a good correlation of the VPM and RGBM [15]. The fundamentals of the MTM are the exchange of inert gas with varying perfusion rates of compartments driven by the gas gradient. Relevant

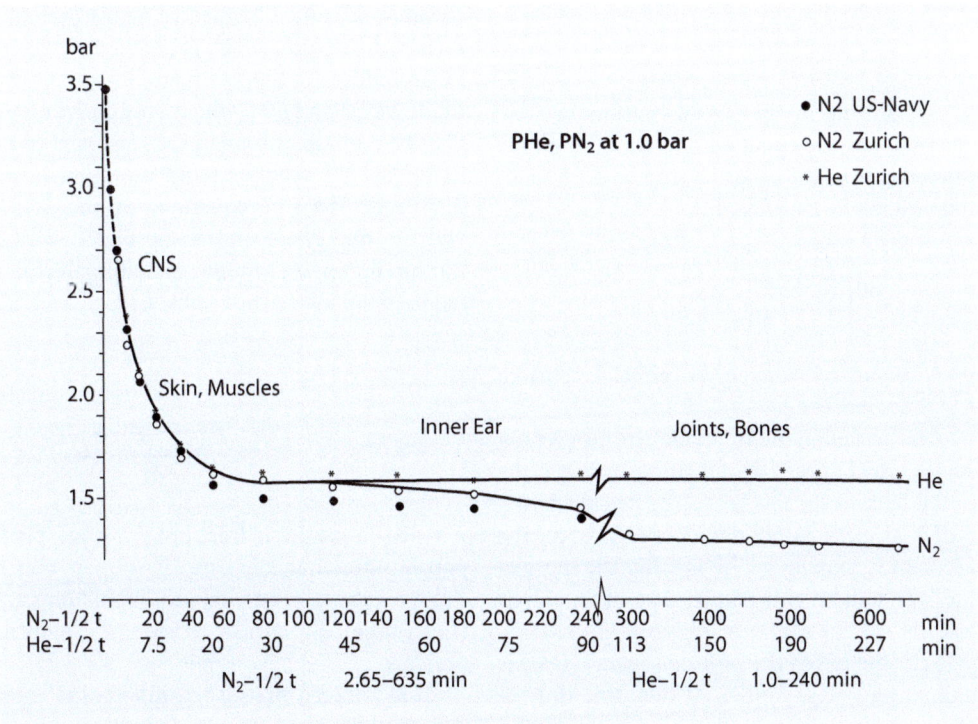

 Fig. 9.5 Tolerated inert gas partial pressure at ambient pressure of 1 bar as a function of nitrogen and helium halftimes in correspondence to different compartments. (Bühlmann, 1984)

gas gradients are the initial tissue pressure (p_{it}), the tissue pressure (p_t) and the pressure in the arterial blood (p_a).

The differential perfusion rate equation is

$$\frac{\partial p_t}{\partial t} = -k\left(p_t - p_a\right)$$

p_t = tissue tension; p_a = arterial tension; k = perfusion constant

with dissolved gas build-up and elimination

$$p_t - p_a = \left(p_i - p_a\right)\exp^{(-kt)}$$

p_t = tissue tension; p_a = arterial tension; p_i = initial tension; k = perfusion constant

The perfusion constant λ is linked to the tissue halftime employing the compartment with 1, 2.5, 5, 10, 20, 40, 80, 120, 240, 360, 480 and 720 min:

$$k = \frac{\ln 2}{T_{1/2}}$$

$T_{1/2}$ = halftime; k = perfusion constant

With a tissue equation, the remaining time t before a stop, the time at a stop or the surface interval can be calculated:

$$t_r = \frac{1}{k}\ln\left[\frac{p_t - p_a}{M - p_a}\right]$$

p_t = tissue tension; p_a = arterial tension; t_r = time remaining

The calculation is made in sequential stages, which means the finishing tension is the initial tension for the next step. By calculating a dive as close as possible to the surface, the gradient is maximized by making the most of the rate uptake and elimination of dissolved gas.

Like the MTM the *diffusion model (DM)* is a dissolved phase model. At the same time of Haldane, Hill presented a more structured alternative to bulk multitissue transfer equations. They were modified by Hempleman in the mid of last century. The inert gas exchange happens via diffusion according to their local gradient and concentration. The sum of the effective tissue compartments with a time constant is influenced by the diffusion and the boundary conditions:

$$p_t - p_a = \left(p_i - p_a\right)$$

$$\sum_{n-1}^{\infty} \frac{8}{\left(2n-1\right)^2 \pi^2}\exp\left(-\omega_{2n-1}^2 Dt\right)$$

p_t = tissue tension; p_a = arterial tension; p_i = initial tension; $\omega_{2n-1}^2 Dt$ = time constant; D = diffusion coefficient; ω = separation constant (eigenvalue)

The DM is the bases of British technical and recreational diving tables.

The *split phase gradient model (SPGM)* divides the gradient in two components, the free-blood and the dissolved-blood gradient. This model is the base of the neo-Haldanian decompression parameters for commercial software. It can be applied to MTM and adds further deep stops, which make them safer. The SPGM addresses the free phase in comparison to the MTM and DM, which only deal with the dissolved phase. It implies that one part of the tissue gas has separated and the other is still dissolved. The rate equation for the SGBM with its free phase and tissue partition fractions in unit tissue volume, including the internal pressure inside the bubble (free phase), is

$$\frac{\delta\left(p_t - p_a\right)}{\delta t} = -\gamma_t k\left(p_t - p_a\right)$$

$$-\gamma_p \frac{\delta\left(p_t - P - \delta\right)}{\delta t}$$

γ_t = tissue partition fraction; γ_p = free-phase partition fraction; p_t = tissue tension; p_a = arterial tension; p_b = internal gas bubble pressure (free phase); δ = surface tension; P = ambient pressure

It is a linear, first-order, differential equation. For the free-dissolved gradient $(p_t - p_b)$ and the surface tension (δ), the dynamics of the free phases in tissue and blood with its bubble kinetics, bubble numbers and bubble film structures need to be respected. By doing that, decompression schedules, critical tension, critical free-phase volume and their interactions can be employed. The partition fractions γ_t and γ_p equal 1.

The *linear-exponential model (LEM)* employs exponential uptake and linear-exponential elimination tissue functions. By applying that, the inert gas uptake is slower than the elimination, consider that the perfusion rate of the tissue is the same. It doesn't use the usual halftimes. The LEM incorporates a characteristic tissue-blood flow timescale (τ):

$$\frac{\delta\left(p_t - p_a\right)}{\delta t} = -\tau^{-1}\left(p_t - p_a\right)$$

p_t = tissue tension, p_a = arterial tension, δ = surface tension, t = time, τ = tissue-blood flow timescale

With $p_t = p_i$ at $t = 0$

$$\left(p_t - p_a\right) = \left(p_i - p_a\right)\exp\left(-\tau^{-1}t\right)$$

p_t = tissue tension; p_a = arterial tension; p_i = initial tension; τ = tissue-blood flow timescale; t = time

However, at a certain tissue tension (p_c), outgassing is clamped, which makes the difference between the tissue and arterial tensions constant. Hence, the gas elimination on decompression is assumed to be linear. The clamping is usually in the early decompression. Later on the elimination becomes exponential again:

$$\frac{\partial p_t}{\partial t} = -\tau^{-1}\left(p_c - p_a\right)$$

τ = tissue-blood flow timescale; p_c = clamped tissue tension; p_a = arterial tension; p_t = tissue tension; t = time

with $p_t = p_c$ at $t = 0$

$$p_t = -\tau^{-1}\left(p_c - p_a\right)t + p_c$$

τ = tissue-blood flow timescale; p_c = clamped tissue tension; p_a = arterial tension; p_t = tissue tension; t = time

The time constant λ doesn't correlate to the MTM halftime (τ) but has the same inverse time units. The perfusion constant, which could be applied in the LEM, is

$$k = \tau^{-1} = \frac{dp_t}{dt}\frac{\pi_b}{\pi_t}$$

k = perfusion constant; τ = tissue-blood flow timescale; π_b = partition fraction of blood; π_t = partition fraction of tissue; p_c = clamped tissue tension; p_a = arterial tension; p_t = tissue tension

The *asymmetric tissue model (ASTM)* includes a possible lengthening of tissue halftimes, caused by gas bubbles in the tissue and the blood vessels. This affects bubble elimination, tissue perfusion and gas transfer across boundaries. That means that the tissue halftimes for elimination are longer than the uptake and hence become asymmetric. This adds greater conservatism to the calculations. Outgassing halftimes (τ_{out}) are slower than ingassing halftimes (τ_{in}) by the inverse fraction (β):

$$\tau_{out} = \beta^{-1}\tau_{in}$$

The tissue equation for ingassing is

$$\left(p_t - p_a\right) = \left(p_i - p_a\right)\exp^{\left(-\lambda_{in}t\right)}$$

The tissue equation for outgassing is

$$\left(p_t - p_a\right) = \left(p_i - p_a\right)\exp^{\left(-\lambda_{out}t\right)}$$

p_t = total pressure; p_a = arterial pressure; p_i = initial pressure; λ = time constant; t = time

The ascent times are converted from symmetric (t_a) to asymmetric ascent times (t_{aa}) by (β^{-1}) for nonstop diving:

$$t_{aa} = \beta^{-1}t_a$$

The ASTM is included in many neo-Haldanian decompression models.

The *thermodynamic model (TM)* combines diffusion and perfusion equations. In this model cylindrical symmetry around the blood vessels is assumed. From blood vessels (a) gas diffuses in the boundaring extravascular region (b). This represents the Krogh's cylinder. The boundaries have the same conditions, the same tissue tension (p_t) and arterial tension (p_a). The diffusion equation is

$$D\frac{\partial^2 p_t}{\partial r^2} + \frac{D}{r}\frac{\partial p}{\partial r} = \frac{\partial p_t}{\partial t}$$

and solving yields

$$p_t - p_a = (p_i - p_a)\sum_{n=1}^{\infty} x_n U_0(\varepsilon_n r)\exp(-\varepsilon_n^2 Dt)$$

p_a = arterial tension; p_t = tissue tension; p_i = initial tension; D = diffusion coefficient; t = time; x_n = constant satisfying initial conditions; U_0 = cylinder functions; ε_n = eigenvalues averaging in the tissue regions $a \leq r \leq b$

$$p_t - p_a = (p_i - p_a)\frac{4}{(b/2)^2 - a^2}\sum_{n=1}^{\infty}\frac{1}{\varepsilon_n^2}\frac{J_1^2(\varepsilon_n b/2)}{J_0^2(\varepsilon_n a) - J_1^2(\varepsilon_n b/2)}\exp(-\varepsilon_n^2 Dt)$$

p_a = arterial tension; p_t = tissue tension; p_i = initial tension; D = diffusion coefficient; t = time; x_n = constant satisfying initial conditions; U_0 = cylinder functions; ε_n = eigenvalues; J_1 and J_0 = Bessel functions, order 1 and 0

According to Hennessey the perfusion is limited as a boundary condition through venous tension by enforcing a mass balance across the vascular and cellular regions. It represents the complex feedback loop combining tension, gas flow, solubility, diffusion and perfusion:

$$\frac{\partial p_v}{\partial t} = -\kappa(p_v - p_a) - \frac{3}{a}S_p D\left[\frac{\partial p_t}{\partial r}\right]_{r=a}$$

p_a = arterial tension; p_t = tissue tension; p_v = venous tension; D = diffusion coefficient; t = time; S_p = ratio of cellular to blood gas solubilities; r = radius; a = vascular radius; κ = perfusion constant

The thermodynamic trigger point for decompression sickness is the volume fraction (χ) of separated gas. The estimated gas fraction of zero gas elimination is

$$\chi P_{N_2} = S_c(p_t - P_{N_2})$$

p_t = tissue tension; χ = volume fraction; S_c = cellular gas solubility; P_{N_2} = separated nitrogen partial pressure

The injection pressure (δ) can be related to the separated gas fraction (χ) through the tissue modulus (K):

$$K\chi = \delta$$

The TM created the base of the VPM and RGBM:

The *varying permeability model (VPM)* was developed by D.E. Yount, Strauss R.H. and M.M. Hoffman. It has 3 parameters for the formation of gas bubbles and 1 decompression parameter, which replaced the conventional M-values as the ascend-limiting factor:

- Gas *nuclei* are the origin of gas bubbles.
- Gas nuclei are always present, and gas bubbles only develop if a certain radius of the gas nuclei is exceeded (*organization hypothesis*).
- *Exponential distribution* of bubbles or gas nuclei according to their size.

The theory was validated by in vitro experiment with galantine as a medium. This theory postulates that there are always microscopic gas nuclei in fluids. They are so small (up to maximum of 1 μm) that they remain freely in a solution without moving upwards and resist to collapse. These gas nuclei are assumed to have a porous, elastic cover (surfactant), which has a varying permeability for gases. The surface tension of the boundary layer prevents the gas nucleus to collapse. By neglecting the electrostatic forces, the formula of Laplace for ordinary gas bubbles is depending on the ambient pressure of the surfactant:

$$p_{in} = p_{amb} + \frac{2\gamma}{r}$$

P_{in} = internal gas pressure; P_{amb} = ambient hydraulic pressure; γ = surface tension; r = radius; $2\gamma/r$ = surface pressure

This formula suggests that P_{in} in gas bubbles is always larger than P_{amb} of the surrounding. That means the gas inside the gas bubble has always the tendency to diffuse from the inside to the outside. However, VPM gas nuclei differ from ordinary gas bubbles as the surfactant creates a skin tension which opposes the surface tension. The surfactant offsets the surface tension. Hence, the formula for gas nuclei is

$$p_{in} + \frac{2\xi}{r} = p_{amb} + \frac{2\gamma}{r}$$

P_{in} = internal gas pressure; P_{amb} = ambient hydraulic pressure; γ = surface tension; r = radius; $2\gamma/r$ = surface pressure; ξ = surfactant tension; $2\xi/r$ = surfactant pressure

This formula suggests that forces effective on gas nuclei are neutral as the surfactant tension offsets the surface tension as well as P_{in} and P_{amb}. Both formulas show us that the surface tension increases with ambient pressure and decreases with increasing radius, assuming that ζ remains constant:

> In other words, the greater the bubble is the faster it can expand.

There are two theories about the structure and function of the surfactant layer [8, 20–23]. The theory from T. Kunkle postulates that with varying sizes, the surfactant layer of the gas nucleus either emits molecules or absorbs them from its environment and thus is able to adapt

to changes. The other theory from D.E. Young states that the molecules of the surfactant shear off and stay within the active layer. Gas nuclei seem to be held neutral by both the Laplace tension and surfactant tension.

> The smaller the radius the greater is the surface tension, and conversely the greater the radius, the smaller is the surface tension.

Cohesive forces of molecules are holding the liquid together. In liquid, molecule forces equally pull in a circular way, so that the net force equals zero (1). At a surface the pulling isn't circular as it is disrupted by the boundary of the air phase. Hence, the pulling force is directed towards the liquid (2). The forces of a small gas nucleus are neutral (3). If the bubble gets too small and the molecules of the liquid come too close, the adhesion forces of the liquid might cause a collapse of the bubble (1). This can be caused by crushing and by spherical or deformed bubbles (◘ Fig. 9.6).

Yount assumed that the pressure within gas nuclei is variable, which means it can be positive or negative. On rapid compression the boundary layer initially contracts, which makes it become rigid and therefore impermeable to gases. This process is dependent on the compression rate and is called crushing. The "crushing" is also termed denucleation. Nuclei can also disintegrate completely. A once denucleated liquid requires higher supersaturations than usual to induce new bubble growth. As the crushing is caused mainly by fast not by slow compression, the influence of this in diving might not be significant, but it has been suggested as a mechanism of acclimatization in diving. Another assumption that gas bubbles reduce in size during compression is the gas exchange with its surrounding. The saturation gradient is reversed compared to the decompression. During a rapid compression, the surfactant molecules of the gas nuclei move together and impede gas or pressure equalization with its surrounding. If the

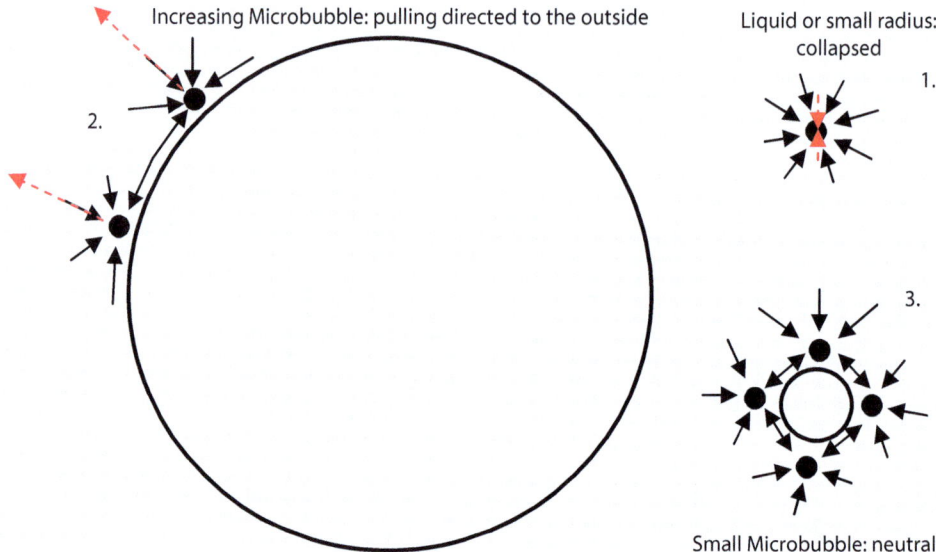

☐ **Fig. 9.6** Adhesion forces in liquids, big bubble, small bubble and liquid itself

ambient pressure increases slowly, the pressure in gas nuclei increases at similar rate. During the compression nitrogen enters the body and accumulates there. When the maximum depth is reached, at isopression, the gas nuclei are already adjusted to ambient pressure. During isopression more and more nitrogen enters the body. During decompression, gas nuclei increase in size, as they absorb excess gas from the surrounding supersaturated tissues. The inside conditions of gas nuclei are dependent on gas diffusion and ambient pressure. The diffusion of each gas needs to be seen individually as they don't diffuse as a bulk but according to their individual partial pressure. Partial pressures of gas nuclei or bubbles adjust to the surrounding partial pressures. But the development of gas nuclei and bubble size does not really correspond to the Boyle's law and is not included in the regular VPM. However, VPM-B (Boyle's law adjustment) respects Boyle's law. The growth or contractions of gas nuclei are more complex than it is in normal bubbles. A Boyle's modifier

(ξ) modifies Boyle's law in regard to molecular membrane of gas nuclei:

$$\xi_i P_i V_i = \xi_f P_f V_f$$

i = initial; f = final; ξ = Boyle's modifier; P = pressure; V = volume

As the gas nuclei are subject to the EOS, the formula for the radius is

$$\xi r = \left[\frac{nRT}{P} \right]^{1/3}$$

ξ = Boyle's modifier; R = universal gas constant; T = temperature; P = pressure; r = radius

The increase of bubbles is dependent on supersaturation (difference of tissue pressure and ambient pressure). Gas nuclei serve as vesicles to transport the excess gas within the liquid. It is similar to opening a bottle of sparkling wine, where excess carbon dioxide create bubbles and exit the liquid at the surface. In the body of course, it is a little more complex. Nitrogen diffuses in different rates out of the various compartments with different perfusion and diffusion rates. Then it is transported in blood and exhaled via the lungs. Various parameters affect this process. If the respiration capacity of the lungs is exceeded, nitrogen bubbles can't be exhaled completely and go through the entire bloodstream again. This leads to accumulation of more nitrogen in blood. Some of the bubbles get filtered out in the lung capillaries and get intercepted. These bubbles reduce the blood flow in the lung capillaries and thus reduce additional nitrogen elimination. Also bloodstream, blood contents and blood vessels themselves affect bubble growth. Therefore, the release of excess gas in humans is a rather complicated process in comparison to a bottle of sparkling wine (▢ Fig. 9.7).

Surface tension counteracts expansion. At decompression, this force must be overcome before gas nuclei can grow. Bubbles grow from gas nuclei when they exceed a "critical" size or

radius. The critical radius (r_c) can be calculated and is dependent on the surface tension (γ) of the liquid in its environment and the saturation gradient (P_{SS}):

$$r_c = \frac{2\gamma}{P_{ss}}$$

The surface tension decreases with increasing size. This means gas nuclei grow exponentially to their radius. Like inflating a balloon, it's initially hard and then suddenly eases. In other words, the larger the gas bubble is, the faster it grows. At decompression supersaturation tension increases. Bubbles are growing, if supersaturation tension is greater than $2\gamma/r$.

The collapse rate of bubbles is quite different to this. Smaller bubbles collapse faster than larger bubbles. But in larger bubbles, the reduction is rather driven by outgassing diffusion

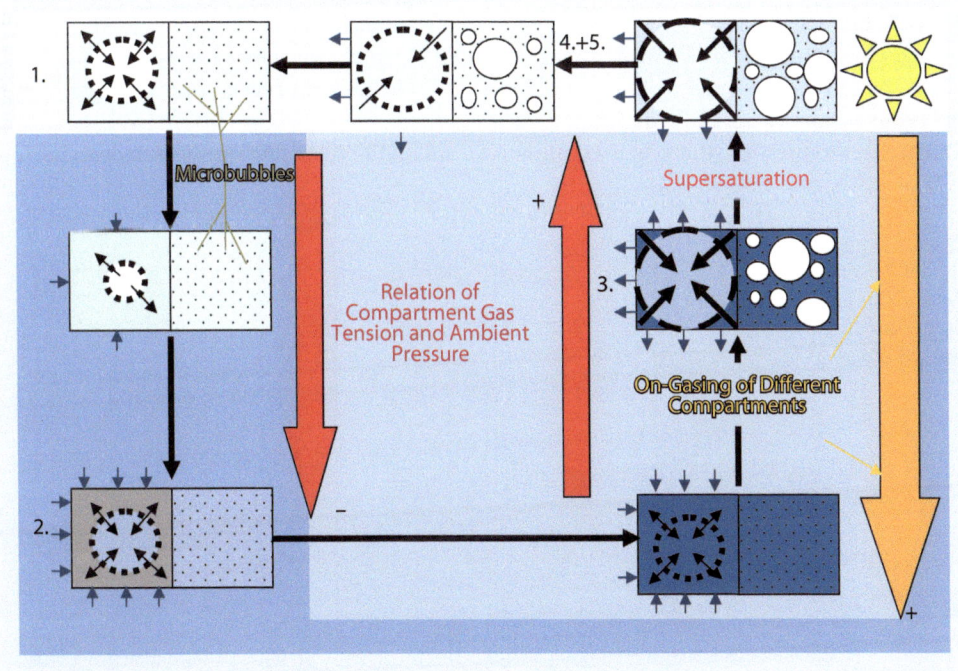

▢ **Fig. 9.7** Inert gas exchange of gas nuclei during symbolised repetitive dives; left box: extension or contraction of gas bubbles, right box: concentration in the tissue compartment and development of free phase

gradients, and smaller bubbles collapse rather due to their constrictive surface tension forces.

Gas nuclei are not growing simultaneously at the same rate. Usually there are more small gas nuclei in comparison to large ones, and their number decreases with increasing size. There is an exponential distribution of the number of gas nuclei or bubbles depending on their size in a stable environmental state. The steepness of the exponential curve is dependent on ambient pressure and the excitation gradient (difference between initial and final depth) (◘ Fig. 9.8) [7].

This exponential distribution can be applied to almost all physiological conditions. During decompression the distribution shifts to more and larger bubbles and less gas nuclei, and the exponential curve flattens out. The formula for the distribution of the bubbles is

$$N_{(r)} = N_0 e^{-k \cdot r}$$

N_0 = total amount of bubbles; r = radius; $N_{(r)}$ = bubbles in dependency to their radius; k = Boltzmann constant

Excess nitrogen of compartments can either be released as bubbles into the blood or creates bubbles directly in tissues itself. During decompression there is a continuous

production of bubbles in the body, but they are eliminated through breathing continuously at the same time. The body itself has a physiological gas volume. This increases during decompression. The gas volume after decompression depends on dive time, depth and surface intervals from previous dives. The gas volume is crucial for the development of a DCI. To a certain degree, the body tolerates a certain number of gas bubbles (N_{safe}) and is independent to gradients of inert gases. The number of gas bubbles can exceed N_{safe}. The degree of excess gas bubbles determines the probability of a DCI. The excess gas volume is proportional to the excess of gas bubbles ($N_{actual} - N_{safe}$) at a new larger supersaturation pressure. The total volume of gas in the body should never exceed the critical gas volume (V_{crit}):

$$\int_0^t P_{ss}(t) \cdot (N_{actual} - N_{safe}) dt \le \alpha V_{crit}$$

P_{ss}= new supersaturation pressure; t = time; N_{actual} = actual bubble numbers; N_{safe} = safe bubble number; V_{crit} = critical gas volume; dt = time interval; α = constant of proportionality

The new supersaturation pressure P_{ss} is the gradient between the current inert gas pressure and the ambient pressure of each dive. The VPM

◘ **Fig. 9.8** Schematic distribution of gas nuclei or bubbles; normal (*yellow*), during decompression (*red*)

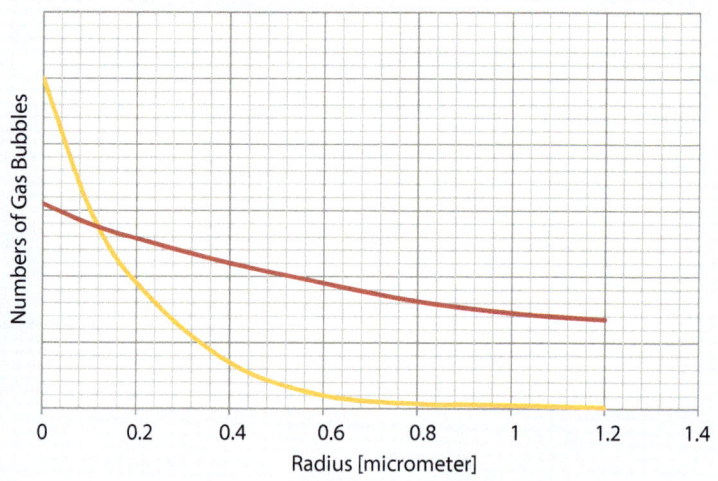

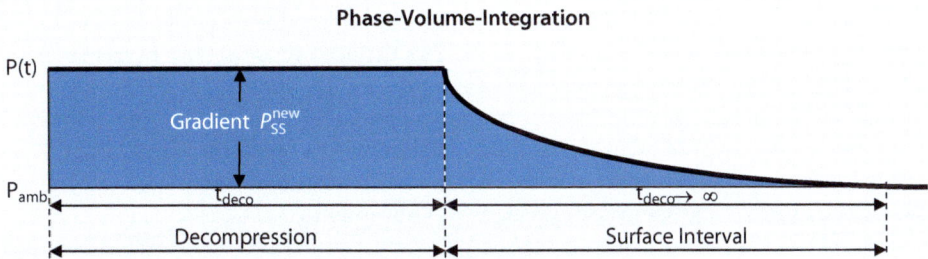

◻ Fig. 9.9 Phase-volume integration

assumes that this gradient is constant during the decompression and then decreases exponentially after the decompression (◻ Fig. 9.9) [1].

The formula for in-water portion is

$$\alpha V_{crit} = \left(N_{actual} - N_{safe} \right)$$

$$\left[\int_0^{t_{deco}} P_{ss}^{new} \left(t \right) dt + \int_{t_{deco}}^{\infty} P_{ss}^{new} \left(t \right) dt \right]$$

The formula for the surface portion is

$$\alpha V_{crit} = \left(N_{actual} - N_{safe} \right) \cdot P_{ss}^{new} \cdot \left(t_{deco} + \frac{1}{\kappa} \right)$$

The VPM takes the dissolved and free-phase gas transfer mechanisms into account by not breaking down the entire body into various compartments. That is not required in the VPM and thus facilitates the calculation of dive profiles. In the VPM deco stops are mainly at shallow depths. For dive planning software calculations, the VPM is complex and hence is only used for some technical diving software.

Another model is the *RGBM* (*reduced gradient bubble model* [9–19]). This model was developed by Dr. Bruce Wienke. It is used in dive computers like Suunto and Mares. It was developed at the same time as the VPM but differs as follows:

- Unlike the VPM the bubbles were not tested in galantine.
- The properties of gas nuclei in vivo are not known. Bubbles in vivo may arise directly of supersaturated tissues or of gas nuclei.

- RGBM deduces bubble persistence timescales from lipid or aqueous seed skin structures, not only as assumed in the VPM's long-term persistence.
- Gas nuclei relate to the biophysical equation of state (EOS).
- Gas transfer between the gas nuclei and the surrounding environment is always possible.
- Diffusion and perfusion is included in calculations.

The RGBM couples perfusion and diffusion as a two-step flow process. The perfusion represents the boundary condition for the gas penetration by diffusion. Whether perfusion or diffusion is dominating is dependent on different factors. However, it is assumed that perfusion in general dominates. Dive computer algorithms of the RGBM incorporate dissolved and free gas. The calculation of the ascent rate prohibits that the collective volume of gas bubbles exceeds the phase volume limit. This controls the inflation rate of gas bubbles. The dissolved gas is located in different compartments, which absorbs and emits inert gas at different rates. It is assumed that the free gas mainly is located in blood vessels but also in body tissues itself. The driving force for the elimination of free gas increases with increasing depth in contrast to the dissolved gases, where it decreases with increasing depth. Bubbles stay either in the tissue or are transported via the blood. For their elimination they either dissolve in the tissue or in the blood, or they are filtered by the lungs and then continuously exhaled.

The RGBM assumes that the formation of bubbles in blood vessels and the development of DCI symptoms are not always related. Many factors, such as quantity of dissolved inert gases, the actual size of the body parts that are exposed to gas, supersaturation of body tissues, deformation and occlusion of surrounding tissues, excitation and growth of bubbles, aggregation of smaller bubbles to larger ones (coalescence), etc., influence the occurrence of DCI. In recreational diving the RGBM limits follow the Haldane model.

The RGBM subdivides the different gas phases and its effects (◘ Figs. 9.10 and 9.11):
1. Nucleation and stabilization (free-phase inception)
2. Supersaturation (dissolved gas build-up)

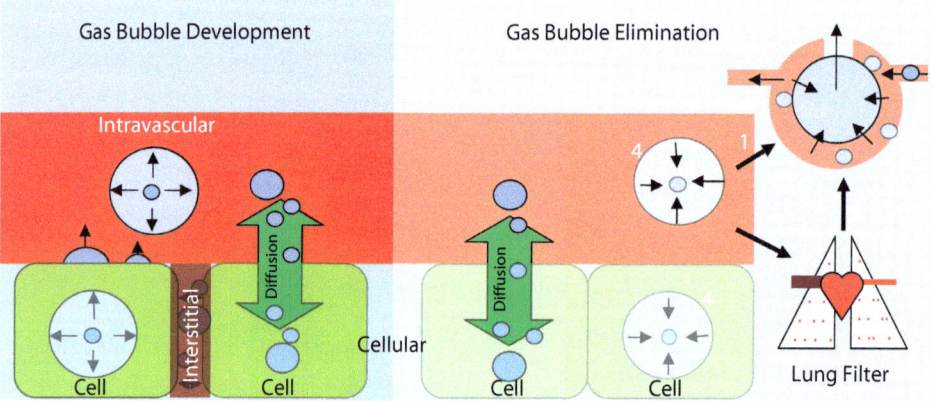

◘ **Fig. 9.10** Formation and elimination of bubbles (intravasal, intracellular and intercellular); 1, normal gas bubble elimination in the alveolae; 2, gas bubble elimination reduced by accumulation in the lungs (lung filter); 3, slow gas bubble elimination; 4, gas bubble decrease by a falling N_2-gradient

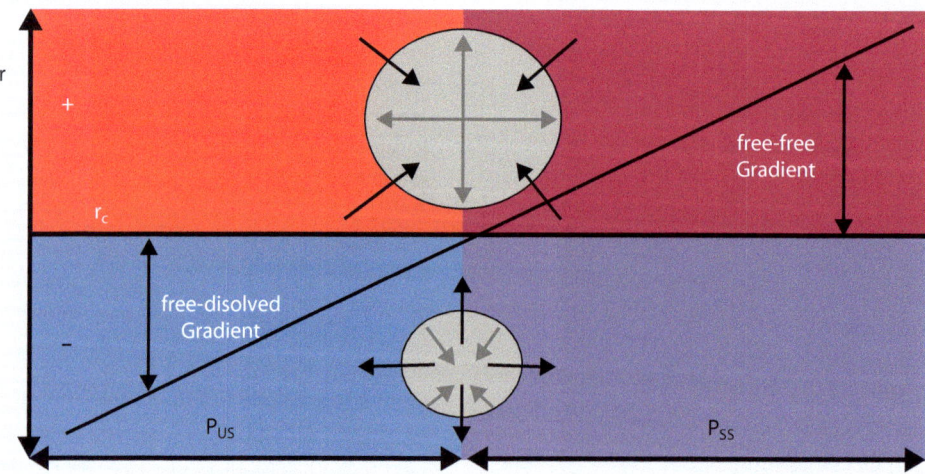

◘ **Fig. 9.11** Gas bubble radius at super- and undersaturation

3. Excitation and growth (free-dissolved phase interaction)
4. Coalescence (bubble aggregation)
5. Deformation and occlusion (tissue damage and ischemia)

r = radius; P_{US} = undersaturation gradient; P_{SS} = supersaturation gradient; r_c = critical radius; black arrows, gas flow direction; black arrows, change of the size of the gas bubble

The growth of bubbles is described as a free-free gradient and the shrinking as a free-dissolved gradient. These gradients describe how gas interacts between gas bubbles and their surroundings, either forming gas bubbles or physically dissolving. In the equilibrium, the neutral position of gas bubbles, the surface tension in combination with the internal pressure of the gas bubble equals the ambient pressure of the tissue. If the ambient pressure is greater than the pressure inside the gas bubbles' boundary layer, the gas flows into the gas nucleus or bubble. If the ambient pressure of the tissue is less, gas flows from the interior of the gas nucleus or bubble in the environment and dissolves there physically. The timescale of changes in bubble size is within milliseconds.

The formation of gas bubbles is best explained by nucleation and cavitation. Cavitation is the process of vapour phase formation of a liquid by pressure reduction. Cavitation in terms of diving can have various causes:

- Flow cavitation (Reynolds nucleation)
- Frictional cavitation (tribonucleation)

The cavitation in a flowing liquid was described by Euler. He defined the cavitation number κ as an indication or a tendency to cavitate.

There are vaporous and gaseous cavitations. The vaporous cavitation mainly takes place in rapid decompression and leads to a rapid bubble growth. The gaseous cavitation is dependent on diffusion and rather a slow process. The gaseous cavitation is not dependent on the decompression rate as it follows the physical process of diffusion. However,

the maximal bubble size is dependent on the duration of the pressure reduction. The stability of the bubble is influenced by the bubble size. The smaller the bubble the faster it can disintegrate. For example, a bubble of 10 µm resolves within 6 seconds. Smaller bubbles require a shorter time and bigger bubbles take longer to resolve. DCI probably is a combination of vaporous and gaseous cavitation.

The cavitation index is present in any flow and is dependent to the temperature as the vapour pressure changes. The more the index is reduced the more bubbles will be produced. However, in reality it is a combination of vapour and gas inside the bubbles, and vapour pressure (p_v) will be replaced by the vapour-gas pressure (p_{vg}):

$$\kappa = 2\frac{p_f - p_{vg}}{\rho u^2}$$

κ = cavitation number; p_f = fluid pressure; p_{vg} = vapour-gas pressure; ρ = fluid density; u = stream velocity

Reynolds described different flow patterns known as laminar and turbulent flow. The Reynolds number describes this flow pattern. With increasing velocity or fluid density, the Reynolds number gets bigger and with increasing viscosity smaller:

$$Re = \frac{\rho u a}{2\eta}$$

Re = Reynolds number; ρ = fluid density; u = velocity; a = cavitation void radius; η = viscosity

The major factor for cavitation under physiological conditions during diving is assumed to be tribonucleation. Boundaries, like particles in the blood or tissue as hydrophobic and hydrophilic surfaces, are linked to the formation of voids and cavitation seeds. Viscous adhesion, or also described as negative tension, easily generates in fluids. For example, the vapour pressure of water is 0.03 bar. Pulling two plates in water apart

9

which are separated by a 0.1 mm gap can cause such a pressure:

$$\tau = \xi \frac{\eta \upsilon A}{V}$$

τ = hydrostatic tension; ξ = constant; η = fluid viscosity; υ = velocity of separation; A = contacting surfaces; V = separation volume

Hence, "friction" could be also involved in various physiological processes in the bloodstream but also in other body parts, which have partially already negative pressures (e.g. joints, muscles, pericardium, interstitial spaces especially of the lung, subcutaneous tissue, epidural space). However negative pressures within the body are not constant and vary greatly under physiological conditions. Micronuclei can be also produced by rapidly narrowing of tissue surfaces followed by widening. This can happen in muscles but also blood vessels or other tissues. It is a dynamic process and occurs very locally. Tribonucleation occurs in a timescale of seconds, but the nuclei may last for hours.

The bubbles seem to have a "memory", which is called *cavitation hysteresis*. That means bubbles, which are once excited, react differently, even if the ambient pressure is restored. The initial cavitation nuclei (κ_i) differ from the new set of cavitation nuclei (κ_n). The difference between them is called hysteresis index (κ_h):

$$\kappa_h = \kappa_i - \kappa_n$$

Cavitation hysteresis might influences diving adaption and bubble formation in repetitive dives.

There is homogenous and heterogeneous nucleation. In homogenous nucleation, temporary microscopic voids form within the liquid by thermal motions. These nuclei rupture and produce macroscopic bubbles [4]. However, this is only limited to thermal motion and in reality it is a far more complex process. The heterogeneous nucleation causes a major weakness at the boundary layers between liquid and solid, even particles. Cervices in the endothelium seem to be a preferred place for that. Homogenous

nucleation is a simplified model for liquids. Intermolecular forces hold molecules together to prevent large spaces in the liquid. The result is a defined bubble with surface tension which rather should be called surface energy. It is not a property of the bubble itself, rather of the liquid at the boundary to the bubble. The interior bubble pressure is dependent on the surface tension, the ambient pressure and the bubble radius:

$$\phi - P = \frac{2\gamma}{r}$$

ϕ = internal bubble pressure; r = radius; P = ambient pressure; γ = surface tension

In homogenous nucleation, the sum of the energy of the nucleus surface is called Gibbs free energy. It can be calculated by including the effective pressure difference across the bubbles ($p_b - p$):

$$G = 4\pi r^2 \gamma - \frac{4}{3}\pi r^3 \psi$$

r = radius; γ = surface tension; $\psi = (p_b - p)$ = effective pressure difference across the bubbles (internal bubble pressure = p_b, external fluid pressure = p)

If included into data like an equation of state (EOS), ψ is

$$\psi = \sum_{n=0}^{N} \alpha_n (p_b - p)^n$$

α = radius; p = fluid tension; p_b = bubble tension; ψ = effective pressure difference across the bubbles ($p_b - p$)

In heterogeneous nucleation, the equation for the Gibbs free energy change is

$$G = 4\pi r^2 \gamma_{lv} - \frac{4}{3}\pi r_0^2 (\gamma_{vs} - \gamma_{ls})$$

r = radius; γ_{lv} = surface tension liquid-vapour interfaces; γ_{ls} = surface tension liquid-solid interfaces; γ_{vs} = surface tension vapour-solid interfaces; ψ = effective pressure difference across the bubbles ($p_b - p$)

If gas bubbles touch a surface, the contact angle (θ) changes according to a hydrophobic or hydrophilic surface:

$$\gamma_{lv}\cos\theta = \gamma_{vs} - \gamma_{ls}$$

when hydrophilic

$$\gamma_{vs} - \gamma_{ls} > 0$$

when hydrophobic (■ Fig. 9.12) [3]

$$\gamma_{vs} - \gamma_{ls} < 0$$

During diving both free gas elimination and dissolved gas elimination are equally important. The important aspect of the RGBM is the understanding of diffusion and perfusion. The perfusion plays a profound role in most of the models as it facilitates the computer calculations. The perfusion influences free or dissolved inert gas transport to and from the tissues. This varies greatly depending on the load and the compartments. The compartments vary greatly in their blood supply and their ability to adjust the perfusion to the current demand. The free and the dissolved forms behave differently. The free form, as bubbles, is better reduced in greater depth. The dissolved form is rather reduced closer to the surface. However, both diffusion and perfusion have characteristic rate constants. When the diffusion rate constants are smaller than perfusion rate constants, diffusion dominates the gas exchange and vice versa. The diffusion is usually only dependent to the concentration and therefore virtually constant. Therefore, perfusion is assumed to be the dominant factor. The RBGM includes also physiological tissue and blood undersaturations (caused by oxygen, which binds mainly to haemoglobin) into its calculation. The metabolic oxygen consumption influences subtly the inert gas transfer and hence bubble growth. Oxygen consumption causes a drop in oxygen tension of tissues, which is lower than the levels in alveoli. Moreover, oxygen in the blood is bound to haemoglobin and hardly goes into physical solution. Therefore, blood and tissue are significantly undersaturated on oxygen compared to dry air at 1 bar. It seems that undersaturation of tissues and blood increases linearly with increasing pressure of constant composition breathing mixture (oxygen window). Like the VPM it also assumes the existence of gas nuclei. But in contrast to the VPM, the bubbles and gas nuclei are subject to the EOS (equation of state). The EOS incorporates the pressure, volume and temperature and incorporates the gas diffusion length:

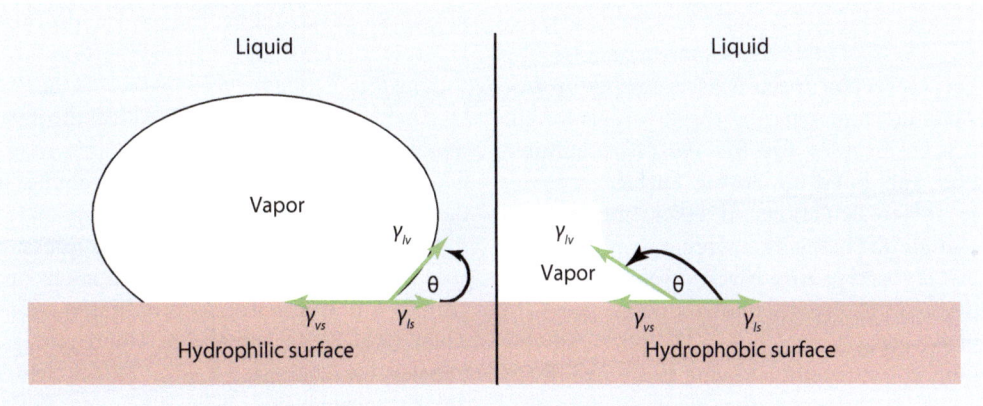

■ **Fig. 9.12**   Properties of gas bubbles on hydrophilic and hydrophobic surfaces

$\xi PV = nRT$

ξ = Boyle's modifier; n = number of bubbles; P = pressure; T = temperature; V = volume; R = universal gas constant

Other than the VPM, the RBGM allows the assumption that the gas nucleus wall can be penetrated by gas at all times, even under compression. The mass coefficient (DS) influences the gas transfer. N_2 has with 56.9×10^{-6} μm^3/fsw a three times higher DS than He (18.4×10^{-6} μm^3/fsw). It is also assumed that the gas bubbles undergo a Boyle-like expansion and contraction.

The volume constraint equation is

$$\phi = \left[\frac{\partial V}{\partial t} \right]_{diffusion} + \left[\frac{\partial V}{\partial t} \right]_{Boyle} + \left[\frac{\partial V}{\partial t} \right]_{excitation}$$

Gas nucleus walls are stabilized with a surfactant (lipid or aqueous) for estimable timescales of hours. Gas nuclei are distributed differently throughout the body. As well as the VPM, the RBGM postulates an exponential distribution of gas nuclei and bubbles depending on their size. Excitation radii in the RGBM range from 0.01 to 0.05 μm compared to 1 μm of the VPM or TBDM. RBGM decompression rate calculates the diving profile so that the total volume of the growing gas bubbles never exceeds a certain gas-phase volume limit. Depending on the gas mixture, RBGM refers to a wide range of compartments (1–720 /min). The main focus is on the phase transition and the formation of gas bubbles in the slow tissue to make repetitive dives more predictable. If decompression speed is exceeded, extra deco stops are integrated in the dive profile. The RBGM includes also free gas-phase elimination and build-up during surface intervals in their calculations. It takes into account altitude above sea level, diving depth of previous dives, repetitive dives, dives on the same day and risk profiles of dives, which keeps the phase separation ϕ below the phase volume limit ϕ_{max}. Repetitive diving in trained divers seems to cause the phenomenon of adaptation. Some studies suggest that divers with

regular exposure are less affected by decompression accidents compared to divers with only sporadic diving exposure. This can be explained either by physical or physiological adaptation. In general, surface intervals are often too short on repetitive dives. This leads to an inadequate elimination of bubbles and an accumulation of new bubbles during the next dive. The RGBM includes this in its estimate and in general integrates deco stops already in greater depth. Thus, calculations of dive profiles are more conservative than that of the VPM.

RGBM and VPM set the nonstop time limits t_n with 122 msw $min^{1/2}$. The US Navy uses 152 msw $min^{1/2}$ and Spencer 142 msw $min^{1/2}$. The formula for the depth-time exposure limitation with the approximate $122 \leq H \leq 152$ msw $min^{1/2}$ ($400 \leq H \leq 500$ fsw $min^{1/2}$) is

$$dt_n^{1/2} = H$$

The *tissue bubble diffusion model (TBPM)* assumes a transport in and out of the gas bubble via diffusion. Radius, gas tension, ambient pressure and surface tension of gas bubbles are hereby linked. Bubbles grow, if gas tension exceeds the ambient pressure and the surface tension and vice versa:

$$\frac{\partial r}{\partial t} = \frac{DS}{r} \left[\Pi - P - \frac{2\gamma}{r} \right]$$

r = bubble radius; t = time; D = diffusion coefficient; S = gas solubility; P = ambient pressure; Π = total gas tension; γ = surface tension

The *linear-exponential phase model (LEPM)* by Thalmann and others extended the USN dissolved gas models with using either modified M-values or separated bubble volume. In this model it is assumed that gas remains in solution at all times during decompression accommodating gas bubble formation and growth. Rate changes of dissolved gas in tissues equal rates of gas uptake in blood and gas transfer into bubbles. It is a model, which doesn't include gas nuclei dynamics and is based on correlation with USN data and was statistically modified. The LEPM uses reduced M-values (MR), which are different to the usual M-values:

$$\frac{\partial D}{\partial t} = -4\pi r^2 \alpha_t D_t \left[1 - \frac{p_t}{p_b}\right]\left[\delta + \frac{1}{r}\right]$$

r = bubble radius; t = time; D_t = compartmental bulk diffusion coefficient; S = gas solubility; p_b = reduced bubble internal pressure; p_t = tissue tension; δ = penetration length; α_t = tissue partition fraction

References

1. Baker EC. Derivation with explanation of the VPM dynamic critical volume algorithm of Yount & Hoffman. 1986.
2. Baker EC. Understanding M-Values. Immersed. 1998;3(3).
3. Blatteau JE, Souraud JB, Gempp E, Boussuges A. Gas nuclei, their origin, and their role in bubble formation. Aviat Space Environ Med. 2006;77(10):1068–76.
4. Brennen CE. Cavitation and bubble dynamics. Oxford: Oxford University Press; 1995.
5. Bühlmann AA, Voelmm EB, Nussberger P. Tauchmedizin, Barotrauma, Gasembolie, Dekompensation, Dekompensationskrankheit. 5th ed. Berlin: Springer; 2002.
6. Haldane JS. Respiration. Oxford: Oxford University Press; 1935.
7. Kaluza M. VPM the inner workings. 2005.
8. Kunkle TD, Beckman EL. Bubble dissolution physics and the treatment of decompression sickness. Med Phys. 1983;10:184–90.
9. Wienke BR. Technical diving in depth. Flagstaff: Best Publishing Company; 2002.
10. Wienke BR. Basic decompression theory and application. 3. Edition: Best Publishing Company; 2008.
11. Wienke BR. Diving decompression models and bubble metrics: modern computer synthesis. Comput Biol Med. 2009;39(2009):309–31.
12. Wienke BR. Basic decompression theory and application. Flagstaff: Best Publishing Company; 2001.
13. Wienke BR. Bubble number saturation curve and asymptotics of hypobaric and hyperbaric exposures. Int J Biomed Comput. 1991;29:215–25.
14. Wienke BR. Computational decompression models. Int J Biomed Comput. 1987;21:205–21.
15. Wienke BR. Equivalent multitissue and thermodynamic decompression algorithms. Int J Biomed Comput. 1989;24:227–45.
16. Wienke BR, O'Leary TR. Statistical correlations and risk analysis techniques for a diving dual phase bubble model and data bank using massively parallel supercomputers. Comput Biol Med. 2008;38:583–600.
17. Wienke BR. Reduced gradient bubble model. Int J Biomed Comput. 1990;26:237–56.
18. Wienke BR. Tissue gas exchange models and decompression computations: a review. Undersea Biomed Res. 1989;16:53–89.
19. Wienke BR. Diving decompression models and bubble metrics: modern computer syntheses. Comput Biol Med. 2009;39:309–31.
20. Yount DE, Hoffman DC. Decompression theory: a dynamic critical-volume hypothesis. In: Bachrach AJ, Matzen MM, editors. Underwater physiology VIII: proceedings of the eighth symposium on underwater physiology. Bethesda: Undersea Medical Society; 1984. p. 131–46.
21. Yount DE, Hoffman DC. On the use of a bubble formation model to calculate diving tables. Aviat Space Environ Med. 1986;57:149–56.
22. Yount DE, Maiken EB, Baker EC. Implications of the varying permeability model for reverse dive profiles. In: Lang MA, Lehner CE, editors. Smithsonian Institution. D.C. pp: Washington; 2000. p. 29–61.
23. Yount DE. Skins of varying permeability: a stabilization mechanism for gas cavitation nuclei. J Acoust Soc Am. 1979;65:1431–9.

Suggested Reading

Ball R, Schwartz SL. Kinetic and dynamic models of diving gases in decompression sickness prevention. Clin Pharmacokinet. 2002;41(6):389–402.

Kuch B, Bedini R, Buttazzo G, Sieber A. Mathematical platform for studies on VPM and Buhlmann decompression algorithms. In: Proc. Of the 35th Annual Scientific Meeting of the European Underwater and Baromedical Society (EUBS 2009), Aberdeen, August; 2009. p. 25–8.

Bubble Flow

© Springer International Publishing AG, part of Springer Nature 2018
O. Rusoke-Dierich, *Diving Medicine*, https://doi.org/10.1007/978-3-319-73836-9_10

Blood flow in our vascular system is quite slow and allows laminar flow patterns in most areas. The critical bubble size not interfering with laminar flow regimes can be estimated, if 0.5 as a rough estimate cut-off Reynolds number for laminar bubble flow is taken [1].

$$\mathrm{Re} = \frac{\rho u a}{2\eta} \leq 0.5$$

then

$$a = \frac{2*0.5\eta}{\rho u} \leq 0.0004\,\mathrm{cm}\ \text{or}\ 4\,\mu m$$

where Re = Reynolds number, a = cavitation void radius, u = stream velocity, η = fluid viscosity, ρ = density of the fluid.

Several studies and calculations were done of bubbles in tubes of various flow patterns and positions [1]. These can be taken as a rough guidance of how bubbles might react in vivo. The vascular system and blood are however variable in flow rate, density, viscosity, surfactants, vascular morphology and interaction of impurities like other cells affecting flow. Bubble flow is defined as a *two-phase flow* where bubbles are dispersed or suspended in a liquid. They can be distinguished in:

- Ideally separated bubble flow (◙ Fig. 10.1)
- Interacting bubble flow
- Churn turbulent bubble flow
- Clustered bubble flow
- Slug bubble flow

10.1   Bubble Flow Patterns

The *ideally separated bubble flow* allows laminar flow as bubbles are too small to interact directly or indirectly with each other. Once bubbles and/or density becomes enlarged, bubbles start to interact due to collision or effects of wakes by other bubbles. This represents the *interacting bubble flow*. Still laminar flow is expected. The void fraction between ideally separated, interacting and churn turbulent bubble flow is roughly 0.1–0.6. After the size and density of bubbles increase further, so-called sickle-shaped cap bubbles form. The laminar flow brakes down to a *churn turbulent bubble flow*. This is a mixture of bigger and smaller bubbles, which are highly interacting. Larger bubbles can form clustered bubbles or gas slugs and lead to *clustered bubble flow* or *slug bubble flow*. The flow pattern of clustered bubbles is similar to the gas slugs [1].

Bubbles in a vertical upwards flow tend rather to be closer to the wall, in contrast to a downwards flow, where bubbles tend to be located in the centre of the tube. The more and the bigger bubbles get, the more they seem to move from the wall-orientated position to the more central position. In horizontal flow, bubble flow is expected to react differently in blood vessels, where the flow rate is slow. In faster flow rates, horizontal flow is similar to vertical flow patterns. Gas slugs can overcome the flow rate of the liquid [2]. They can either travel faster or even against the flow rate of the liquid. For the development of DCI symptoms, it means that venous gas slugs might travel against the blood flow and reach retrograde cranial regions in an upright position as described in iatrogen cerebral venous air gas embolism (CVGE) [3].

Bubbles aren't rigid spheres. They are flexible and very dynamic within their environment. Smaller bubbles hardly get distorted, whereas bigger bubbles tend to change shape during blood flow. They become club or cup shaped and somehow dysmorphic. Interaction between bubbles itself and interfaces increase, which cause more turbulence. At a certain size, bubbles can break apart. The bubble flow fracture is depended on the flow rate and the surface tension pressure. The lower the flow rate is, the bigger bubbles can be without breaking apart. Gas slugs in capillaries add to the already existing decrease of pressure along capillaries, which can result in significant pressure but also flow rate loss [4]. In physiological term, this can be translated that bubbles can inter-

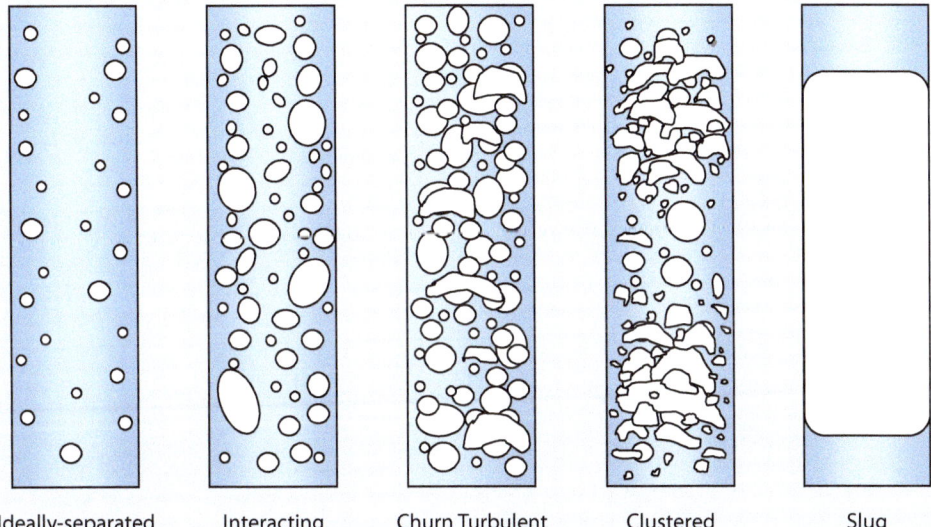

| Ideally-separated | Interacting | Churn Turbulent | Clustered | Slug |

☐ **Fig. 10.1**   Bubble flow patterns

fere significantly with perfusion pressure and resulting ischaemia, despite minimal flow rate:

$$\Delta p_t = \Delta p_s + \Delta p_b$$

Δp_t = total pressure drop; Δp_s = single phase pressure drop; Δp_b = pressure drop by gas bubbles.

For DCI the transition from stable, organised bubble flow to unstable chaotic bubble flow has a major impact. Turbulence causes reduced blood flow and additionally a pressure drop caused by bubbles. The tissue perfusion pressure can be significantly compromised by this.

References

1. Kataoka I, Serizawa A. Bubble flow. http://www.thermopedia.com/content/8/DOI:10.1615/AtoZ.b.bubble_flow. Accessed 25 Oct 2017.
2. Fabre J, Line A. Slug flow. http://www.thermopedia.com/content/38/ Accessed 21 Dec 2017.
3. Schlimp CJ, Bothma PA, Brodbeck AE. Cerebral venous air embolism: what is it and do we know how to deal with it properly? JAMA Neurol. 2014;71(2):243. https://doi.org/10.1001/jamaneurol.2013.5414.
4. Wals E, Muzycha Y, Walsh P, Egan V, Punch J. Pressure drop in two phase slug/bubble flows in mini scale capillaries. Int J Multiphase Flow. 2009;35(1):879–84.

Archimedes' Principle

© Springer International Publishing AG, part of Springer Nature 2018
O. Rusoke-Dierich, *Diving Medicine*, https://doi.org/10.1007/978-3-319-73836-9_11

Archimedes looked for a solution on how he could test the crown of King Hiero of Syracuse on its content of gold. He previously noticed how his body extruded water out of a tub and simultaneously seemed to become "lighter". A body is experiencing a reduction in the down-force (G) in fluid. He compared the crown and an equally heavy lump of gold on a scale immersed in the water. Since the lump of gold in the water was heavier than the crown despite having the same weight above water, he realised that the crown may not consist of pure gold. Archimedes found out that the buoyancy, or the reduction of the downforce in a liquid, equals the weight of the displaced fluid. An object placed in the water begins either to swim or to sink. This property is determined by density (ρ) of an object. If the density of the object (ρO) is lower than that of the fluid (ρFl), it has buoyancy and floats. If it is higher in comparison to the fluid, it sinks. This phenomenon can as well be described with the downforce F_G and the lifting force F_A. According to that, buoyancy is depending on the density of the body itself and on the

density of the liquid in which the body is in (◘ Fig. 11.1).

The simplified formula for the density of an object is

$$\rho = \frac{m}{V}$$

where ρ = density; m = mass; V = volume

Example

Air has a lower density compared to water and is therefore suitable for adjusting buoyancy. Under water the buoyancy can be adjusted with the BCD. During diving with a diving suit made out of neoprene, the strong lifting force caused by trapped air bubbles must be overcome. This can be achieved with a weight belt. With increasing depth, air inclusions in the diving suit are compressed (Boyle's law). That's why the loss of buoyancy at increasing depth has to be balanced out by inflating the BCD. Since the density of salt water is higher than that of freshwater, buoyancy is greater in the sea, and more weights are required to balance this out.

11

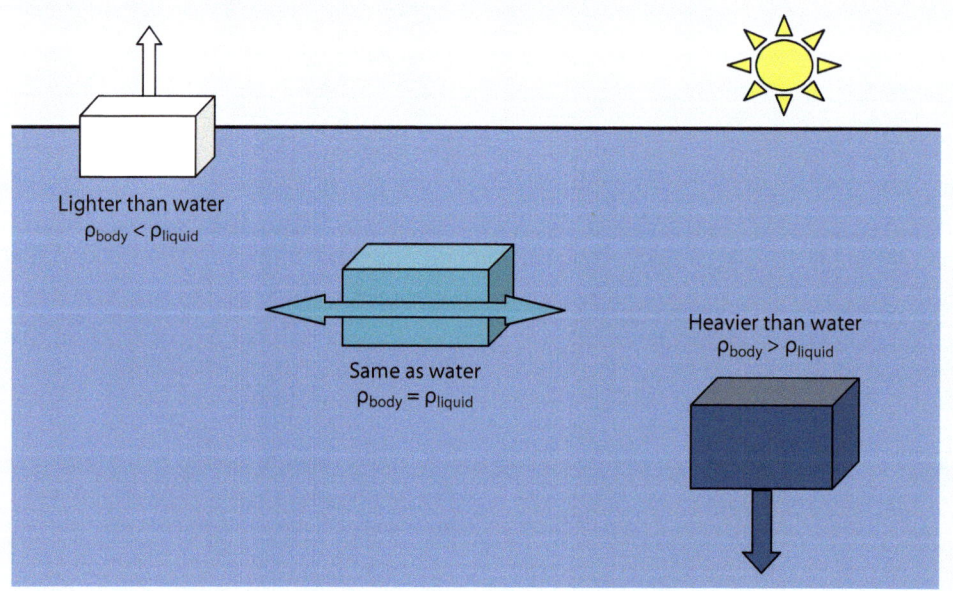

Lighter than water
$\rho_{body} < \rho_{liquid}$

Same as water
$\rho_{body} = \rho_{liquid}$

Heavier than water
$\rho_{body} > \rho_{liquid}$

◘ **Fig. 11.1** Properties of bodies with different density immersed in water

Optical and Acoustic Changes Underwater

Suggested Reading – 90

© Springer International Publishing AG, part of Springer Nature 2018
O. Rusoke-Dierich, *Diving Medicine*, https://doi.org/10.1007/978-3-319-73836-9_12

Sound conductivity of water is greater than that of air (■ Table 12.1). It is caused by the closer proximity of molecules of water compared to air. Thus, sound conducts faster.

Discrimination of the sound direction under water becomes more difficult than on air. The sound travels faster and farther. For the diver this means that the sound sources can appear closer, and the direction it comes from cannot be detected (■ Fig. 12.1).

The human ear is used to conditions in its natural environment, the air. The recognition of the sound direction is caused by the sound arriving at the different times in both ears. At a velocity of 332 m/s and only approximately 20 cm distance between both ears, this is an enormous feature of nature to determine where the sound is coming from. At minimum deviation of direction with 4° angulation, the time difference of the sound reaching both

ears is only about 10^{-5} s. The speed of sound is increased under water. Therefore, the sound source can't be localized under water as this time difference is too small to be processed by the brain.

Optical conditions are changing under water too. Water has a different index of refraction than air. The refractive index of water (1.33) compared to the air (1.000292) is 4/3. Thus, objects appear approx. 1/3 *larger and* 1/4 *closer* than they really are. It is partly caused by the different refractive indices but also due to the adaptation of the brain to the optical distortion.

Diving masks are required to see under water. The eye, which mainly contains water itself, breaks the incoming light that previously crossed the air. The eye is used to this angle of refraction, and the eyes are in focus, so that everything appears clearly (■ Fig. 12.2).

Water is a different medium and changes the refraction at the interface to the eye compared to the air. The angle of refraction is different, and everything seems to be out of focus. That's why a mask is required to see clearly under water to restore the usual medium air in front of our eyes. The mask itself creates refraction even before the eyes (at the interception

■ **Table 12.1** Speed of sound

Air	332 m/s
Water	1450 m/s

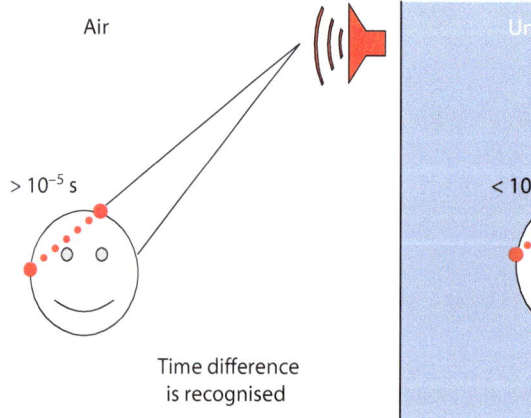
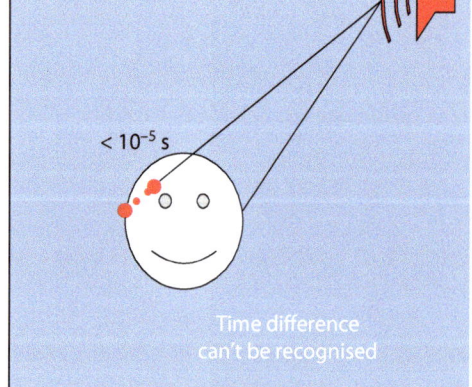

Air

> 10^{-5} s

Time difference
is recognised

Under Water

< 10^{-5} s

Time difference
can't be recognised

■ **Fig. 12.1**   Sound above and under water

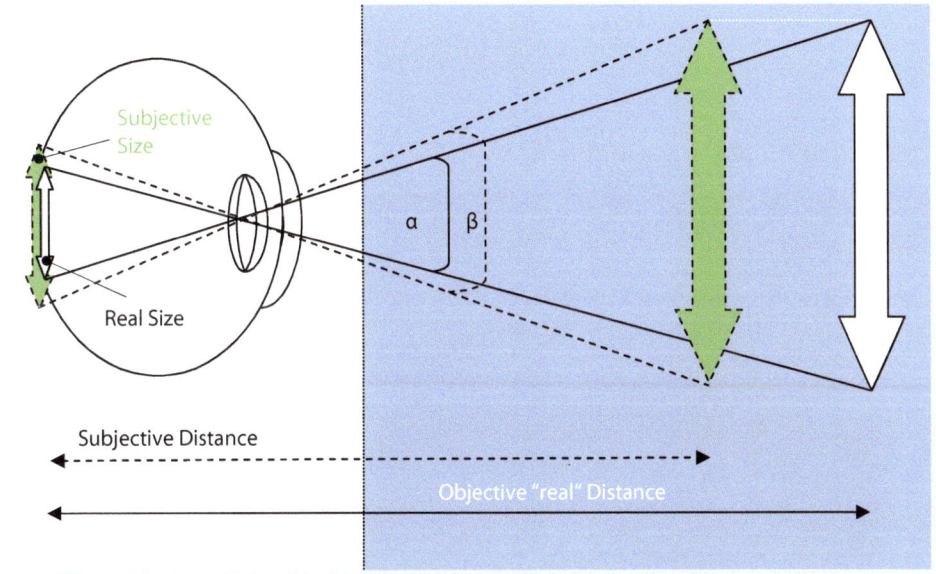

■ **Fig. 12.2**   Vision under and above water

of glass and water). Therefore, things seem to appear differently in size and distance. Objects under water (blue arrow) appear ¼ closer than at air (white arrow). The light of perceived objects is broken in the lens of the eye, and a mirror image is reflected onto the retina. The refraction angle under water (β) of the falsely closer object is greater than that of the real object (α) which you would have above water. Therefore, the image on the retina is larger and is perceived as such.

Due to the higher density of water, the different light waves are filtered in a certain pattern. First the long wavelength light waves are absorbed and then the short wavelength. Therefore, everything appears greenish bluish in 30 meters depth of clear water, because these are the only wavelengths of the natural light, which are reaching this depth. Red, orange and yellow appears brownish as they are filtered out. Original colours can be seen in greater depths with the help of a flashlight (■ Fig. 12.3).

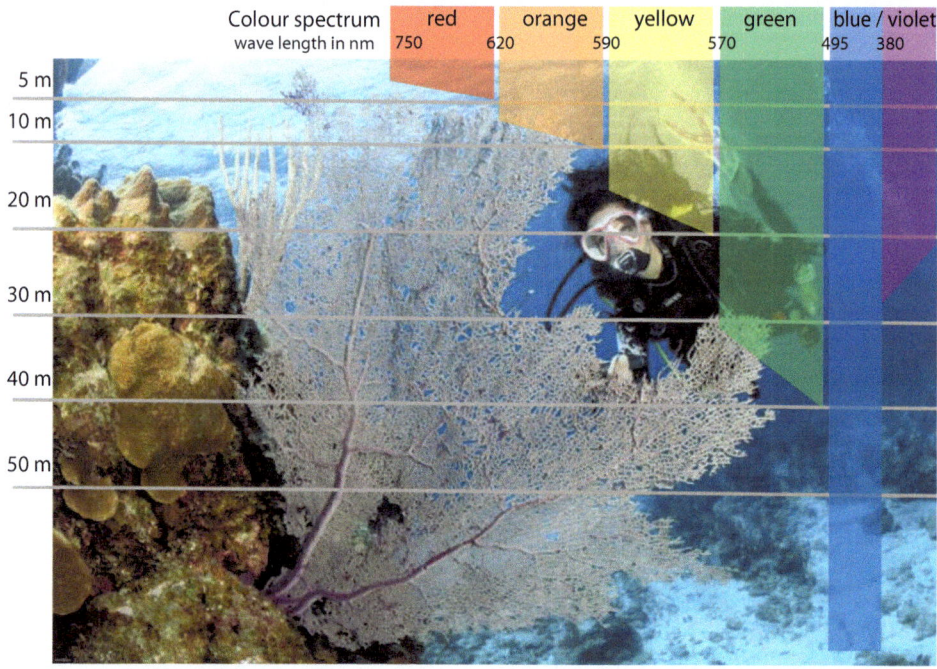

Colour spectrum	red	orange	yellow	green	blue / violet
wave length in nm	750 620	590	570	495	380

■ **Fig. 12.3**   Light absorption under water. (With kind permission of Mares)

Suggested Reading

Ross HE, Nawaz S. Why do objects appear enlarged under water? Arq Bras Oftalmol. 2003;66:69–76.
Silbernagel S, Despopuluos A. Taschenatlas der Physiologie, 7. Auflage. Thieme: Stuttgart; 2007.

Thermal Conductivity

© Springer International Publishing AG, part of Springer Nature 2018
O. Rusoke-Dierich, *Diving Medicine*, https://doi.org/10.1007/978-3-319-73836-9_13

Different materials have different thermal conductivities (■ Table 13.1). Thermal conductivity means that if a specific point of a material heats up or cools down, thermal transfer within this material takes place. Gases in general have bad thermal conductivity and are therefore also good insulators (e.g. air bubbles in wetsuits, yarns such as wool which have a loose structure). Water has a good thermal transfer, and heat or cold can be easily distributed. In the air however, only the immediate point of contact is heated or cooled, because the thermal transfer is poor. When two different materials (e.g. water/air) with different temperatures meet, heat exchange occurs. The temperature exchange is also known as convection. The greater the thermal conductivity is, the faster heat energy can be absorbed. Water has a tenfold higher thermal conductivity compared to air and extracts the heat energy from the air far quicker.

This means that heat from water quickly is transferred to air, but vice versa heat transfer from water to air is slow. The human body produces heat, to keep an almost constant body temperature of 37 °C. This works quite well on air. In contrast, water extracts heat from the body. Diving suits protect against heat loss. They reduce direct contact of the skin with water. The wetsuit has tiny air bubbles in its rubbery material. The rubber itself and air pockets insulate the body against the environment. A film of water between the body and the wetsuit is trapped. The temperature of the water film adjusts quickly to the body temperature. The water trapped in the wetsuit should be exchanged as little as possible with the water of the environment, to reduce heat loss by convection. However, this heat loss can't be entirely avoided as there is always a gradual exchange of water. That's why wetsuits should sit tight and not too loose to reduce the degree of that exchange. The improvement of a wetsuit is the semidry suit that is even tighter and has less zippers and tight arms and legs cuffs. Another variation to protect against heat loss is the dry suit. With the dry suit, a contact with water will be completely avoided. Because air has a lower thermal conductivity such as water, the insulation effect is better than the one of the wetsuits. All parts of the body, which are covered by the dry suit, remain dry. To achieve an insulating effect, warm clothing must be worn for insulation. So, the dry suit is preferred in cold water temperatures.

Example

Immerse in water at 35 °C as heat is still removed from the body, and it has to produce it again. The body starts freezing and shivering to produce heat through the muscle activity to achieve the desired temperature. Outside the water, with the same temperature, sweat is produced to transfer heat out of the body. By sweating, heat is removed from the body as water absorbs heat quickly. The evaporation of sweat removes heat eventually from the body and the body is cooling down.

13

■ Table 13.1	Thermal conductivity
Air	0.09
Water	0.9
Copper	1400

Conversion Tables for Physical Units

© Springer International Publishing AG, part of Springer Nature 2018
O. Rusoke-Dierich, *Diving Medicine*, https://doi.org/10.1007/978-3-319-73836-9_14

▫ Table 14.1   Units of pressure

	Bar	Atm	PSI	kPa	mmHg = Torr	mmWC
1 bar	1	0.987	14.7	100	750	10.02
1 atm	1.013	1	14.89	101.32	760	10.33
1 PSI	0.068	0.067	1	6.802	51.02	0.6816
1 kPa	0.01	0.099	0.147	1	7.5	0.102
1 mmHg/Torr	0.00131	0.00132	0.0195	0.133	1	0.1336
1 mmWC	0.099	0.097	1.455	0.98	7.48	1

Units for pressure, *atm* physical atmosphere, *kPa* kilo pascal, *mmHg* millimeter mercury, *mmWC* millimeter water colum

▫ Table 14.2   Units of length

	Meter	Feet	Inch	Stat. mile	Naut. mile	Yard
Meter	1	3.28	39.37	0.00062	0.00054	1.09
Feet	0.305	1	12.01	0.00019	0.00016	0.33
Inch	0.0254	0.083	1	0.00016	0.00014	0.03
Stat. mile	1610	5263	62,500	1	0.87	1755
Naut. mile	1852	6250	71,428	1.15	1	2016
Yard	0.914	3.03	33.33	0.00057	0.0005	1

m meter, *f* feet, *stat. mile* statistical mile, *naut. mile* nautical mile

14

Box 14.1   Units of Temperature
- *°Fahrenheit/°Celsius*
  $°C = (°F − 32)·5/9; °F = °C·1.8 + 32$
- *°Celsius/Kelvin*
  $0 °C = +273 K; 0 K = −273 °C$

°F conversion of Fahrenheit, *°C* Celsius, *K* Kelvin

▫ Table 14.3   Units of speed

	m/s	km/h	miles/h	Knots
m/s	1	3.6	2.22	6.66
km/h	0.28	1	0.621	1.86
miles/h	0.45	1.61	1	3
Knots	0.15	0.54	0.33	1

m meter, *km* kilometer, *s* seconds, *h* hours

Diving Physiology and Anatomy

As highly specialised creatures human beings have adapted to their habitat. Thanks to their ability to understand correlations in nature and to use their knowledge creatively, humans expanded their habitat into the underwater world. With the help of technical support, they created an artificial environment, which enables them to be in the otherwise hostile environment for a limited time. Without this, it would be not possible to enjoy the miracles under water.

Physiology is the study of life processes within the body. This section of the book discusses those organs and their functions that are relevant for diving. The following chapter outlines the necessary physiological and anatomical basic knowledge for diving.

Contents

Diving Physiology and Anatomy

© Springer International Publishing AG, part of Springer Nature 2018
O. Rusoke-Dierich, *Diving Medicine*, https://doi.org/10.1007/978-3-319-73836-9_15

As highly specialised creatures, human beings have adapted to their habitat. Thanks to their ability to understand correlations in nature and to use their knowledge creatively, humans expanded their habitat into the underwater world. With the help of technical support, they created an artificial environment, which enables them to be in the otherwise hostile environment for a limited time. Without this, it would be not possible to enjoy the miracles under water.

Physiology is the study of life processes within the body. This section of the book discusses those organs and their functions that are relevant for diving. The following chapter outlines the necessary physiological and anatomical basic knowledge for diving.

15.1 Cardiovascular System

Various substances have to be absorbed, transported and eliminated to maintain vital functions. Unicellular organisms, such as bacteria, have a direct exchange with their environment. In multicellular organisms, like humans, transport systems are needed to provide for individual cells. Oxygen and nutrients from our environment are transported to the entire body, and metabolic waste products are eliminated.

15.1.1 Heart

The heart is usually located in the left chest cavity behind the sternum and between the two lungs. It is an average 12–14.5-cm long and 10-cm wide and weighs 200–300 g. The size and weight depend on the workload. For example, by doing sports or having high blood pressure, the heart is exposed to a higher workload, and it might grow in size and weight. A weight over 500 g is considered pathological. However, athletes might exceed this weight due to excessive exercise. The heart is supplied with oxygenated blood via the coronary arteries, which originate from the ascending part of the aorta and lead back to the right atrium.

The heart is divided into right and left atrium, as well as right and left ventricle. The atria collect the blood from the body's periphery and the lung. The blood is then redirected to the chambers and ejected from there. The circulatory system of the body periphery represents the large circulation and of the lungs the small circulation. The blood, which enters the small circulation, will be ejected from the right heart, the one that enters the large circulation from the left heart (◘ Figs. 15.1 and 15.2).

The heart transports the blood through the body perpetually through ongoing coordinated

15

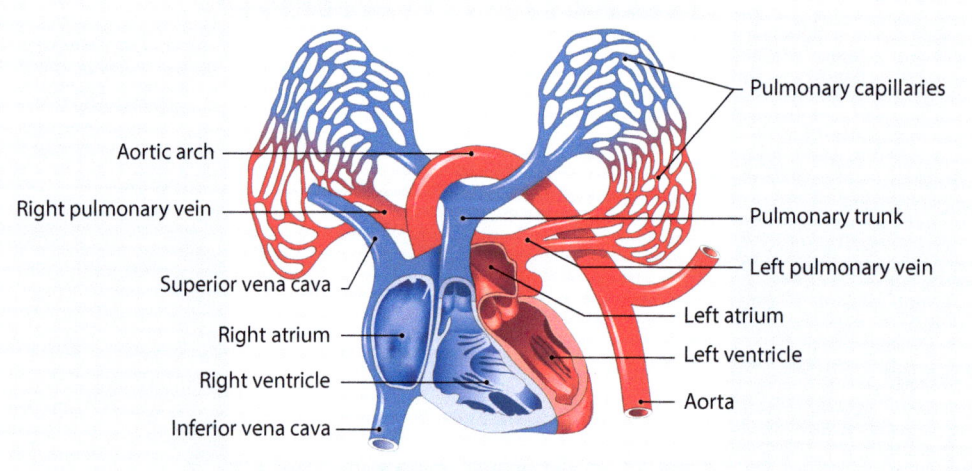

Aortic arch
Right pulmonary vein
Superior vena cava
Right atrium
Right ventricle
Inferior vena cava

Pulmonary capillaries
Pulmonary trunk
Left pulmonary vein
Left atrium
Left ventricle
Aorta

◘ **Fig. 15.1**   Heart anatomy (From Spornitz 2002 [3])

contractions (systole) and relaxations (diastole). During the filling period, the expansion increases tension to the individual muscle fibres. The greater the tension is at the end of the filling period, the greater is the ejection fraction of the heart (inotropy).

> **The lower the tension is at the end of the filling period, the lower is the ejection fraction and the higher is the venous return to the heart.**

This mechanism ensures a continuous flow of the blood without cutting off the blood flow. This phenomenon is known as the *Frank-Starling mechanism*. Thus, the ejection fraction of the heart adapts to the different conditions (◘ Fig. 15.3).

The underlying unit of the cardiac muscle is known as sarcomere. These are long, fibrous proteins that can move against each other. With expansion of the heart, calcium sensitivity of individual muscle cells is increased. Calcium is one of the most important electrolytes in the excitation of muscle cells.

> **The more fibres of the heart are extended, the higher is the calcium sensitivity and thus its contractility.**

The heart has different layers. The inner layer is called the endocardium. The endocardium covers the interior of the heart with a smooth layer of the squamous epithelium. The frictional resistance is lowered through its surface and ensures an undisturbed blood flow within the heart. The myocardium is composed of striated muscles and helps with the contraction of the heart. The epicardium is located on the outside of the heart. The heart itself is surrounded with a rigid collagen fibre-rich connective tissue sheath called the pericardium. The epicardium and pericardium together form the pericardial sac. They are not fused together and therefore can move smoothly against each other.

On the interception of the atria, chambers and major arteries valves are located. These valves ensure a unidirectional blood flow.

There are four valves all together:

— *Tricuspid valve*: Between the right atrium and ventricle
— *Pulmonary valve*: Between the right ventricle and blood vessels of the small circuit
— *Mitral valve*: Between the left atrium and ventricle

◘ **Fig. 15.2** Big and small circulation. (From Zilles and Tillmann 2010 [2])

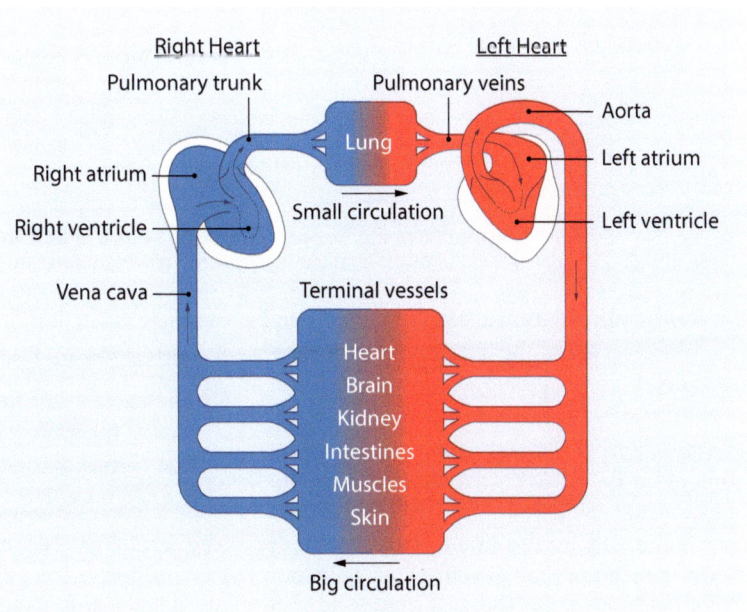

Right Heart
Pulmonary trunk

Left Heart
Pulmonary veins

Aorta

Lung

Right atrium

Left atrium

Small circulation

Right ventricle

Left ventricle

Vena cava

Terminal vessels

Heart
Brain
Kidney
Intestines
Muscles
Skin

Big circulation

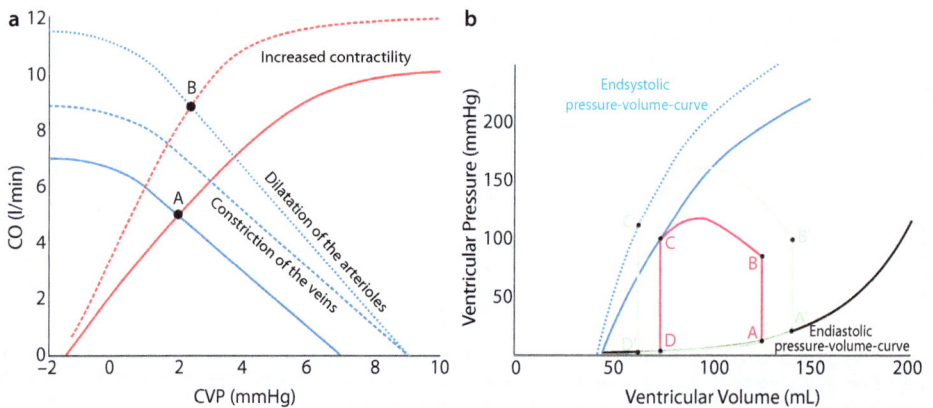

◻ Fig. 15.3 Illustration of Frank-Starling mechanism under different physiological conditions and activity; **a** Frank-Starling curve, **b** ventricular pressure-volume relationship, (From Schmidt, 2010)

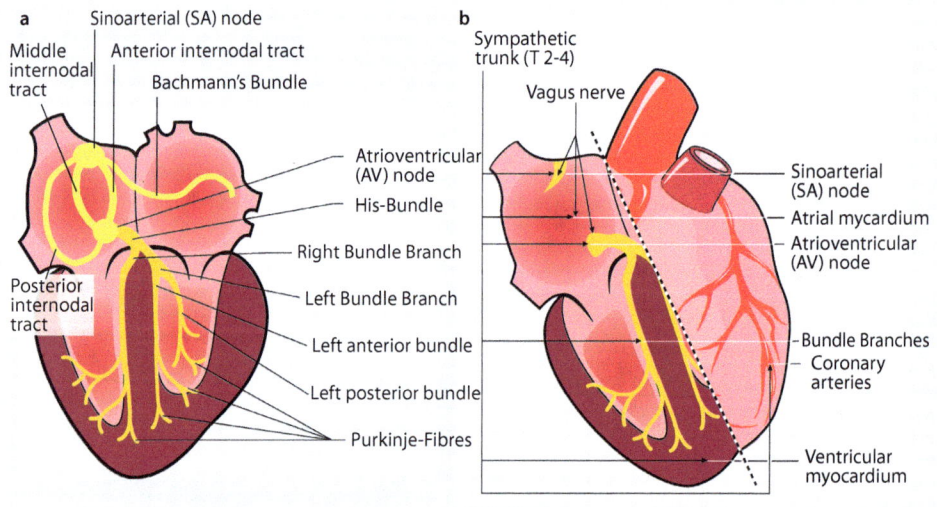

◻ Fig. 15.4 Schematic display of **a** conduction pathways of the heart; **b** innervation of heart structures by the sympathicus and vagal nerve. (Modified by Rusoke-Dierich 2017 (From Spornitz 2002 [3]))

— *Aortic valve*: Between the left ventricle and blood vessels of the big circuit (ascending aorta)

Contractions of the heart are caused by excitation of cardiac muscle cells. While for targeted movement excitations of skeletal muscles are controlled by the brain, cardiac muscles have their autonomous centres of excitation. This means that the heart can independently generate excitation of cardiac muscles without any direct external influences of the brain.

⟩ Each area in the heart has its own pacemaker function. If a superior centre fails, the corresponding next lower laying centre can take on the pacemaker function.

The frequency becomes less, the more inferior the centre is located within the heart. The physiological pacemaker is the sinoatrial (SA)

15

node. It is located in the right atrium and primarily regulates the heart rate. From there the excitation spreads across the atria. There are several bundles in the atria itself. The internodal bundles are located in the right atrium and the Bachmann's bundle in the left atrium. The atrioventricular (AV) node is the next pacemaker centre, which is located between the atria and ventricle (■ Fig. 15.1). The atrioventricular node has a filter function for heart conduction. It regulates the conduction from the atrium to the ventricles and hence determines the heart rate. The His bundle is divided into the right and left bundle, providing the left and right ventricle from the atrioventricular node with excitation. From these two bundles, the Purkinje fibres branch off. Additionally, from the left bundle, the left posterior bundles branch off. The autonomic nervous system regulates not only frequency (chronotropy) but also conduction speed (dromotropy), contractility (inotropy) and excitability (bathmotropy).

The sinus and atrioventricular node are subject to the autonomic nervous system, which allows that frequency can be increased or decreased depending to its needs. Via baroreceptors in the aortic arch and carotid sinus, located at the bifurcation of the carotid arteries, blood pressure and heart rate are detected. By means of a feedback mechanism with the autonomic nervous system, the heart rate is then regulated through interference with the sinoatrial and the atrioventricular node.

The contractility of the heart is produced by contractions of the muscle fibres. The heart moves up and down in the pericardium like a piston. The separation layer, the so-called cardiac valvular plane, is located between the atria and ventricles. The cardiac valvular plane rises and falls, causing the blood to be ejected into the blood vessels.

Exercise raises stroke volume as well as heart rate. This increases turnover of blood volume and supply of oxygen-rich blood. Cardiac output is blood volume ejected per time unit. In an untrained person, adaptation to higher demand is due to an increase in heart rate. In trained athletes, it is caused by increasing of

stroke volume. Changes in stroke volume are much more effective than increase of heart rate on its own.

At rest the heart beats about 60–80 times per minute. At an average heart volume of 500–900 mL, approx. 5 L are circulated per minute. That corresponds roughly to the total blood volume of an average adult person. The rate can rise to 150–180 beats per minute during sport activities. After exercise, the heart rate should normalise again after 15 min. An approximate estimate of the maximum heart rate in a healthy heart is: 220 – age = maximum heart rate.

Slow heart rates are called bradycardia. Heart rate above normal is called tachycardia. Cardiac arrhythmias can cause extremely high pathological rates. In extreme cases, an arrhythmia can lead to ventricular tachycardia (VT) or ventricular flutter (VF) (■ Table 15.1). Due to the Frank-Starling mechanism, cardiac output and end-diastolic blood pressure are reduced with increasing heart rates.

■ **Overview of Classification of Different Heart Rates**

During diving the cardiovascular system has to adapt to some changes. Gravitation under water is almost non-existent. Hence, the blood is differently distributed in the body under water compared to above the surface. The blood that normally accumulates in the lower limbs is now distributed evenly throughout the body. The blood volume in the lower limbs can be up to 500 mL, which represents approximately 10% of the total blood volume. In cold environment, such as underwater, additional narrowing of cutaneous blood vessels occurs to protect from

■ **Table 15.1** Classification of different heart rates

Brady- cardia	Normal heart beat	Tachy- cardia	VT	VF
<60	60–90	>100	150–250	>250

external heat loss. This leads to a central blood shift from the body periphery and thus relatively increases the central blood volume. The Frank-Starling mechanism causes an increased cardiac output during immersion by up to 32%. Changes in blood volume will be detected in the walls of venous blood vessels and in the right atrium. A change of blood pressure will be detected in the carotid node and the aortic arch. Increased blood pressure and volume in return trigger excretion of ANP and BNP and a reduction in ADH. ADH, BNP and ANP are hormones that help regulate the body's fluid balance via renal fluid excretion. After diving, the blood redistributes again. However, the volume already secreted by the kidney is "missing", which results in dehydration.

Immersion in cold water alone causes a reduced heart rate and peripheral vasoconstriction. The intensity of this reflex is more pronounced in colder water. Partial pressures seem to influence the heart rate. An increase of oxygen and inert gas partial pressure seems to be able to reduce the heart rate up to 10 beats per minute.

Valsalva manoeuvres are typically performed to equalise pressure in the ears during descending. This can increase the intrathoracic pressure for a short time and partially reduce blood flow. During the Valsalva manoeuvre, the blood is ejected additionally from the lungs (afterload), and the subsequent venous blood flow (preload) increases initially the blood pressure. Shortly after, the blood pressure drops again due to the reduced cardiac output. There is a compensatory initial heart rate reduction, which is followed by an increased heart rate. These factors could affect the diver during diving and should be kept in mind in the cardiac assessment for diving fitness, particularly in divers with cardiovascular diseases.

15.1.2 Vascular System

The vascular system is a closed system. It is used for transporting the blood. All vessels arising from the heart are called arteries. They split up into smaller vessels, arterioles and capillaries. In the latter, the transfer of gas and substances between the body tissue, lungs and blood takes place. The blood is transported back over venules and veins to the heart.

Blood vessels have three layers. The *intima* is the inner layer with endothelial cells. In addition, veins have venous valves, which prevent a backflow of the blood. Vascular muscles are located in the next layer (*media*). In correlation to veins, arteries have a thicker layer of muscles. The *adventitia* is the outermost layer, which contains mainly connective tissue, which stabilises the blood vessels. In addition, larger veins have their own blood supply. Capillaries consist only of the endothelium. Blood vessels in general are not like a closed tube, rather more a close-meshed network, allowing the exchange with its surrounding tissue. Exemption for this is the blood supply of the CNS. Tight junctions are an important factor in the blood-brain barrier. Tight junctions close the endothelial gaps of cerebral blood vessels and selectively restrict paracellular diffusion.

The blood flows from the left ventricle into the aorta. The aorta is the largest arterial blood vessel. It has high elasticity, which balances the initially high pressure and speed of the blood flow and evenly distributes it during the ejection phase. This feature of the aorta is called bag pipe function. Blood vessels closer to the heart are more elastic. The further the distance of the arteries is from the heart, the more smooth muscles are contained in their walls. The increase of muscles results in a reduction of elasticity. The aorta is followed by smaller arteries, which further continue to branch. The next smaller vessels are called arterioles. They have significant influence on blood pressure, due to the ability to contract and dilate and hence influence resistance. The smallest blood vessels are called capillaries. This is where the exchange of gas and metabolic substances to tissues takes place. The branching of blood vessels increases significantly the total surface area. The parallel blood flow also reduces pressure and flow rate (◘ Table 15.2 and ◘ Fig. 15.5).

15

	Aorta	Arteries	Capillaries	Veins	Vena cava
Diameter [cm]	2.6	0.3–0.06	0.0009	0.15–0.7	3.2
Common cross section [cm²]	4	20	3000	100	6
Filling volume [cm³]	180	250	300	1500	250
Flow rate [cm/sec]	20	15	0.03	8	11
Median blood pressure [mmHg]	100	20–100	15–20	12–15	5–12

◼ **Table 15.2** Specifications of different parts of the vascular system

◼ **Fig. 15.5** Distribution of blood pressure, total diameter and mean flow in the cardiovascular system (From Schmidt 2010 [1])

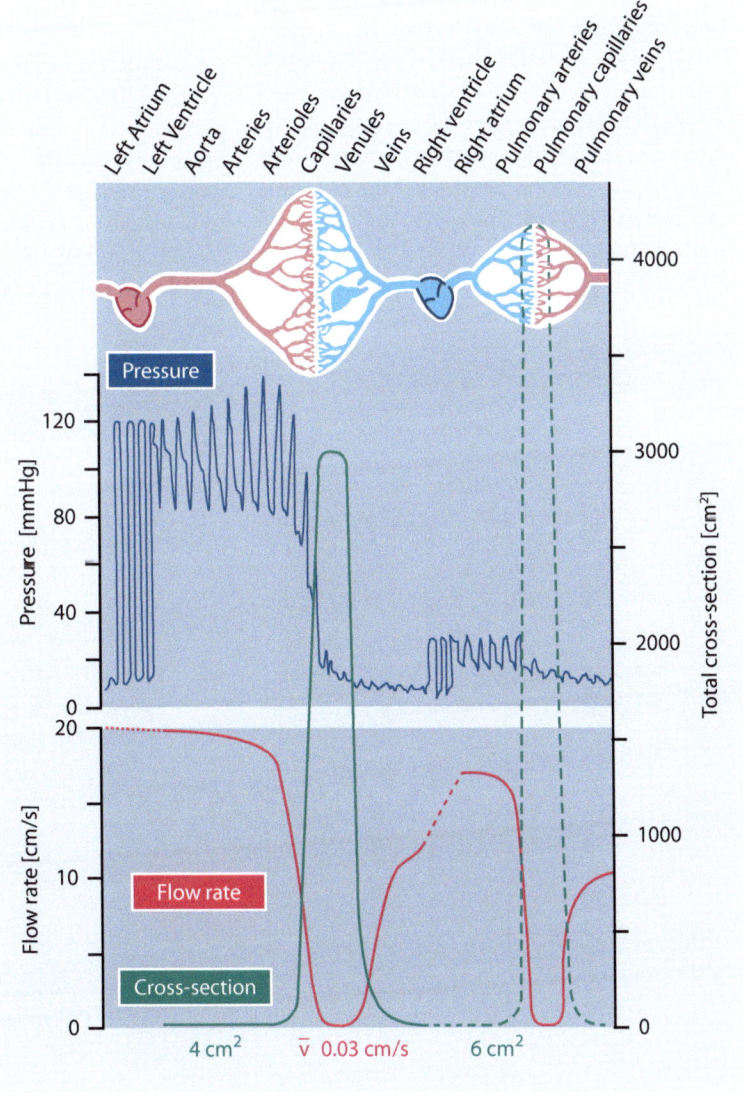

■ **Overview of the Different Blood Vessels**

The blood returns in venules and veins back to the heart. Unlike arteries, veins have flexible walls and therefore only have a minor impact on blood pressure. Veins are often in close anatomical relationship with arteries. The pulsation of arteries helps with the blood flow of veins. However, venous return is rather the effect of suction caused by the heart, breathing (filling of blood vessels in the lungs during exhalation), as well as by contracting muscles (muscle pump) and sympathetic stimulation-induced contraction of the veins. Venous valves, which are located mainly in veins of the lower extremities, prevent the blood from going in the wrong direction and ensure the blood flows in the direction to the heart. Veins, right heart and pulmonary vessels form together the low-pressure system. The low-pressure system functions as a blood reservoir and can hold approximately 80% of the total blood volume at rest. The high-pressure system consists of the arteries and the left heart (■ Fig. 15.6).

15.1.3 **Perfusion**

The body needs sufficient amount of the blood for oxygen transport. Cardiac output and vascular tone are responsible for blood flow and supply. Vascular tone is affected by chemical or hormonal signals.

Myogene effects are arising from muscles in the vessel wall. If the vessel walls extend due to increased blood pressure, vascular muscles and blood vessels themselves respond with vasoconstriction. Pulmonary or cutaneous blood vessels are an exception to this.

Blood vessels are affected by several *exogenous and endogenous factors* (■ Table 15.3). In general, lack of oxygen in tissues is a vasodilator to offset the oxygen deficit by increased perfusion. Oxygen deficiency in lung tissues however causes the contrary. Increased oxygen partial pressure triggers vasodilatation of pulmonary vessels. Hence, perfusion of the lungs can be directed into areas, which are better ventilated and rich on oxygen. An increase in

■ **Fig. 15.6** Venous valves (From Schmidt 2010 [1])

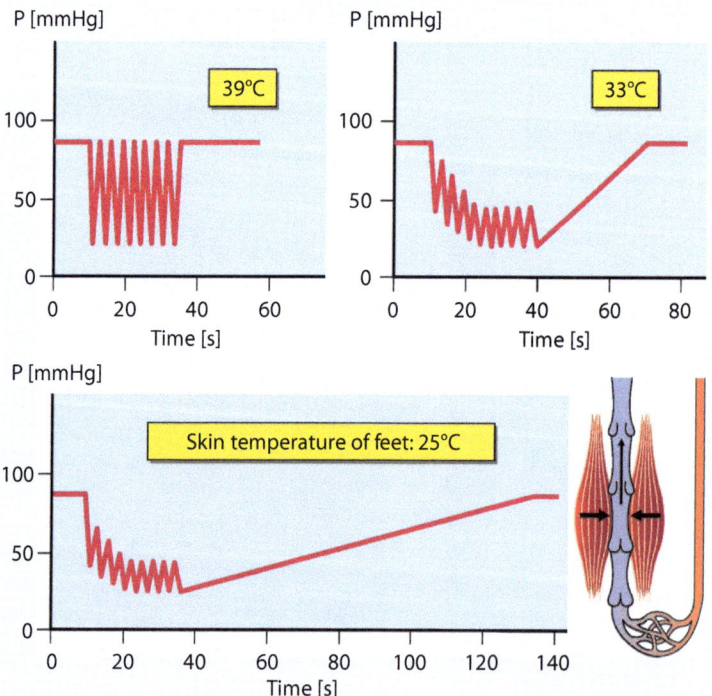

◧ **Table 15.3**   Overview of factors affecting vasoconstriction and dilatation

Vasoconstriction	Vasodilatation
Noradrenaline (alpha-receptors)	
High adrenaline concentrations (alpha-receptors)	Low adrenaline concentrations (beta-receptors)
Angiotensin II	Inflammatory mediators (quinine, histamine, etc.)
Decreased pO_2 (lungs only)	Increased pO_2 (lungs only)
Increased pO_2 (other blood vessels)	Decreased pO_2 (other blood vessels)
Low pCO_2	High pCO_2
Low H^+ concentrations	High H^+ concentrations
Myogene effects	Prostaglandin (e.g. cortisone)
Serotonin	NO = EDRF = endothelium-derived relaxing factor
ADH = adiuretin	AMP, ADP, ATP, adenosine, pyruvate
Aldosterone	

concentrations of some metabolites (e.g. CO_2, H^+ -ions, ATP, AMP, ADP, pyruvate, adenosine) has vasodilatory effects. But also, some vascular active substances have an influence on blood vessel diameters.

Changes of diameter in blood vessels result in changes in intravascular flow resistance, flow rate and pressure. Dilation of blood vessels decreases blood pressure and flow rate and vice versa. Blood viscosity is mainly dependent on length, diameter, flow rate, pressure, as well as temperature. By reducing flow rate, for example, viscosity increases. This means that the blood becomes "thicker". Viscosity, pressure, flow rate, temperature and flow resistance affect the flow properties of the blood. Under physiological conditions, a laminar flow prevails in almost all sections of blood vessels. This is the best condition for an almost smooth and turbulence-free blood flow. Disruptions of the laminar flow, caused, for example, by arteriosclerosis, blood clots, embolisms and nitrogen bubbles or during shock, result in turbulent flow.

Nervous and hormonal influences also affect the blood pressure. The sympathetic nervous system of the autonomic nervous system has the main control over the vascular tone. Stress hormones (catecholamines), like adrenaline and noradrenaline, are produced in the adrenal glands and delivered from there into the blood stream. Noradrenaline is also produced and stored in knotty distensions of nerves along blood vessels. The effects of catecholamines are mediated by alpha- and beta-receptors. Noradrenaline mainly shows an affinity for alpha-receptors. Adrenaline mainly has an affinity for alpha-receptors in lower concentrations and to beta-receptors in higher concentrations. The activation of alpha-receptors causes vasoconstriction and the activation of beta-receptors vasodilatation.

The interaction of these factors allows a fast, localised but also long-term and comprehensive control of circulation.

15.1.4 **Blood Pressure**

Maintaining a constant blood pressure is a requirement for continuous blood flow and thus sufficient blood supply to all body parts. Generally, the term blood pressure describes the arterial blood pressure. It varies between a maximum (systolic blood pressure) and a minimum value (diastolic blood pressure). It varies also in different parts of the vascular

◘ Table 15.4 Blood pressures in the vascular system

Vessel type	Median pressure in mmHg
Aorta	100
Artery	80–70
Arteriole	70–35
Capillary	35–10
Venole	15–10
Veins	<10

system (◘ Table 15.4) The systolic value corresponds to the blood pressure of the ejection phase of the heart and the diastolic blood pressure to the one of the filling phase. Blood pressure is measured usually in a sitting or lying position on the upper arm. As the blood pressure is affected by orthostatic forces, the cuff should be at the same level as the heart. It is usually 120/80 mmHg at rest. Values over 160/95 mmHg are considered as high blood pressure (hypertension). Systolic values under 100 mmHg are classified as hypotension. Generally, blood pressure in arteries decreases with greater distance to the heart. Blood pressure is detected by receptors (presso-, tension- and chemoreceptors) in the high- and low-pressure system. The response is passed on by afferent nerve pathways to the autonomic nervous system in the brain stem, where blood pressure is controlled. Via efferent nerves, heart and blood vessels are influenced to regulate blood pressure. Sympathetic, parasympathetic nervous system, angiotensin II produced by the kidneys and NO (=EDRF) produced by vascular endothelial cells are the main influencing factors of blood pressure.

15.1.5 Blood

The total blood volume is approx. 4.5–5.5 L, which is about 6–8% of the total body weight. Cells in the blood are originated from progenitor cells in the bone marrow. Transport of substances and gases, thermal regulation, buffering of the acid-base household, signal transmission through hormones, blood clotting and the immune defence are some functions of the blood.

Blood Components:
- *Erythrocytes* (oxygen and carbon dioxide transport)
- *Leukocytes* (immune defence)
- *Thrombocytes* (clotting)
- *Proteins* (transport, defence and transmission of information; osmotic force for the fluid regulation between tissue and blood vessels)
- *Electrolytes* (cellular metabolism)

Due to increased alveolar oxygen, partial pressure oxygen diffuses into the pulmonary capillaries. Haemoglobin (Hb) of red blood cells binds oxygen reversibly. One haemoglobin molecule can bind up to four oxygen molecules. This process is called oxygenation. The oxygenated blood is measured in percent as oxygen saturation via pulse oximetry. During normal breathing, the blood almost completely saturates (97–99%). The ability of haemoglobin to bind oxygen changes, depending on various factors. Oxygen binding to Hb can be graphically displayed by the oxygen dissociation curve. It has a sigmoid (s-shaped) curve and is mainly depended to pH, pCO_2 and partially to temperature as well as of 2,3 DPG. Any changes of these factors can cause an alteration of oxygen affinity to Hb. A right shift causes a decrease of oxygen affinity and facilitates the release of oxygen from haemoglobin. Metabolic products, such as CO_2, lactate and lowering of pH-levels cause a right shift, resulting in an increase of O_2 extraction from haemoglobin by up to 20%. With endurance training, O_2 extraction may increase up to 35%. On the other hand, a left shift means an increased oxygen affinity. After oxygen binds to haemoglobin and CO_2 is eliminated by the lungs through exhalation in return, the pH increases, which leads then to the left shift.

This optimises oxygen transport. With increasing age, the ability of the lung to absorb oxygen subsides, and also the capacity of the haemoglobin to bind oxygen is reduced.

Carbon dioxide is one of the major metabolic products. There are three ways CO_2 is transported in blood. Carbon dioxide (CO_2) is mainly transformed to bicarbonate by chemical processes. Through further processes, bicarbonate is split to a bicarbonate ion (HCO_3^-) and a hydrogen ion (H^+) and can be therefore transported in the blood stream. CO_2 and H^+ affect the affinity of haemoglobin for oxygen which is reflected in the oxygen-haemoglobin dissociation curve. An increase of CO_2 and H^+ lowers the oxygen affinity and vice versa. This process is called *Bohr effect* (◻ Fig. 15.7).

$$CO_2 + H_2O \rightleftharpoons H_2CO_3 \rightleftharpoons H^+ + HCO_3^-$$

This usually slow process is catalysed by carbonic anhydrase, an enzyme inside erythrocytes. Carbon dioxide (CO_2) diffuses into erythrocytes. There it converts together with water and accelerated by carbonic anhydrase to carbonic acid (H_2CO_3) and then to bicarbonate ions (HCO_3^-) and hydrogen ions (H^+). Hydrogen ions can't leave the erythrocytes. Bicarbonate ions pass readily through cell membranes and enter the plasma in exchange with chloride ions. The chloride shift is also known as the *Gibbs-Donnan equilibrium* or *Hamburger effect*. The H^+ − ions are buffered by reduced haemoglobin, and hence the pH changes only slightly. Reduced haemoglobin is made available when oxygen is released. Reduced haemoglobin is less acidic than oxygenated haemoglobin and facilitates therefore the binding of hydrogen ions. Approximately 90% (arterial) and 60% (venous) of CO_2 are transported this way. Carbon dioxide is bound only partially to haemoglobin in erythrocytes. A small portion of carbon dioxide is held in carbamino form and binds mainly to haemoglobin and to other proteins (~5% arterial, ~30% venous). The rest, about 5% (arterial) and

◻ **Fig. 15.7** Oxygen dissociation curve. (From Schmidt 2010 [1])

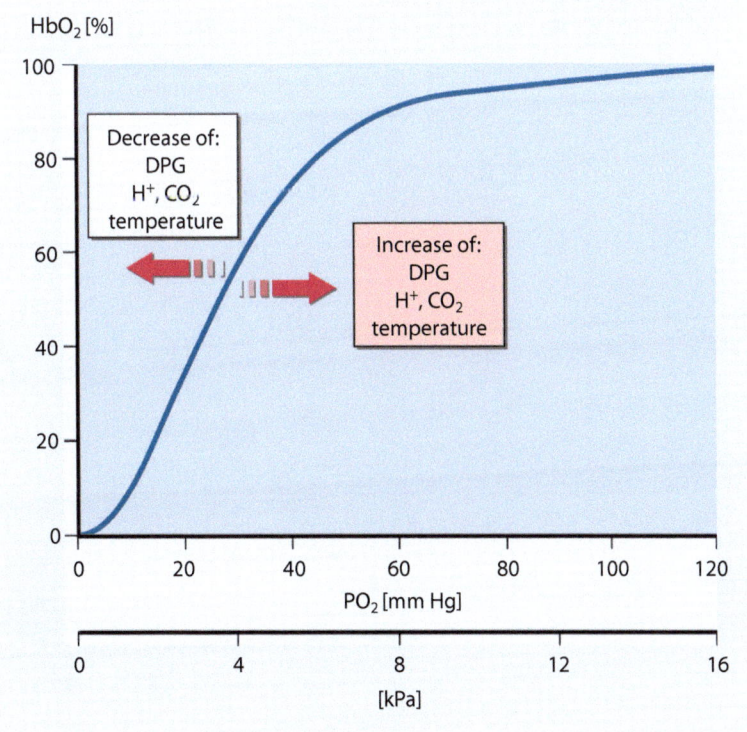

10% (venous), is physically dissolved in blood. The CO_2 dissociation curve is different to the O_2 dissociation curve. It doesn't have a sigmoid shape but rather a hyperbolic shape. It is to a lesser degree influenced by haemoglobin but however sensitive to pH level changes. Hence, CO_2 has different distributions in venous and arterial blood. As reduced haemoglobin is less acidic than oxygenated haemoglobin, in the lungs CO_2 is forced out of the haemoglobin binding. Hydrogen ions and bicarbonate together are converted to carbonic acid and then to carbon dioxide and water. CO_2 can thus be eliminated via exhalation over the lungs. The process is reversed in tissues as oxygen is release and haemoglobin is reduced. The ability of haemoglobin to store H^+ and CO_2 decreases

with increasing arterial pO_2 and is known as the *Haldane effect*. It is important to have sufficient haemoglobin as well as functional red blood cells. During apnoea CO_2 rises by 0.4–0.8 kPa/min (3–6 mmHg/min). In 1 min pCO_2 is expected to rise from 5.3 to 6.1 kPa (40–46 mmHg) and pO_2 to fall from 14 to 5.3 kPa (105–40 mmHg) in 1 min. Preoxygenation with 100% oxygen can defer the decline of oxygen. This is due to relatively high oxygen levels within the lungs but also a higher dissolved pO_2 in the blood. Carbon monoxide (CO) has a 200 times higher affinity to haemoglobin as oxygen and therefore can dislodge it from its bond to haemoglobin. Thus oxygen cannot be transported sufficiently in the blood to meet demands (◘ Figs. 15.8 and 15.9).

◘ **Fig. 15.8** Chemical reaction in erythrocytes during gas exchange in tissues ("internal respiration") and in the lungs ("external respiration"). **a** gas exchange tissue (internal respiration); **b** gas exchange lungs (external respiration). (From Schmidt 2010 [1])

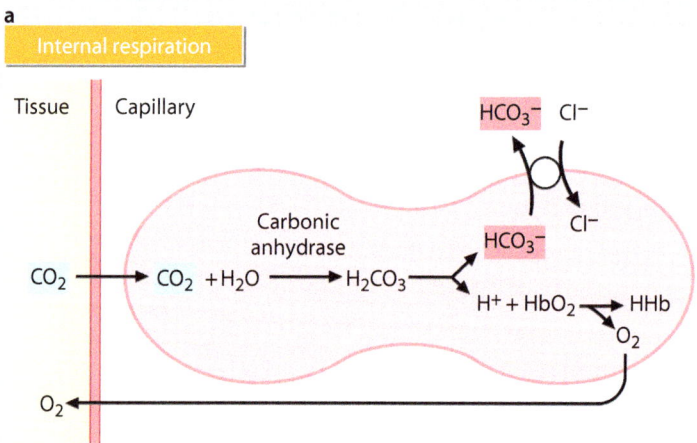

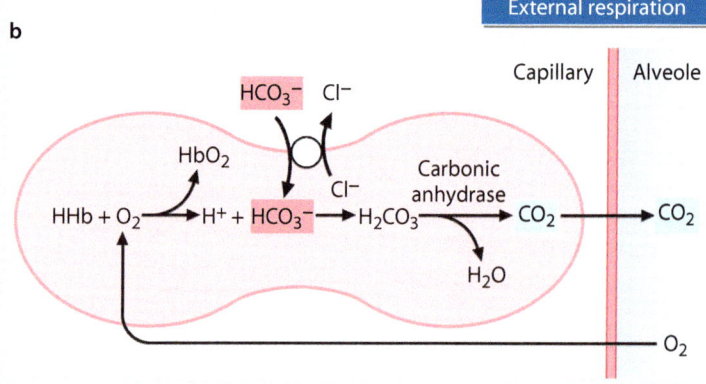

■ **Fig. 15.9** CO_2 transport in the blood. **a** carbon dioxide content in oxygenated and deoxygenated blood; **b** distribution of carbon dioxide in blood. (From Schmidt 2010 [1])

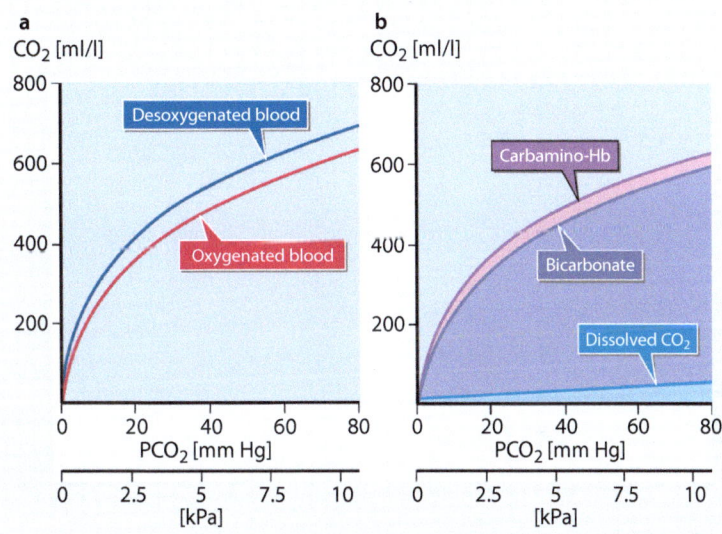

References

1. Schmidt RF, Lang F, Heckmann M. Physiologie des Menschen. 31st ed. Berlin: Springer; 2010.
2. Zilles K, Tillmann BN. Anatomie. Berlin: Springer; 2010.
3. Spornitz UM. Herz-Kreislauf-System, 3. Auflage. Berlin: Springer; 2002

Suggested Reading

Geers C, Gros G. Carbon dioxide transport and carbonic anhydrases in blood and muscle. Physiol Rev. 2000;80(2):681–715.

Moll KJ, Moll M. Anatomie. 18th ed. München: Elsevier; 2006.

Moss RL, Fitzsimons DP. Frank – Starling relationship; long on importance, short on mechanism. Circ Res. 2002;90:11–3. American Heart Association.

Silbernagel S, Despopuluos A. Taschenatlas der Physiologie. 7th ed. Stuttgart: Thieme; 2007.

Solaso RJ. Mechanism of Frank – Starling law of the heart. The beat goes on. Biophys J. 2007;93(12): 4095–6.

Respiration

© Springer International Publishing AG, part of Springer Nature 2018
O. Rusoke-Dierich, *Diving Medicine*, https://doi.org/10.1007/978-3-319-73836-9_16

In general, breathing represents the process of gas exchange of organisms with their environment. In the human body, air is conducted via the upper, bigger airways to the smallest airways, the alveoli, where gas exchange takes place. During the passage of the upper respiratory tract, air is cleaned, warmed and saturated with water vapour before entering the alveoli.

The lung is the organ where gas exchange takes place. The gas exchange in the lungs is also referred to as external respiration. Internal respiration refers to oxygen metabolism inside cells. Breathing facilitates oxygen absorption, carbon dioxide elimination as well as inert gas in- and outgassing. Few other metabolic products, such as alcohol, are eliminated via the lungs too. The entire respiratory tract is divided into upper and lower airways. The nose, mouth and pharynx belong to the upper airways. The trachea, stem bronchus, bronchioles and alveolar ducts belong to the lower airways. Airways are considered small, if their diameter is less than 2 mm. The smallest non-gas-exchanging airways and the terminal bronchioles have a diameter of 0.5 mm. The airways consist of mucosa, basement membrane, smooth muscle matrix and predominantly fibro-cartilaginous of fibro-elastic connective tissue. Cellular elements, like mast cells, but also macrophages, activated T lymphocytes, eosinophiles, neutrophils and basophiles are responsible for the mediator release. Stretch as well as irritant receptors and cholinergic receptors influence the smooth muscle and glandular unit response. During the passage through the airways, the air is cleaned and enriched with water vapor (◨ Figs. 16.1 and 16.2).

16.1 Lungs and Respiratory Mechanics

The right and left sides of the lung are located within the chest cavity. The right side is divided into three, the left into two lobes. Air enters via the bronchial tubes. The right main bronchus is slightly steeper than the left and is therefore more prone to aspiration. The lung is separated from its surrounding tissue by the pleural gap and can freely move. Due to negative pressure in the pleural gap and

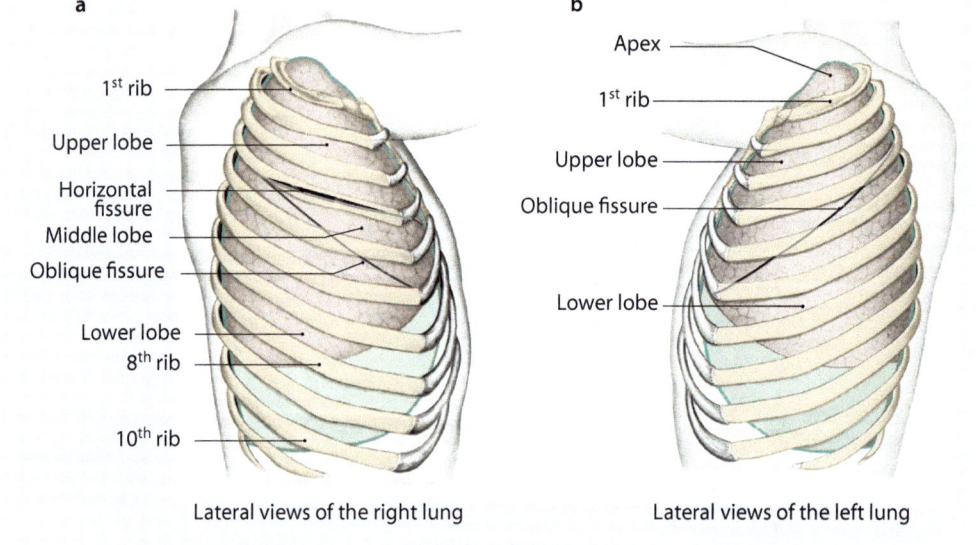

Lateral views of the right lung   Lateral views of the left lung

◨ **Fig. 16.1** Lung anatomy; **a** lateral views of the right lung, **b** lateral views of the left lung, (From Guellich and Krueger 2013 [1])

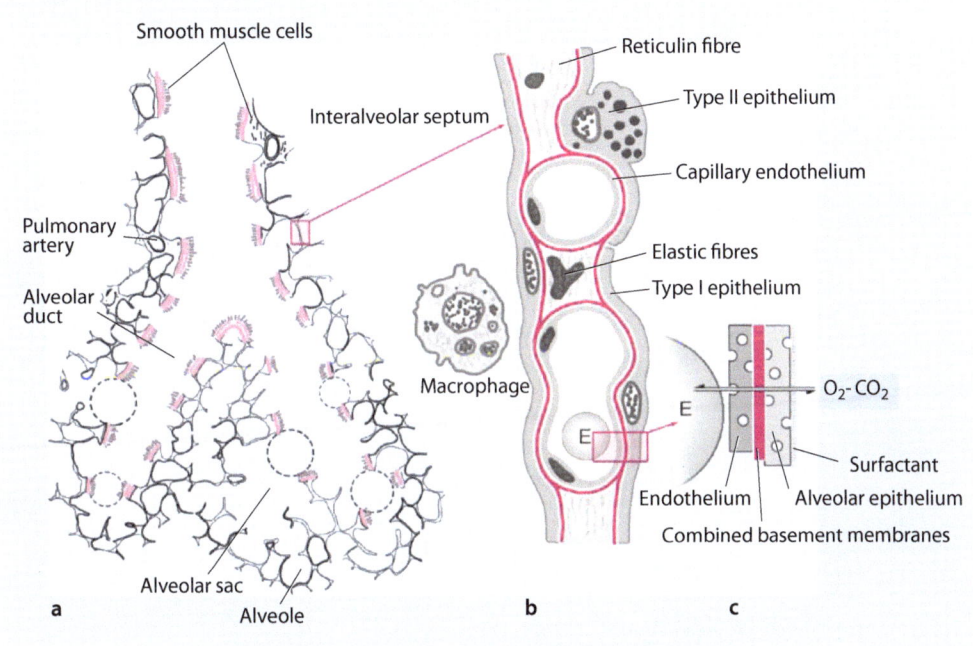

□ **Fig. 16.2**   Alveolar anatomy; **a** histological structure our the gas exchanging system, **b** alveolar septum, **c** alveolar basement membrane, (From Guellich and Krueger 2013 [1])

adhesion forces, the lung is prevented from collapsing. It is the same mechanism as when two wet glass panes are pressed together. They can be moved against each other, but can't be pulled apart. The lung has two separate vascular systems. One supplies blood to the lung tissue itself, the other is used for gas exchange. Blood vessels of the small circulation are not only responsible for gas exchange but also to filter small thrombi out of the blood and hence prevent arterial embolisms entering the large circulation, e.g. like the brain or other vital organs, preventing strokes or other organ damage.

The lung functions like bellows when breathing in and out. Flattening of the diaphragm and simultaneously raising of the ribs increases the volume in the chest cavity. The vacuum, which is created during inhalation, forces the air to be sucked in. On exhalation the curvature of the diaphragm increases and the ribs are getting pulled down. This causes the air to be pressed out during exhalation.

16.2 Respiratory Regulation

The respiration is regulated by the CNS (medulla oblongata). Inhalation and exhalation are caused by alternate activation of inspiratory and expiratory neurons. Partial pressures of oxygen and carbon dioxide are important factors in the regulation of respiration. Chemoreceptors located in the CNS itself as well as in the body's periphery are used for pO_2 and pCO_2 detection. Peripheral arterial chemoreceptors measure mainly oxygen partial pressures. They are located in the aortic arch and the carotid artery (□ Fig. 16.3).

Central chemoreceptors rather respond to changes of carbon dioxide partial pressure and of pH levels. They are found in the medulla oblongata. In healthy individuals respiration is mainly regulated through pCO_2. Respiration can be increasingly influenced by pO_2, in chronic lung diseases, which interfere with pulmonary gas exchange. In addition to these main factors, there are still a number of other factors,

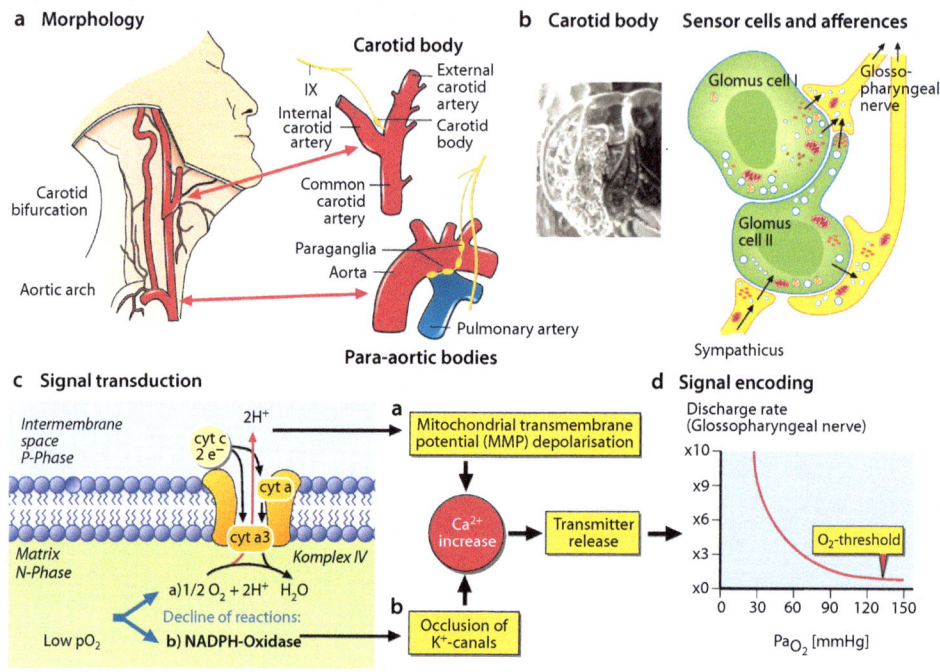

◼ Fig. 16.3 Arterial chemoreceptors; **a** morphology, **b** carotid body/sensor cells and afferences, **c** signal transduction, **d** signal encoding (From Schmidt 2010 [2])

which affect respiration. Mechanoreceptors in muscles and tendons are excited during exertion and result in increased respiratory activity. In a trained person this trigger is less effective. Additionally, influences from higher CNS centres, such as psychological arousal, arbitrary breathing, pain or reflexes such as coughing, sneezing and yawning, affect the respiration as well. Hormones such as adrenaline or steroids influence breathing too. Cool ambient temperatures trigger increased respiration. Presso-receptors are excited when blood pressure drops, resulting in increased respiratory activity. Stretching of rib muscles receptors affects breathing. Full exhalation or free diving more than 15–20 m, where the chest wall is compressed, triggers an inspiratory reflex. For deep diving, it is therefore better to fill the lungs completely, as air volume in the lungs decreases during compression. On the other hand, full inspiration leads to an expiratory reflex. Therefore, for distance diving at the same level, better results are achieved by avoiding maximum inhalation (◼ Fig. 16.4).

16.3 Alveolar Gas Exchange

Gas exchange takes place in the alveoli (diameter 0.3 mm). The surface for gas exchange is enlarged as respiratory units branch continuously, ending up in air sacs (alveoli). The entire lung surface would cover more than 100 m². Gas has to pass through the surfactant, cells of alveoli, interstitial fluid, cells, connective tissues and endothelium of capillaries to reach the blood. Although, the entire diffusion distance between the alveoli and the lung capillaries is only 0.0002 mm. The capillaries surround closely the alveoli like a net. The contact time of blood with alveoli is 0.75 s, but gas exchange usually takes less than 0.25 s. Driving forces for diffusion is the difference of partial pressures of individual gases in alveoli and blood. Gases

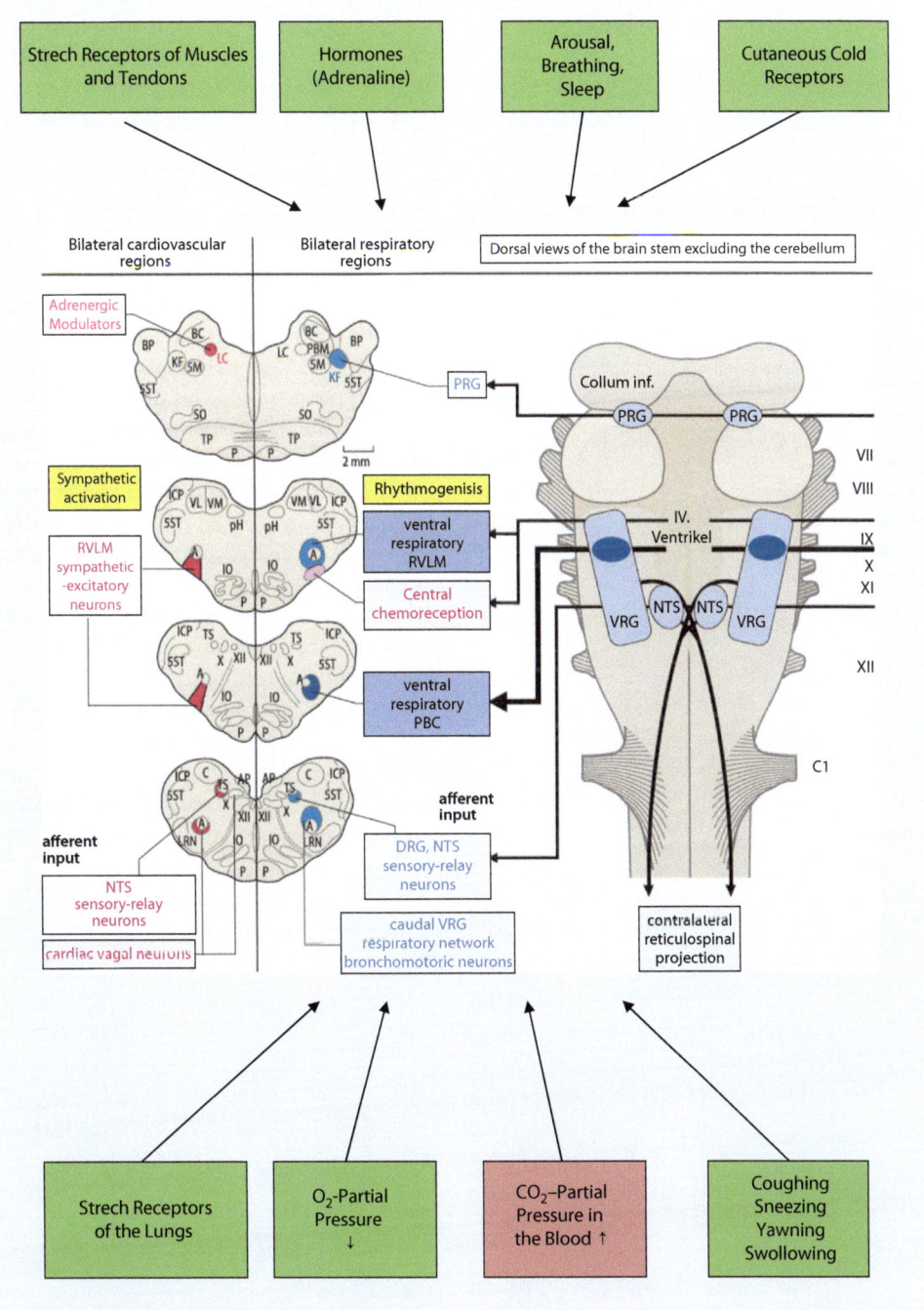

Strech Receptors of Muscles and Tendons

Hormones (Adrenaline)

Arousal, Breathing, Sleep

Cutaneous Cold Receptors

Bilateral cardiovascular regions

Bilateral respiratory regions

Dorsal views of the brain stem excluding the cerebellum

Adrenergic Modulators

Sympathetic activation

RVLM sympathetic-excitatory neurons

afferent input

NTS sensory-relay neurons

cardiac vagal neurons

Rhythmogenisis

ventral respiratory RVLM

Central chemoreception

ventral respiratory PBC

afferent input

DRG, NTS sensory-relay neurons

caudal VRG respiratory network bronchomotoric neurons

Collum inf.

IV. Ventrikel

contralateral reticulospinal projection

Strech Receptors of the Lungs

O_2–Partial Pressure ↓

CO_2–Partial Pressure in the Blood ↑

Coughing Sneezing Yawning Swollowing

▣ **Fig. 16.4** Respiratory regulation of the medulla oblongata (*green*, peripheral factors; *red*, central factors), (Modified by Rusoke-Dietrich 2017, from Schmidt, 2010)

diffuse from the place of higher pressure or concentration to the place of lower pressure or concentration (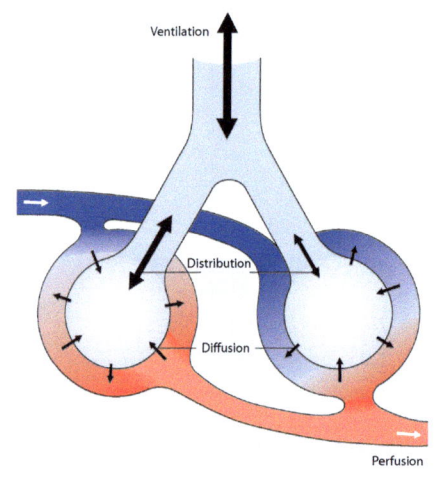 Fig. 16.5).

Inspirational air (STPD) has an oxygen content of about 21% and 0.03% carbon dioxide. Expirational air has an oxygen content of only 15–18% but 2.5–6% of carbon dioxide. Gas fractions change within the airways as air

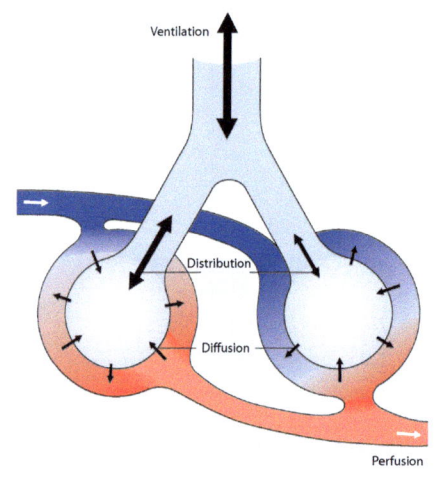

Ventilation
Distribution
Diffusion
Perfusion

Fig. 16.5 Alveolar gas exchange. (From Schmidt 2010 [2])

gets warmed and saturated with water vapour. Air is fully warmed and saturated in the trachea at the level of the bifurcation. Hence, partial pressures from gases are reduced from STPD to BTPS. This is explained in detail in the ► Chap. 25. The average oxygen partial pressure (pO_2) is 145 mbar (14.5 kPa or 109 mmHg) in the alveoli and 53 mbar (5.3 kPa or 40 mmHg) in the pulmonary artery. The carbon dioxide partial pressure (pCO_2) in the blood of the pulmonary artery is 61 mbar (6.1 kPa or 45 mmHg) with an alveolar pCO_2 of 53 mbar (5.3 kPa or 40 mmHg) Table 16.1). Partial pressures of gases in pulmonary arteries adjust to the partial pressure of the gases in the alveoli. The partial pressure of the inhaled air depends on the ambient pressure (Table 16.2). Oxygen diffuses into the blood and carbon dioxide out of the blood. Gases entering the bloodstream are either bound chemically or physically. Oxygen, carbon monoxide and the small amount of carbon dioxide are bound chemically to haemoglobin in the erythrocytes. All other gases, especially nitrogen, as the main component of air, are only dissolved physically in the blood. According to Henry's law, gases only can be dissolved to a certain level in liquids depending on their

Table 16.1 Comparison of partial pressures in alveoli and pulmonary artery

	PCO_2		PO_2	
Pulmonary artery	45 mmHg	0.061 bar	40 mmHg	0.053 bar
Alveoli	40 mmHg	0.053 bar	109 mmHg	0.145 bar

Table 16.2 Partial pressures of gases (STPD) at different depths

Gas content (STPD)	Partial pressure in bar					
	0 m	10 m	20 m	30 m	50 m	60 m
Oxygen (21%)	0.21	0.42	0.63	0.84	1.26	1.68
Nitrogen (78%)	0.78	1.56	2.34	3.12	4.68	6.24
Carbon dioxide (0.03%)	0.0003	0.0006	0.0009	0.0012	0.0018	0.0024

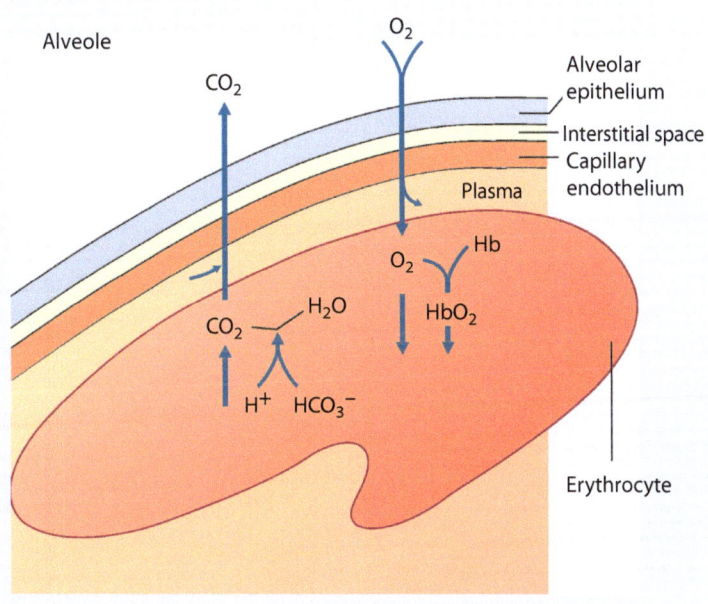

■ **Fig. 16.6** O_2 and CO_2 transport pathways during the pulmonary gas exchange. (From Schmidt 2010 [2])

solubility. Likewise in a glass of water when adding salt, only a certain amount is resolved. The rest of the excess salt is visible in its original solid form. Gases behave the same way in liquids when the saturation capacity is exceeded. The ability of fluids to bind gases depends on ambient pressure and partial pressure. Higher ambient pressure results in a higher amount of gases to be dissolved in liquids and vice versa in pressure reduction. Usually excess nitrogen is exhaled. If there is more nitrogen in blood and tissues that can be exhaled, decompression sickness might occur (■ Fig. 16.6).

Gas exchange may be disturbed by various factors:
- Aspiration, such as drowning, can cause airways to be blocked.
- Reduction of the alveolar perfusion, for example, in a pulmonary infarction. Thus, in some sections of the lungs, perfusion decreases, resulting in decreased oxygen uptake.
- In some chronic lung diseases, such as emphysema, or toxic gas inhalation, the alveolar membrane may thicken, which inhibits the gas exchange.

- Arteriovenous shunts in the lungs, which are bypassing the blood within the lungs, can cause a reduced oxygen or nitrogen absorption.

16.4 Internal Respiration

Oxygen binds reversibly to haemoglobin. This process is called oxygenation. Haemoglobin is also responsible for the red colour of our blood. It contains a haem prosthetic group that has an iron atom at its centre. Oxygenated blood is red (oxyhaemoglobin) and deoxygenated blood is blue-red. One haemoglobin can bind up to four oxygen molecules. This is the reason that oxygen is able to be transported in such high concentrations throughout the body. Oxygen is released from haemoglobin by low tissue pH. The blood's pH is primarily lowered by carbon dioxide and lactic acid. Tissue oxygen partial pressures adjust to vascular oxygen partial pressures and are utilised in cells for energy production. This energy is produced by intracellular oxidative processes, which require oxygen, glucose and fatty acids. A number of chemical processes are involved in this. Glycolysis is one of them, which is processed in the cytoplasm. It provides pyruvate for the citric acid cycle. The Krebs cycle is located in the matrix of mitochondria. The end products are NADH and $FADH_2$, both energy-rich compounds (◘ Fig. 16.7).

The respiratory chain is located in the mitochondrial wall. Hereby, a controlled oxy-hydrogen reaction takes place, which reduces O_2 to H_2O. Carbon dioxide is the metabolic product of this reaction. ATP is produced from ADP + P. ATP is extremely energetic and provides energy for many intracellular processes. This process is called oxidative phosphorylation. Oxygen consumption varies from tissue to tissue and is dependent on the demand. Oxygen consumption of skeletal muscles, for example, can rise 20 times from rest compared to exercise. The increased oxygen consumption is balanced by increased respiratory minute volume, with increased respiratory rate and tidal volume. Since red blood cells have no cell nuclei and no mitochondria, they consume almost no oxygen and thus have only transport function.

16.5 Lung Perfusion/Ventilation

The right ventricle ejects in average as much blood into the pulmonary vessels as the left heart pumps through the whole large circulation. Both chambers of the heart are coordinated to ensure a continuous blood flow (Frank-Starling mechanism). The pulmonary vessels are highly elastic and have therefore also a reservoir function for blood. In an upright position the blood shifts mainly due to gravity to lower regions of the lung. This results in reduced ventilation in these parts. In contrast the ventilation increases from the base up to the top. To avoid extreme values in ventilation/perfusion ratio, blood flow has to be regulated in individual lung areas. Oxygen regulates the diameter of blood vessels. A lack of oxygen causes vasoconstriction. Thus, blood flow decreases in the lower lung sections, and blood is directed into the upper sections of the lung. In the upper sections, a relative high

proportion of oxygen is leading to vasodilatation. As a result blood vessels expand and perfusion increases. There is an intrapulmonary shunt caused by anatomic connections of pulmonary veins and arteries. Deoxygenated blood of pulmonary arteries enters pulmonary veins, and thus blood gets mixed with the oxygen-rich blood. Usually the intrapulmonal (IP) shunt is approximately 2%. Under exercise it can rise to 5%. Bronchioli and alveoli are the only parts of the airways, which are capable of exchanging gas. The proportion of the respiratory tract, which doesn't take part in gas exchange, is referred to as dead space. The dead space is distinguish between anatomical and functional (= physiological) dead space. The anatomical dead space includes the entire upper respiratory tract with trachea and bronchi. The functional dead space includes the whole area of the respiratory tract, where no gas exchange takes place. Typically the anatomical dead space matches the functional. Usage of snorkels or diving helmets however causes the functional dead space to increase. A common calculation of the physiological dead space is the *Bohr equation*:

$$\frac{V_D^{phys}}{V_T} = \frac{F_{A_{CO_2}} - F_{E_{CO_2}}}{F_{A_{CO_2}}}$$

or

$$V_D^{phys} = V_T \times \left(1 - \frac{F_{E_{CO_2}}}{F_{A_{CO_2}}}\right)$$

V_D^{phys} = physiological dead space, V_T = tidal volume, $F_{E_{CO_2}}$ = expired CO_2, $F_{A_{CO_2}}$ = alveolar CO_2

This equation shows that with unchanged tidal volume the dead space increases with increasing alveolar CO_2. This is the case at depth greater than 40 m, as the density increases and laminar flow turns into turbulent flow (◘ Figs. 16.8 and 16.9).

The total lung capacity, which includes the total pulmonary gas volume is usually around 6–8 L. After complete exhalation, only about 1.5 L remain in the lung. The maximum inhalation from a neutral respiratory position is up to 3 L (inspiratory reserve volume). The

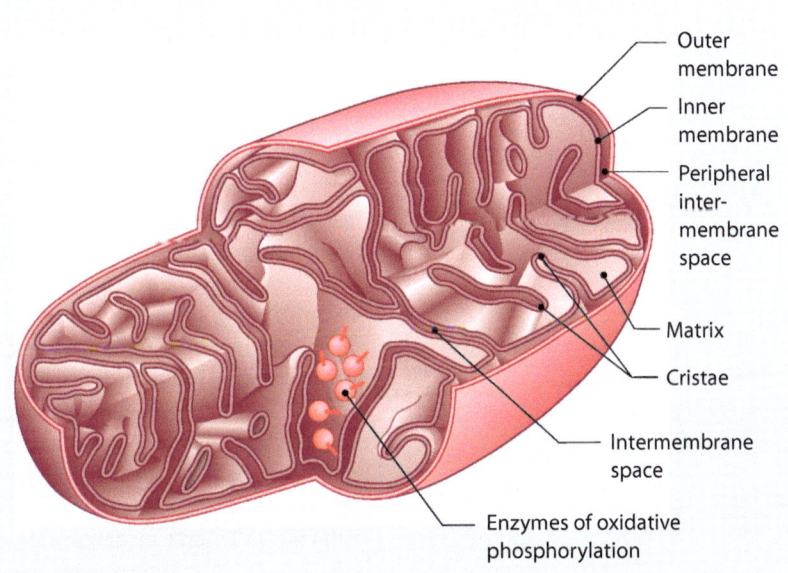

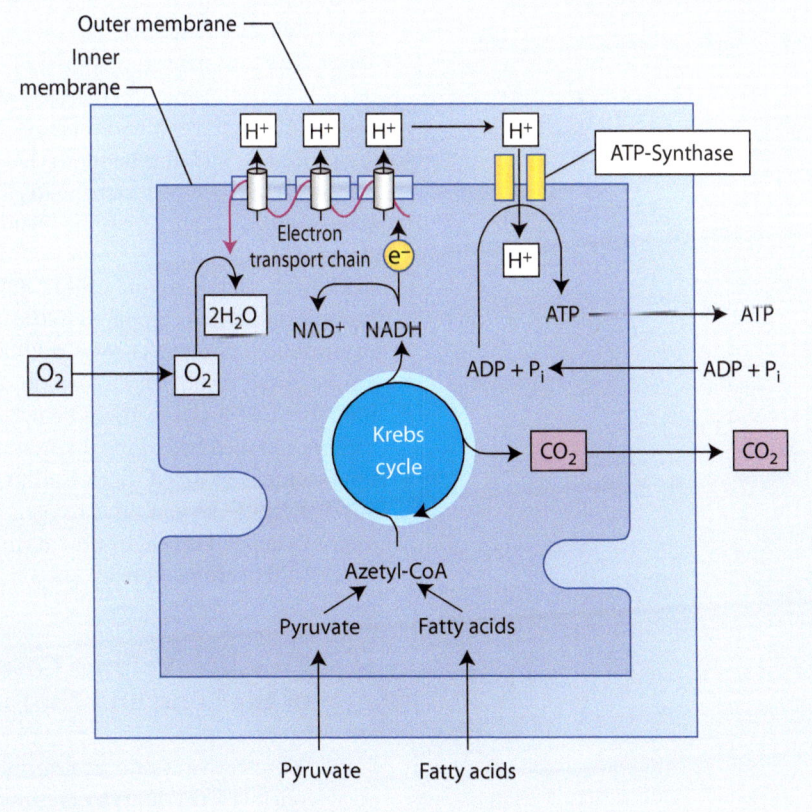

■ **Fig. 16.7** Mitochondrial structure and function; Krebs cycle, (From Schmidt 2010 [2])

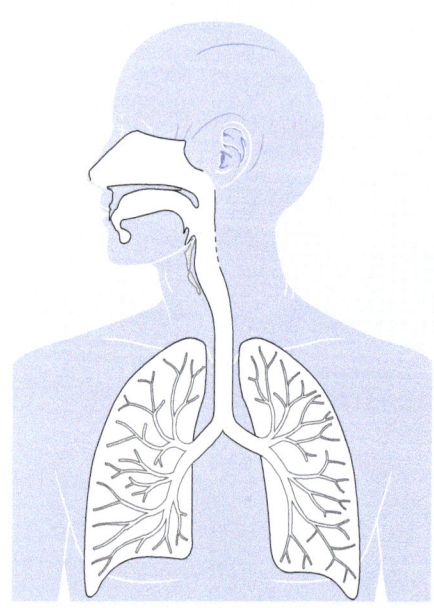

Fig. 16.8   Anatomical dead space (Ecomed)

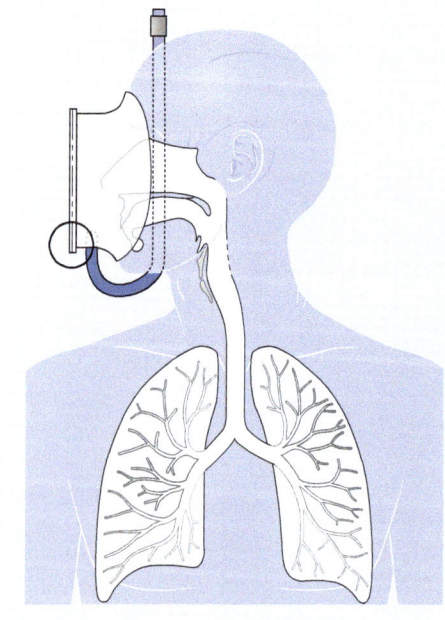

Fig. 16.9   Functional dead space (Ecomed)

maximum exhalation is approximately 1.5 L (expiratory reserve volume). The remaining volume is called residual volume. The normal tidal volume is about 0.5 L at rest. Tidal volume and expiratory and inspiratory reserve volume when combined are called vital capacity (approx. 4.5–7 L). All these parameters are depending on age, gender, size, weight and fitness. The vital capacity decreases with increasing age. In athletes the vital capacity may be up to 10 L. Throughout normal breathing, laminar flow prevails in the airways. Forced respiration however increases flow rate. In scuba diving at greater depths, gas density is increasing and the gas mixture becomes "thicker" and laminar flow may become turbulent. Turbulences of the air can result in insufficient ventilation. This again causes a reduction of efficient gas exchange and therefore deterioration of oxygen utilisation. Also, carbon dioxide may be exhaled inadequately, which can lead to an excess of carbon dioxide (hypercapnia) remaining in the lungs. The turbulent flow results in inadequate gas exchange despite unchanged tidal volume (euvolemic hypoventilation) (Fig. 16.10).

Generally said, it is better to change breathing depth and not respiratory rate. The expiration should be longer than the inspiration. The flow resistance on inspiration is lower than on expiration, as the airway calibre during inspiration is increased compared to the one during expiration. Pathological conditions can lead to an increased respiratory afford. In obstructive lung diseases, airways might be narrowed (e.g. asthma). In restrictive lung diseases, functional lung tissue is reduced. Both lead to a reduced absorption of oxygen. The oxygen utilisation seems to depend on environment (in or out the water) and personal fitness.

16.6 Pressure: Volume Correlation of the Lung and Thorax

Elastic connective tissue and surface tension of alveoli force the lung to contract. Alveoli would shrink like an emptying balloon. However, the alveolar walls are lined with a

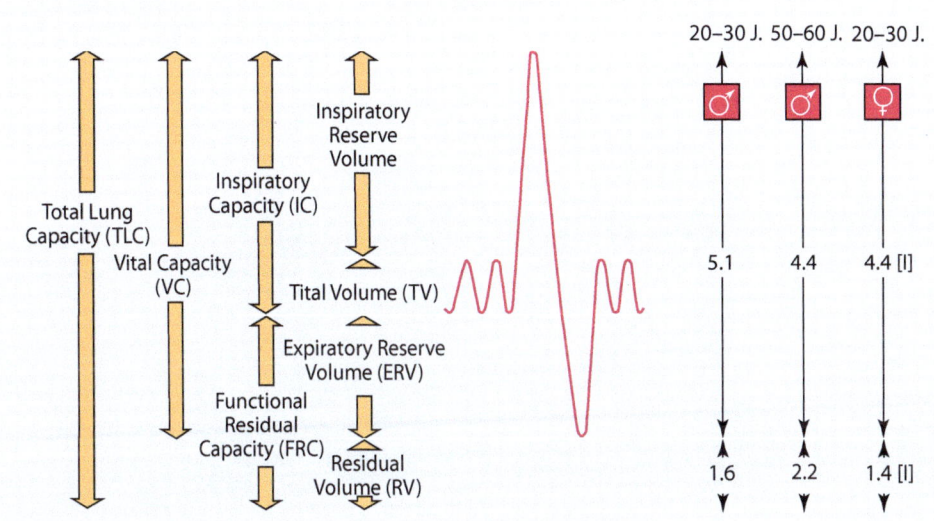

☐ **Fig. 16.10**   Lung volume and capacity. (From Schmidt 2010 [2])

surfactant, which reduces surface tension. Also, adhesion force of the lung and pleura prevent the lung to collapse. For gas exchange, it is necessary that carbon dioxide-rich air is transported out and oxygen-rich air into the lung. The supporting mechanism for this is the changing pressure within the lungs. After normal exhalation, the lung and thorax are in a resting end-expiratory position. The resting end-expiratory position represents a steady state in which forces of expansion of the thorax and adhesion forces of the lung are neutralised. The pressure in the lung (intrathoracic) equals the external pressure (extra-thoracic). During inhalation a negative intrapulmonary pressure (approx. -25 mbar) develops with expansion of the chest wall and diaphragm. As a result air is sucked into the lungs. On exhalation this mechanism is reverse. Increased interpulmonary pressure of approximately 40 mbar is created, which forces the air out.

On exhalation three different mechanisms limit airflow [3]. The first 25% are driven by respiratory muscles and are dependent on the generated force. The following 50% are independent of the effort but limited by the airway walls in regard to laminar and turbulent airflow. Here, the airflow is inversely related to the square root of the gas density. When exhaling the last 25% small airways start to collapse as the pleural pressure exceeds the intrapulmonary pressure of some of the small airways. The main factor in this phase is related to the viscosity of the gas and not to its density (☐ Fig. 16.11).

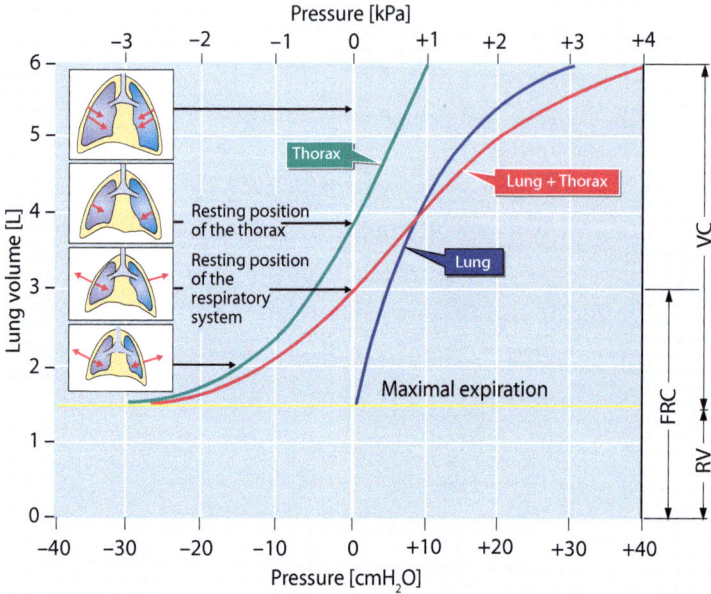

◘ Fig. 16.11 Pressure-volume correlation of lung and thorax. (From Schmidt 2010 [2])

References

1. Guellich A, Krueger M. Sport: Berlin: Springer; 2013.
2. Schmidt RF, Lang F, Heckmann M. Physiologie des Menschen. 31st. ed. Berlin: Springer; 2010.
3. Segadal K, Gulsvik A, Nicolaysen G. Respiratory changes with deep diving. Eur Respir J. 1990;3:101–8.

Suggested Reading

Arthurs GJ, Sudhakar M. Carbon diaoxid transport. Contin Educ Anaesth Crit Care Pain. 2005;5(6):207–11.

Geers C, Gros G. Carbon dioxide transport and carbonic anhydrases in blood and muscle. Physiol Rev. 2000;80(2):681–715.
Moll KJ, Moll M. Anatomie. 18th ed. München: Elsevier; 2006.
Silbernagel S, Despopuluos A. Taschenatlas der Physiologie. 7th ed. Stuttgart: Thieme; 2007.
West JB. Respiratory physiology. 5th ed: Williams & Baltimore: Wilkins; 1995.
Zilles K, Tillmann BN. Anatomie: Berlin: Springer; 2010.

Nervous System

© Springer International Publishing AG, part of Springer Nature 2018
O. Rusoke-Dierich, *Diving Medicine*, https://doi.org/10.1007/978-3-319-73836-9_17

To adapt to new conditions, the body must constantly be in communication with its environment. Stimuli are absorbed and emitted. Movements have to be targeted and coordinated. Reflexes and essential life processes such as breathing, heart activity or digestion need to be continuously adjusted according to their demand. For all these processes internal and external stimuli are sensed via receptors, transmitted to the brain via neural pathways, processed and again redirected to the effector organs. Failure in each single part of the nervous system usually causes significant malfunction, mainly manifested by disturbed sensory perception (pain, temperature, sensitivity), paralysis, poor coordination or inability to speak properly.

17.1 Nerve Cells

Nerve cells (neurons) are the structural and functional unit of the nervous system. It consists of a cell body (soma), dendrites and axons. Signals from other cells are received by dendrites and transmitted via axons to other nerves, glands or muscle cells. The axon itself distributes several branches. While the so-called collaterals only cover short distances, axons themselves can be up to 1 meter long. The junctions between nerve cells are called synapses. At the synapses electrical signals are converted into chemical ones. Some synapses in the CNS are electronic synapses, which electronically transmit the signals via gap junctions. A synaptic unit consists of the axon terminal, presynaptic membrane, synaptic cleft, postsynaptic membrane and the dendritic spine. Via the synaptic cleft, the signal is passed on to the postsynaptic membrane of another neuron. Most of the transmissions are chemically with carrier substances such as acetylcholine, glutamate, norepinephrine, GABA, etc. (◘ Figs. 17.1, 17.2, 17.3, and 17.4).

Cholinergic synapses with acetylcholine as transmitter substance are an example for typical synapses. The stimulation of an axon terminal results in Ca^{2+}-influx. That again leads to an emptying of neurotransmitters filled vesicles into the synaptic cleft. Neurotransmitters reaching the receptors of the postsynaptic membrane cause Na^+ influx and thus trigger a reaction. Then the neurotransmitter is immediately split into its components again and reabsorbed in the axon terminal. Therefore, the response at the postsynaptic membrane is time-limited. Synapses are distinguished in excitatory and inhibitory synapses. Each cell has about up to 10,000 synaptic inputs. Activation of excitatory synapses causes an increase of the electric potential of cells (excitatory postsynaptic potential = EPSP) and activation of inhibitory synapses to a reduction (inhibitory postsynaptic potential = IPSP). All these activations sum up, and depending on which of the two will dominate, there is an action potential, if the threshold is exceeded. Transmission speed of nerve cells is dependent on type and diameter of the individual nerve fibre. In the peripheral nervous system, axons are covered with lipid-containing Schwann cells. These form myelin sheaths in concentric layers around axons. The myelin sheaths are interrupted about every 1.5 mm at the Ranvier's node. Nerve signals are therefore not continually transmitted. They "jump" from one Ranvier's node to the other. This transmission is called saltatory transmission. Schwann cells increase the transmission speed and due to its insulating effect enable transmissions over longer distances with only little loss of energy. The equivalent in the CNS to the axons with Schwann cells of the peripheral nervous system are the oligodendrocytes. Neurons themselves are "adaptive". Through creation of new excitatory and inhibitory synapses, signal transmission can be increased or decreased according to its demands.

■ **Fig. 17.1** Neuron
(From Zilles and
Tillmann 2010 [3])

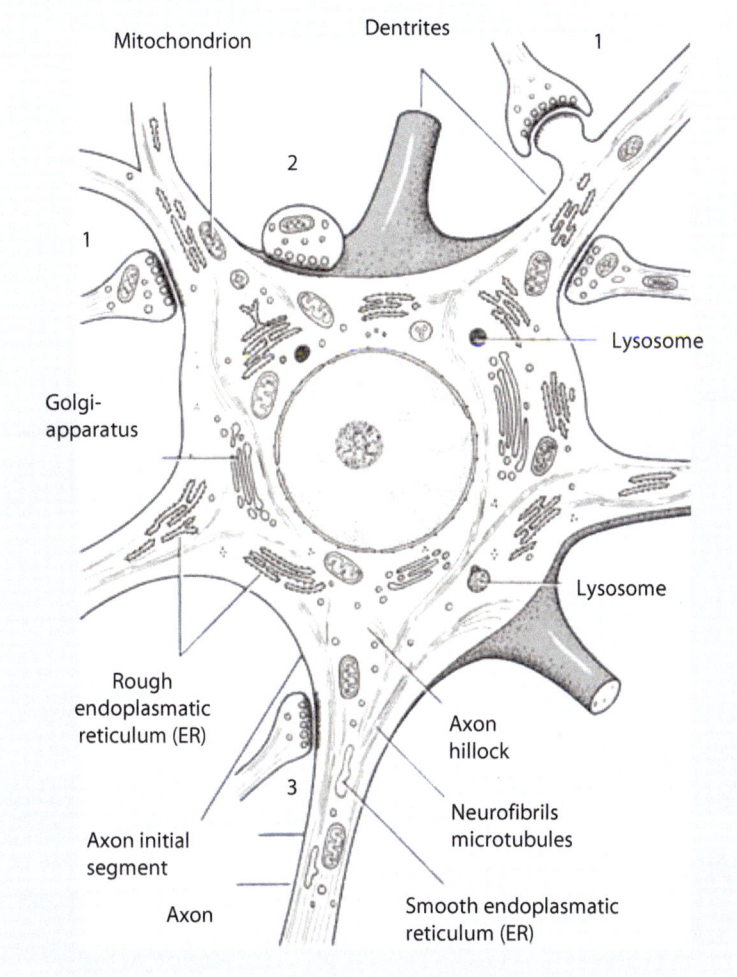

Mitochondrion

Dentrites

1

2

1

Lysosome

Golgi-
apparatus

Lysosome

Rough
endoplasmatic
reticulum (ER)

Axon
hillock

3

Neurofibrils
microtubules

Axon initial
segment

Axon

Smooth endoplasmatic
reticulum (ER)

17.2 Resting Membrane Potential/ Action Potential

Between the inside and outside of cell membranes, there is an electrical potential difference. The electrical disbalance is caused by uneven ion distribution between intra - and extracellular fluid (ICF and ECF). Depending on cell types of muscle and nerve cells, it varies between 50 and 100 mV. Hereby, intracellular fluid is negatively charged. To help maintain electrical disbalance, ions are transported actively or passively through cell membranes. $Na^+ - K^+ -$ pumps can be mainly held responsible for this (■ Table 17.1). There is a continuous flow of $Na^+ -$ ions out of cells and $K^+ -$ ions into cells. The ratio of Na^+ for K^+ in $Na^+ - K^+ -$ pumps is 3:2. This enables ions to be transported against their chemical gradient. Passive transport of ions is promoted by

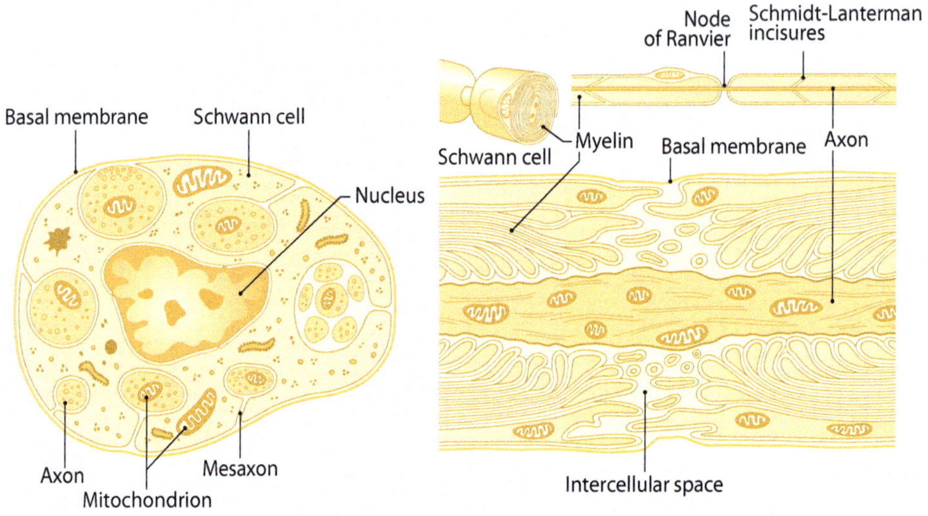

Node   Schmidt-Lanterman
of Ranvier incisures

Basal membrane   Schwann cell

Nucleus

Myelin   Basal membrane   Axon

Schwann cell

Axon   Mesaxon

Mitochondrion

Intercellular space

■ **Fig. 17.2**   Unmyelinated and myelinated nerve fibre (From Zilles and Tillmann 2010 [3])

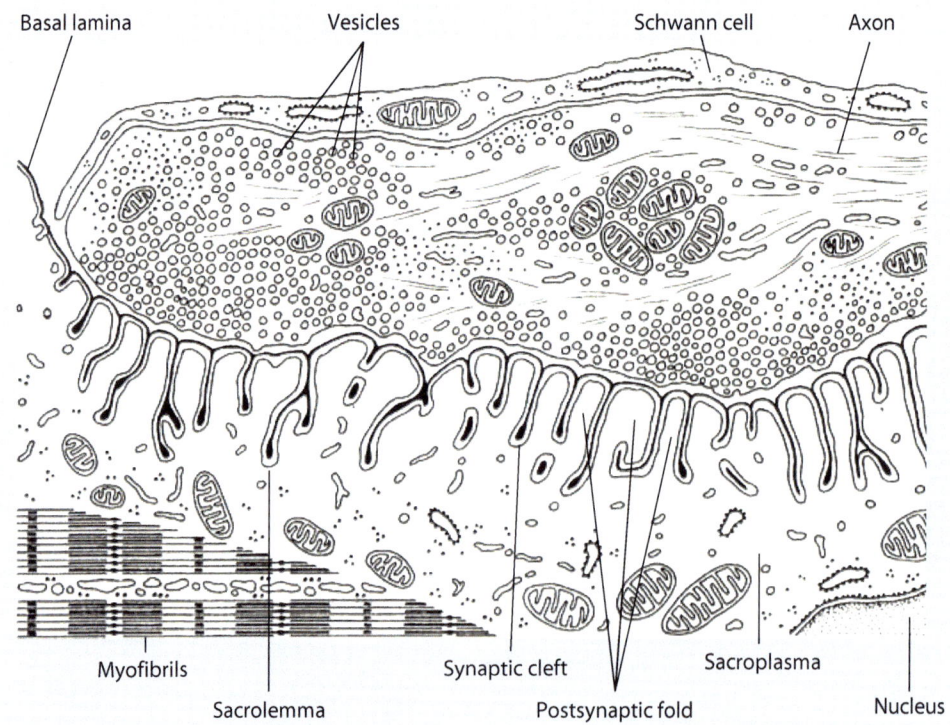

Basal lamina   Vesicles   Schwann cell   Axon

17

Myofibrils   Synaptic cleft   Sacroplasma

Sacrolemma   Postsynaptic fold   Nucleus

■ **Fig. 17.3**   Example of a synapsis with motoric end plate (From Zilles and Tillmann 2010 [3])

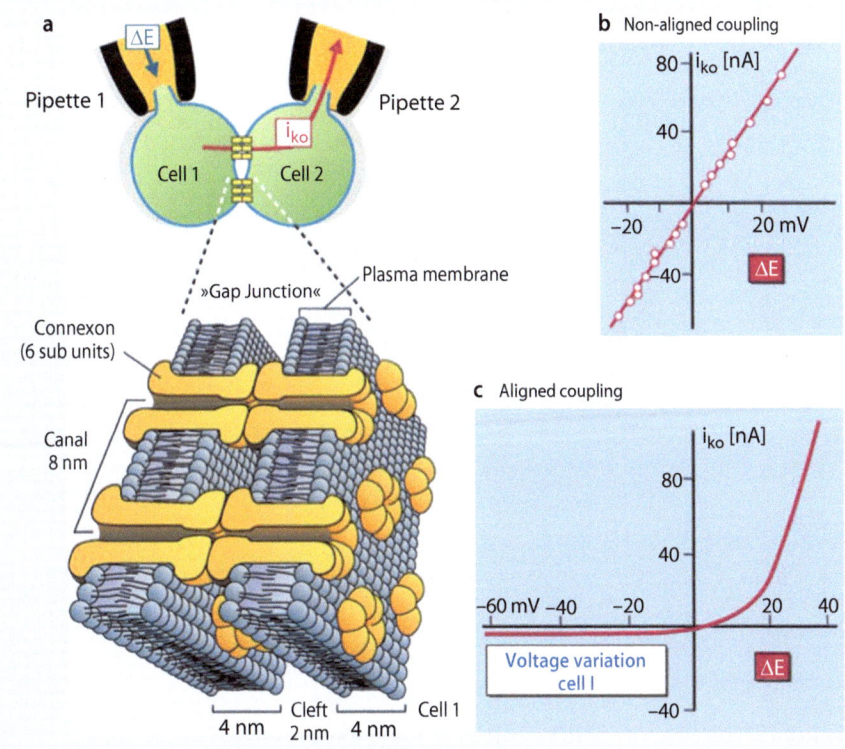

Fig. 17.4 **a** Electrical synapsis, **b** non-alligned coupling, **c** alligned coupling (From Schmidt 2010 [2])

Table 17.1 Ion concentration in extracellular fluid (ECF) and intracellular fluid (ICF) of skeletal muscles

Ions	ECF	ICF
Potassium (K+)	4.5	160
Sodium (NA+)	144	7
Chlorid (CL−)	114	7
Bicarbonate (HCO$_3$−)	28	10

diffusion through specific channels located in cell membranes. Ions diffuse as long to the other side until their potential on both sides is equal, as similar charged ions usually act like magnets with the same pole. They expel each other (**Fig. 17.5**).

The "+" or "−" specifies positive or negative charge of ions. If excitable cells are stimulated, ionic conductivity and thus membrane potential change. If the stimulus is strong enough, an action potential is generated. The ion concentration must exceed a certain threshold to make that happen. Once the threshold is exceeded, an action potential is followed according to the all-or-nothing principle. This results in a rapid sodium ion conductivity increase and a simultaneous potassium ion conductivity decrease. The sodium ion conductivity increase causes depolarisation. This means that the negative resting membrane potential increases towards 0. Depolarisation reaches even positive values, which is called "overshoot". At the same time the slowly increasing potassium ions are causing repolarisation. The repolarisation exceeds briefly

Fig. 17.5 Action potential and changes in sodium and potassium conductivity (From Schmidt 2010 [2])

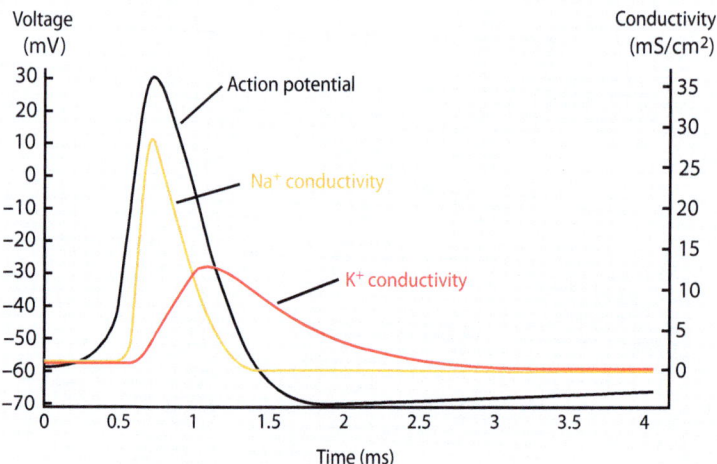

Fig. 17.6 Phases of the action potential (From Schmidt 2010 [2]) I, initiation phase; IIa + IIb, depolarisation with overshoot; III, repolarisation; IV, after-hyperpolarisation

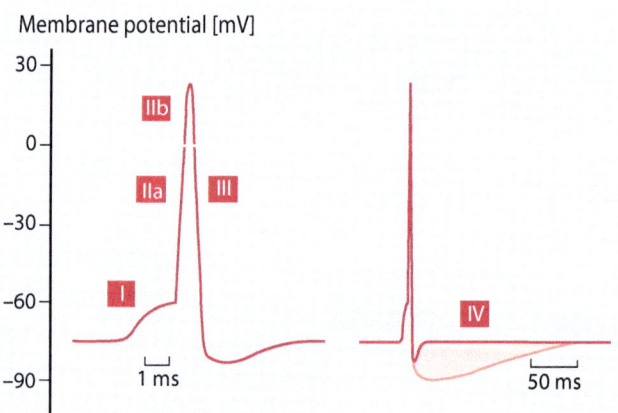

the initial level (hyperpolarisation) before settling again to the original level (**Fig. 17.6**).

Shortly after an action potential, cells can't be excited again, even not by large stimuli (absolute refractory period). Some cells can have an action potential with only low-intensity and slow increase in slope (relative refractory period) shortly after excitation. Single action potentials of different cells vary in their duration (**Table 17.2**).

Table 17.2 Refractory period

Cells	AP in ms	Absolute	Relative
Nerves	1	1	/
Skeletal muscle	10	2	/
Cardiac muscle	250	200	50

17.3 Peripheral Nervous System (PNS)

The peripheral nervous system is made up of nerve fibres, receptors and neurons. Nerves themselves are composed of a number of nerve fibres. They are divided into 12 cranial nerves and 31 spinal nerves, which are branching the further they get into the periphery. These are classified as sensitive (touch, temperature and pain sense), motor (muscle) and sensory (taste and smell) nerve cells. Stimuli are mediated by receptors from the periphery. They then get transmitted to the central nervous system (CNS). There, information is processed and sent back to individual organs. Nerves leading towards the CNS are called afferent pathways (sensory and sensitive pathways). Nerves leading from the CNS are called efferent pathways (motor pathways).

17.4 Central Nervous System (CNS)

The central nervous system includes the brain and spinal cord. The brain can roughly be divided into telencephalon, diencephalon, mesencephalon and rhombencephalon. A grey and white substance is present in the entire central nervous system. The grey substance consists mainly of cell bodies. The white matter consists mainly of myelin sheath containing nerve fibres. Axons, which transmit information between cells, are within the white matter. The CNS is responsible for the coordination of movements, the hormonal regulation, control of emotions, thinking and the learning processes (via the limbic system) and maintaining vital functions such as breathing, heart rate and temperature regulation. All parts of the brain are directly or indirectly connected (🔵 Figs. 17.7 and 17.8).

17.4.1 Telencephalon

The telencephalon consists of cerebrum, telencephalon nuclei and rhinencephalon, the oldest part of the brain. It represents the largest portion of the brain with over 85% of the volume and is divided into two hemispheres, which are connected by the corpus callosum. Centres, which are responsible for specific functions, are located in different areas of the cerebral cortex. It is mainly responsible for motor coordination such as movement of arms and legs or muscles involved in the speaking process.

17.4.2 Diencephalon

The diencephalon is composed of thalamus, subthalamus, metathalamus, epithalamus, hypothalamus, and pineal gland. Their function consists of coordinating stimuli between afferent musculoskeletal or sensory pathways and the brain, control of the autonomic nervous system, temperature control, interface to the limbic system and regulating the hormonal system.

17.4.3 Mesencephalon

In the mesencephalon muscle movements are interconnected between optical and acoustic senses and vestibular senses. Also, important pathways of the musculoskeletal system, spinal cord, brain and pain perception are linked (pyramidal and extrapyramidal system).

17.4.4 Rhombencephalon

The rhombencephalon consists of the pons, cerebellum and medulla oblongata. Almost all cranial nerves arise from the medulla oblongata

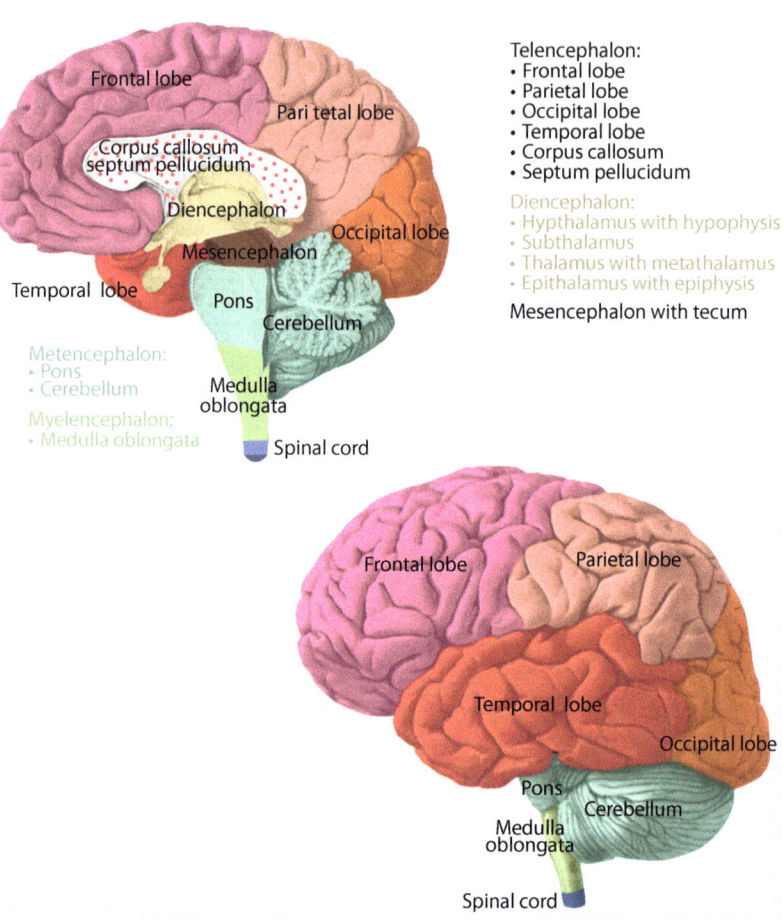

Telencephalon:
• Frontal lobe
• Parietal lobe
• Occipital lobe
• Temporal lobe
• Corpus callosum
• Septum pellucidum

Diencephalon:
• Hypthalamus with hypophysis
• Subthalamus
• Thalamus with metathalamus
• Epithalamus with epiphysis

Mesencephalon with tecum

Frontal lobe
Pari tetal lobe
Corpus callosum
septum pellucidum
Diencephalon
Occipital lobe
Mesencephalon
Temporal lobe
Pons
Cerebellum

Metencephalon:
• Pons
• Cerebellum
Myelencephalon:
• Medulla oblongata

Medulla oblongata

Spinal cord

Frontal lobe
Parietal lobe
Temporal lobe
Occipital lobe
Pons
Cerebellum
Medulla oblongata
Spinal cord

◻ **Fig. 17.7**   Brain (From Zalpour 2014 [4])

◻ **Fig. 17.8**   Cortex of a human brain (From Schmidt 2010 [2])

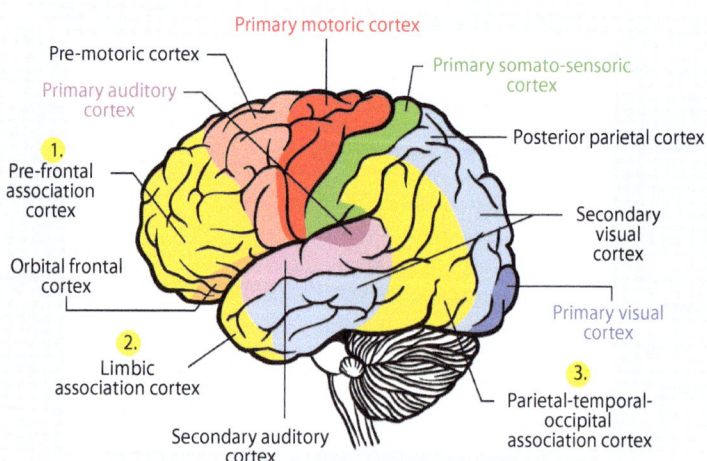

Primary motoric cortex
Pre-motoric cortex
Primary somato-sensoric cortex
Primary auditory cortex
Posterior parietal cortex
1.
Pre-frontal association cortex
Secondary visual cortex
Orbital frontal cortex
Primary visual cortex
2.
Limbic association cortex
3.
Parietal-temporal-occipital association cortex
Secondary auditory cortex

and pons. Cerebral nuclei of the medulla oblongata and pons are an interface between the cerebrum, cerebellum and spinal cord. There are also a number of centres included in this area, which are necessary for regulation of vital functions, such as respiration, heartbeat, blood pressure and digestion. The medulla oblongata and pons are also described as midbrain. The cerebellum is mainly responsible for the fine motor skills.

17.4.5 Spinal Cord

The spinal cord is located in the spinal canal of the spine. It is approx. 40–50 cm long and about 1–1.5 cm in diameter. It is divided into cervical, thoracic, lumbar and sacral cord. However, the subdivision of the spinal cord doesn't necessarily correspond to the actual location of each spinal section. Except the first spinal nerve, all others exit below the corresponding vertebrae. It contains motor and sensory nerve fibres going to and from all body parts. The spinal cord is sheeted with the same three layers (pia, arachnoid and dura) similar to the brain.

The spine consists of 24 vertebral bodies:
- 7 cervical vertebrae
- 12 thoracic vertebrae
- 5 lumbar vertebrae
- Sacrum
- Coccyx (◼ Fig. 17.9)

Structure of a spinal vertebra:
- Vertebral body (carries the body weight)
- Neural arch (surrounding the spinal cord)
- Spinous and transverse process (point of attachment for the spinal muscles)
- Spinal canal (opening for the spinal cord)
- Intervertebral foramen (entry and exit of nerves and blood vessels) (◼ Fig. 17.10)

Each of the 31 spinal nerves emerges from the spinal cord on both sides. The spinal nerves are entry and exit pathways of sensitive, motor and vegetative nerves. In a cross section through the spinal cord, the butterfly-shaped grey matter in the centre and the white matter in its surrounding are visible. The white matter contains predominantly nerve fibres with myelin sheaths as extensions of neurons.

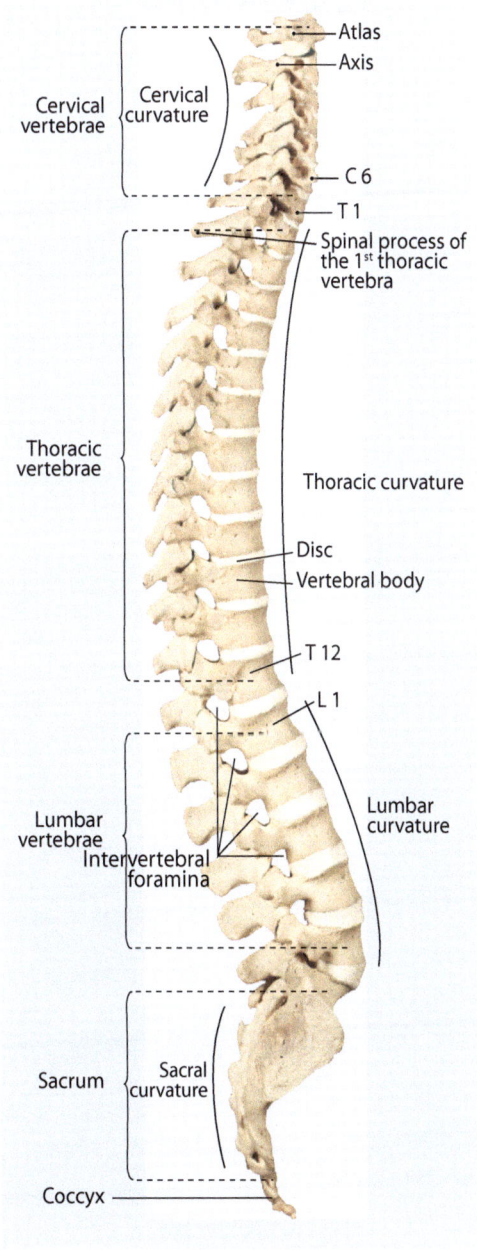

◼ **Fig. 17.9**   Spine (From Zilles and Tillmann 2010 [3])

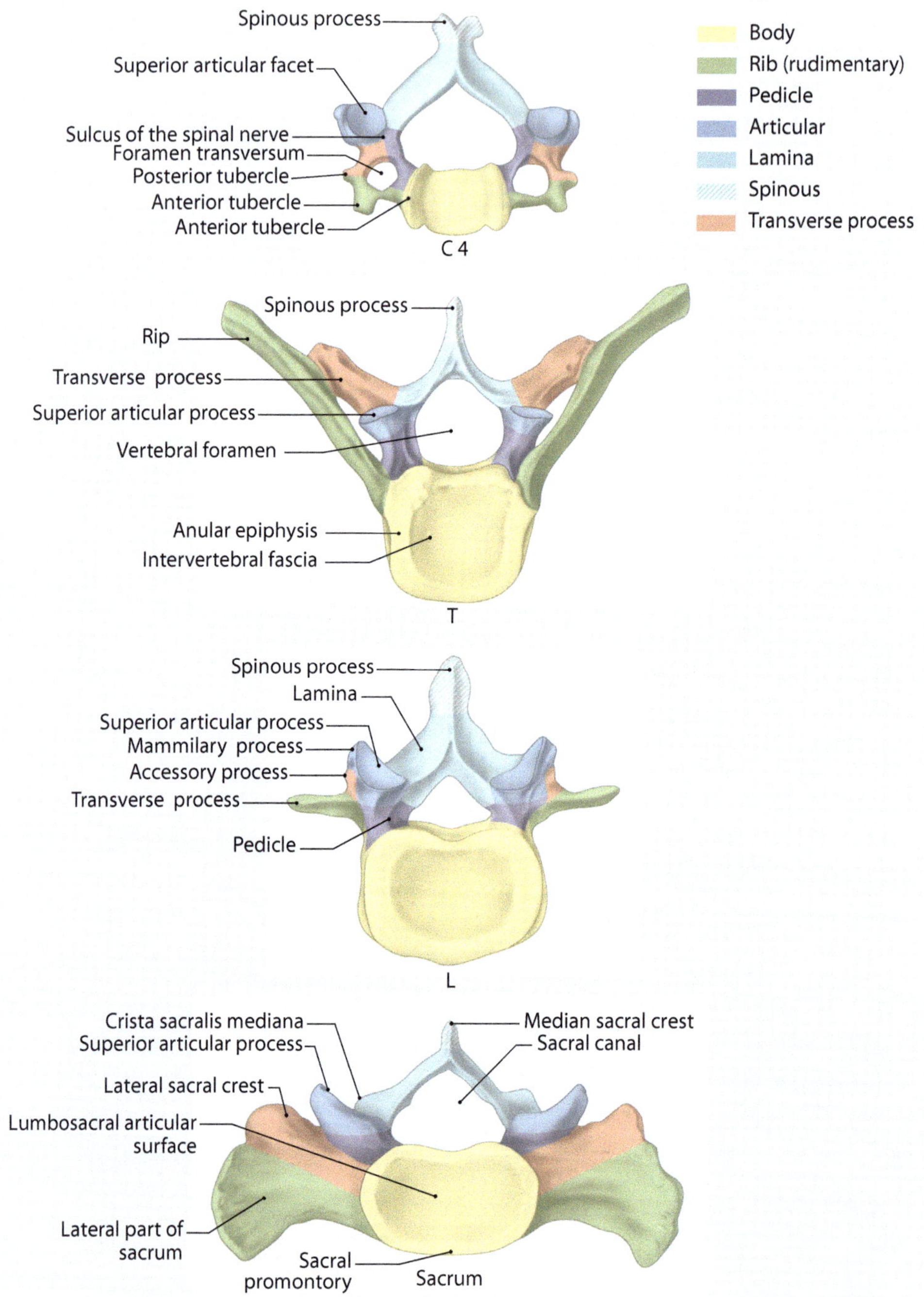

Spinous process

Superior articular facet

Sulcus of the spinal nerve
Foramen transversum
Posterior tubercle
Anterior tubercle
Anterior tubercle

C 4

Body
Rib (rudimentary)
Pedicle
Articular
Lamina
Spinous
Transverse process

Spinous process

Rip

Transverse process

Superior articular process

Vertebral foramen

Anular epiphysis
Intervertebral fascia

T

Spinous process
Lamina
Superior articular process
Mammilary process
Accessory process
Transverse process

Pedicle

L

Crista sacralis mediana
Superior articular process

Lateral sacral crest

Lumbosacral articular
surface

Lateral part of
sacrum
Sacral
promontory
Sacrum

Median sacral crest
Sacral canal

17

🔲 **Fig. 17.10**   Spinal vertebra (From Zilles and Tillmann 2010 [3])

The white matter is divided into:

— *Ventral column*
— *Dorsal column*
— *Lateral column*

The grey matter contains:

— *Ventral horn*
— *Dorsal horn*
— *Intermediate substance (lateral horn)*
   (■ Fig. 17.11)

Ascending (afferent) pathways are mainly in the dorsal column but also to an extent in the ventral and lateral column of the white matter. Descending (efferent) pathways are only in the ventral and lateral column of the white matter. The grey matter is mainly composed of Golgi type I and Golgi type II nerve cells. The long Golgi type I nerve cells enter into the ventral spinal roots or the fibre tracts of the white matter. The short Golgi type II nerve cells remain within the grey matter. They are divided in three categories: root cells, column or tract cells and the propriospinal cells. The root cells are located in the ventral and lateral horn either feed skeletal muscles or build the preganglionic autonomic axons. The column and tract cells and their processes are mainly located in the dorsal horn and are entirely confined within the CNS. They receive their information from the root ganglia. The root ganglia are collections of sensory afferent nerve cell bodies of the periphery (with exemption of the head). They mainly end in the brain stem, cerebellum or diencephalon. The propriospinal cells are interspinal neurons confined in the spinal cord. They count up to 90% of all cells in the spinal cord. The interneurons have mainly efferent motor function. The grey substance itself is divided into ventral, dorsal and intermediate substance. The thoracic vertebra and partially the lumbar vertebrae have also a lateral horn as a part of the intermediate substance. In the dorsal horn are mainly sensory nuclei that receive and process incoming sensorimotor information.

■ **Fig. 17.11** Cross section of the spinal cord at different levels (From Schmidt 2010 [2])

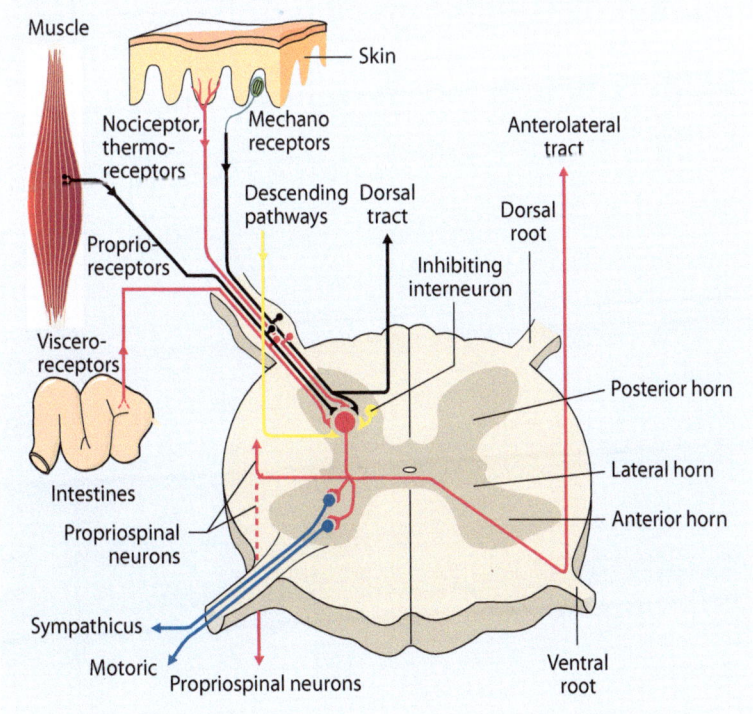

They forward information to the midbrain and diencephalon via emerging ascending pathways. Pyramidal and extrapyramidal pathways innervating skeletal muscles end in the ventral horn. The lateral horn and intermediate substance are neurons of the autonomic nervous system innervating visceral and pelvic organs (◻ Fig. 17.12).

Different parts of the body receive nerves of corresponding segments of the spinal cord.

For example, nerves of the legs arise from the lumbar and sacral level and nerves of the arms from the cervical level. If any damage or disorder of the spinal cord is present, body functions below that level are affected. One-sided damages of the spinal cord cause loss of motor function on the same side of the body and loss of sensitivity on the opposite side (Brown-Séquard syndrome) (◻ Fig. 17.13).

Arterial blood supply of the spinal cord arises mainly from the anterior spinal artery and the two posterior spinal arteries. In the upper parts of the spinal cord, they are derived from the vertebral artery and the posterior cerebellar arteries or from the subclavian artery

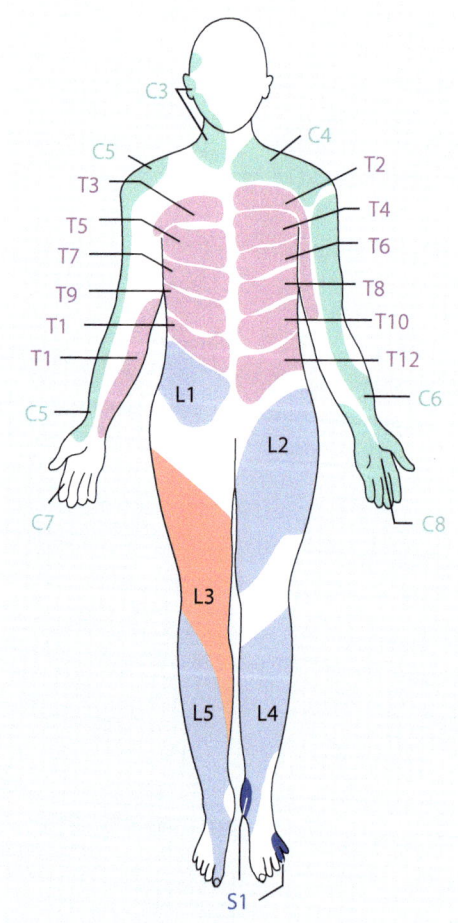

◻ **Fig. 17.12**   Pyramidal tract (From Schmidt 2010 [2])

◻ **Fig. 17.13**   Dermatome (From Schmidt 2010 [2])

via the cervical radicular arteries. The posterior spinal arteries are paired posteriorly of the spinal cord arising from the posterior inferior cerebellar arteries. At the level of the foramen magnum, two branches of the vertebral arteries form a single anterior spinal artery, which lies in the anterior median fissure. The upper thoracic spine gets its supply from the anterior and posterior thoracic radicular artery via the posterior intercostal arteries, which are arising from the aorta. In the lower parts, they get their supply from the anterior and posterior radicular arteries, also via the posterior intercostal arteries out of the aorta. One major branch of the anterior radicular artery is the artery of Adamkiewicz. This artery arises usually at the T9–T11 level but can range from T7 to L4. At a high uptake of the artery of Adamkiewicz, the blood of the lower spinal cord is supplied by the iliac arteries. Along the spinal cord the anterior and posterior spinal arteries form an anastomotic chain around the spinal cord the so-called vasocorona or pial plexus. The vasocorona supplies the periphery of the spinal cord. From the anterior spinal artery, the sulcal arteries branch off to supply the majority of the spinal cord's inside (◘ Figs. 17.14 and 17.15).

Venous blood of the spinal cord drains horizontally via the sulcal veins. The sulcal veins also have axially (vertical) and longitudinally interconnections. The part inside the spine is also referred as the intrinsic spinal venous system. The extrinsic spinal venous system is mainly located in the intradural space. But the axial interconnections in the periphery of the spinal cord also belong to the extrinsic system. After exiting the spinal cord, blood enters the longitudinal posterior and anterior spinal veins. The anterior and posterior spinal veins are interconnected and form the pial

◘ **Fig. 17.14** Arterial blood supply of spine. **a** longitudinal views, **b** cross section (From Zilles and Tillmann 2010 [3]); Ab = abdominal aorta, Aic = common iliac artery, Ara = anterior radicular artery, ArmA = great anterior radiculomedullary artery or artery of Adamkiewicz, As = subclavian artery, Asc = sulcal artery, Aspa = anterior spinal artery, Aspp = posterior spinal artery, Ath = thoracic artery, Av = vertebral artery, Ic = cervical intumescent, Ii = lumbar intumescence, Tth = thyrocervical trunk, Vc = vasocorona

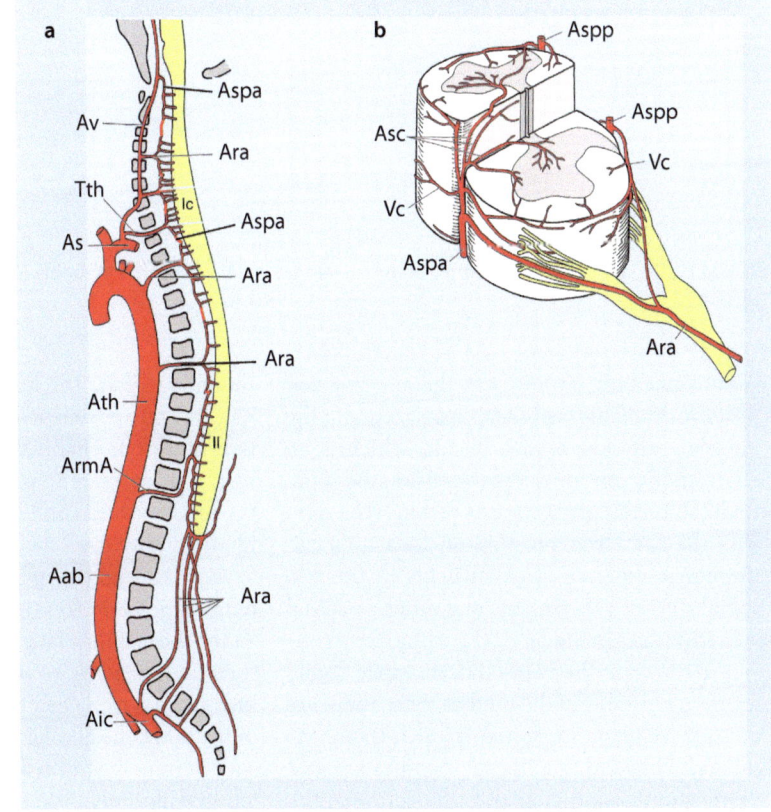

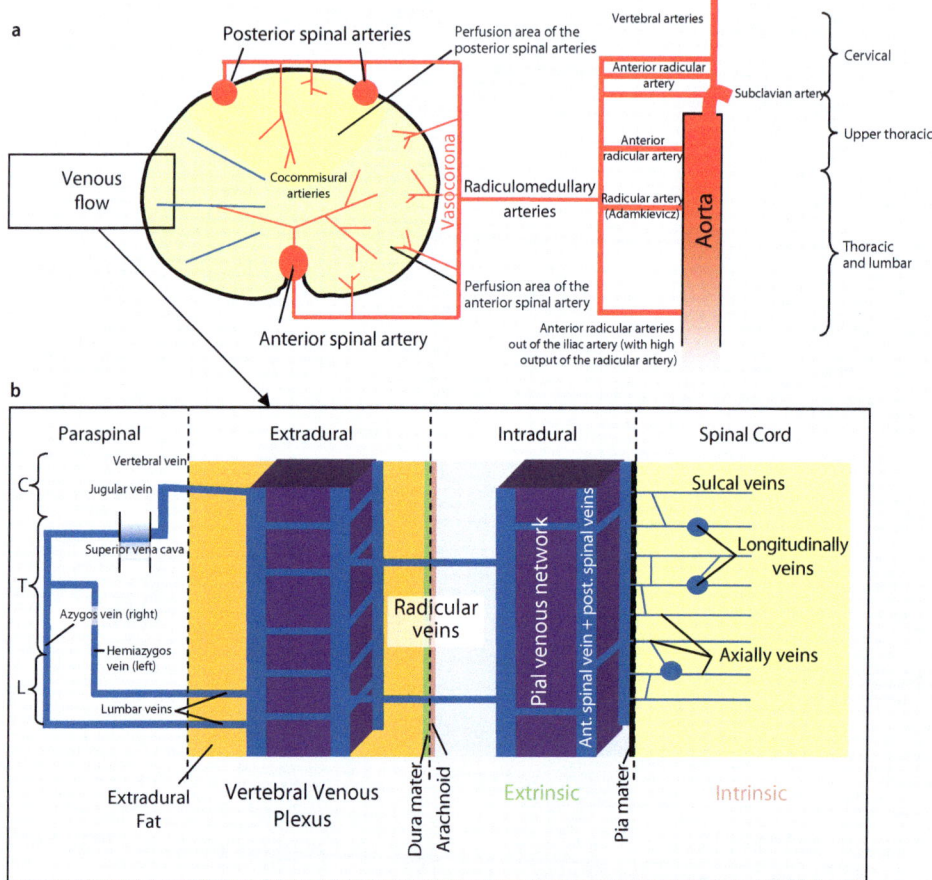

□ **Fig. 17.15** **a** Arterial blood supply of the spinal cord and **b** venous blood supply of the spinal cord in a cross section

venous network. From there the anterior and posterior radiculomedullary veins feed into the internal vertebral venous plexus, which is an anastomotic venous network outside the dura. Radiculomedullary veins exit through the dura with the nerve roots in 60% of cases. 40% exit through a separate foramen between the two spinal nerves [1]. Usually, one anterior spinal vein triplicates in the cervical area and then converges to two in the upper thoracic area, finally forming one vein in the lumbar area. There are up to three posterior spinal veins in the cervical area, converging in the cervicothoracic and thoracolumbar junction and triplicating in the

thoracic region. The lumbosacral region again has only one posterior spinal vein. The triplication of venous channels in the thoracic region results in decreased venous flow and may lead to venous stasis and engorgement [1]. The blood drains over the lumbar veins into the azygos vein (on the right side of the spine) and hemiazygos vein (on the left side of the spine). At the thoracic level the hemiazygos vein drains then into the azygos vein, which in turn drains into the inferior vena cava. In the upper part of the body, the hemiazygos vein runs as accessory hemiazygos vein and enters then into the left brachiocephalic vein. The anterior internal vertebral venous plexus communicates with the intercranial sigmoid, basilar venous sinuses, basivertebral vein, occipital vein and the azygos system. From there the blood reaches the heart over the internal jugular vein, the right brachiocephalic vein and the superior vena cava. The venous back flow is mainly triggered by the respiration.

The epidural space, where the internal vertebral plexus is located, has a high fat content. Also nerve roots in the intradural space contain a high amount of fat. The combination of poor venous flow, limited space and high fat content make this to a likely area, where spinal DCI may develop. Additionally, the venous system of the epidural space is prone to develop negative pressure, which might promote tribonucleation effects. The veins of the internal vertebral venous plexus have no valves. Hence, the distribution of the venous blood flow is dependent on the positioning of the body, the intra-abdominal and intrathoracic pressure. The venous pressure usually varies between 0.7 and 7 mmHg but could be also negative in upright position in the cranial segments.

17.5 Autonomic Nervous System

The autonomic nervous system regulates all vital functions. In general, the sympathetic nervous system is responsible for flight and fight. The parasympathetic nervous system is rather responsible for functions of relaxation and food intake. In contrast to the central nervous system, it can't be directly influenced. Pain stimuli and irritation of mechano- and chemoreceptors from the medulla oblongata, lung, vascular system, etc. are forwarded via afferent fibres to the autonomic nervous system. The reflex response to the effector cells (smooth muscle, glands and cells of the AV node of the heart) is mediated via efferent fibres. The interaction of the parasympathetic nervous system and sympathetic nervous system, by means of excitation and inhibition, establishes a balance in the body's functions. Efferent fibres of the sympathetic and parasympathetic nervous system are interconnected twice. The first interface is the ganglion. Depending on their localisation in regard to the ganglion, the fibres are called pre- or postganglionic fibres. The preganglionic fibres arise from the corresponding vegetative centre of the CNS. Via specific mediators the information is transferred from the preganglionic to the postganglionic membrane of the synapsis. The second interface is at the effector organ (◘ Figs. 17.16 and 17.17).

The synaptic transmission is adrenergic (adrenaline and noradrenaline) or cholinergic (acetylcholine). There are two different types of acetylcholine receptors (nicotinic and muscarinic). Both respond to acetylcholine. The nicotinic receptors respond also to nicotine, e.g. of cigarettes, the muscarinic receptors to muscarine, e.g. of a poisonous mushroom. The adrenergic receptors have alpha-receptors (α_1 and α_2) and beta-receptors (β_1 and β_2). Both respond to adrenergic substances (epinephrine and norepinephrine). They differ in their effects on effector organs or cells and are either exciting or inhibiting. Centres of the sympathetic nervous system are located in the thoracic and lumbar mark. The preganglionic fibres end on the chain ganglia, right next to the spine. There, the signal transmission is mediated with acetylcholine. The postganglionic fibres reach the effector organs and the transmission there is mediated adrenergic. Alpha-receptors are generally inhibitory and the beta fibres generally excitatory to the effector organs/cells. The ratio of preganglionic to postganglionic fibres is 1–20. Autonomic centres of the parasympathetic nervous system are located in the brain stem and the sacrum. The preganglionic fibres end up close to the effector organs and the mediator is acetylcholine. The ratio of preganglionic to postganglionic fibres is 1–1. An important parasympathetic nerve is the vagal nerve. He has inhibitory affects to the heart rate. The vagal nerve has also influence on the larynx, trachea, kidney, spleen, liver and parts of the gastrointestinal tract.

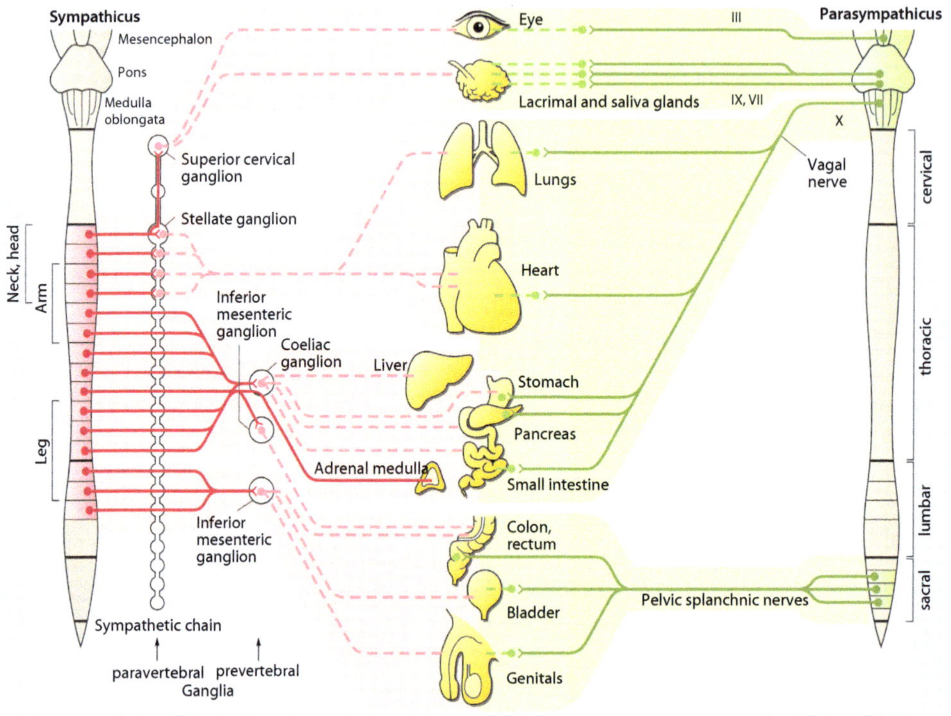

Sympathicus
Mesencephalon
Pons
Medulla
oblongata

Superior cervical
ganglion

Stellate ganglion

Neck, head
Arm

Inferior
mesenteric
ganglion
Coeliac
ganglion

Leg

Adrenal medulla

Inferior
mesenteric
ganglion

Sympathetic chain

paravertebral   prevertebral
Ganglia

Eye
III
Parasympathicus

Lacrimal and saliva glands   IX, VII
X

Lungs   Vagal
nerve

Heart

Liver

Stomach

Pancreas

Small intestine

Colon,
rectum

Pelvic splanchnic nerves

Bladder

Genitals

cervical
thoracic
lumbar
sacral

□ **Fig. 17.16**   Overview of the sympathetic and parasympathetic nervous system (From Schmidt 2010 [2])

□ **Fig. 17.17**   Transmitters
and receptors in the autonomic
nervous system (From Schmidt
2010 [2])

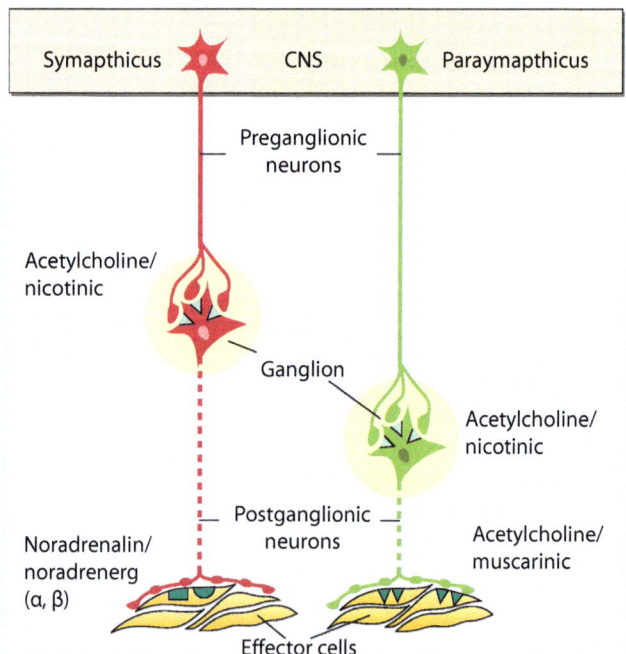

Symapthicus   CNS   Paraymapthicus

Preganglionic
neurons

Acetylcholine/
nicotinic

Ganglion

Acetylcholine/
nicotinic

Noradrenalin/
noradrenerg
(α, β)

Postganglionic
neurons

Acetylcholine/
muscarinic

Effector cells

References

1. Griessenauer CJ, Raborn J, Foreman P, Shoja MM, Loukas M, Tubbs RS. Venous drainage of the spine and spinal cord: a comprehensive review of its history, embryology, anatomy, physiology, and pathology; Wiley Online Library. Clin Anat 2015;28:75–87.
2. Schmidt RF, Lang F, Heckmann M. Physiologie des Menschen. 31st ed. Berlin: Springer; 2010.
3. Zilles K, Tillmann BN. Anatomie. Berlin: Springer; 2010.
4. Zalpour C. Springer Lexikon Physiotherapie. 2nd ed. Berlin: Springer; 2014.

Suggested Reading

Anaesthesia UK; spinal cord. www.frca.co.uk/article.aspx?articleid=100360. Accessed 30 Jan 2016.

Moll KJ, Moll M. Anatomie. 18th ed. München: Elsevier; 2006.

Silbernagel S, Despopuluos A. Taschenatlas der Physiologie. 7th ed. Stuttgart: Thieme; 2007.

Sensory Organs

© Springer International Publishing AG, part of Springer Nature 2018
O. Rusoke-Dierich, *Diving Medicine*, https://doi.org/10.1007/978-3-319-73836-9_18

Sensory organs are responsible for receiving information from the environment. External stimuli activate receptors and transmit the information via nerves to the brain. All information will be processed and coordinated, so that a useful response is generated. Hence, sensory organs are an important connection to the environment.

18.1 Eyes

The eye is the organ of visual perception. Light entering the eyes, passes through cornea, anterior chamber, lens and orbital body before it hits the receptors of the retina on the back of the orbita. Eyes need to be lubricated. Lacrimal fluid is produced in the lacrimal glands, which are on the lateral side of the eyelid. In the area of the eyelashes, tarsal glands produce oily substances. Together the lacrimal fluid and the oily substances form a protective layer. The fluid runs off into the lacrimal duct, which is located on the medial side of the eye and drains into the nasal cavity. The retina covers the back of the orbita. There are two types of receptors,

rods and cones. Rods are responsible for black-and-white vision and hence for light perception. Cones are responsible for colour perception. The point of the best vision is the fovea centralis. In this area there are almost only cones. The blind spot, where the optic nerve passes through, has no receptors at all (◘ Fig. 18.1).

The eye is able to adapt to brightness and distance of objects. To adapt to changing distances from objects, the curvature of lenses can be changed by ciliary muscles. By changing the curvature, the refraction changes and hence vision can be adjusted and focused (◘ Fig. 18.2).

With dilatation and constriction of the pupil, the eye can adopt to different brightness. The receptors themselves can adapt to brightness too, but that is rather a slow process, and the maximum of adaptation is achieved after 30 min. The vision underwater is blurred as the eye is not used to the different refraction underwater. By using a diving mask, the normal medium air is reinstated to allow clear vision. However, due to the series of several mediums, water and air, subjects appear 1/3 bigger and 1/4 closer as they are (◘ Fig. 18.3).

◘ **Fig. 18.1** Anatomy of the eye and refraction. (From Schmidt 2010 [1]) G, object; L, lens; B, inverted image; α, visual angle; g, object distance; b, image distance

18

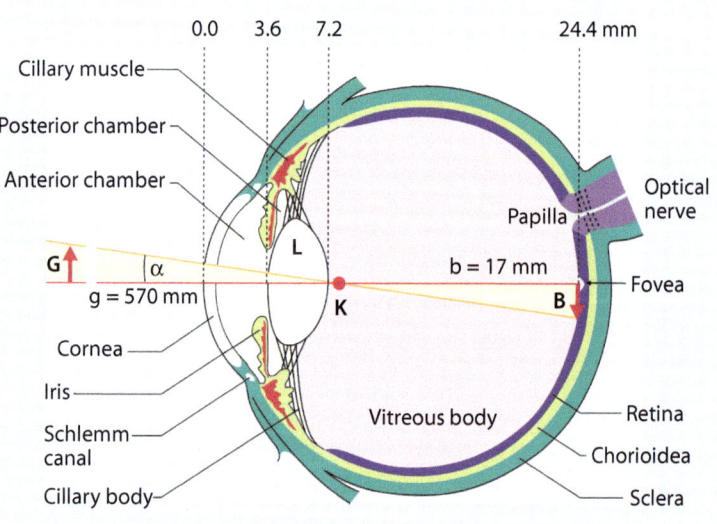

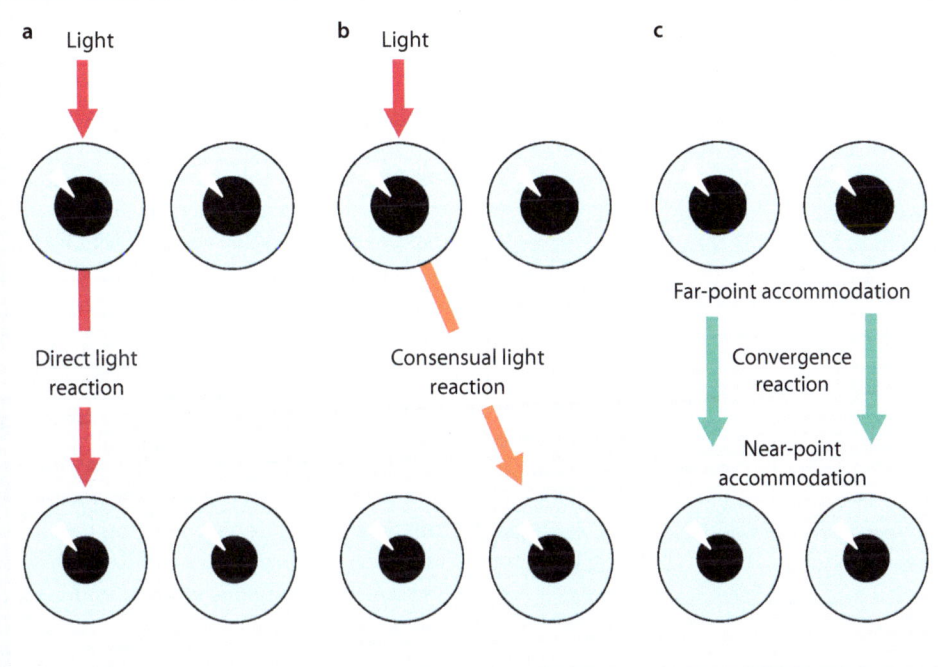

🔹 **Fig. 18.2** Reaction of the pupils. **a** direct light reaction, **b** consensual light reaction, **c** convergence reaction (From Schmidt 2010 [1])

🔹 **Fig. 18.3** Light adaptation of the human eye. (Form Schmidt 2010 [1])
a and **b**, curve of the normal mean value (red, cone; yellow, rod); **a** and **c**, curve of normal dark adaptation; **d** and **b**, curve of dark adaptation of a patient with complete monochromasy

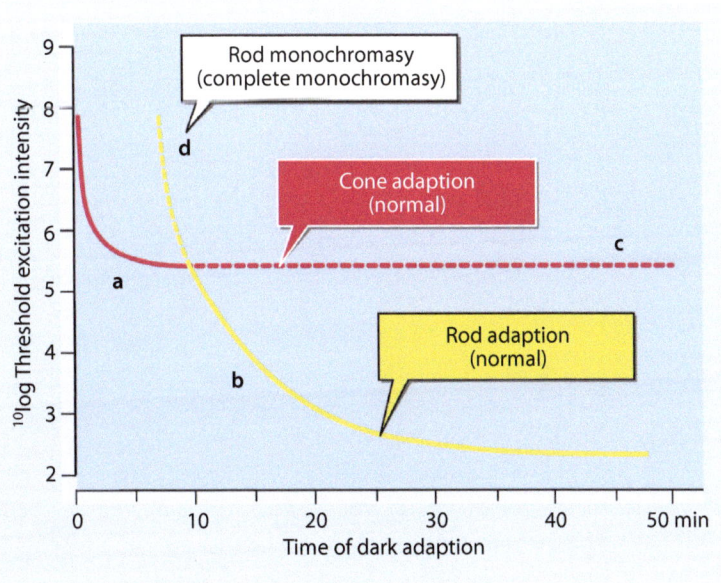

18.2 **Ears**

Ears have two functions, sound reception and keeping balance. The ear is subdivided into outer ear, middle ear and inner ear. The outer ear consists of auricles and ear tubes. The skin of the ear canal produces an oily substance for its protection, which we know as ear wax. With the help of hair inside the ear canal, the wax is transported to the outside. If too much ear wax is produced, it can occlude the ear canal. If the outer ear is occluded by wax, a perfect breeding ground for pathogens is created. If the ear canal is completely occluded by ear wax, barotrauma during the descent may occur during diving, as vacuum may develop. The tympanic membrane is only 0.03–0.12 mm thick and divides the outer ear from the middle ear. Located in the air filled middle ear, ossicles transmit the sound from the tympanic membrane to the oval window of the cochlea. In the lower part of the middle ear, the Eustachian tube connects the ear with the nasopharynx. The entire tube has a mucous membrane. The shorter part, close to the ear, is embedded in bone. The larger cartilaginous musculous part is close to the nasopharynx. The bony part is usually always open and can be opened arbitrarily or automatically.

Sound enters the auricles and ear canal and hits the tympanic membrane. The vibration of the tympanic membrane is transmitted to the ossicles, which again transmit that vibration to the oval window of the cochlea. With help of the smallest muscle of the body, the stapedius muscle, ossicles are able to amplify or reduce sound. In the cochlea the mechanical trigger is transformed into an electrical one. The vibration of the oval window causes a travelling wave in the perilymph of the scala vestibuli. The rigidity of the cochlear canal is increasing through its course. This results in shortening and increasing the amplitude of the travelling wave. Just after reaching the maximal amplitude, the travelling wave diminishes. Each frequency has a specific location in the cochlea, where its maximum appears. A change of sound intensity changes the amplitude, but doesn't affect the location of the maximal amplitude. Therefore, each frequency can be distinguished (◘ Fig. 18.4).

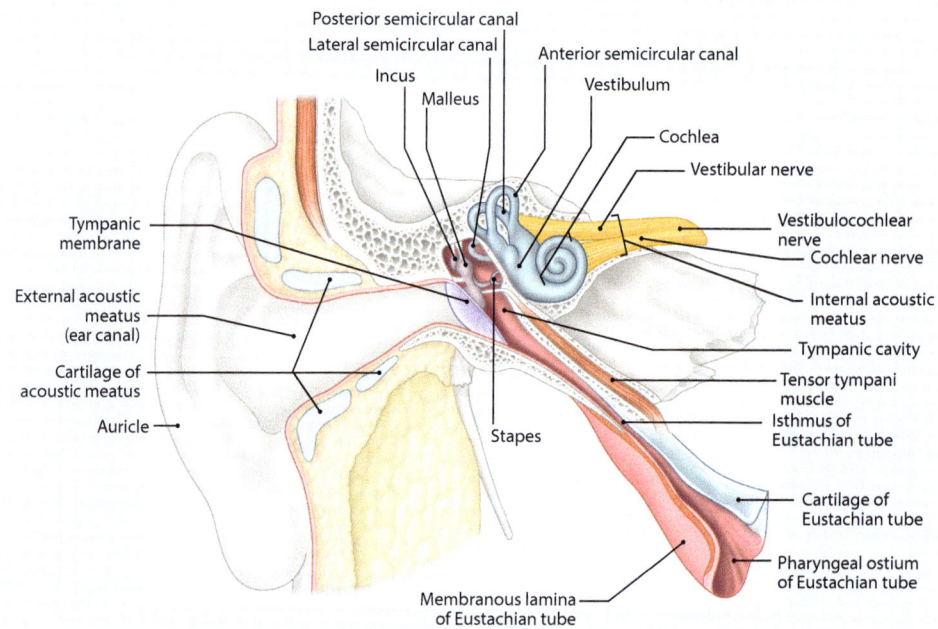

◘ **Fig. 18.4** Ear anatomy. (From Zilles and Tillmann 2010 [2])

Fig. 18.5 Travelling wave. (From Schmidt 2010 [1])

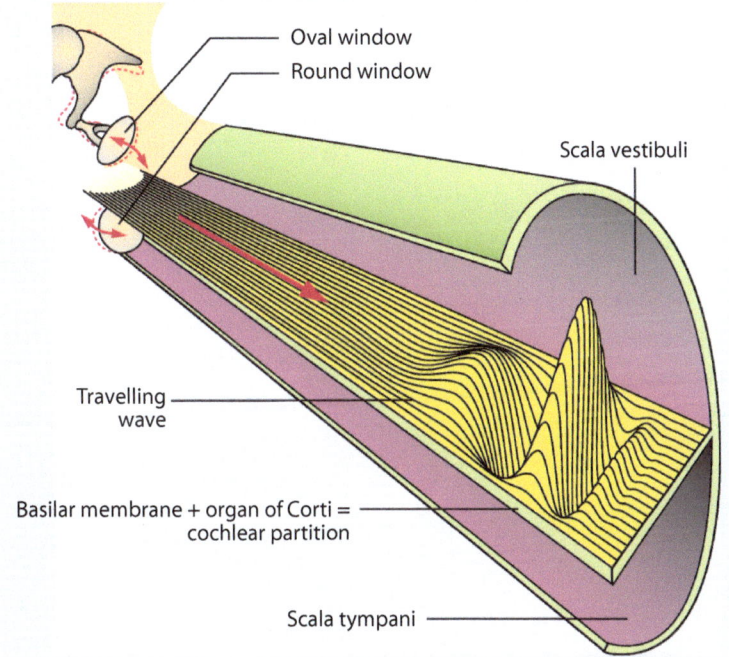

Oval window
Round window
Scala vestibuli
Travelling wave
Basilar membrane + organ of Corti = cochlear partition
Scala tympani

If sound waves reach the ear in an oblique direction, sound reaches the tympanic membrane to different times and intensity. The minimum deviation in direction, which can be recognised, is 4, which equals a time difference of 5–10 ms, of sound reaching each tympanic membrane. Underwater sound travels 4 times faster and hence sound reaches the tympanic membranes faster too. As the time difference between the both tympanic membranes becomes too short, sound can't be located. Therefore, potential hazards underwater can't be located by sound either (**□** Fig. 18.5).

The balance organ is used for orientation in space. It is located in the inner ear and consists of three semicircular canals (vertical and horizontal), containing endolymph. By the inertia of the endolymph, the change of direction causes a subtle change of the flow in the semicircular canals. This flow causes shearing of receptors in the semicircular canals. The balance organ and the eyes are connected with each other in the superior colliculi of the midbrain. Therefore, disturbances of the balance organ reduce dra-

matically the ability of visual orientation. For example, underwater, particularly at night or when diving in murky water without landmarks, orientation might become difficult. Cold water in the ear canals can lead to an irritation of the balance organ and cause acute vertigo.

18.3 Skin

The total skin surface is approx. 1.5–1.8 m². It is sensitive to tactile, pressure, vibration and pain stimuli. The skin is a barrier against mechanical, chemical and thermal damage. With 1% it is responsible for the gas exchange of the body. The epidermis is on average 0.05 mm thick. The epidermis of the heal can reach up to 1 mm. It consists of keratinising squamous epithelium, whose top layer is expelled every day. The entire epidermis is renewed within 30 days. The bottom layer of the skin is the basal layer (stratum germinativum). In this area, skin cells are produced. Increasingly, from the top layer to the deeper

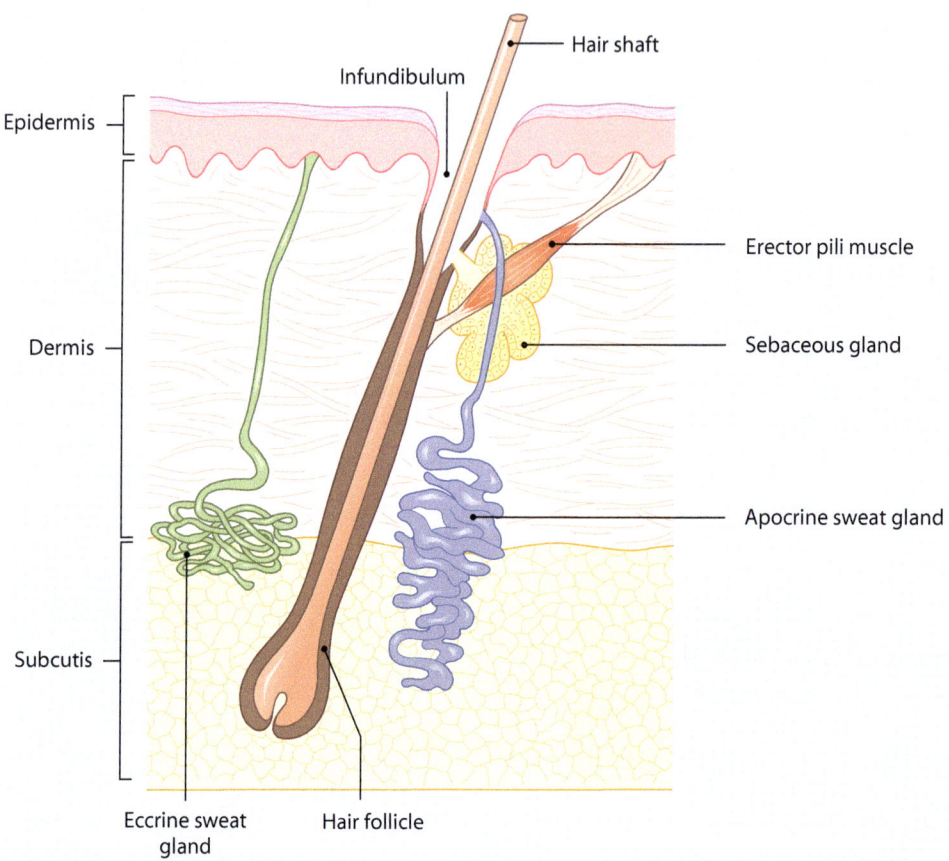

○ **Fig. 18.6**   Skin anatomy. (From Zilles and Tillmann 2010 [2])

layers of the epidermis, cells have fewer nuclei. Melanocytes are located in the basal layer. They produce melanin, the skin dye. Depending on the skin type or sun exposure, melanocytes produce their melanin. However, the number of melanocytes is independent of skin colour. The more melanin the skin has, the darker it becomes. Melanin protects the skin from UV radiation. The dermis consists of two layers, the reticular region and papillary region. The stratum has small papillary spines, which protrude into the stratum basal of the epidermis. Next to these processes, containing capillary loops, which serve skin perfusion and heat regulation, various skin receptors are found. The dermis with its connective tissue provides strengths to the skin (○ Fig. 18.6).

In addition to the protection function, the skin has other functions, like the perception of pressure, vibration and touch receptors that represent tactile perception. Thermoreceptors are responsible for the body heat regulation. There are hot and cold receptors. Their quantitative distribution is depending on the region of the body. The largest number of cold sensors is located in the facial skin. Cold receptors are activated for temperatures below 36 °C, and heat receptors are activated for temperatures above 36 °C. The maximum increase in impulse ranges between 20 and 36 °C and 36 and 43 °C. The lower or higher temperatures are, the higher is the pulse frequency of the receptors. After extreme values are exceeded, the pulse frequency decreases rapidly. In the range of 20–40 °C, the skin rapidly adapt to changing temperatures. The impulse frequency subsides, and the body's response becomes weaker.

The skin perfusion mainly is regulated by thermoreceptors. When surface temperatures are falling, cutaneous blood vessels constrict. They expand again with increasing temperature. Blood vessels of the scalp are an exception for that. Temperature-induced regulation of capillary vessels of the head remains unchanged at temperatures ranging from −28° to +32°. The inability of a temperature-induced vasoconstriction of the scalp results in significant heat loss. Approximately 30% of the body's heat loss is related to the head. Therefore, it is better to use a wetsuit with a hood, even if the water is relatively warm, to avoid excessive heat loss, in particular when diving every day. In contrast to other receptors, pain receptors can't adapt to triggers. The number of pain receptors is significantly higher compared to other receptors.

The skin has different glands to its protection or for signal transmission:

— *Sebaceous glands* (protective barrier of the skin)

— *Sweat glands* (water and electrolyte excretion, regulation of the body heat through cooling with the help of evaporation, control of the pH level of the skin)

— *Scent gland* (nonverbal signal transmission)

Continuous washing in particular with soap destroys the protective barrier of the skin and dries it out. The barrier and normal pH-levels can be altered by this, resulting in increased risk of pathogens like bacteria, viruses and fungi entering the skin and causing infections.

References

1. Schmidt RF, Lang F, Heckmann M. Physiologie des Menschen. 31st ed. Berlin: Springer; 2010.
2. Zilles K, Tillmann BN. Anatomie. Berlin: Springer; 2010.

Suggested Reading

Decraemer WF, Funnell WRJ. Anatomical and mechanical properties of the tympanic membrane: chronic otitis media. In: Pathogenisis-orientated therapeutic management. The Hague: B. Ars © Kugler Publications. p. 51–84.
Silbernagel S, Despopuluos A. Taschenatlas der Physiologie. 7th ed. Stuttgart: Thieme; 2007.
Moll KJ, Moll M. Anatomie. 18th ed. München: Elsevier; 2006.

Energy Balance

© Springer International Publishing AG, part of Springer Nature 2018
O. Rusoke-Dierich, *Diving Medicine*, https://doi.org/10.1007/978-3-319-73836-9_19

The body uses energy for all life processes. The energy is provided by nutrition like fats, proteins, carbohydrates, vitamins, trace elements, minerals as well as oxygen. Through various biochemical processes, organic materials and oxygen are converted into energy (ATP, GTP, NADH, NADPH, etc.) to be directly utilised by the body's metabolic processes. Depending on the demand, the body needs a certain amount of energy. *ATP* is a powerful energy source. Each mole of ATP releases 7.3 kcal (30.7 kJ). However, ATP stores in muscles last only for 1–2 s after onset of exercise and have to be resynthesised again after being used. As some enzymes only can use energy of ADP and inorganic phosphate (P_i) together, ATP has to be hydrolysed:

$$ATP + H_2O \xrightarrow{\text{ATPase}} ADP + P_i + \text{Energy}$$

The *phosphocreatine system* lasts a bit longer. It contributes quantitatively most and lasts for up to 10 s. It creates a buffer for short high-intensity activities. Phosphocreatine (*PCr*) and ADP produce ATP and creatinine, which then can be utilised:

$$PCr + ADP \xrightarrow{\text{creatine phosphokinase}} ATP + \text{Creatinine}$$

A smaller component for short-term energy supply is the *adenylate kinase reaction*, which converts 2 molecules of ADP into 1 AMP and 1 ATP:

$$2 ADP \xrightarrow{\text{adenlyate kinase}} 1 AMP + 1 ATP$$

A longer-lasting energy source is the anaerobic glycolysis, which lasts up to a minute and the aerobic glycolysis up to multiple hours. One glucose or glycogen produces two pyruvate molecules. In anaerobic glycolysis, *lactate* is produced via lactate dehydrogenase (LDH) and with the help of hydrogen in a timescale of microseconds:

$$\text{Pyruvate} + 2H \xrightarrow{\text{LDH}} \text{Lactate}$$

Lactate is later converted back to pyruvate again. Pyruvate is used in aerobic glycogenesis, which provides hydrogen carrier for the electron transport chain. Pyruvate can be produced directly from glucose or glycogen and from lactate. If all oxygen is used, lactate is formed from glycogen. This process yields only 3 mol ATP per molecule of glycogen but is available within seconds. In contrast, the complete breakdown of glycogen via *aerobic glycolysis* including Krebs cycle and respiratory chain yields 39 mol per molecule of glycogen. However, oxygen is required for this process. Aerobic glycogenesis develops approximately after 1 min. If the energy supply of aerobic processes is insufficient, deficits can be compensated with additional *anaerobic processes*.

Fatty acids also can enter the Krebs cycle and contribute to aerobic energy production. It yields approximately 129 molecules of ATP for a typical fat, but their rate of ATP resynthesis is so slow that it is not of great importance for high-intensity activities (◘ Fig. 19.1).

The components for energy from food or from endogenous storage (e.g. fat or glycogen from the liver) are taken to meet the demand. If the demand in energy increases, more energy-rich sources are required. If there are no reserves of energy sources left, the body turns to energy from ketone bodies, which are produced in the liver. Brain and muscles cells can adjust to catabolic metabolism such as starvation or extreme physical exertion and produce enzymes to use these ketones as an energy source for their cells.

Energy consumption of different physical activities can be specified in either Watt or MET (◘ Table 19.1) [2]. Although diving seems to be relaxing, the energy consumption is pretty high. The energy consumption corresponds to skiing, playing football or cycling. Thus, the fatigue after a day of diving is understandable.

■ **Energy Consumption During Different Exercises**

Another description of energy consumption is the metabolic equivalent of task (*MET*). It is defined as the resting metabolic rate,

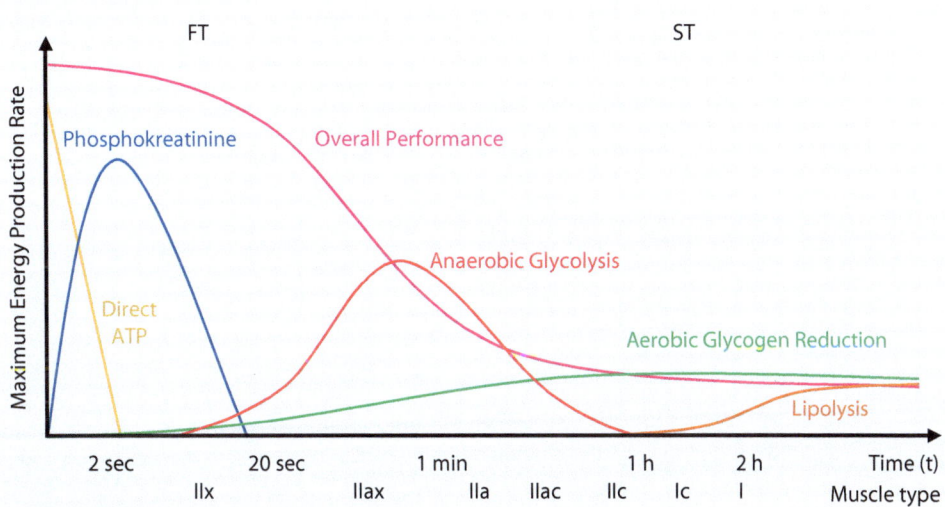

□ **Fig. 19.1**   Schematic overview of energy production in relation to time

□ **Table 19.1**   Energy consumption on METS of different exercises

Exercise	Energy consumption in Watt	METS
Scuba diving	70–193	4–11
Swimming with fins at the surface	70–105	4–6
Swimming	53–158	3–9
Cycling	53–175	3–10
Rowing	123–228	7–13

Jette et al. [2]

where approximately 3.5 ml O_2/kgbw/min are consumed. Hence, 2 MET represent 7.0 mL O_2/kgbw/min, etc.:

$$1\ MET = 3.5\ ml\,O_2/kgbw/min$$

Perfusion and oxygen consumption of different organs during exercise vary (□ Table 19.2) [1]. While perfusion during exercise of some organs like the brain remains unchanged, oth-ers like muscle experience a dramatic increase in perfusion. This is particular in diving form interest as inert gas absorption and elimination is dependent of perfusion.

There are two types of muscle fibres [3]. Both have different metabolic properties [4]. Type I muscles (slow-twitch) utilise the aerobic system as the main energy source. They are involved in endurance activities, have a high blood supply and a high number of mitochondria, which means they can produce a lot of energy via aerobic glycolysis. Type IIa fibres (fast-twitch) are fast oxidative fibres, which are a hybrid of type I and type IIb fibres, which can utilise aerobic and anaerobic metabolism. Type IIb fibres (fast-twitch) are fast glycolytic fibres, which utilise mainly the anaerobic system for their energy supply. They have less perfusion and mitochondria. These muscles are mainly utilised for short high-intensity activities. The contribution of these muscles varies in location and is affected by training or hereditary differences [4].

During exercise normal ventilation of 5–6 L/min can increase to more than 100 L/min, as oxygen consumption increases linearly to increasing work rate at submaximal intensities. Resting oxygen consumption of 250 mL/min

Table 19.2 Distribution of cardiac output to the various organs and oxygen consumption of organs at rest and during exercise

Organs	Weight	Perfusion (L/min/kg)		Oxygen consumption (mL/min)	
		At rest	Exercise	At rest	Exercise
CNS	1.7	0.5	0.5	40	40
Kidney	0.3	4.0	3.0	20	20
Stomach, intestine, liver	1.5	0.8	0.6	65	65
Heart	0.3	0.7	2.0	25	165
Muscles	30	0.04	0.4	60	2000
Joint, bones	14	0.03	0.06	15	25
Skin and fatty tissue	12	0.04	0.1	15	50
Others	10			10	135
Total	75			250	2500

Bühlmann [1]

Table 19.3 Comparison of approximate heart rate and stroke volume in trained or untrained person

	Stroke volume [ml][a]	Heart rate [beats/min][a]
At rest		
Untrained	70	70
Trained	100	50
Maximum exercise		
Untrained	110	190
Trained	160	180

[a]Approximate

can increase during very high-intensity activity to 5000 mL/min. The ventilation increases by increasing respiratory rate and tidal volume to match oxygen intake and elimination of carbon dioxide. The VO_2max [mL O_2/kgbw/min] is the measure of the maximum oxygen, which can be used. It varies between gender, age and fitness level (Table 19.3). Poor VO_2max in male is between 20 and 35 depending on age and in female 17–25. For diving a VO_2max of 40 should be reached.

During exercise muscles require increased blood flow. During rest it is around 2–4 mL/min in 100 mg muscle. During maximal activity it may rise to 100 mL/min per 100 mg muscle. The increased blood flow is affected by increased cardiac output but also by localised vasodilatation of precapillary sphincters in muscles, mediated by AMP, H^+, K^+ and PO_4^{3-}. Moreover, decreased pH caused by lactic acid and increased temperature during exercise causes a right shift of the oxygen dissociation curve, making oxygen more available for muscles. The cardiac output of a trained person increases mainly by the increase of the stroke volume compared to an untrained person.

The cardiovascular function is the limiting factor for oxygen delivery of tissues. Diving like other sport activities has an increased energy demand.

19

References

1. Bühlmann AA. Decompression/decompression sickness. Berlin: Springer; 1984.
2. Jette M, Sidney K, Blümchen G. Metabolic equivalents (METS) in exercise testing, exercise prescription and evaluation of functional capacity. Clin Cardiol. 1990;13:555–65.
3. Scott W, Stevens J, Binder-Macleod SA. Human skeletal muscle fiber type classifications. Phys Ther. 2001;81:1810–6.
4. Zierath JR, Hawley JA. Skeletal muscle fiber type: influence on contractile and metabolic properties. PLoS Biol. 2004;2(10):1523–7.

Suggested Reading

Burton DA, Stokes K, Hall GM. Continuing education in anaesthesia. Critical Care Pain. 2004;4(6):185–8.

Kenney WL, Wilmore JH, Costil DL. Physiology of sport and exercise. 5th ed. Champaign: Human Kinetics; 2012.

Kerem D, Melamed Y, Moran A. Alveolar PCO2 during rest and exercise in divers and non-divers breathing O2 at 1 ATA. Undersea Biomed Res. 1980;7:17–26.

Schmidt RF, Lang F, Heckmann M. Physiologie des Menschen. 31st. ed. Berlin: Springer; 2010.

Spomedial. 2003. URL: www.vmrz0100.vm.ruhr-uni-bochum.de; 2009-09-18.

Nutrition

© Springer International Publishing AG, part of Springer Nature 2018
O. Rusoke-Dierich, *Diving Medicine*, https://doi.org/10.1007/978-3-319-73836-9_20

The body requires energy for its metabolism and the regulation of cell processes. Some substances which the body cannot produce have to be supplemented by food. This includes unsaturated fatty acids, essential amino acids and some of the vitamins. The required amount depends on the individual needs and energy metabolism.

The former unit for energy metabolism was calories. A calorie is defined from the amount of heat quantity needed to heat 1 g of chemically pure water of 14.5–15.5 °C. The new unit is Joule:

$$1\,\text{Calorie} = 4.1868\,\text{Joules}$$

By metabolising nutrition together with O_2 to CO_2 and H_2O, their resulting energy content equals their calorific value (R). Fats and carbohydrates have the physical and physiological calorific value. Proteins need to be metabolised, and their physiological calorific value is smaller than the physical one. The physiological and physical average caloric value determines the respiratory quotient (RQ). The RQ describes the CO_2 elimination/O_2 absorption ratio. For carbohydrates and fat, RQ = 1. For proteins the RQ = 0.8. The average RQ = 0.82.

Diet should contain certain components (◘ Table 20.1), and energy supply should be balanced and adapt to the demand (◘ Table 20.2). Vitamins can be fat- and water-soluble. Vitamins A, D, E and K are fat-soluble vitamins. All fat-soluble vitamins are only absorbed in the presence of additional fat provided in food. Therefore, a certain amount of fat should be included in the normal diet. Fat soluble vitamins may cause symptoms of intoxication when taken excessively. The remaining vitamins are water-soluble and are eliminated, if taken more than needed. Essential vitamins are A, D, K, E, B1, B2, B6, B12, C, niacin, folic acid, pantothenic acid and biotin. Essential means that they must be supplemented as food, because they cannot be synthesised by the body itself. The vitamin B complex is mainly found in meat, fish and whole wheat bread. Vitamin C-rich foods are fresh fruits, especially kiwi fruit. Vitamin E can be found in oils, like nuts, or in oily fish, such as salmon. Vitamin D is produced mostly in the skin by sunlight and is responsible for the calcium balance and the strength of bones and muscles. Vitamin A is especially in red or orange fruits or vegetables, as in carrots or pawpaw. Fats are divided into saturated and unsaturated fatty acids. The saturated or multiple saturated fatty acids are most valuable. They are present in vegetable oils. Unsaturated fatty acids can be found mainly in animal fats. Unsaturated fatty acids adversely affect cholesterol and play a role in the development of coronary heart disease and stroke. Unsaturated trans-fatty acids are particularly unfavourable. Multiple heating of other fatty acids, in particular, processed foods (junk food), causes even "good" fats to turn into trans-fatty acids. Sugars and fats are used directly as energy sources. The glycemic index (GI) is a measure of how fast energy of food is made available. A high GI value means that the type of food is converted quickly into energy. An initial energy peak is reached but then quickly declines again. With high GI it is possible that more energy will be provided than needed. Hence, excess sugar is stored as fat in the body. A low GI slowly increases blood sugar levels but is longer available. Therefore, foods with low GI value are preferable. There

◘ **Table 20.2**   Energy requirement

Resting	7000 kJ/day
Light workout	11,000 kJ/day
Heavy workout	15,000–20,000 kJ/day

◘ **Table 20.1**   Requirement of food components per day

Food component	Requirement in g/day
Fat (25%)	65
Protein (12%)	70
Carbohydrate (63%)	370

are different kinds of sugar, like glucose, fructose, lactose, dextrose, sucrose and maltose. All these different sugars are absorbed easily by the body and can be used directly as energy sources. Some foods, such as starch (wheat products or potatoes), can only be transformed by digestive processes into sugar. Fructose, or fruit sugar, is naturally present in fruits. Fructose can be absorbed in excess by fruit juices or blending, like in many processed foods. This leads not only to excess supply of carbohydrates but also increases triglycerides and cholesterol. This can cause health issues like atherosclerosis, fatty liver and diabetes (◘ Figs. 20.1 and 20.2).

■ **Fig. 20.1** Schematic illustration of the effects of GI on utilization and fat production

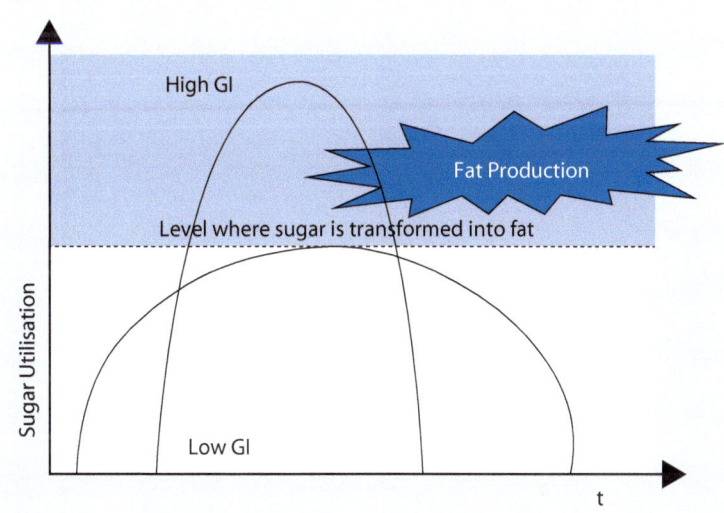

■ **Fig. 20.2** Nutrition pyramid

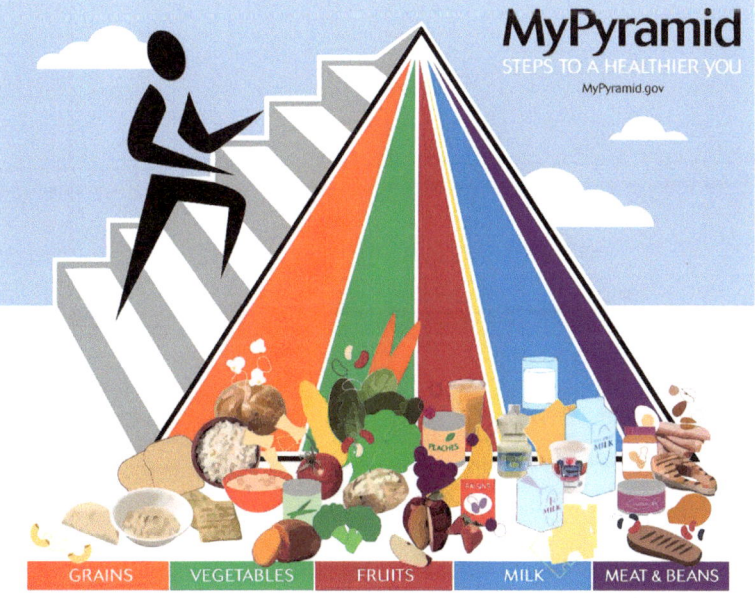

Temperature Regulation

© Springer International Publishing AG, part of Springer Nature 2018
O. Rusoke-Dierich, *Diving Medicine*, https://doi.org/10.1007/978-3-319-73836-9_21

21

For the body's enzymes and biological processes, a certain body temperature is necessary. In humans, the temperature optimum is from 36.4 °C to 37.4 °C. A slight rise of the temperature can increase body processes for a short time. Temperatures above 39.5 °C could affect the body negatively. If these temperatures persist longer, it might result in heat-related injuries. It can cause seizures, destruction of muscle tissue (rhabdomyolysis), hypotension, shock, etc. Temperatures above 43 °C are usually fatal. In body temperatures below 36.4 °C, body processes slow down. 26 °C and 28 °C are regarded as critical benchmarks, as heart arrhythmias and CNS changes may occur.

To maintain the required temperature, the body has to adapt to changing situations. The control centre of the thermoregulation is located in the hypothalamus. The information about the body's core temperature is sensed in the hypothalamus itself and also in thermoreceptors of the skin and spinal cord. In the thermoregulatory centres of the hypothalamus, actual temperatures are compared with desired temperatures. Desired values represent temperatures, which are currently needed (e.g. waking and sleeping, fever, etc.). If actual and desired values differ, the body adjusts the temperature as needed. If the temperature has to be increased, muscle contracts, which is perceived as muscle tremors. Chemical processes of muscle activity are responsible for the increase in body temperature. Excess heat is compensated via heat emission through increased blood circulation to the skin or via evaporative cooling by means of perspiration.

Acid-Base Balance

© Springer International Publishing AG, part of Springer Nature 2018
O. Rusoke-Dierich, *Diving Medicine*, https://doi.org/10.1007/978-3-319-73836-9_22

22

To ensure normal body function, specific pH levels need to be maintained. In average it is about 7.4 (◘ Table 22.1). The pH level reflects the effective H^+-ion concentration or H^+-ion activity. Increase of H^+-ions and decrease of OH^--ions result in a shift of the pH level towards the acid range and vice versa to the alkaline range (H^+-ions = acid ions; OH^--ions = base ions). The formula for the pH level is

$$pH = -\log\left[H^+\right]$$

In particular respiration and enzyme activity is dependent on the pH level. A shift of the pH from physiological values of 7.37–7.43 towards the alkaline range is called alkalosis, and towards the acidic range, acidosis. pH levels outside 7.0 and 7.8 are regarded as life-threatening (◘ Fig. 22.1).

To keep pH levels constant, various buffering systems balance changing H^+- or OH^--ion concentrations. The bicarbonate buffering system has the largest share of the pH buffering.

◘ **Table 22.1**   Standard values of a standard arterial blood gas

pH	7.37–7.45
PO_2	75–100 mmHg
PCO_2	35–45 mmHg
HCO_3^-	21–26 mmol/L
Base excess (BE)	−2 bis+2
Anion gap	3–11 mmol/L

Together with H_2O (water), H_2CO_3 and H^+ and HCO_3^- are formed from CO_2.

■ **Bohr Effect**

$$CO_2 + H_2O \leftrightharpoons H_2CO_3 \leftrightharpoons H^+ + HCO_3^-$$

Haemoglobin in red blood cells as well as plasma proteins contributes to the protein buffering system. The buffering properties of proteins (mainly albumin) are determined by ionizing groups of amino acids. The main part of this buffering system falls on haemoglobin, since it has high concentrations in blood. The phosphate buffering system is composed of organic phosphates. However, concentrations in blood are so low that it is hardly involved in the regulation of pH.

The main organs that regulate the pH are the kidney and lungs. The lungs have the ability to influence the pH by changing CO_2 levels. The kidney regulates the pH level with the secretion of acids and bases. A pH change due to breathing is called respiratory, and all other causes are called metabolic alkalosis or acidosis. The pH level can be compensated only to a certain extent. It is referred to as compensated alkalosis or acidosis. If the imbalance can't be compensated, it is classified as a noncompensated alkalosis or acidosis.

■ **Metabolic Acidosis** (◘ Table 22.2)
Causes
— Renal failure
— Increased H^+-ion absorption (fruit acid, protein, increased urea production of the liver in liver failure)

◘ **Fig. 22.1**   pH level; red, acidic; blue, alkaline

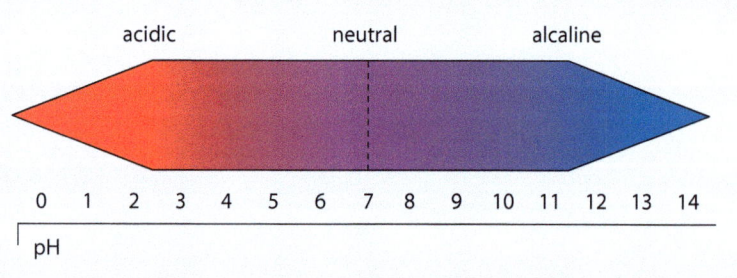

- Oxygen deficiency (lactate production)
- Ketoacidosis (diabetes, starvation)
- Diarrhoea
- Medication (metformin, salicylate)

■ **Respiratory Acidosis** (🔲 Table 22.3)
Causes
- Pulmonary diseases (pneumonia, tuberculosis, COPD)
- Depressed respiration (drowning, intoxication, e.g. alcohol or drugs

■ **Metabolic Alkalosis** (🔲 Table 22.4)
Causes
- Vomiting (loss of gastric acid)
- Medication (diuretics, bicarbonate)
- Mineralocorticoid excess (Conn syndrome, medication)

■ **Respiratory Alkalosis** (🔲 Table 22.5)
Causes
- Hyperventilation

🔲 **Table 22.2** Metabolic acidosis

Compensated (increased respiration)	pH normal $HCO_3^- < 21$ mmol/L $pCO_2 < 35$ mmHg
Decompensated	pH < 7.37 $HCO_3^- < 21$ mmol/L pCO_2 normal

🔲 **Table 22.4** Metabolic alkalosis

Compensated (reduced respiration)	pH normal $HCO_3^- > 26$ mmol/L $pCO_2 > 45$ mmHg
Decompensated	pH > 7.45 $HCO_3^- > 26$ mmol/L pCO_2 normal

🔲 **Table 22.3** Respiratory acidosis

Compensated (reactive increase of respiration, H^+-ion renal secretion)	pH normal $HCO_3^- > 26$ mmol/L $pCO_2 > 45$ mmHg
Decompensated	pH < 7.37 HCO_3^- normal $pCO_2 > 45$ mmHg

🔲 **Table 22.5** Respiratory alkalosis

Compensated (reduced respiration, HCO_3^-, renal excretion)	pH normal $HCO_3^- < 21$ mmol/L $pCO_2 < 35$ mmHg
Decompensated	pH > 7.45 $HCO_3^- >$ normal $pCO_2 < 35$ mmHg

Diving Medicine

Diving has become a popular recreational sport. With increasing numbers of people who are enjoying this sport, diving accidents increasingly occur. Therefore, it is important for physicians to be informed about injuries and dangers related to diving. The chapter "Diving Medicine" tries to outline aetiology, symptoms, treatments and prevention detailed but also in a hopefully understandable way. In this book a new classification of barotraumas is included, whether the damage is due to increasing or decreasing pressure (hyper-/hypobaric or positive/negative pressure barotrauma).

Contents

Barotrauma

© Springer International Publishing AG, part of Springer Nature 2018
O. Rusoke-Dierich, *Diving Medicine*, https://doi.org/10.1007/978-3-319-73836-9_23

Damages to divers caused by pressure changes are called barotrauma. Barotraumas are quite common in diving. It can affect any air-filled spaces of the body. With increasing and decreasing pressure, gas volumes are changing in confined spaces (Boyle's law) (■ Tables 23.1 and 23.2). Ascending increases gas volume and decreases during descending. In this book I described damage as a result of increased pressure as *hyperbaric barotrauma* (*ppBT = positive-pressure barotrauma*) and injuries caused by vacuum as *hypobaric barotrauma* (*npBT = negative-pressure barotrauma*). This allows a better differentiation between the causes and a better prediction of the damage that might have occurred (■ Fig. 23.1).

The first 10 meters below the surface is the area in which pressure changes are most prominent. As seen in ■ Table 23.1, gas volume changes increasingly towards the surface. This means the biggest risk of barotrauma is predominantly in the first 10 meters below the surface (■ Fig. 23.2).

- **Formula for Gas Volume and Pressure Changes**

$$\frac{P_1}{P_2} \cdot V_1 = V_2$$

P_1 = initial ambient pressure; P_2 = current ambient pressure; V_1 = initial gas volume; V_2 = current gas volume

Barotraumas occur when gas is entrapped in air-filled body cavities and its pressure can't adjust to the ambient pressure. Pressures in closed cavities will rise or fall accordingly and cause damage to the surrounding tissue. All

■ **Table 23.2** Equations for volume and partial pressures during compression and decompression

Factor x for change in	Volume	Partial pressure of gases
Compression	$\frac{P_1}{P_2} = x$	$\frac{P_2}{P_1} = x$
Decompression	$\frac{P_2}{P_1} = x$	$\frac{P_1}{P_2} = x$

P_1 = initial ambient pressure; P_2 = current ambient pressure

■ **Table 23.1** Gas volume changes with changing ambient pressure

Depth in [m]	Volume change [L] during ascending and descending	Pressure In [bar]
0	10	1
10	5	2
20	3.3	3
30	2.5	4
40	2	5
50	1.6	6
60	1.4	7
70	1.25	8
80	1.1	9

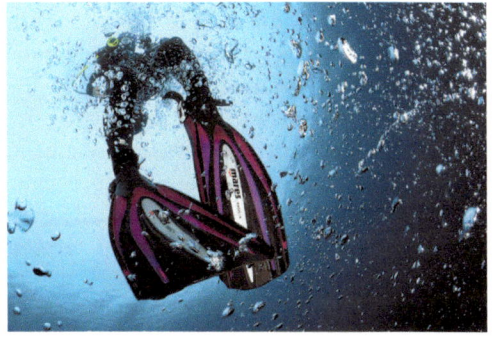

■ **Fig. 23.1** Risk of barotrauma due to high ascent rates (With kind permission of Mares/A. Balbi)

23

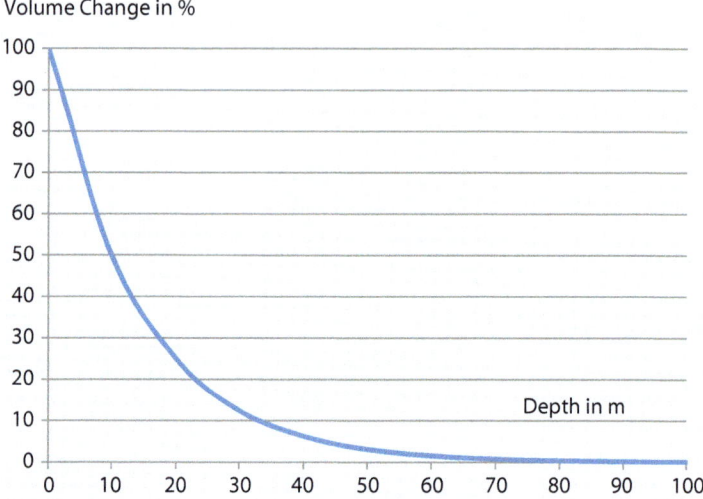

■ **Fig. 23.2** Volume changes in correlation to the diving depth

cavities in the body are connected to the environment via ducts. These ducts are either permanently open or can be automatically or arbitrarily opened. Thus, gas can flow in and out. Hence, the pressure inside the cavity remains neutral. If the duct is blocked, either increased pressure or vacuum develops, and barotrauma with varying severity might occur (■ Fig. 23.3).

Cavities of the body are commonly lined with mucous membranes. Mucous membranes have the ability to produce secretions or to swell by increasing perfusion. Cavities, such as the lung or middle ear, can be closed and opened with the help of muscles of the mouth, the larynx or the Eustachian tubes arbitrarily and automatically. Other cavities such as the sinuses are constantly open. Is a cavity closed by muscles or swelling of mucous membranes, increased pressure or vacuum can build up. Vacuum can be partially offset by fluid secretions, bleeding and mucous membrane swelling, as this reduces the gas volume inside the cavity. This mechanism is mainly seen at barotraumas of rigid-walled cavities (sinuses). Cavities with elastic walls (alveoli and intestines) have the ability to compensate pressure to some extent due to their elasticity of its tissue.

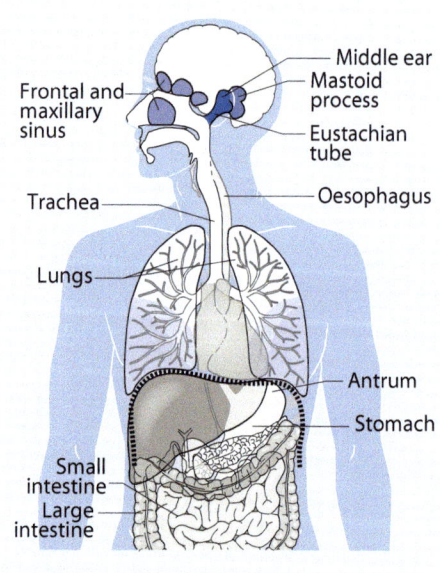

■ **Fig. 23.3** Gas-filled cavities in the body (Ecomed)

Pain associated with barotraumas is caused by space limitation and reduction with associated damage to the surrounding tissue. Mucous membranes or tissues have pain receptors, which respond to pressure or damage. Acute pain that is caused by pressure or tissue damage is superficial, pungent and sharp in its quality. The subacute pain starts with certain latency after a trauma and is more a sign of wound healing, oedema or inflammatory reaction. Its quality is dull, deep and diffusely distributed at the damaged area.

Barotraumas of sinuses and ears are usually characterised by increasing pain, which suddenly subsides, when membranes or mucous membranes rupture. Easing of the pain is a result of the elimination of the triggering stimulus on tissues. In the case of the eardrum, a perforation stops the strain on the eardrum and pain subsides. In case of sinus barotraumas bleeding or secretion can fill the air-filled space and replace the gas volume with liquid. Volumes of liquid are independent of pressure changes in comparison to gas volumes. Hence, pressure neutralises and membranes or mucous membranes are no longer irritated by the vacuum. In regard to the lungs and skin, however, pain is rather caused by tissue damage and bleeding or swelling of the interstitial space. This kind of pain won't ease off quickly.

23.1 Barotrauma of the Ear

The ear consists of outer, middle and inner ear. Over the auricle, acoustic signals are captured and redirected via the s-shaped ear canal to the eardrum. In adults, the external ear canal is about 3.5 cm in length, approximately 0.5 cm in diameter and 1 cm high. Its pathway is directed to the inside and slightly ventral. The cartilaginous part forms the smaller outer section. The larger inner section is formed by the bony part. The middle ear is an air-filled space in the lateral bone of the skull. It contains the auditory ossicles, which serve for sound transmission from the tympanic membrane to the oval window. The inner ear contains the cochlea and the labyrinth for hearing and balance.

Eardrums divide the middle ear from the outer ear. The Eustachian tube opens and closes arbitrarily or automatically and thus helps in equalising the pressure inside the middle ear via connections to the nasopharynx. Usually,

there is a pressure difference in the middle ear to the ambient pressure ranging from 0.0049 up to −0.0049 bar (4.9 mbar to −4.9 mbar). Through connections to the nasopharynx secretions also can be drained. The approximately 3–4 cm long Eustachian tube consists of a small petrous and a larger cartilaginous-muscular part. The transition from the bony to the cartilaginous-muscular is the narrowest point, the isthmus tubae. The orifice to the nasopharynx has two lips, which are closing the Eustachian tube. The cartilaginous portion consists of a U-shaped plate, which consists of elastic cartilage and opens face down and laterally. This part is also embedded in the skull bone. The open side facing down is bordered by a membrane. The tube muscles (levator veli palatine muscle and tensor veli palatine muscle) run longitudinal and open the tube by approximately 3 mm (Fig. 18.4).

23.1.1 Aetiology and Pathogenesis

■ **Tympanic Barotrauma (TBT)**
Usually the Eustachian tube is slightly closed. Pressure equalisation takes place through arbitrary (Valsalva manoeuvre) or automatic opening (swallowing, yawning) of the tube. While descending, the Eustachian tube is sucked together and thus prevents equalisation between the middle ear and nasopharynx. A vacuum builds up within the tympanic cavity. This pulls the eardrum inward. The vacuum stretches the tympanic membrane and creates suction on the lining of the middle ear, which causes pain and irritation of eardrums and mucous membranes. This vacuum may lead in extreme cases to the rupture of the tympanic membrane. This can be described as *hypobaric tympanic barotrauma* (*npTBT = negative-pressure tympanic barotauma*) or middle ear barotrauma. A complication of the TBT could be a dislodgement of the ossicles. Barotraumas of the eardrum and damage to the middle ear occurs rather on descending than ascending. In general, an increased pressure in the tympanic cavity leads to the opening of the tube. A vacuum, however, inevi-

23

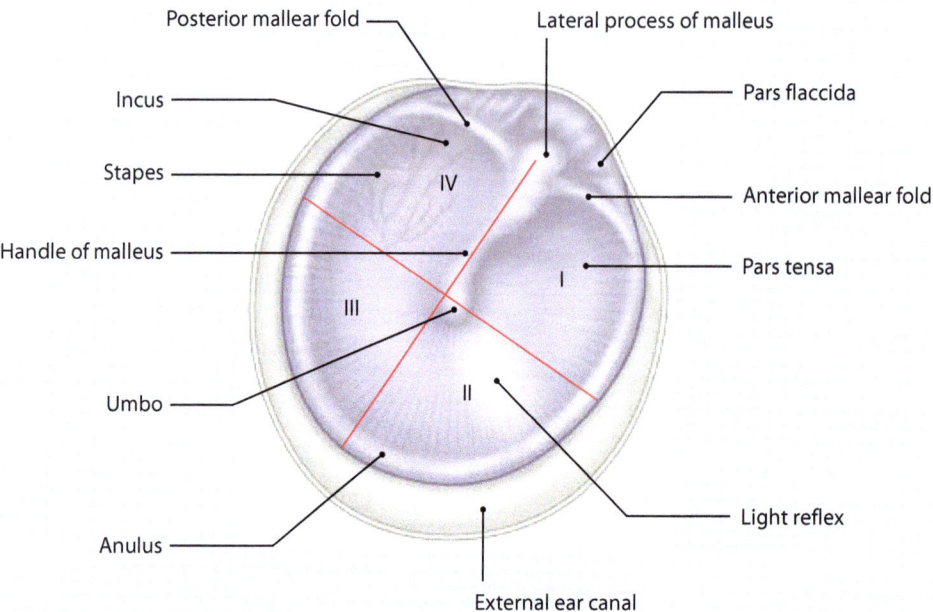

□ **Fig. 23.4** Tympanic membrane (From Zilles and Tillmann 2010 [18])

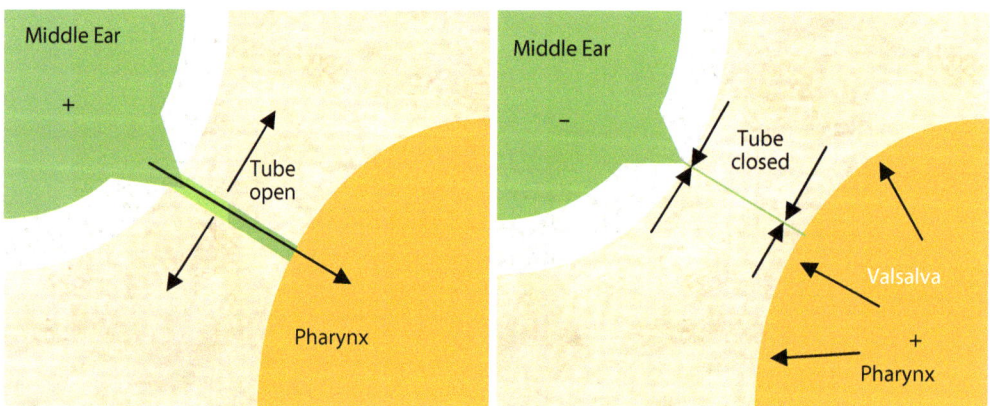

□ **Fig. 23.5** Eustachian tube with changing pressure

tably leads to the closure of the tube, since the walls along the tube are collapsing. The vacuum leads to an increased perfusion of the tubal mucous membranes, which reinforced the closure of the tube. The stronger the vacuum in the middle ear is, the stronger also is the pulling on the Eustachian tubes. By attempting a forced equalisation, pressure increases in the nasopharynx. The consequence of this is that due to the slight expansion of the nasopharynx, the tube additionally will be compressed from this end, hindering equalisation even further (□ Figs. 23.4 and 23.5).

■ **Inner Ear Barotrauma (IEBT)**

The Barotrauma of the inner ear can be subdivided in a hypobaric (*npIEBT = negative-pressure inner ear barotrauma*) or a hyperbaric barotrauma (*ppIEBT = positive-pressure inner ear barotrauma*). A study on guinea pigs suggested that the risk of a barotrauma of the inner ear seems more likely in the round window compared to the oval window [9]. The oval window seems to be more protected by stabilisation by the ossicles and their ligamentous attachments. There a two theories about the development of IEBT [4, 10, 11].

- **ppIEBT (Implosive)**
  - *Forced equalisation* with sudden opening of the Eustachian tube can cause a *rupture of the round window* in the direction to the inner ear during compression. If the tube is occluded by bleeding, mucus secretions or polyps and equalisation between the middle ear and nasopharynx is not possible, the round window can rupture during decompression as well.
  - Sudden increase of pressure due to equalisation can cause a *dislocation of the ossicles with perforation of the oval window*.

- **nplEBT (Explosive)**
  - *Vacuum* in the middle ear created by an occluded Eustachian tube during compression, making equalising impossible. It may cause a *rupture of the round window* in the direction to the middle ear. The bulging of the round window in the direction of middle ear can additionally be reinforced by a *forced equalisation*. The inner ear has a connecting duct (Aquaeductus cochleae) to the cerebral ventricles. A forced equalisation can cause a temporary increase of the cerebrospinal fluid pressure and thus of the anatomically connected perilymph of the inner ear. By this, the round window can be assumed to bulge out towards the direction of the tympanic cavity. The simultaneously existing vacuum in the middle ear has a pulling effect on the round window, which enhances the push of the inner ear from the other side. If the pressure difference exceeds a certain point, the membrane is at risk of rupturing.

- *Vacuum* in the middle ear can cause the dislocation of the ossicles, resulting in a *rupture of the oval window* by pulling forces.

23.1.2 Symptoms

The tympanic membrane can be more or less affected (◘ Tables 23.3 [4] and 23.4). Barotraumas to the eardrum cause increasing stabbing pain of the affected ear during changes in ambient pressure. This pain subsides suddenly, if the eardrum ruptures. It is associated with acute sensorineural hearing loss. At the same time [13], acute temporary disorientation, vertigo, nausea, vomiting and spontaneous nystagmus may develop. Triggers for these symptoms are the caloric stimulation of the semicircular canals through the influx of cold water into the tympanic cavity.

Rupture of the oval or round window produces similar symptoms. This may present with

◘ **Table 23.3** Modified TEED classification of tympanic barotrauma

Grade 0:	Homogenous greyish-yellowish discoloration of the tympanic membrane; slight protrusion, subjective symptoms
Grade I:	Slight injection and swelling of the tympanic membrane around the malleus
Grade II:	Increased diffuse injection with loss of contours of the malleus of the tympanic membrane; inversion of the tympanic membrane
Grade III:	Intense injection of the entire tympanic membrane, blistering of the tympanic membrane
Grade IV:	Blood blisters of the tympanic membrane; haematotympanum
Grade V:	Perforation; muffled tympanic membrane

Edmonds et al. (2016) [4]

23

■ **Table 23.4** TEED classification of tympanic barotrauma

I	Injection of the tympanic membrane margins
II	Injection of the entire tympanic membrane
III	Blood blisters and excretion of the tympanic membrane
IV	Blood blisters and perforation of the tympanic membrane

acute or progressing sensorineural hearing loss only or be associated with vestibular symptoms. Both symptoms seem to persist for an unusual prolonged time. Disturbance of the balance is caused by the loss of perilymph into the middle ear resulting in a quantitative imbalance against the endolymph. The loss of the perilymph causes a long-lasting irritation of the semicircular canals compared to the brief caloric irritation after rupturing the tympanic membrane.

A differential diagnosis to both, tympanic or inner ear barotrauma, is the inner ear DCS. In absence of clinical finding and in combination with dive profiles, which may carry a risk of DCS, this should be considered. Important clues in regard to the differentiation between BT and DCS can be obtained by the patient's history and the diving profile. Urgent assessment by an ENT specialist might be required when in doubt in regard to management, as inner ear DCS requires HBOT, and on the other hand IEBT is a contraindication for HBOT.

23.1.3 Treatment

■ **Tympanic Barotrauma**

With stage I and stage II, TBT diving might still be possible. But even if diving is allowed, it might be better to postpone it until complete healing is achieved. A temporary absolute unfitness for diving exists from stage III on. Diving restrictions allow time for regeneration of eardrums and give a certain protection against otitis media and externa.

Uncomplicated *tympanic membrane perforations* heal within 1–4 weeks. However, diving and swimming is contraindicated for 6–8 weeks. Dirty, bacteria-rich water may cause secondary infections, resulting in significant delay in healing. Eardrum splinting or tympanoplasty might be necessary in some cases. Antibiotic prophylaxis in form of ear drops or orally and short-term administration of nose decongestants are recommended. Local infrared light application of tympanic membranes promotes wound healing. If the eardrum heals without complications, a whitish scar, which lies in the level of the tympanic membrane, is visible. In this case fitness of diving can be attested. Usually, the hearing is back to normal. If there is a poor healing of the tympanic membrane after a perforation, a slight protrusion of a bluish atrophic scar appears above the level of the tympanic membrane. Atrophic scars easily can perforate and represent a permanent weakness of the tympanic membrane. Therefore, diving is contraindicated. Marginal perforations may cause damage to the ossicles. Complicated perforations, like marginal perforations, atrophic scars or chronic perforations, always require ENT review, as they might require surgery.

■ **Inner Ear Barotrauma**

A *barotrauma of the inner ear* is relatively rare. As consequential damages may result in lifelong hearing loss or tinnitus, these require specific treatment and follow-up by specialists. An initial treatment with high doses of oral prednisolone (1 mg/BWkg daily for 3 days with tapering of over 18 days) or intravenous steroids might be considered. This should be commenced as soon as possible. If necessary, in particular if a perilymphatic fistula is suspected, a tympanotomy could be performed to cover of the round window. The patient should avoid coughing, crunches and Valsalva attempts to prevent further leakage of the perilymph, as these manoeuvres cause an increase of the cerebral blood pressure. Strict bed rest with head elevation is advisable. Inner ear barotrauma is a contraindication for HBOT and diving.

■ **Therapy**

Tympanic membrane perforation

– Diving and swimming restrictions till complete healing is achieved (usually 6–8 weeks)
– Local infrared light irradiation of the tympanic membrane
– Eardrum splinting, possibly tympanoplasty
– Antibiotic prophylaxis (amoxicillin with or without clavulanic acid; ciprofloxacin, if pseudomonas is suspected) and nasal decongestants (oxymetazoline)

Inner ear barotrauma

– Bed rest with head elevation could be considered.
– Tympanotomy.
– Avoid increase in cerebral blood pressure (no Valsalva manoeuvre, no
– exercise, crunches, coughing, sneezing and constipation).
– HBOT and diving is *contraindicated.*

If a dislodgement of the ossicles or perilymphatic fistula is expected, a HRCT of the temporal bones should be performed and ENT review be sought. Further testing with cervical vestibular-evoked myogenic potentials (cVEMP) and electronystagmography (ENG) can be considered, if inner ear damage is expected.

23.1.4 Prophylaxis

The easy way to avoid barotraumas of the ear is to equalise. There are different methods available for this (■ Fig. 23.6).

■ **Valsalva method**

The Valsalva manoeuvre is as an attempt to exhale against a closed nose with otherwise close airways. The thereby increasing pressure in the nasopharynx causes a temporary opening of the Eustachian tube. The pressure increases to approximately 53 mbar (40 mmHg) in the nasopharynx. The tube is thus opened by positive pressure of the nasopharynx, similar to blowing up a balloon.

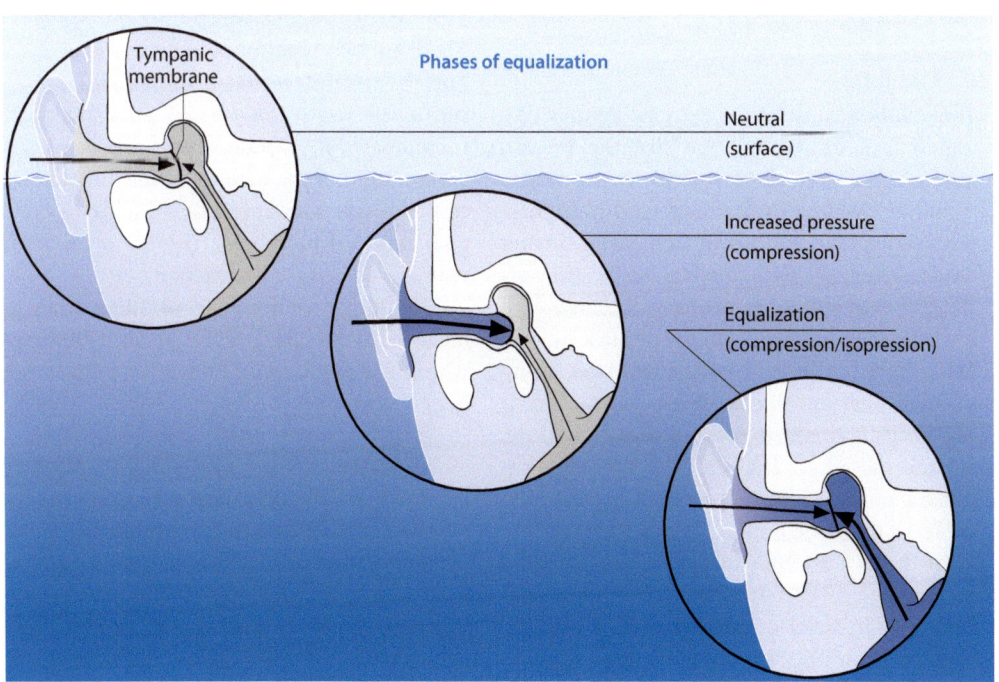

■ **Fig. 23.6** Phases of equalisation (Ecomed)

23

■ **Frenzel method**

Barotraumas of the ear were common in pilots of the German Luftwaffe as one of their manoeuvres in a specific plane ("Stuka") were rapid descents. In 1939, H. Frenzel introduced a hand-free equalisation method to prevent barotrauma of the ear. Thereby, the nose has to be closed as with the Valsalva method, commonly with a nose clip. In contrast to the Valsalva method, the increased pressure is not created by exhalation but by pressure of the tongue and mouth floor muscles against the palate. The glottis is hereby closed and doesn't allow air flow into the lungs, and pressure increases only in the nasopharynx. The pressure resulting from this method is approximately® 119 mbar (90 mmHg) and is thus greater than the Valsalva method. Hence, the Frenzel method seems to be more efficient. It particularly is used in apnoea diving.

■ **Swallowing/Yawning**

For some divers, it is sufficient to make sipping, yawning or chewing movements or simply moving the jaw to equalise. These movements open the Eustachian tube by activation of its own muscles.

■ **Mouthfill**

This method is useful for extreme apnoea diving. It is a similar method like the Frenzel method. However, on greater depth, the diminishing air volume in the lungs and nasopharynx might prevent the diver from going further down. To ensure that equalisation is still possible, the nasopharynx needs to be filled with the little remaining air volume of the lung, just before that resource is exhausted. After filling the nasopharynx the diver closes the glottis and keeps it closed to avoid a backflow of the air into the lungs. That ensures that equalisation beyond that critical point is still possible.

In all these methods, it is important to perform the first attempt to equalise right at the surface before even descending. This avoids subsequent forced equalisation. Pressure differences of only 60–80 mbar (corresponding to a depth of 60–80 cm) are enough to close the

Eustachian tube, making it difficult or impossible to open it again. This is due to the vacuum and strong suction effect in the middle ear. If there are difficulties with equalising, the diver has to ascend few meters till equalisation is possible. Diving beginners or divers at the start of their diving holiday might find it particularly hard to equalise. This is often due to the irritation of the tube through water, particularly salt water, or the lack of training. Positioning might influence the ability to equalise. Sometimes equalisation can be more easily achieved when the diver is in an upright position.

The use of earplugs during diving is absolutely contraindicated. By this a vacuum between earplugs and eardrum develops, which can lead to the rupture of the eardrum either directly through the earplugs getting sucked in or indirectly through the vacuum building up between eardrum and ear plugs. The same can happen by ear wax occluding the ear tube.

23.2 Pulmonary Barotrauma (PBT)

There are two types of pulmonary barotrauma. Lung tissue damage arising from increased pressure is referred to as *hyperbaric pulmonary barotrauma* (*ppPB = positive-pressure pulmonary barotrauma*). If the damage of the lung tissue is caused by vacuum, it is referred to as *hypobaric pulmonary barotrauma* (*npPB = negative-pressure pulmonary barotrauma*).

The lung's weight is about 400 g. They are located in the chest cavity and fill the space within the chest wall. Lungs have three borders:
- *Diaphragm* separates the lungs from the abdomen.
- *Ribs* form the outside of the chest wall.
- The *medial side* is in front of the spine and the mediastinum.

Lungs are almost completely separated from the chest cavity and can therefore freely move. The smallest anatomical units of the lung, in which also the gas exchange takes place, are the alveoli. They have a diameter of approximately 0.3 mm. The 0.0022-mm-thick alveolar wall, allowing the diffusion of respiratory gases, consists of alveolar epithelium, a fibrous supporting structure made of elastic and collagen fibres and the capillary wall. It is elastic and covered with a phosphorus lipid layer, the surfactant. The surfactant reduces the surface tension and prevents a collapse of the alveoli. The capillaries of the lung, where gas exchange takes place, are located in the alveolar wall. The alveoli, which are grape-like structures, are connected to the outside via the airways. The upper portion of the airways in the lungs contains horseshoe-shaped cartilage segments. The epithelium consists of goblet cells which produce mucus and bind foreign bodies and ciliated epithelium, which steadily transports mucus and foreign bodies to the outside. In the bronchial tubes and bronchioles, cartilaginous components are replaced by smooth muscles. This enables the bronchioles to alter their diameter by contracting or relaxing. There are no glands that produce mucus in the bronchial tubes and bronchioles.

23.2.1 Hyperbaric Barotrauma of the Lungs (ppPBT = Positive-Pressure Pulmonary Barotrauma)

23.2.1.1 Aetiology and Pathogenesis

Hyperbaric pulmonary barotrauma is one of the most serious accidents, which can occur during diving. It occurs mainly in near-surface sections or immediately after reaching the surface. It leads to the most serious symptoms. This type of damage with lung distension has often fatal consequences (fatality rate 20–30%). It represents next to DCI the biggest risk to divers.

Hyperbaric pulmonary barotrauma occurs during the ascent, if air in the lungs is entrapped and is unable to escape. The pulmonary barotrauma with mechanical ventilation is also referred as volutrauma. It seems that rather the volume expansion than the pressure is responsible for pressure-related lung injury [8], even if both are involved in the process. Observation of trumpet players suggested that short time airway pressures of about 150 mbar can be achieved without resulting in lung damage. Peak airway pressure of 14 mbar has no effect on the lung. With increasing pressure or volume, lung damage becomes more likely. Transpulmonary pressure gradients of about 95–110 mbar seem to lead to alveolar rupture [2]. However, peak airway pressure is not always related to alveolar pressure, as airway pressure is greatly influenced by airflow resistance. Only at zero airflow airway opening pressure is assumed to be equal to alveolar pressure. The degree of alveolar distension is determined by the pressure gradient across the alveoli, which is reflected by the transpulmonary pressure. The transpulmonary pressure (p_{tp}) is traditionally defined as airways opening or static airway pressure (p_{saw}) minus pleural pressure (p_{pl}).

$$p_{tp} = p_{saw} - p_{pl}$$

The elastic recoil pressure (p_{er}) is

$$p_{er} = p_{alv} - p_{pl}$$

Acute and chronic inflammatory processes, as well as changes in anatomical structure, pose in general an increased risk of pulmonary barotrauma. In diving, lung damage is mainly due to volume and pressure increase over a short period of time. This can occur during ascent or by excessive overinflating the lungs with techniques like buccal pumping or lung packing at apnoea diving.

Another phenomenon is the so called "air trapping". Bronchiolar obstruction leads to air trapping distal to the affected bronchiole.

There are various reasons for a reduced air flow:
- Excessive ascent rate
- Poor exhalation during the ascent
- Pathological pulmonary changes

23

■ **Excessive Ascent Rate**

Air, which is located in the alveoli, expands during the ascent. As the diameter of the alveoli and distal respiratory airways is approximately 0.3 mm, only a limited amount air flow is possible due to its size. During the ascent, the pulmonary air volume increases. Usually, a significant increase in gas volume is prevented by steady breathing, so lung tissue won't get injured. However, if certain ascent rates are exceeded, air may not be able to escape fast enough out of small airways, which might cause tissue injury. Maximum air inlet speed is depending on gas densities and mixtures.

■ **Missing Exhalation During Ascending**

There are two main reasons that the diver can't exhale during ascent. One is simply to forget to breathe or holding the breath due to panic and stress. The other reason is a laryngospasm, where the larynx occludes. A laryngospasm could be, for example, provoked by inhalation of water (water aspiration). It leads to a complete airway obstruction. After a loss of consciousness the spasm usually resolves spontaneously.

A brief example explains the impact of volume increase due to pulmonary pressure changes. At 10 m depth the diver has a total assumed gas volume of approximately 3.5 L (residual volume + expiratory reserve volume + tidal volume) with normal breathing. The total lung capacity is estimated with 6 L. If the diver holds his breath, even without additional deeper inhalation during the ascent, the lung volume would be 7 L at the surface and thus exceeds its total capacity by 1 L! (■ Fig. 23.7).

■ **Pathological Changes**

Following pathological lung disorders may lead to a ppPBT:

- Constriction, increased mucus production and airway obstruction (e.g. obstructive respiratory diseases such as asthma)
- Irritation of the bronchoalveolar tissue (such as bronchitis)
- Pathological changes of the respiratory tract (e.g. tuberculosis, emphysema, bullae, pleural adhesions, cysts, tumours)

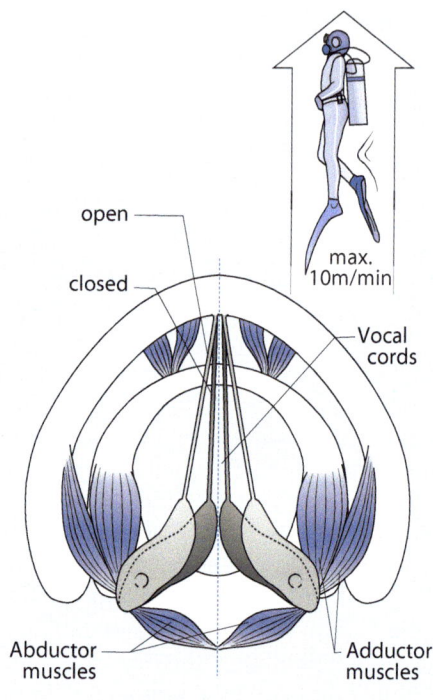

■ **Fig. 23.7** Laryngospasm and/or exceeding the maximal ascend rate in surface-near areas (With kind permission of Ecomed)

❯ **Air trapping!**

Acute lung injury (ALI) is well described in literature. The term is now included in ARDS (Berlin 2011) [6]. ARDS is an acute respiratory condition, which develops within a week. It shows on CXR bilateral opacities in at least three quadrants, without having cardiogenic origin, or is related to fluid overload, pleural effusion, atelectasis and nodules. There is a mild, moderate and severe form of ARDS, which is defined by the PaO_2/FiO_2 ratio with PEEP or CPAP of more than 5 cmH_2O.

- Mild 200–300
- Moderate 100–200
- Severe <100

ARDS could be a complication of chokes or AGE resulting from lung injury. The mechanism of pulmonary barotrauma with parenchymal tissue damage might be quite similar to ventilator-induced lung injury (VILI). However, in diving, the pressure and volume increase is far more important than the time factor. On rapid ascent, gas volumes expand or pressure increases at fast rate. Additionally, dissolved inert gas turns into bubbles. These bubbles get trapped and cause VGE of the lungs and may affect significantly the pulmonary perfusion and cause lung damage.

There are several mechanisms related to VILI [8, 15], which may also contribute to diving-related injuries. Increased volume may lead to physical disruption (stress failure). In particular, high volumes (volutrauma) cause damage in the blood-gas barrier, probably related to increased longitudinal forces acting on the blood vessels. Alveoli and terminal bronchioles share common wall structures. Forces are thereby transferred to neighbouring lung units. This is called interdependence. Under physiological conditions, this is believed to help in maintaining uniformity of alveolar size and surfactant function. However, if the lung is unevenly expanded, these forces vary considerably. When alveoli collapse and reopen, the transpulmonary pressure could be theoretically enhanced by more than fourfold. In recruitment-derecruitment, occluded alveoli require higher airway pressure to restore patency. The pressure related to reopen occluded airways is inversely proportional to first diameter. The resulting shear stress may damage the airways. During a rapid ascent in diving, all the above might contribute to the injury, as in addition to pulmonary changes increased gas volumes and hence pressure are to be expected. Experimental models of VILI described interstitial oedema and alveolar flooding as well as endothelial damage. It seems to release a variety of proinflammatory mediators like thromboxane B_2, platelet activating factor and cytokines. These might exert the damaging effect, which led to the term "biotrauma".

If pathological changes reduce pulmonary air flow, lung distension during ascent may be possible. The expanding air can't or can only partially escape. The thin alveolar skin might tear by overstretching the alveoli. Usually it is not a single large defect but a number of small defects' summation causes the symptoms of ppPBT. Particularly lung distensions in central areas are a common cause of pulmonary barotrauma. This acute lung injury can result in mediastinal emphysema, pericardial emphysema, subclavian emphysema, peritoneal emphysema or pneumothorax. The release of gas into the intercellular space seems to be purely mechanical and easy to understand. The release of gas into the vascular system is another assumed mechanism in diving accidents, leading to arterial gas embolisms. The theory behind this is that a tear in alveoli may lead to a direct flow of gas bubbles into the vascular system, which eventually end up in the arterial system. Gas bubbles can reach organs like heart and central nervous system and cause serious damage. However, AGE in combination of PBT and rapid ascent is probably a rather complex process and not solely related to simple overexpansion of the lungs and air entry of gas bubbles into the vascular system. AGE via intrapulmonary shunt or retrograde CVGE need to be considered to be involved in this process too.

Gas bubbles entering the bloodstream have usually a small radius. The accumulation of small gas bubbles leads to a formation of larger bubbles. The gas bubbles can cause an embolic occlusion of the arterial vessels (arterial gas embolism = *AGE*) resulting in reduced blood supply of affected tissues (ischaemia). Usually, the smaller arterial or capillary vessels are affected. Small air bubbles can pass through capillaries and are transported through the venous system to the lungs, where they are finally eliminated. Occlusions of a blood vessel result in tissue damage (ischaemic hypoxydosis). In addition, haemorrhaging and oedema formation cause further reduction in local perfusion and affect the remaining perfusions of collaterals. Tissues become irreversibly damaged and necrotic by ineffective perfusion. Depending on location and function of the damaged organ, effects are more or less severe. Damages in the *peripheral* lung can lead to gas entering the pleura or mediastinum. Hereby, air remains outside the blood vessels (extravascular). This may result in mediastinal emphysema or pneumothorax. Mediastinal emphysema is gas formation within the mediastinum. Gas usually travels to the skin

23

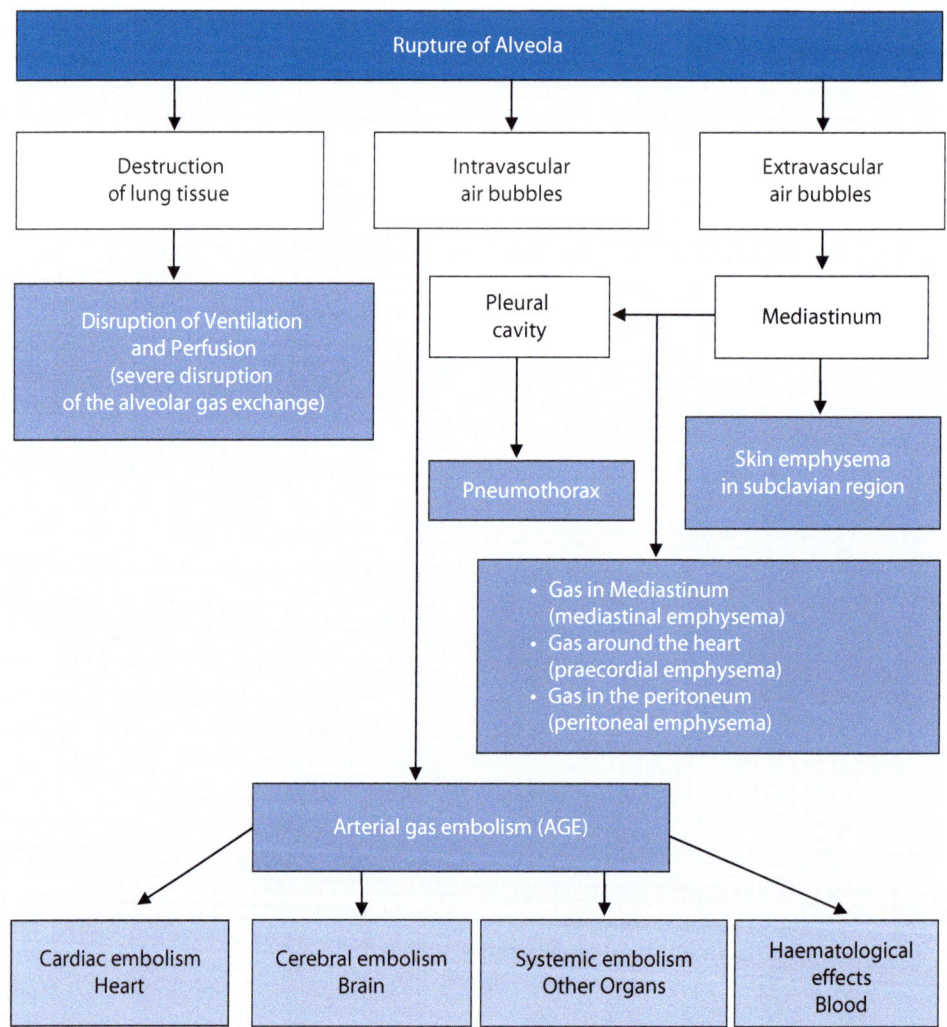

□ **Fig. 23.8**   Overview of damaging effects of positive-pressure pulmonary barotrauma

above the clavicle, resulting in a percutaneous emphysema. Due to the massive destruction of alveoli in a pulmonary barotrauma, ventilation and perfusion are commonly disrupted, as pulmonary gas exchange is severely reduced (□ Fig. 23.8).

23.2.1.2 **Symptoms**

■ **Destruction of lung tissue**

Pulmonary barotrauma may cause an explosive exhalation and a sudden high-pitched scream after reaching the surface. Damaged lung tissue may also cause coughing, breathing difficulties (dyspnea) and haemoptysis. The most severe form of hyperbaric pulmonary barotrauma can cause air to enter the bloodstream (see also AGE). The result of destruction of normal lung tissue and of bleeding in the functional lung tissue (parenchyma) disrupts gas exchange (ventilation) and pulmonary perfusion. Serious respiratory problems, lowering of SaO_2 in pulse oximetry, altered level of

Fig. 23.9 Occurrence of AGE during ascent, upon and after surfacing

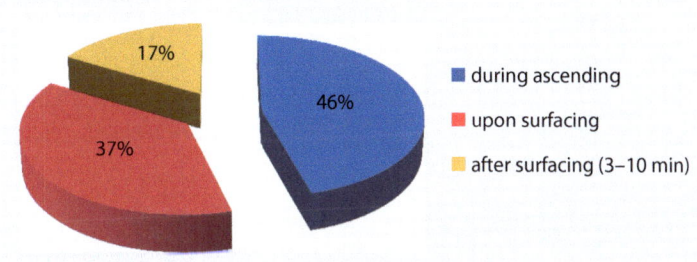

- 17%
- 37%
- 46%
- during ascending
- upon surfacing
- after surfacing (3–10 min)

consciousness and cardiovascular effects are symptoms related to this.

Arterial Gas Embolism (AGE)

Symptoms of gas embolisms may vary, since the clinical picture depends on the affected organ. Usually, the central nervous system and heart are affected. In a small case study with only a small number ($n = 24$), 4 mild cases occurred 3–10 min after surfacing, 11 during ascending and 9 upon surfacing. The more severe cases were either during ascending or just after surfacing within 1 min [7]. Even if these cases were related to submarine escape training, this data of AGE might be able to be transferred to diving (Fig. 23.9).

Arterial gas embolisms can occur in hyperbaric pulmonary barotrauma as well as in DCS. They may differ in their aetiology, but are very similar or identical in their symptoms.

Cerebral Arterial Gas Embolism (ceAGE)

Cerebral blood supply arises from the left and right common carotid arteries and the left and right vertebral arteries. The carotid arteries split up into the internal and external carotid artery. The external carotid artery supplies mainly scalp and face. The internal carotid artery supplies blood to 3/5 of the cerebrum, except parts of the temporal and occipital lobes. The vertebral arteries supply blood the other 2/5 of the cerebrum, parts of the cerebellum and brainstem. The cerebellar arteries arise mainly from the vertebral arteries, but also from the basilar arteries. The two vertebral arteries form together the basilar arteries. The posterior cerebral arteries arise from the basilar arteries. The vertebral and carotid arteries form at the base of the brain the circle of Willis. From there the main three cerebral arteries arise and supply other parts of the brain (Fig. 23.10).

Supply Areas of the Cerebral Arteries

- *Anterior cerebral artery (ACA)*: medial cortex, frontal lobe, parts of the temporal lobe, thalamus, anterior internal capsule, basal ganglia, corpus callosum, anterior hypothalamus and commissure
- *Medial cerebral artery (MCA)*: parts of the frontal lobe, temporal lobe, parietal lobe, parts of the occipital lobe, anterior commissure, basal ganglia and motor cortical fields
- *Posterior cerebral artery (PCA)*: parts of the occipital lobe, temporal lobe, thalamus, pons, hypothalamus, internal capsule, tectum, tegmentum and choroid plexus
- *Lenticulostriate arteries (deep penetrating arteries)*: pallidum, putamen, thalamus, caudate, pons and internal capsule
- *Choroid artery*: choroid plexus (produces the liquor), amygdala, insular cortex and cortex areas of voice and hearing centres

If blood supply to the brain is compromised, extra - and intracranial anastomoses offer collateral blood supply bypassing the occluded vessels.

23

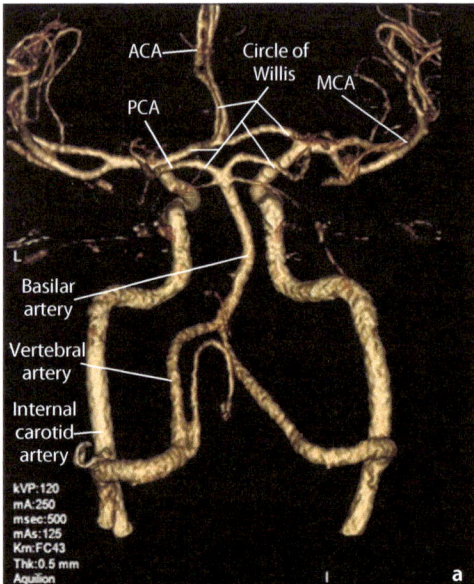

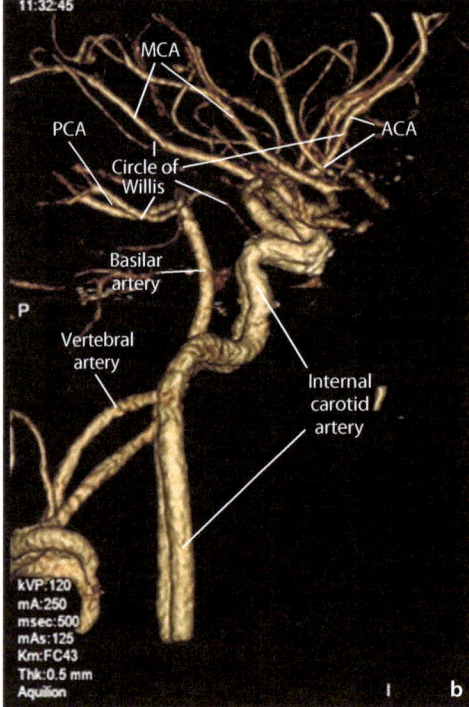

□ **Fig. 23.10   a, b** CT angiogram of cerebral arteries. a frontal view, **b** side view. ACA anterior cerebral artery, MCA medial cerebral artery, PCA posterior cerebral artery

- ■ **Additional Damaging Factors to Contribute to Cerebral Ischaemia**
- — Cerebral oedema
- — Reperfusion syndrome
- — Increase intracranial pressure

The lack of perfusion results in a complex biochemical cascade. This cascade evolves within a few seconds to minutes and continues normally for 2–3 h, sometimes for days, even if normal blood flow is restored. Due to impaired perfusion, there is a lack of oxygen (ischaemia) and reduced glucose supply in brain cells. These energy sources are necessary for upkeeping ion gradients and hence for neural activity. ATP starts to decline. ATP is responsible for the cell's energy exchange. The energy failure by itself is not the main cause for cell death. An ATP deficit of 5–10 min is usually tolerated. The loss of ATP in the affected neurons causes a disruption of the Na^+-K^+-ATPase, Ca^{2+}-H^+-ATPase. This leads to a reversal of Na^+-Ca^{2+} transporter resulting in increase in intracellular Na^+, Ca^{2+} and Cl^- concentrations and efflux of K^+. Embolic events of the CNS don't commonly result in a complete loss of perfusion but in a partial one. A long-standing poor energy supply causes brain cells to change to anaerobic metabolism. By-products like lactate and hydrogen ions (H^+) accumulate. In particular the H^+ facilitates the ferrous-iron-mediated free-radical mechanism, which leads to irreversible neural damage. Increased intracellular calcium leads to a release of glutamate. Glutamate itself stimulates AMPA and NMDA receptors, which promote water and calcium transport into cells. Increased Ca^+-accumulation and accompanied inflow of water causes rapid swelling of the neurons (cytotoxic oedema). Excess calcium, sodium and ADP leads to an increased activity by proteases and lipases, high levels of mitochondrial reactive oxygen species (mtROS) and increased use of ATP, resulting in the destruction of cells (excitotoxicity). Additionally, Ca^{2+}-dependent activation of nNOS (neuronal nitric oxide synthase) leads to increased NO production, contributing to the oxidative stress and excitotoxicity. Another isoform of NOS, the iNOS (induced nitric oxide synthase), seems to play a role in the ischaemia-reperfusion injury and the development of apoptosis [17]. Under normal conditions, iNOS seems to be only minimally expressed. However, due to ischaemia-related cell damages, iNOS might be increased [5, 16]. iNOS increases NO, which in return causes further cell damages. The third isoform, eNOS (endothelial nitric oxide synthase) promotes neutrophil adherence in the endothelium. The isoform eNOS is the major component in in the NOS group. Gas embolisms cause a significant damage to the endothelium. Vascular endothelial growth factor (VEGF) seems to be involved in the development of ischaemia reperfusion injury (IR injury) and oedema in ischaemic tissue. VEGF activates eNOS and hence promotes NO production during ischaemia and the early phases of ischaemic-reperfusion injury. Excessive NO promotes mtROS resulting in cell damage. But NO also seems to form together with the oxygen radical O_2^- peroxynitrite (ONOO⁻). ONOO⁻ has also cell-damaging effects. Damage to the endothelium leads to leukocyte adhesions mediated by neutrophil β-2 integrin causing intracellular adhesion molecule ICAM-1 activation on the leukocyte surface. This mediates leukocyte adhesion to the endothelium, via interaction with the neutrophil CD 18 molecules [1, 14]. Inhibition of iNOS as well as nNOS seems to be neuroprotective and inhibition of eNOS neurotoxic (◘ Fig. 23.11).

Accumulated toxins cause damage to adjacent nerve cells. In addition, disrupted perfusion causes oedema in the adjacent tissues, leading to further damage. The cerebral oedema can be differentiated into two categories. *Cytotoxic oedema* can be caused by hypoxia, ischaemia-reduced energy supply, hypotonic hyper-hydration, hepatogenic encephalopathy, intoxication (e.g. CO, cyanide) or microbial toxins. A diving accident falls also under this category. There is a loss of Na^+-K^+ pump. Sodium and water thus accumulate in cells and cause damage. The blood-brain barrier is hereby intact. *Vasogene oedemas* are caused by damage to blood vessels (vascular lesions), which increases permeability of cerebral capillaries. Large molecules can penetrate the blood vessel wall for up to an hour and small molecules for up to 24 h. The molecules, mainly proteins, pull the water into the extravascular space by osmotic forces. The blood-brain barrier is disrupted. Vasogenic oedemas usually follow the cytotoxic oedema within hours to days. The cytotoxic and the vasogenic oedema can increase intracranial pressure and structures of the brain, could be trapped and may cause a herniation of the cerebellar tentorium.

Ischaemia of the brain is divided in two zones, the *core ischaemic zone* and the *ischaemic penumbra*. The core ischaemic zone is the area with severe ischaemia (perfusion below 10–25%). The loss of glucose and oxygen depletes rapidly energy stores and leads to necrosis. The penumbra is mild to moderate ischaemic but still has viable cerebral tissue for several hours. The penumbra still gets some blood supply from collateral arteries. If the perfusion is not restored, the tissue in the penumbra will die as well.

During the *reperfusion syndrome* (*post-ischaemic anoxia*), metabolism and perfusion increase in surrounding intact brain tissues (rebound effect). The result of this is an extraction of blood supply of intact tissue from the damaged tissue (*intracranial steal syndrome*). This and increased metabolic changes of affected brain tissue cause additional damage.

Intracranial blood pressure increases with injuries of brain tissue. As a result, *intracranial pressure* increases mainly due to increased cerebral blood pressure. With elevated intracranial pressure, cerebral blood pressure increases again. Thus, a vicious circle evolves. Signs of increased intracranial pressure are

23

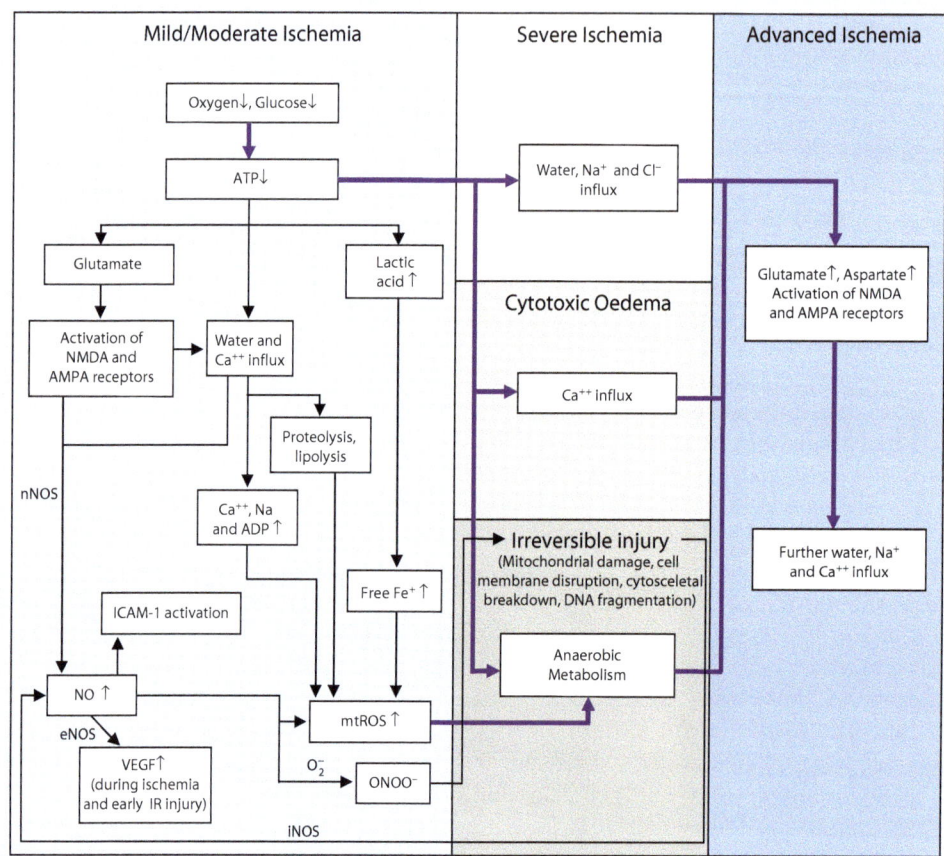

■ **Fig. 23.11**   Ischaemic biochemical cascade: AMPA α-amino-3-hydroxy-5-methylisoxazole-4-propionic acid, NMDA N-methyl-D-aspartate, NO nitric oxide, NOS NO-synthase, ROS reactive oxygen species, VEFG vascular endothelial growth factor

increasing, sometimes severe headaches, vomiting, simultaneous hypertension and bradycardia and various neurological symptoms. Embolic cerebral occlusions cause various unspecific symptoms. Often fatigue and malaise are common signs. A reduced perfusion may cause a dysregulation of the autonomic nervous system, particularly if the brainstem is affected. The implications of this are pronounced cardiovascular and respiratory effects. Cerebral gas embolisms often result in a temporary loss of consciousness. Further symptoms are depending on which cerebral segment is affected by the gas embolism. The symptoms mainly tend to occur unilaterally.

■ **Symptoms of Gas Embolisms in the Brain**
— Headache
— Visual field defect
— Monocular or binocular visual loss
— Diploplia
— Loss of consciousness
— Hemisensory defects
— Hemiparesis, monoparesis and quadriparesis (rare)
— Slurred speech
— Perceptual disorder
— Ataxia
— Vertigo
— Dysarthria

- Abnormal fatigue, malaise and sudden decrease of consciousness
- Hyperreflexia in the acute phase
- Anisocoria
- Facial drop
- Fine motor skills disturbance/dysdiado-chokinesia (cerebellar involvement)

■ **Overview of the Symptoms of the Blood Supply Regions**
- *Anterior cerebral artery*: contralateral hemiparesis (especially legs), apathy, confusion, incontinence, apraxia and mental symptoms (akinetic mutism, mania, delusions, delirium, depression, diminished affect)
- *Medial cerebral artery*: contralateral hemiparesis, aphasia (inability to speak or understand spoken words), apraxia, dysarthria, contralateral homonymous hemianopia, monocular vision loss, unawareness of deficits and nonverbal memory impaired (right-sided MCA only)
- *Posterior cerebral artery*: contralateral homonymous hemianopia, one-sided contralateral cortical loss of vision, colour blindness, failure to see to and fro movements, memory loss, unilateral third brain nerve palsy, verbal dyslexia and hemiballism
- *Vertebrobasliar artery*: single-sided or double-sided brain nerve failures (nystagmus, vertigo, dysphagia, dysarthria, diplopia, blindness, deafness, tinnitus), double hemisensory or hemiparesis, spastic paresis, sensory disturbance with contralateral paralysis, intractable vomiting, decline in consciousness and coma
- *Lacunar infarction*: unilateral motor losses (hemiparesis, hemiplegia of face, arm or leg), ataxic hemiparesis (develops often with delay over hours and days), dysarthria and clumsy hand or sensory impairment and mixed sensorimotor stroke (hemiparesis/hemiplegia) with ipsilateral sensory impairment

Midbrain and brainstem involvement usually leads to coma and significant cardiovascular and respiratory symptoms. Increased intracranial pressure by oedema and bleeding causes initially strong headaches. Subsequently, stuporous and comatose symptoms will develop.

■ **Staging with Secondary Brainstem and Midbrain Involvement**
Stage I:
- Extension of legs and plantar flexion induced by pain stimulus of the feet.
- Small pupils with decreased light response, reduced oculocephalic reflex (ipsilateral deviation in caloric stimulation with cold water) and switch from divergence-convergence position.
- Breathing and pulse rate are significantly accelerated; body temperature and blood pressure increase.

Stage II (Midbrain Syndrome):
- Generalised spasmodic flexion of the limbs and trunk
- Absence of the oculocephalic reflex (ipsilateral deviation in caloric stimulation with cold water, tonic-tonic dissociated)
- Tachypnoea (superficial and regularly "machine-like")

Stage III (Bulbar Brain Syndrome):
- Reduced to vanished muscle tone
- Maximum wide, light rigid pupils
- Cessation of spontaneous breathing

■ **Cardiac Arterial Gas Embolism (caAGE)**
Coronary arteries arise from the aorta and supply the heart with oxygen-rich blood. Cardiac blood vessels are muscular-type blood vessels and hence produce uniform blood supply by adjusting perfusion via vasoconstriction and dilatation. Coronary blood vessels also have anastomoses. If vessels get occluded and cannot meet the blood supply of a particular area of the heart, blood could be partially supplied via these anastomoses. However, due to their small diameter blood, this collateral blood supply is limited. A reduction in perfusion can lead to ischaemia and destruction of affected heart muscles. Cardiac arterial gas embolisms

23

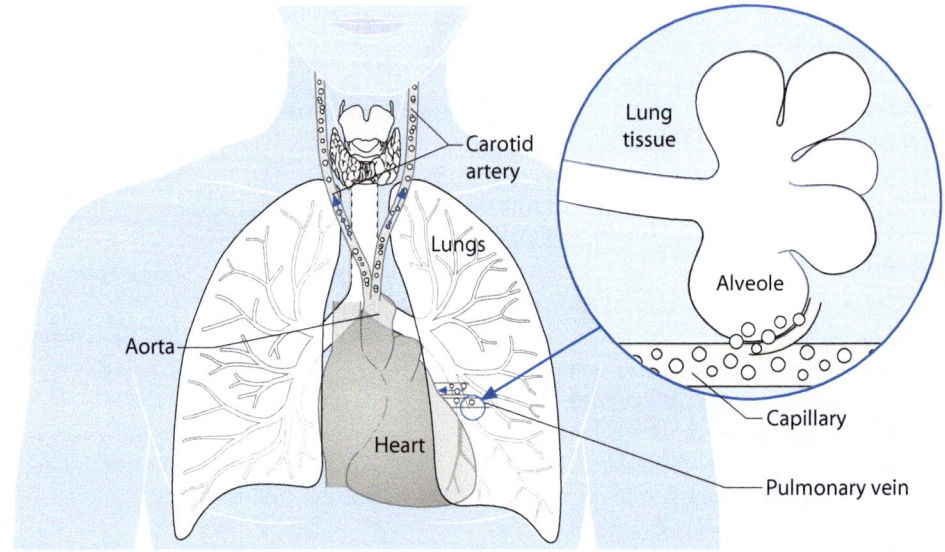

Carotid
artery

Lung
tissue

Lungs

Alveole

Aorta

Capillary

Heart

Pulmonary vein

◻ **Fig. 23.12**   AGE/ arterial gas embolism (With friendly permission of Ecomed)

are rare. But in case of chest pain, even if it is associated with other causes like pneumothorax or chokes, an ECG and serial troponins should be obtained.

Typical signs of a cardiac gas embolism are similar to acute myocardial infarction and vary in their intensity. Patients usually complain of severe pain behind the sternum. The pain can be described as crushing or heavy. However, any pain or discomfort in the chest area should be considered to be of cardiac origin, till proven otherwise. Depending on the location of the coronary embolus, pain can radiate to the neck, to the arm (especially the left side) or in the upper abdomen. Simultaneously diaphoresis, impending doom, nausea, vomiting, general feeling of weakness, pallor, restlessness and shortness of breath are often associated with cardiac chest pain. In general, approximately 20% of myocardial infarctions are "silent". This means that no pain symptoms at all are experienced. However, this mainly is a feature associated with diabetic neuropathy. An exclusion of a myocardial infarction requires a normal ECG and negative troponins (specific cardiac enzyme in myocardial infarction). Troponins need to be

repeated approximately 6–8 h after onset of the initial symptoms. If there is a suspicion of coronary heart disease, investigations should be initiated at a later stage (EST, thallium scan, stress ECHO, angiogram), even if acute myocardial infarction is ruled out (◻ Fig. 23.12).

▪ **Symptoms**
– Pain/discomfort behind the sternum radiating to the left arm and neck or upper abdomen
– Shortness of breath
– Anxiety
– Fear of death
– Nausea and vomiting
– Pallor
– Diaphoresis
– Weakness

▪ **Pneumothorax**
Symptoms are depending on the extent of the pneumothorax. The air flow in a pneumothorax is directed out of the lungs into the pleural cavity, which is the intermediate gap between pleura and lung. A small pneumothorax causes a slight detachment of smaller parts. Usually

no other symptoms exist apart from dyspnea. Chest pain, especially on deep inspiration or coughing, might be another sign. The pain is sharp and localised increased. Shortness of breath increases according to the extent of the displacement of the lung tissue. On the side of the detachment, the respiratory sounds are diminished and percussion is hyper-resonant. A larger pneumothorax can cause hypotension, increased heart rate and decreased oxygen saturation. If the lung collapses completely, pneumothorax can even become life threatening. A severe complication is the *tension pneumothorax*. Air flows via a valve mechanism from the lungs into the pleural gap and gets trapped. The incoming air in the pleural gap is increasingly displacing the lung even to the unaffected other side. The increasing pressure moves heart, trachea and the unaffected lung to the opposite side. The displacement leads to a compression of the intact lung, vena cava and heart. This causes an increase of resistance of pulmonary vessels, which results in a decreased venous blood supply of the vena cava and cardiac output as well as an increase of venous pressure. As a result blood pressure drops rapidly. Severe progressive symptoms are expected with a tension pneumothorax. Acute-onset respiratory distress directly after the dive, with unilateral thoracic pain radiating into the shoulder and sometimes into the abdomen may develop. Shortness of breath is expected to increasingly intensify. On examination tachycardia, cyanosis (blue lips and fingernails) and hypotension are typical signs. Increased jugular venous pressure (JVP) with visible neck veins in a position with >30 degrees elevation of the upper body associated with shock symptoms and a deviation of the trachea can be observed. Percussion of the affected side compared to the normal side is hyper-resonant. On auscultation, a lack of respiratory sounds on the affected side can be noted. The unaffected side is normal on examination. The investigation of choice is an USS or an inspiratory and expiratory CXR. After exhalation, a pneumothorax is more pronounced on CXR. A demarcation of the parenchyma of the lung and the

absence of lung vessels are typical radiological signs. A small pneumothorax can be missed on an inspiratory CXR, but may be visible on an expiratory CXR. M-mode USS seems to have a higher sensitivity than CXR. Moreover, it can be not only used for diagnostic but also for therapeutic purposes. Absence of signs of the normal aerated lung like "lung sliding", "B-lines", "comet tail artefacts", and the presence of "A-lines" and "lung point sign" are indicative signs in ultrasonography of a pneumothorax. CT has the highest sensitivity and is the gold standard but is in clinical settings often not feasible to use (■ Figs. 23.13, 23.14, 23.15 and 23.16).

■ **Symptoms of a Tension Pneumothorax**
- Shortness of breath
- Chest pain
- Tachycardia
- Hypotension
- Cyanosis
- Side difference on percussion
- Side difference in breath sounds
- Shock symptoms
- Increased JVP
- USS or CXR (expiratory)

■ **Mediastinal Emphysema**
In general, an expansion of tissue due to gas is called emphysema. Mediastinal emphysemas are extremely rare. The main cause of it is an excessive intrapulmonal pressure. Statistics showed that there is a slight increased risk for divers, which are breathing against increased respiratory resistance at a nearly empty scuba tank at shallow dives and normal ascent rate. Gas may enter the interstitial pulmonary space when alveoli rupture. Along the bronchi, gas reaches the mediastinal space via the hilum region. The hilum area is a transition area between lungs and mediastinum, in which large airways as well as blood and lymphatic vessels are present. From the lung defect, free gas enters regions above the clavicle and form a skin emphysema. Gas can also accumulate in the peritoneal cavity and the heart (precardiac space). Symptoms of mediastinal emphysema

23

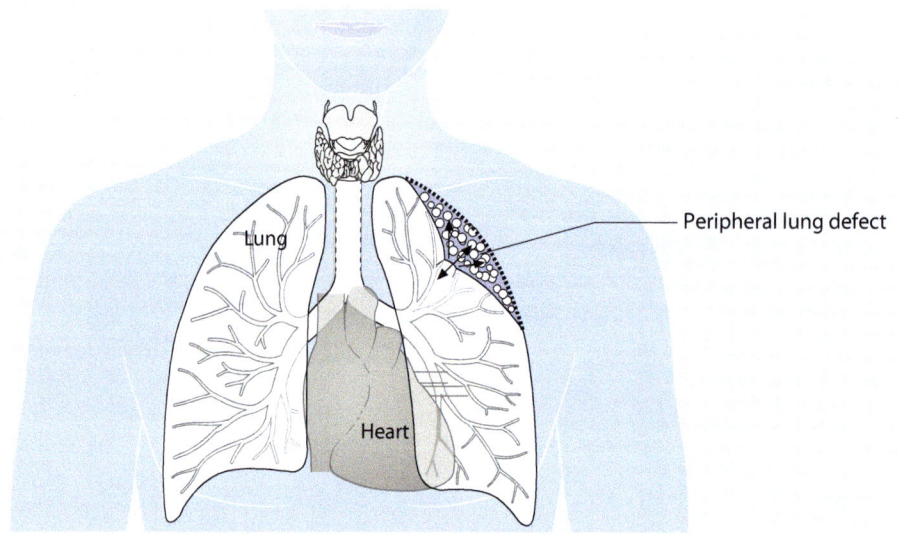

Peripheral lung defect

Lung

Heart

◘ Fig. 23.13 Pneumothorax (With kind permission of Ecomed)

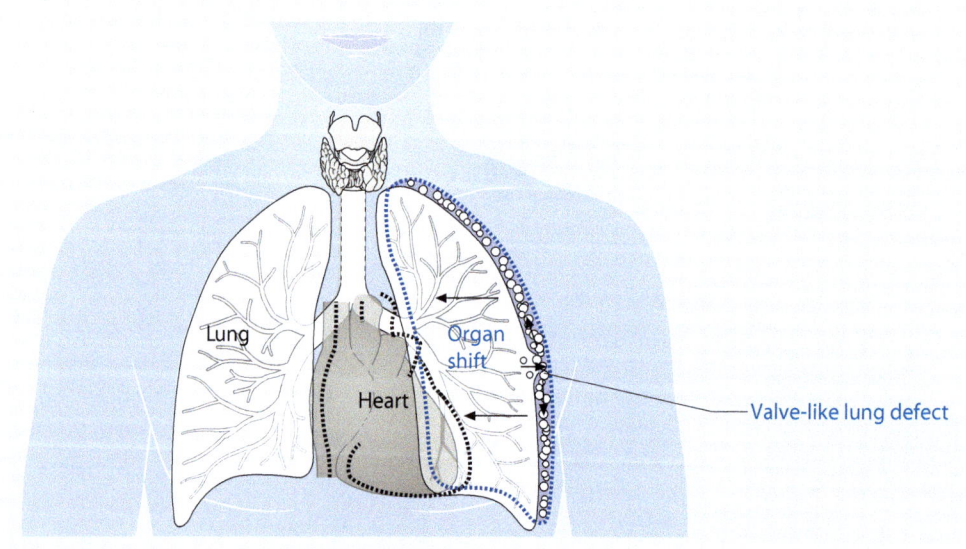

Lung

Organ shift

Heart

Valve-like lung defect

◘ Fig. 23.14 Tension pneumothorax (With kind permission of Ecomed)

can occur immediately or delayed by few hours. Symptoms are subtle changes of voice or hoarseness, dyspnoea, dysphagia, retrosternal pressure, tachycardia, loss of consciousness, shock, cyanosis and low blood pressure. Skin emphysema in the subclavian region expresses with swollen skin that discreetly crackles when touched (◘ Figs. 23.17 and 23.18) [3].

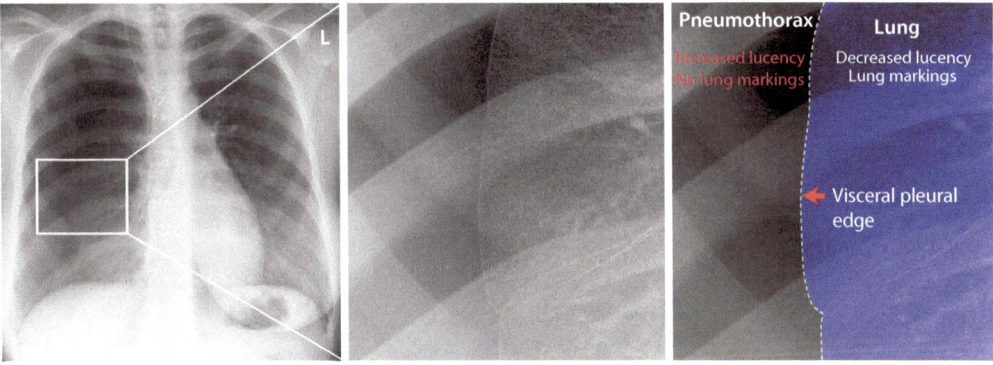

Fig. 23.15 Pneumothorax. (From Tilmann 2010)

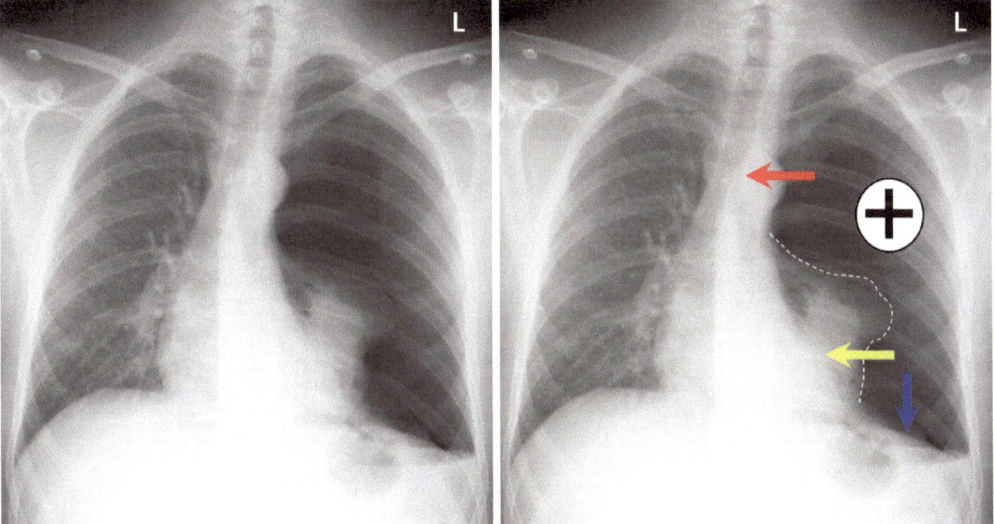

Fig. 23.16 Tension pneumothorax with right-sided tracheal deviation (*red arrow*). (From Tilmann 2010)

- **Symptoms of the Mediastinal Emphysema**
- Hoarseness
- Dyspnoea
- Dysphagia
- Retrosternal pressure
- Tachycardia, hypotonus
- Crackling skin emphysema
- Oedematous swelling of the skin of the subclavian region
- XR shoes dark, radiolucent line along the heart contour

With exemption of the mediastinal emphysema, all pulmonary barotraumas occur during or within minutes of ascending to the surface!

23.2.1.3 Treatment

See decompression sickness/treatment for the treatment of *AGE* due to a hyperbaric pulmonary barotrauma.

Patients with *pneumothorax* should be positioned on the side of the affected lung, so that the still functional lung can unfold freely. A small pneumothorax with asymptomatic

23

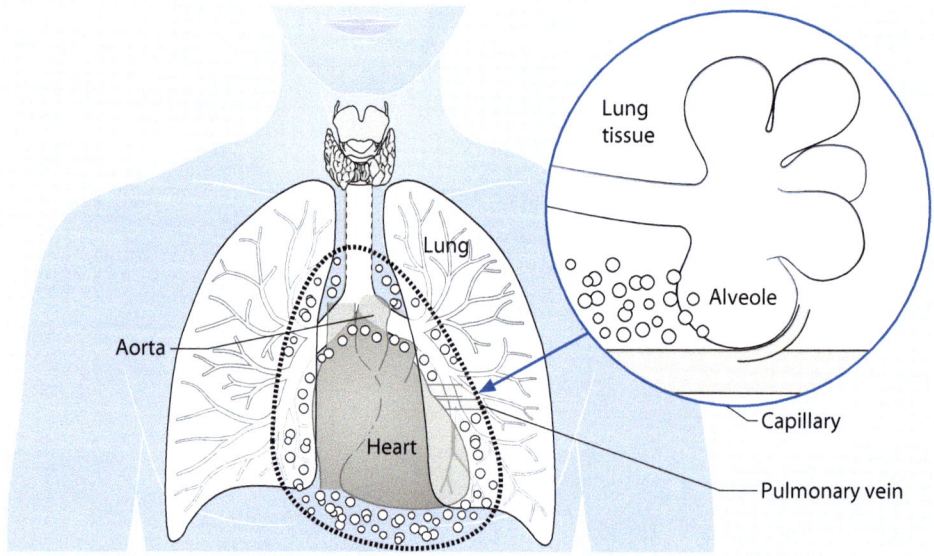

■ **Fig. 23.17**   Mediastinal emphysema. (With kind permission of Ecomed)

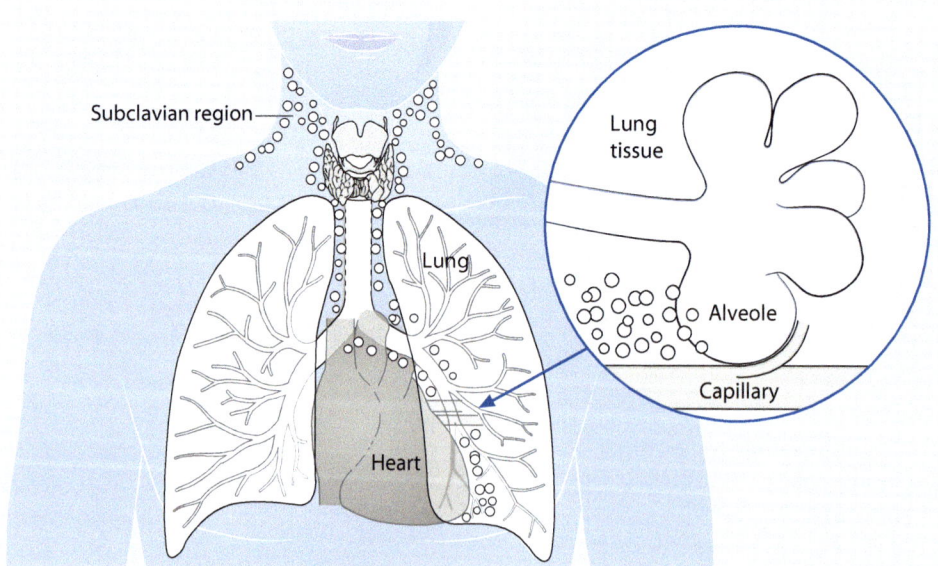

■ **Fig. 23.18**   Skin emphysema of the subclavian region. (With kind permission of Ecomed)

patient might only require watchful waiting, as some are resolving spontaneously without intervention. Symptomatic but stable patients require a small-bore catheter or chest tube. Tension pneumothorax requires immediate treatment with pressure relief via large-bore cannulas or pleural cannulas. The preferred location after Matthys for the immediate interventions is the second ICR (= intercostal) medioclavicular (parallel axis to the vertical body axis in the middle of the collarbone). A pleural suction drainage can be inserted at a later stage. A chest tube or pleural drainage (Bülau) can be inserted in the fourth ICR of the posterior axillary line (parallel to the vertical body axis in the axilla). The other location for the tube insertion in the second ICR of the medioclavicular line (Monaldi) is rarely used. To avoid a damage of the lung and intercostal muscles, only a small incision of the skin is required. Preferably the incision should be 1–2 ICR below the insertion side. The skin then can be moved over the insertion side, and the intercostal muscles can be perforated and widened with a blunt object, like an artery forceps. The insertion side of the chest tube should follow the upper side of the ribs (nerves and vessels are on the lower side of the ribs!). The chest drain is then pushed up to the ICR 1–2. The chest tube can be fixed with sutures (silk) on the site of the insertion to avoid a displacement of the chest tube. Depending on the extent of the pneumothorax, a pigtail catheter can be used instead of a large-bore chest tube. This has the advantage of a relatively easy insertion process with fewer traumas to the tissue.

For uncomplicated cases of *mediastinal emphysema* with asymptomatic course, only observation is required. In a mild course, 6–10 mL/min 100% oxygen via mask over 4–6 h should be applied. In serious cases, when cardiovascular system is affected, intensive medical treatment may be necessary. Mediastinal emphysemas often are associated with pneumothorax or gas embolisms.

Patients with small pneumothorax should have a CXR at 0 and 6 h. If the patient is stable and there is no enlargement of the pneumothorax, the patient can be discharged and followed up with another CT 2 days and 1 month later.

Therapy

■ **AGE**

Initial treatment
- Stabilisation of vital functions
- 100% oxygen by mask (rebreather 6 L/min; non-rebreather 10 L/min)

- Intravenous access, isotonic sodium chloride solution for rehydration, aiming for a urine output of 0.5 mL/kg BW/h) [12]
- Monitoring
- Transport to the nearest recompression chamber

Follow-up treatment (see also decompression sickness/treatment)
- Pressure chamber treatment ASAP aiming for <4 h (exclude pneumothorax before HBOT!):
  - Table 6, minor symptoms (◘ Fig. 24.20)
  - Table 6a or Comex 30, major symptoms (◘ Figs. 24.21 and 24.24)
  - Table 4 or 7, if required (◘ Figs. 24.18 and 24.22)

■ **Pneumothorax**
- Lateral positioning on the affected lung side at an unconscious patient
- Mild pneumothorax: observation only
- Severe pneumothorax: pleural drainage
- Tension pneumothorax: Instant pressure relief of the affected side (e.g. with large-bore cannula in the second ICR in the medioclavicular line, above the ribs) followed by pleural drainage
- 100% oxygen
- No HBOT without thoracotomy

■ **Mediastinal Emphysema**
- 100% oxygen
- Mild: observation only
- Severe: intensive medical treatment

23.2.1.4 Prophylaxis

The risk of hyperinflation of the lungs with accelerated ascent rate mainly occurs near surface. The reason for this is that in the areas near-surface volume changes are more pronounced than in greater depth (◘ Table 23.5). An ascent of 10 meters from 40- to 30-meter depth reflects a volume increase of only 25%. However, an ascent from 10 meters to the surface has a 100% volume increase as a result. This means that the volume has doubled. Ascents from 40 to 30 meters would correspond to a change in volume of an ascent from

23

◘ Table 23.5 Ascent rates in correlation to the depth*	
Depth in m	Ascent rates in m/min
<6	6–9
6–18	8–12
18+	16–18

*Diving computers vary slightly in their ascent alarm rates according to certain diving depths. Some computers have only a single ascent alarm rate

2.5 meters to the surface. Ascents from 70 to 30 meters would correspond to ascents from 10 meters to the surface. Hence, the ascent rate should be adjusted to the according depth. Ascent rates additionally are involved in the development of microbubbles to gas bubbles resulting in decompression illness.

> Especially in near-surface areas, ascent rates should be slow with continuous breathing!

Ascent rates should decrease the closer the diver reaches surface. An approximate rule is that the maximum ascent rate correlates to the formula below:

$$v_{asc} = \frac{(d+x) \cdot (0.6 - d \cdot 0.001)}{min}$$

v_{asc} = Ascent rate; d = depth; x = 10 (meter) or 33 (feet)

For example the ascent rate corresponds at 40 m to 28 m/min and at 18 m to 16 m/min. However, the ascent rate may be reduced when decompression time due to supersaturation is included in the calculation. Ascending the last 5 meters to the surface should generally take 3–4 minutes but at least 2 minutes.

If the depth gauge or the dive computer fails, because vison is obstructed by sediments or lack of light, or as various activities (e.g. rescue) hinder to read the depth gauge or dive computer, alternatives to estimate the ascent rate need to be established. The ascent rate of the smallest air bubbles is a good indication for this. The ascent rate of small bubbles is equiva-

lent to approximately 10–18 m/min. Unfavourable events like being unable to release air from the BCD due to positioning or a defect or the loss of the weight belt can lead to an excessive ascent rate. The ascent rate can be minimised by putting out fins, arms and legs, which increase friction.

If a diver notices that his dive buddy stopped breathing and begins to swim erratically to the surface, action needs to be taken quickly. Initially, the dive buddy should be addressed via hand signals, asking if everything is OK and reminding to slow down. If the buddy is not responding or continues ascending, his or her ascent needs to be slowed down to a safe rate. At first, it is important to prevent the excessive ascend rate by reducing buoyancy (exhale, emptying the BCD). A person in panic is a potential hazard for everyone surrounding them. Therefore, an approach to that diver from the back could be considered, if safe.

Rule number one when diving is never hold your breath, always breathe!

23.2.2 Hypobaric Pulmonary Barotrauma (npPBT = Negative-Pressure Pulmonary Barotrauma)

23.2.2.1 Aetiology and Pathogenesis

Critical reductions in lung volume due to rapid descent or extreme levels of freediving can result into hypobaric pulmonary barotrauma. Hypobaric pulmonary barotrauma commonly occurred in helmet divers or in diving bells, which have their own enclosed air space. On rapid pressure reduction or rupture of a hose, for example, vacuum in the lungs is compensated by the collapse of lung tissue itself or by secretions produced by the lung (pulmonary oedema or bleeding). Acute pulmonary oedema results in acute right heart failure. Hypobaric pulmonary barotrauma can also affect freedivers exceeding the freediving limit ("divers squeeze"). Diving with a snorkel longer than 100 cm may cause an inability of the

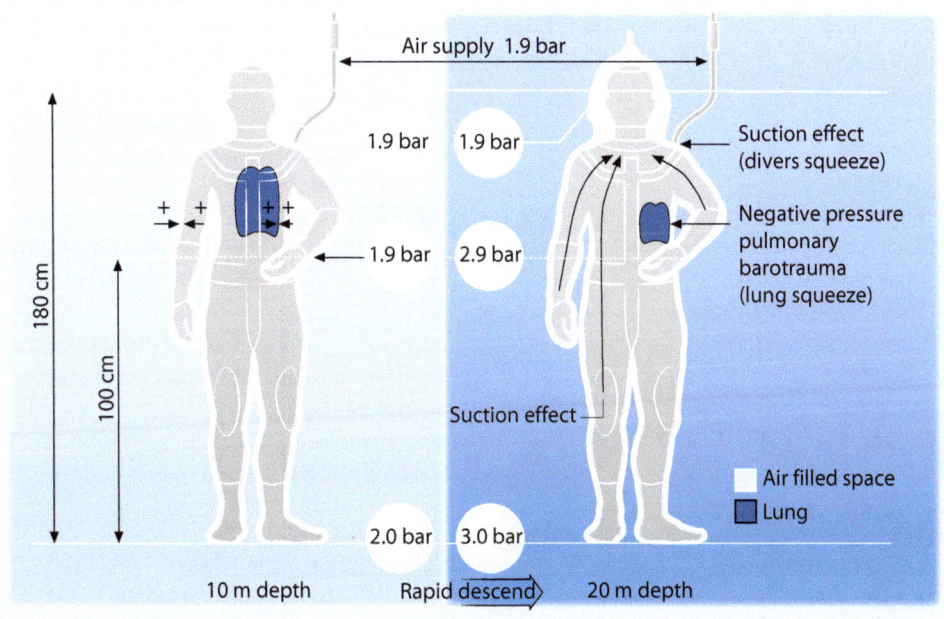

Air supply 1.9 bar

1.9 bar   1.9 bar   — Suction effect
(divers squeeze)

1.9 bar   2.9 bar   — Negative pressure
pulmonary
barotrauma
(lung squeeze)

Suction effect —

☐ Air filled space
■ Lung

2.0 bar   3.0 bar

10 m depth   Rapid descend▷   20 m depth

180 cm   100 cm

◼ Fig. 23.19 Pressure changes of a helmet diver during a rapid descent (With kind permission of Ecomed)

lungs to expand against the ambient pressure. Hypobaric pulmonary barotrauma can develop by using such a snorkel (◼ Fig. 23.19).

- ◼ **Causes that Can Lead to a Hypobaric Pulmonary Barotrauma During Diving**
  - ▬ Freediving beyond 30–50 meters
  - ▬ Snorkelling with a snorkel longer than 1 meter
  - ▬ Sudden pressure reduction in helmet divers or diving bells

23.2.2.2 Symptoms

Hypobaric pulmonary barotrauma is a result of growing vacuum in the lungs caused by increased ambient pressure. It is caused by volume reduction of gas-filled cavities in the lungs. Therefore, the chance of hypobaric pulmonary barotraumas is only given on descending. Damages to the lung can be partially prevented due to its elasticity. Vacuum can be partially compensated simply by a reduction of the lung volume by its own tissue, increased blood pooling in the pulmonary vessels or increased curvature of the diaphragm. However, reduction of pulmonary gas volume is only guaranteed, if air can flow freely. If the air flow rate in small airways is exceeded, small airways collapse and inhibit air exchange between different parts of airways. In addition, minimal lung volume is reached at the level of residual lung volume. Therefore, compensation mechanisms are limited by following factors:

- ▬ *Restricted air flow* limited by the alveolar diameter of approximately 0.2–0.3 mm
- ▬ *Max. air flow speed*: approximately 0.06 L/s (depending on viscosity of the gas and thus also of depth and utilised gas mixtures)
- ▬ *Min. lung volume*: approximately 1.5 L (residual volume)

If these limitations are exceeded, vacuum in the lung and alveoli builds up, causing airways to collapse. Furthermore, fluid (pulmonary oedema) or blood secretion of alveolar vessels leaks into alveoli and pulmonary interstitial space. Due to damages of the lung tissue, pulmonary hypertension develops. The result is right heart failure. Symptoms are severe shortness of breath, respiratory failure,

23

chest pain, tachycardia, increased JVP, cough with bloody mucous discharge (haemoptysis) and general symptoms of shock. This all can lead to cardiovascular failure.

■ **Symptoms of Right Heart Failure**
  - Tachycardia
  - Hypotension
  - Tachypnoea and haemoptysis
  - Increased JVP
  - Shock symptoms
  - Central chest pain
  - Cyanosis

23.2.2.3 Treatment and Prophylaxis

Mild hypobaric pulmonary barotrauma require only normobaric oxygen via mask. Patients should be closely monitored the following 24 h. Pulmonary oedema is visible on CXRs. Pulsoxymetry or regular blood gas analyses are important to assess the progress of respiratory failure. In severe cases, patients may need to be carefully ventilated with PEEP (positive end-expiratory pressure) or CPAP (continuous positive airway pressure)/BiPAP (bilevel positive airway pressure) and 100% O_2. Oxygen saturations should be >92%. The adjustment of ventilation in right heart failure is quite delicate to avoid adverse haemodynamic effects or iatrogenic barotrauma. Hypercapnia should be avoided. A mild hyperventilation without increasing tidal volume might be even beneficial. Intensive monitoring of vital functions is necessary at all times. For symptom relief pre- and afterload could be reduced with nitrates (GTN) or diuretics (frusemide). Nitrates may be administered as a continuous infusion and titrated up to a level, which still allows an adequate blood pressure (systolic BP > 90). Frusemide could be either given as a continuous infusion or as bolus injections. There seems to be no major difference in high doses versus low doses. However, some patients seem to have a diuretic resistance, and the dosage needs to be adjusted. After stabilisation of acute right heart failure, ACE inhibitors, ARBs and beta-blocker are the drugs of choice and might be considered.

Hypotension is the main feature of right heart failure, and a careful volume challenge of 500–1000 mL of normal saline could be considered to increase the blood pressure. This should be only done in conjunction with invasive or noninvasive assessment of the cardiac output. As the right ventricular function is highly volume dependent, a careful balance between preload and afterload is important. If the fluid challenge has no effect on hypotension, vasopressors/inotropes/inodilators (dobutamine, milrinone, levosimendan, norepinephrine, low-dose vasopressin; avoid dopamine and phenylephrine) can be used to elevate the blood pressure. In addition, antibiotic prophylaxis may be considered to prevent infections.

23.3 Paranasal Sinus Barotrauma (PSBT)

Paranasal sinuses include the maxillary sinuses, the frontal sinuses, the sphenoid sinus and ethmoids. All paranasal sinuses are rigid-walled air-filled body cavities, connected via ducts to the nasopharynx and hence to the ambient pressure. They themselves and the connecting ducts are lined with a mucous membrane. The paranasal sinuses are used for resonance amplification of the sound and the weight reduction of the skull bone (◘ Fig. 23.20).

23.3.1 Aetiology and Pathogenesis

During diving paranasal sinuses become only noticeable when the mucous membranes of the connecting ducts become irritated and swollen (common cold, smoking, allergy) or mechanically blocked (anatomical anomalies and lesions such as septal deviation, polyps, hypertrophy). The orifices of the connecting ducts in the nasopharynx have lips that can close like a valve. The frontal sinuses are most commonly affected. If the connection ducts are blocked, the cavities are isolated from their environment and ambient pressure. Hence, gas and secretions remain in the affected sinuses and

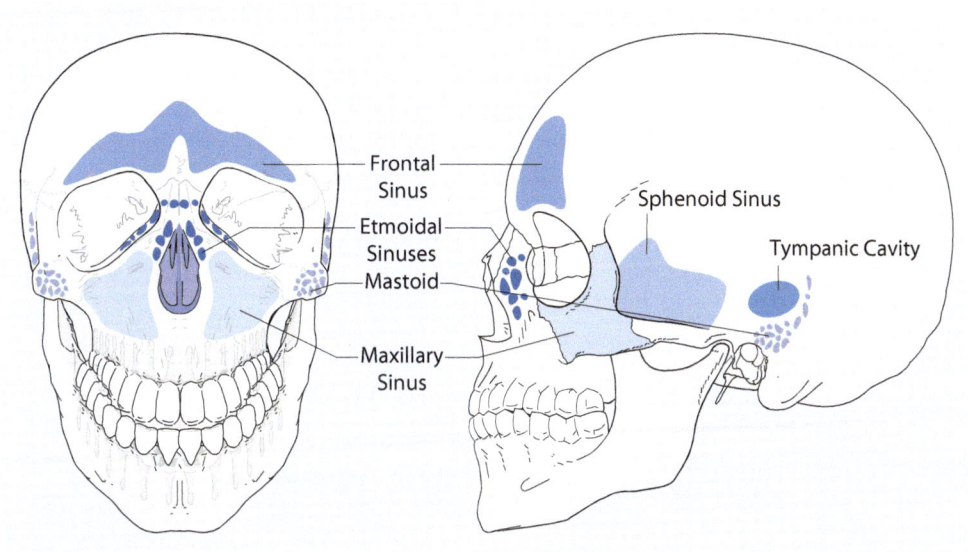

Fig. 23.20 Paranasal sinuses (With kind permission of Ecomed)

pressure can't be equalised. Infectious processes of sinuses can spread to anatomical adjacent structures. Often infections of the frontal sinuses spread to the maxillary sinuses.

Theoretically, paranasal barotrauma can occur during the ascent and descent. Usually it occurs during the descent (*npPSBT = negative-pressure paranasal sinus barotrauma*). Blocked connecting ducts facilitate a vacuum in affected sinuses. As the borders of sinuses are rigid, vacuum causes a pulling effect onto the mucous membranes, which leads to swelling due to the increase perfusion. The result is exudation into the sinuses. At some point, vessels of the mucous membranes may rupture and cause bleeding into the sinus (**Fig. 23.21**).

But it is also possible to develop a sinus barotrauma during the ascent (*ppPSBT = positive-pressure paranasal sinus barotrauma*). Mucous membranes of the connecting ducts can already be swollen while descending, but they are still open and gas exchange is possible. Due to irritation by differences in pressure and salt water connection, ducts may swell during diving and block. During the ascent, air may be trapped and pressure increases within the sinus. A blockage of the

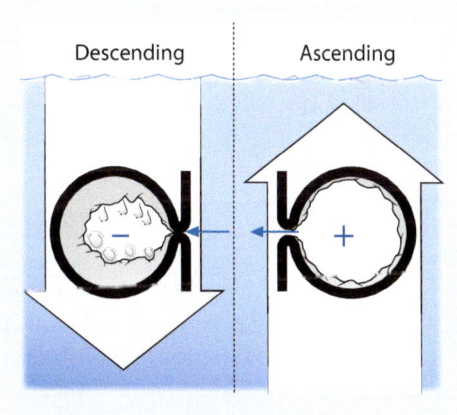

Fig. 23.21 Effects of a vacuum or increased pressure to a sinus during diving (With kind permission of Ecomed)

ducts can also be caused by mucus or anatomical anomalies.

23.3.2 Symptoms

The symptoms of npPSBT are caused by vacuum and of ppPSBT by increased pressure, irritating the sensitive mucous membranes

23

or surrounding tissues and structures. Increasing changes of ambient pressure causes increasing pain. The pain subsides when the pressure or the vacuum is reduced. Vacuum in a PSBT can either be reduced by equalisation, by swelling of mucous membranes, by exudation or by rupturing of vessels of the mucous membranes, filling the cavity with fluid. During the ascent, the increased pressure only can be released by equalisation.

The first symptoms of npPSBT often occur at depths of 2–5 m. Characteristic signs are diffuse headache with dull pain quality. Further increase of pressure results in well-localised, strong, stabbing pain of the forehead or the maxillary sinuses, which may radiate to the surrounding areas. The symptoms of a ppPSBT are similar. However, they can occur at any depth.

If the diver continues descending despite pain and the pain decreases, sudden bleeding into the sinus is most likely. Sometimes damages to the mucous membranes can be even painless. Later, during the ascent blood and exudates may be expressed and enter the mask space, which could be very distressing for the diver. Often, the bleeding continues for some time.

During the ascent, excess gas can usually escape through the connecting ducts. Rarely, these ducts get blocked. A blockage results in increased pressure within the sinuses. Initially, a dull headache is noticed which quickly increases. Usually, excess gas escapes from the sinuses with a squeaking noise through the connecting ducts. If gas can't escape, surrounding structures like for example the thin orbital floor, could be damaged. Air may be trapped under the skull bones (pneumocephalon), which is radiographically detectable. Symptoms are pain on the affected side, periorbital oedema or haematoma, loss of vision, diplopia and a sunken eyeball (enophthalmus). However, ppPSBT is rather rare.

The most common complications of all PSBTs are secondary infections. Symptoms are tenderness over the affected sinus, fatigue, purulent nasal discharge, fever and headache with a certain delay after the trauma.

- **Symptoms of Paranasal Sinus Barotraumas**
  - Initial dull and then stabbing pain on the affected sinus that can radiate in the proximity; improvement or worsening of the symptoms by changing the depth
  - Blood-stained discharge in the mask space during ascending

- **Complications**
  - Pneumocephalon
  - Orbital floor fracture
  - Infections

23.3.3 Treatment

Paranasal sinus barotraumas are usually unpleasant but don't represent a serious injury, even if the discharges of blood and exudates make their way from the nasal cavity to the mask, which might have a quite dramatic appearance. So, there is no reason to panic, if the mask fills up with blood during the ascent. Panic should be strictly avoided to prevent other serious diving accidents. A pneumocephalon and an orbital floor fracture are an emergency and have to be treated in the hospital.

Decongestants (e.g. Otriven®), antibiotics (e.g. amoxicillin with or without clavulanic acid) and red light can be used to prevent secondary infections and relapses. However, the best treatment is prevention. In general, diving should only be performed in good health and the absence of any respiratory or ear, nose and throat infections.

23.3.4 Prophylaxis

If any early symptoms of ppPSBT occur during diving, the dive should be terminated to avoid further damage. If any PSBT occurs, there is a risk that middle ear or lungs might be also affected. This poses a more serious risk of a pulmonary barotrauma. If symptoms occur during the ascent, the diver should try to dive down a few meters, until pain subsides. Then a new attempt to ascend at a reduced ascent rate could be attempted. In case of unexplained PSBT, e.g. in absence of infections, an ENT specialist should be consulted to evaluate, if there are underlying reasons leading to that event, which might require treatment.

23.4 Hypobaric Cutaneous and Ocular Barotrauma (npCBT = Negative-Pressure Cutaneous Barotrauma, npOBT = Negative-Pressure Ocular Barotrauma)

By putting on a helmet, a mask, goggles or a dry suit, artificial air-filled cavities around the body's surface are created. The airspace is necessary for thermal insulation or to facilitate vision and breathing under water.

23.4.1 Aetiology and Pathogenesis

With increasing ambient pressure, a vacuum develops in closed air-filled spaces. If the vacuum can't be neutralised, tissues of affected areas might be damaged. Usually such vacuum is created by descending to a greater depth without sufficient equalisation, for example, when there is insufficient filling of dry suits or masks during the compression phase.

Negative pressure causes suction on affected body regions. To a certain extent, skin or eyes can compensate this by decreasing the volume due to their elastic properties. If the vacuum can't be neutralised, damage occurs by rupturing blood vessels or direct tissue damage. The arising pain is usually caused by rupturing of blood vessels and tissue haemorrhage. The demarcation of the tissue damage is very well defined. Affected are mainly eyes and the skin in the mask area. When diving with goggles, ocular barotrauma is very likely to occur during descending as pressure can't be equalised like in normal diving masks, which have the nose included in their mask space. Episcleral and subconjunctival bleeding are the result of rupturing superficial blood vessels of the eye. Rupture of the vessels between the cornea and iris may also lead to bleeding into the anterior chamber and causes hyphaema. The damage of a barotrauma caused to the skin by a dry suit or a helmet suit can be significant. Due to the large surface area of the body, the blood loss can be extensive and may be haemodynamically significant.

23.4.2 Symptoms

The diver may experience a slight pain in the exposed area due to the suction when diving down. The discomfort rapidly develops into pain, if the diver continues to descend. In contrast to a barotrauma of cavities, the pain doesn't settle after blood vessels rupture as the volume of the blood doesn't compensate the vacuum. Moreover, it infiltrates the tissue. The space occupation of the haemorrhage in tissues themselves can cause pain and leads to bruising. The pain typically persists for a while after diving and is very much localised to the area, which was exposed to the vacuum. If larger areas of the skin are affected, volume shifts to the extracellular/interstitial space and in extensive cases can even lead to hypovolaemia. An accidental rapid descent during helmet diving may affect the entire body area. In this case almost the entire skin of the body may develop a haematoma. This is quite serious and often is associated with hypobaric pulmonary barotrauma. In case of episcleral und subconjunctival bleeding, blood enters the white of the eye. This is commonly painless but might cause some discomfort or irritation. However, the vacuum it causes pain. Bleeding into the anterior chamber (hyphaema) is painful and may affect visual acuity of the affected eye. Hyphaemas due to barotraumas however are rare. Hereby, blood collects in the lower part of the iris and is usually sickle-shaped. The bleeding could be very discrete and not visible to the naked eye. A painful eye always requires slit lamp examination to exclude hyphaema (◘ Figs. 23.22 and 23.23).

23

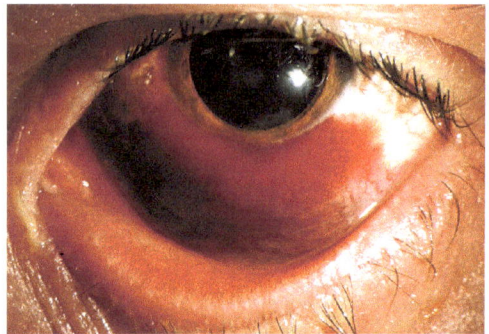

◘ **Fig. 23.22**   Subconjunctival haemorrhage. (From Grehn 2003)

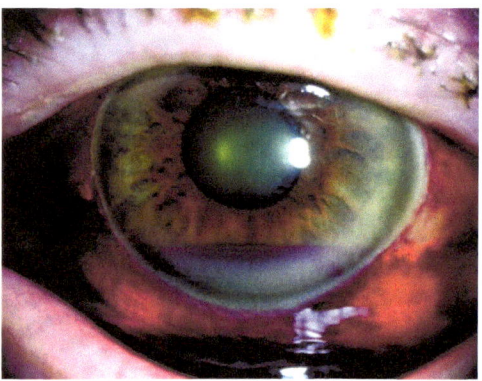

◘ **Fig. 23.23**   Hyphaema. (From Shacknow 2010)

❯❯ Any painful eye should be reviewed by an ophthalmologist.

23.4.3 Treatment

The symptoms can be alleviated by immediate application of cold bandages on the affected skin to reduce additional swelling. If the eyes are affected, laying cool gauze on the closed eyelid may provide symptom relief. Ice should never be applied directly on the skin or the eye to avoid thermal damage. Usually subconjunctival bleeding resolves within days. Absolute bed rest is indicated in hyphaema. In addition, a bilateral cover of the eyes and a topical or systemic administration of steroids may be necessary.

Symptoms suggesting an extensive hypobaric barotrauma of the skin require 24-h

monitoring as potentially associated delayed symptoms of hypobaric pulmonary barotrauma need to be excluded.

23.4.4 Prophylaxis

Diving equipment, which doesn't allow equalisation (e.g. mask without nose part), should not be used for diving. Abrupt descent, especially in the diving helmet and dry suits, should be avoided by all means, as a sudden decrease of pressure can't be balanced out and can lead to serious damage.

23.5 Dental Barotrauma (DBT)

Each of the 32 permanent teeth consists of crown, neck and root. The crown consists of the hard dentine and enamel. Once the teeth are established the enamel can no longer regenerate. The enamel has neither nervous nor collagen fibres. The root of the tooth and the tooth neck are built mainly by dentin. The cementum in the area of the root gives the tooth stability by attaching the periodontal ligaments. Dentin and cement itself can regenerate, as long as the tooth alive. The central part of the tooth contains the nerves containing pulp (◘ Fig. 23.24).

23.5.1 Aetiology and Pathogenesis

Caries is softening of the enamel. The cavities are treated filling with various materials. Gas-filled cavities under the filling may develop after dental treatment due to further tooth decay. Change in pressure (diving, flying) can lead to dental barotrauma. Pressures in the cavity are changing with varying ambient pressure. Commonly, dental barotraumas occur during descending. Main feature is increasing pain during descending. Dental pain can increase during ascending, which is related to the increase of positive pressure in cavities. If the dental filling comes out, pain is expected to disappear suddenly. Dental barotraumas during

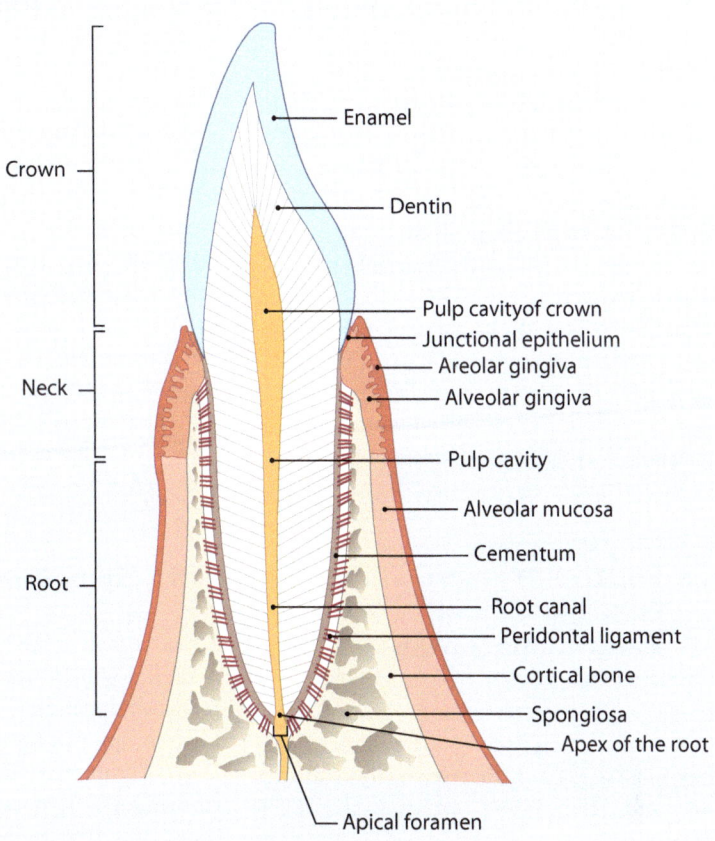

Crown

Neck

Root

Enamel

Dentin

Pulp cavityof crown
Junctional epithelium
Areolar gingiva
Alveolar gingiva

Pulp cavity

Alveolar mucosa

Cementum

Root canal
Peridontal ligament

Cortical bone

Spongiosa
Apex of the root

Apical foramen

ascending, however, are rare. It only can occur if the connection between the cavity under the filling and the oral cavity is occluded during the ascent. During descending, the connection duct might be patent. However, loose particles may dislodge and occlude the duct so that on ascent the pressure can't escape (■ Fig. 23.25).

23.5.2 **Symptoms**

The resulting nerve pain is intense and isolated. The pain might be not localised to the affected tooth only but can be also referred to different areas of the head. Pain increases rapidly with increasing or decreasing pressure and is quickly unbearable. Usually it occurs during the descent. Tooth decay itself usually doesn't cause a dental barotrauma. An open

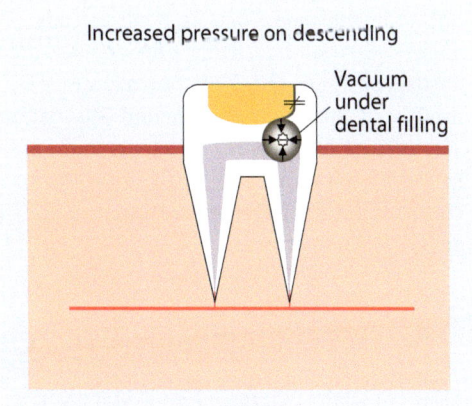

Increased pressure on descending

Vacuum
under
dental filling

■ **Fig. 23.25** Dental barotrauma

connection between the cavity in the tooth and oral cavity leads to permanent pressure equalisation.

23.5.3 Treatment and Prophylaxis

If dental barotrauma occurs while descending, divers should refrain from further descending and return to the surface. Till the dental defect is repaired, further diving should be avoided. If the symptoms arise while ascending, the diver can try to descend again till the pain subsides and retry an ascent at a slower ascent rate again. If the pain reoccurs, the diver still has to ascent despite the pain with the support of the diving buddy. The ascent might result in losing the filling or bursting of the tooth. The main risk is uncontrolled and risky behaviour during diving, which may lead to serious diving accidents. The best prophylaxis is regular dental visits.

23.6 Positive-Pressure Gastrointestinal Barotrauma (ppGIBT)

The gastrointestinal tract is the largest cavity of the body, which is characterised by its elasticity in all areas. It is the area of food absorption and elimination of non-absorbable substances. The gastrointestinal tract is an open system. It starts at the mouth and ends at the rectum. By chewing, intestinal peristaltic and stomach acid, food is mechanically and chemically modified. Thus, nutrients are made absorbable with the help of enzymes of the mouth, stomach, pancreas and duodenum. The absorption of nutrients occurs in the small intestine (jejunum, ileum). In the colon (caecum, colon), the water is removed and the faeces are thickened.

23.6.1 Aetiology and Pathogenesis

Approximately 200 mL of intestinal gas is created by the intestinal bacteria and decomposition per day. The gas production varies individually between 200 and 2000 mL per day. It also depends on the food composition. Cellulose-containing food increases gas formation. The gas consists 99% of CO_2, N_2, O_2, H_2 and CH_4. The smell of gases derives from protein-based degradation products of bacteria (indole, scatole, mercaptan, hydrogen sulphide).

Gases develop either by swallowing air, formation of CO_2 from chemical degradation reactions of food, formation of CH_4 from bacterial breakdown of carbohydrates in the colon or diffusion of gases from the blood plasma. Gases emitted in the GI tract extend during ascending. Because of its elastic properties, volume increase of gases is hardly noticeable. But due to pathological changes such as diverticular disease, adhesions, occlusions or hernias, the volume increase may be noticeable. If the gas can't escape, pain develops. This can particularly be the case in hernias. In severe cases it can even result in a rupture of the GI tract.

23.6.2 Symptoms and Prevention

Barotraumas of the GI tract can lead to strong colic-like pains in the abdominal area. They are localised depending on the affected part of the GI tract but can be referred to the close proximity. Symptoms occur during ascending or immediately after surfacing. Posture changes may reduce the intensity of the pain.

Food causing gas should be avoided before diving. Some diseases such as inflammation of the GI tract, allergies and liver dysfunction or secretion disorders of digestive organs can lead to increased gas formation. Pathologies of the GI tract should be treated before fitness to dive is granted. Hernias should be excluded prior to diving.

References

1. Bergh K, Hjelde A, Iversen OJ, Brubakk AO. Variability over time of complement activation induced by air bubbles in human and rabbit sera. J Appl Physiol. 1993;74:1811–5.
2. Bove AA. Diving medicine. Am J Respir Crit Care Med. 2014;189(12):1479–86.
3. Carloan PL: Pneumomediastinum. http://emedicine.medscape.com/article/1003409-overview. (abgreufen am 4.5.2015).
4. Edmonds CW, Bennett M, Lippmann J, Mitchel SJ. Diving and subaquatic medicine. 5th ed. Mosman: CRC Press; 2016.

5. Elayan IM, Axley MJ, Prasad PV, Ahlers ST, Auker CR. Effect of hyperbaric oxygen treatment on Nitric oxide and oxygen free radicals in rat brain. J Neurophysiol. 2000;83(4):2022–9.

6. Fanelli V, Vlachou A, Ghannadian S, Simonetti U, Slutsky A, Zhang H. Acute respiratory distress syndrome: new definition, current and future therapeutic options. J Thorac Dis. 2013;5(3):326–34.

7. Moses H: Casualties in individual submarine escape, Bureau of Medicine and Surgery, Navy Department Research Project MR005.14–3002-4.17, Report No. 438, 1964.

8. Richard JD, Dreyfuss D, Saumon G. Ventilator-induced lung injury. Eur Respir J. 2003;22(Suppl. 42):2s–9s.

9. Shupak A, Gil A, Nachum Z, Miller S, Gordon CR, Tal D. Inner ear decompression sickness and inner ear barotrauma in recreational divers: a long-term follow-up. Laryngoscope. 2003;113(12):2141–7.

10. Snow JB, Wackym PA.: Ballenger's Otorhinolaryngology: head and neck surgery,. Bc Decker, 2009.

11. Takahashi S. Inner Ear Barotrauma. Bull Tokyo Med Dent Univ. 1985;32(1):19–30.

12. US Navy Diving Manual: www.uhms/images/DCS-and-AGE-Journal-Watch/recompression_therapy_usn_di.pdf. Accessed 04 Oct 2015.

13. Uzun C, Yagiz R, Tas A, Adali MK, Inan N, Koten M, et al. Alternobaric vertigo in sport SCUBA divers and the risk factors. J Laryngol Otol. 2003;117(11):854–60.

14. Van Poucke S, Jorens P, Beaucourt L.: Chapter 1.7 Physiologic Effects Of Hyperbaric Oxygen On Ischemia-Reperfusion Phenomenon, in Handbook on Hyperbaric Medicine Edited by Daniel Mathieu, Springer 2006.

15. Whitehead T, Slutsky AS. The pulmonary physician in critical care: ventilator induced lung injury. Thorax. 2002;57:635–42.

16. Wisløff U, Richardson RS, Brubakk AO. NOS inhibition increases bubble formation and reduces survival in sedentary but not exercised rats. J Physiol. 2003;546:577–82.

17. Zhao Y, Vanhoutte PM, Leung SWS. Vascular nitric oxide: Beyond eNOS. J Pharmacol Sci. 2015;129:83–94.

18. Zilles K, Tillmann BN. Anatomie. Springer; Berlin: 2010.

Suggested Reading

Baumann MH, Strange C, Heffner JE, Light R, Kirby TJ, Klein J. Management of spontaneous pneumothorax: an American College of Chest Physicians Delphi consensus statement. Chest. 2001;119(2):590–602.

Bennett PB, Elliott DH. The physiology and medicine of diving and compressed air work. 2nd ed. Baltimore: Lippincott William & Wilkins; 1975.

Bhardwaj A, Ulatowski JA. Cerebral edema: hypertonic saline solutions. Curr Treat Options Neurol. 1999;1:179–88.

Brain Trauma Foundation. American Association of Neurological Surgeons, joint section on Neurotrauma and critical care: guidelines for cerebral perfusion pressure. J Neurotrauma. 2000;17:507–11.

Bruno A, Williams LS, Kent TA. How important is hyperglycemia during acute brain infarction? Neurologist. 2004;10:195–200.

Bühlmann AA, Voelmm EB, Nussberger P. Tauchmedizin, Barotrauma, Gasembolie, Dekompensation, Dekompensationskrankheit. 5th ed. Berlin: Springer; 2002.

Chang Y, Chen TY, Chen CH, Crain BJ, Toung TJ, Bhardwaj A. Plasma arginine-vasopressin following experimental stroke: effect of osmotherapy. J Appl Physiol. 2006;100:1445–51.

Headache CWP. facial pain in scuba divers. Curr Pain Headache Rep. 2004;8:315–20.

Daley BJ: Pneumothorax. http://emedicine.medscape.com/article/424547-overview. Accessed 21 July 2015.

Decraemer W.F, Funnell W.R.J.: Anatomical and mechanical properties of the tympanic membrane: Chronic Otitis Media. Pathogenesis-Orientated Therapeutic Management, pp. 51–84; edited by B. Ars © Kugler Publications, The Hague, Amsterdam, The Netherlands.

Duplessis C, Hoffer M. Tinnitus in an active duty navy diver: a review of inner ear barotrauma, tinnitus, and its treatment. Undersea Hyperb Med. 2006;33(4):223–30.

Eftedal Hardy KR. Diving-related emergencies. Emerg Med Clin North Am. 1997;15(1):223–40.

Hunter SE, Farmer JC. Ear and sinus problems in diving. In: Bove AA, Davis JC, editors. Diving medicine. 4th ed. Philadelphia: Saunders; 2004. p. 431–59.

Klingmann C, Praetorius M, Baumann I, Plinkert PK. Barotrauma and decompression illness of the inner ear: 46 cases during treatment and follow up. Otol Neurotol. 2007;28:447–54.

Klinsmann C, Tetzlaff K. Moderne Tauchmedizin, Gentner Verlag. 2nd ed; 2012.

Latham E, van Hoesen K, Grover I. Diplopia due to mask barotrauma. J Emerg Med. 2011;41(5):486–8.

Masuda Y, Tanabe T, Murata Y, Kitahara S. Protective effect of edaravone in inner-ear barotrauma in guinea pigs. J Laryngol Otol. 2006;120(7):524–7. Moses H: casualties in individual submarine escape, Bureau of Medicine and Surgery, Navy Department Reserch Project MR005.14–3002-4.17, Report No. 438, 1964.

Neuman TS. Pulmonary barotrauma. In: Bove AA, Davis JC, editors. Diving medicine. 4th ed. Philadelphia: Saunders; 2004. p. 185–94.

Ramos CC, Rapoport PB, Brito Neto RV. Clinical and tympanometric findings in repeated recreational scuba diving. Travel Med Infect Dis. 2005;3(1):19–25.

Decompression Illness (DCI)

© Springer International Publishing AG, part of Springer Nature 2018
O. Rusoke-Dierich, *Diving Medicine*, https://doi.org/10.1007/978-3-319-73836-9_24

Synonyms of decompression illness (DCI) are dysbaric illness (DI), decompression sickness (DCS), decompression accident or caisson disease. As DCS and AGE quite often occur together, these are commonly summarised as DCI or DI which is used as the preferred term for decompression-related accidents. DCS alone is rather subject to inert gas bubbles related to decompression effects as aetiology by itself. Neurological symptoms of DCS might be quite similar to AGE caused by pulmonary barotrauma. However, spinal symptoms are only found in DCS. DCI is a spectrum, which may have no symptoms at all, minor unspecific symptoms like fatigue up to fatal complications.

The development of DCI is a rather complex issue, which exceeds damages solely caused by bubble formation [26]. Bubble formation may lead to arterial as well as venous gas embolism (AGE and VGE) and tissue destruction. But bubbles additionally can also cause haematological effects. The gas mainly responsible for gas bubble formation is nitrogen. Even if we know that inert gas bubbles are the causes of DCI, we still have little evidence why and how this actually happens. This is also reflected in the occurrence of DCI in divers, who adhered strictly to dive tables and dive computers. Bubble growth itself is very dynamic and many other factors influence the development of DCI. One important parameter in gas exchange is perfusion. Perfusion is mainly contributing to saturation and elimination of inert gases in tissues. But also pulmonary perfusion influences off-gassing. Intrapulmonary shunt might prevent off-gassing and lead to accumulation of in particular free phase inert gas.

24.1 Aetiology and Pathogenesis

Inert gas is absorbed and eliminated via the lungs. Inert gas partial pressure adapts in alveolar capillaries to the one of alveoli and vice versa (see chapter "Alveolar Gas Exchange/External Respiration"). Inert gas transfer is limited by the short time of gas exchange between capillaries and alveoli, perfusion and respiratory minute volume. Inert gas, which can't be exhaled, still remains dissolved or undissolved in the blood system. Most of the smaller gas bubbles in the venous system are filtered by the lungs and are eliminated to a large extent. However, if a certain amount of gas bubbles is exceeded, not all gas bubbles can get filtered by the lung. An increase of about 30% in the pulmonary artery pressure is considered enough to cause arterialisation of venous gas bubbles. Some gas bubbles bypass the lung via right-left intrapulmonary shunt and enter the arterial system [6]. Gas bubbles enter either directly from the right to the left heart (septal defects) or by bypassing the capillaries (arteriovenous shunts). Bubbles caught in the lung increase the physiological right-left shunt significantly for the next few hours after diving. As a result, inert gas elimination decreases, which enhances pre-existing gas bubbles (◘ Fig. 24.1).

If gas bubbles enter the arterial system, they can cause gas embolisms, which are referred to as arterial gas embolisms (AGEs). Various other factors contribute to AGEs:

— Accumulation of gas bubbles in pulmonary capillaries can be anticipated for gas bubbles of at least 22 μm [8].
— Connecting blood vessels between pulmonary arteries and veins (arteriovenous anastomosis) of the pulmonary vascular system and increasing intrapulmonary

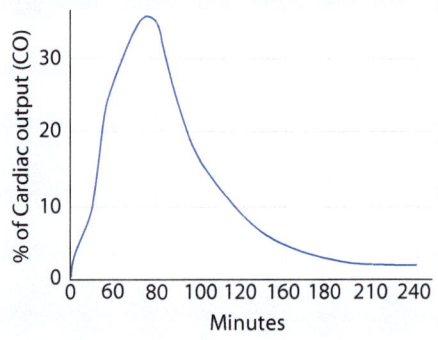

◘ **Fig. 24.1**   Intrapulmonal right-to-left shunt in percent of the cardiac output after diving (From Bühlmann et al. 2002 [7])

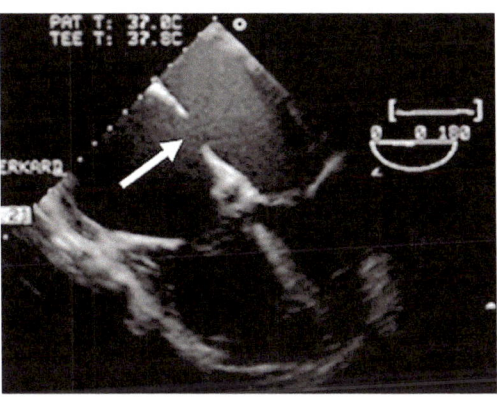
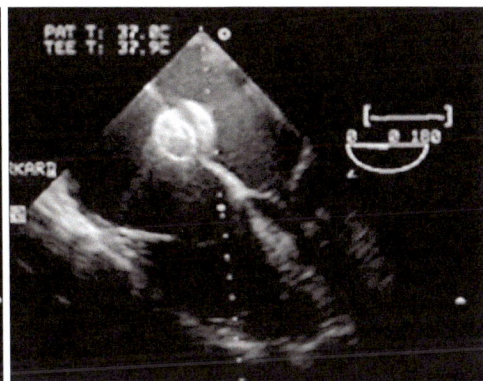

Fig. 24.2 ASD (atrial septal defect) (From Erdmann 2006 [15])

shunt, allowing particles even bigger than 25 μm to enter the arterial system from the venous system [39].

— *Paradoxical embolism*

— Gas bubbles causing pulmonary gas embolism temporarily increase the pulmonary blood pressure and increase right-left shunt via arteriovenous anastomosis. Hence, gas bubbles can be diverted from the venous to the arterial system.

— *Paradoxical embolism*

— Congenital heart defects can result in right-left shunt, e.g. atrial septal defect (ASD) like a patent foramen ovale (PFO), ventricular septal defect (VSD) or ductus Botalli (patent ductus arteriosus (PDA)). A right-left shunt is created, when the right heart pressures are bigger compared to the left heart. This can happen permanently via a pathological pressure reversal of ASD or VSD or temporarily due to physiological increase of the pulmonary perfusion (during coughing, Valsalva manoeuvre or forced respiration) in presence of a PFO or PDA.

— *Paradoxical embolism*

A paradoxical embolism is defined as an embolism entering the arterial from the venous system due to pathological changes (■ Fig. 24.2).

The main component of inert gases is nitrogen, which has its share of 78% of the total gases in normal air. However, all inert gases together

Table 24.1 Bunsen solubility coefficient (a) for O_2, CO_2 and N_2 in blood at 37 °C

Bunsen solubility coefficient (a)	O_2	CO_2	N_2
Blood	0.028	0.47	0.015
Fat	0.12	1.1	0.057
Partition coefficient: n-octanol/water [$logK_{OW}$]	0.65	0.83	0.67

are responsible for development of decompression sickness. O_2 and CO_2 are involved in metabolic processes. Hence, they don't really contribute to gas bubble formation. During diving gases are dissolved in blood as well as in tissues and have increased partial pressures. Additionally, the solubility coefficient determines how much of each particular gas can be dissolved (Henry's law). The solubility coefficient in blood and fat of nitrogen is smaller than the one of oxygen and carbon dioxide (■ Table 24.1). This means that less nitrogen content can get dissolved and less partial pressure changes for nitrogen are required to force it into the free phase.

The n-octanol/water ratio of N_2 is approximately 5:1. This means that the solubility of nitrogen in adipose tissues, lipoids and lipid-containing cells or cell structures (e.g. nerve tissue) is higher than in blood. This also means

24

higher dissolved nitrogen contents in fatty tissue are achieved at equal gas tension compared to water or blood. Hence, nitrogen has higher affinity for lipid-containing cells during the ingassing process. Even tiny structures, like lipid bilayers with its small diameter of approx. 5 nm, need to be considered. Even these small structures take a considerate part in the total body volume due to the cell quantity. Assuming a spherical shape of a cell with an average diameter of 50 µm, the lipid bilayer's surface would be 31,416 µm². The resulting volume of the entire lipid bilayer of the cytoskeleton, excluding the mitochondrial lipid bilayer, would be 125 µm³ per cell. With 10^{13} cells in the body of 80 L, the total sum would be 1.25 dm³ of double lipid bilayer, not including double lipid bilayers of cell structures like mitochondria. This contributes approximately to 1–2% of the total body mass! Keeping in mind, the lipid content of cells and cell structures vary in regard to their lipid content. In average its lipid content is around 50% with the rest resembling protein.

The lipid bilayer is considered to be a two-dimensional fluid layer, which is constantly in movement. Gas molecules have to pass through this structure. The mechanism of passive diffusion via the lipid bilayer is not fully understood. It is only a short distance for molecules to pass, considering gas molecules are only around 0.15 nm. Passive diffusion of gases happens in nanoseconds. At equilibrium, pressure inside bilayers is inhomogeneously distributed, but in overall it reflects the partial pressure of both sides of the membrane and is equal to them [32, 51]. Moreover, cell membranes with their high-fat content are an important component in gas exchange, dividing intracellular space from the extracellular space, including blood and interstitial fluid. Ingassing has little effect in regard to the blood-bilayer interface. The bilayer has a greater capacity to absorb gas molecules compared to blood due to their higher solubility. The lipid content in the bilayers varies between 30 and 80%, as bilayers contain protein structures to various degrees. The gas molecules are then passed on to the intra-cellular space. Assuming the ratio from blood or intracellular fluid and bilayer is 1:4, that means a partial pressure unit equalling 4 gas molecules from the fluid increases the partial pressure of the bilayer by factor 1, which is only 1/4 and vice versa. Each decrease in partial pressure of the bilayer causes an even greater release of free phase gas molecules into the blood due to their solubility differences. Partial pressure and content can't be used together in the same way as they are dependent on the ambient pressure gas, solubility coefficient and fraction:

$$C_{diss_n} = \left(a_n * p_{amb} * f_n \right).$$

- C_{diss} = concentration of dissolved gas$_n$
- a = solubility coefficient
- n = gas
- f_n = fraction of gas$_n$
- p_{amb} = ambient pressure

When fatty and watery solutes come together at constant pressure, the factor for the concentration difference between them would be

$$x = \frac{C_{diss_2} * a_1}{a_2 * C_{diss_1}}$$

- 1 = initial solute, 2 = end solute

The bilayer is an interface between gas-loaded cells and fluids with lower gas tension during decompression. The resulting gradient and the properties of bilayer and blood promote gas bubble development. Fatty cells assumingly have a slower elimination rate than watery cells as more nitrogen is dissolved in these cells, which means it has a higher nitrogen concentration. If the fat content inside the cell is similar to the one of the membrane, the decline of the cell gas tension via the membrane would be slower, as the concentration of the cell via the membrane would adjust at the same rate. The elimination would be along the pressure gradient. In watery cells different concentrations inside and outside the cell are present, divided by a membrane, which has a different affinity

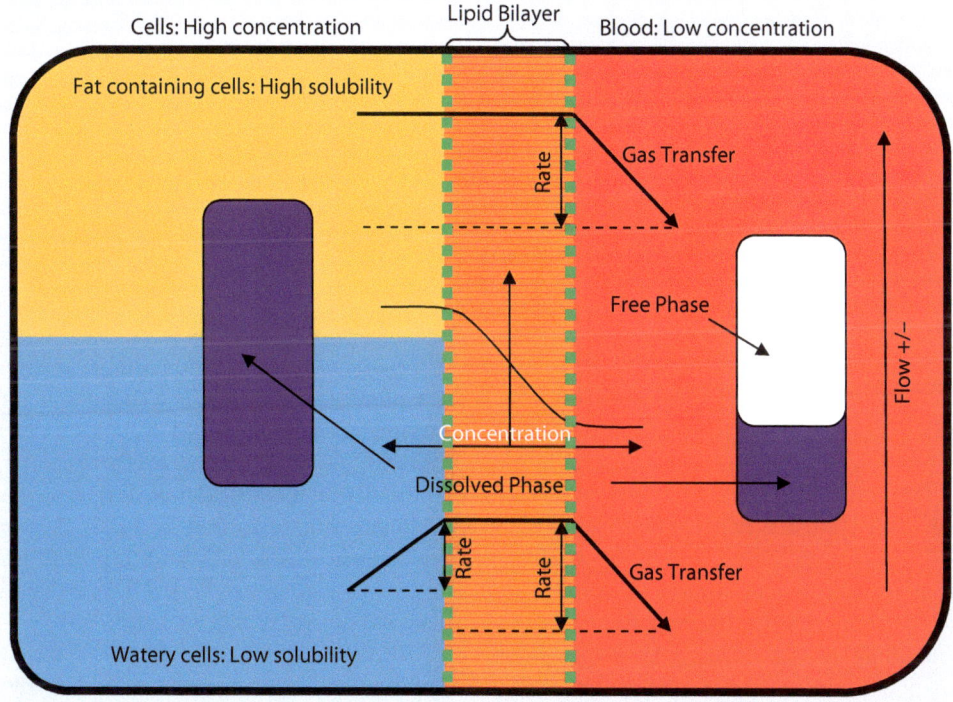

Fig. 24.3   Diffusion of inert gases through the bilipid layer

to nitrogen than the watery solute of the cell's inside and blood. Hence, there are two gradients on the membrane and also two different flow rates, which influence each other. The transport into the cell membrane is expected to be at the same speed as the release of the gas molecules to the blood. Another main limiting factor would be perfusion. The flow and perfusion rate determine gas elimination of individual cells (■ Fig. 24.3).

Different body parts vary in their fat content and perfusion. These parts are described as tissue compartments with different half-lives. Nitrogen is absorbed in tissue compartments, "stored" and released again. Depending on the compartment, it will take more or less time to clear it from excess nitrogen. On repetitive dives these compartments may not off-gas completely. As a result, nitrogen accumulates. On elimination, nitrogen with its relative high dissolved contents in fatty structures can cause gas bubbles when released into compartments with lesser fat content like blood or interstitial fluid. The same content, which was dissolved in the fatty medium, may not be dissolved in the new watery medium. Hence, gas bubbles are likely to form. To allow enough time for nitrogen elimination, appropriate surface times between dives should be kept, and flying directly after diving should be avoided.

Other important points for inert gas intake are *exposure time* and *half-life*, which need to be highlighted. Half-life is a specified time period, in which half of the nitrogen is eliminated. Usually it takes 5–6 half-lives to eliminate 97–98%. The half-life of absorption and release of inert gas is dependent on the type of the tissue. There are fast, medium and slow tissue compartments (■ Table 24.2) [6]. Nerve tissue has a short half-life with only 10–20 min. Medium tissues, like skin, have a half-life of 30–180 min and muscles

Table 24.2 Tissues and their half-lives for absorption and elimination of nitrogen (Bühlmann 1984 [6])

Tissue compartment	Tissue	Half-life in min
Fast	Blood	2–4
	Nerve tissue	10–20
Medium	Skin	30–180
	Muscles	100–240
Slow	Joints, ligaments, bones	300–600

During rapid decompression the neural tissue might be even directly damaged by developing gas bubbles. The tissue saturation highly depends on perfusion. This leads to significant variations in development of a decompression sickness in different tissues. Mainly skin and muscles as medium tissue compartments have significant fluctuations in their perfusion depending on temperature and activity. A cool environment or increased activity causes an increased perfusion and thus accelerated inert gas absorption. Especially muscles are sensible to these changes. Slow tissue compartments are less affected by short-termed changes of ambient pressure but influenced by exposure times. Certainly, in subsequent dives there can be an accumulation in particular of slow tissue compartments due to its long half-life. Therefore, professional divers with long exposure times under water are more affected by this than recreational divers (◘ Figs. 24.4 and 24.5).

Nitrogen is the main factor of the DCI development. During diving the body is exposed to higher ambient pressures and hence to higher partial pressures of nitrogen. Different compartments absorb nitrogen during the exposure time. This is also called ingas-

of 100–240 min. Joints, ligaments and bones have the longest half-lives with 5–10 h. Different tissue compartments group several body structures according to their half-lives.

Nitrogen has a high affinity to fat-containing tissues. That's why obese people might accumulate more nitrogen compared to people with normal BMI. Hence, they theoretically carry a greater risk of decompression sickness. Nerve tissues, in particular fat-containing myelin sheets, are prone to absorb nitrogen.

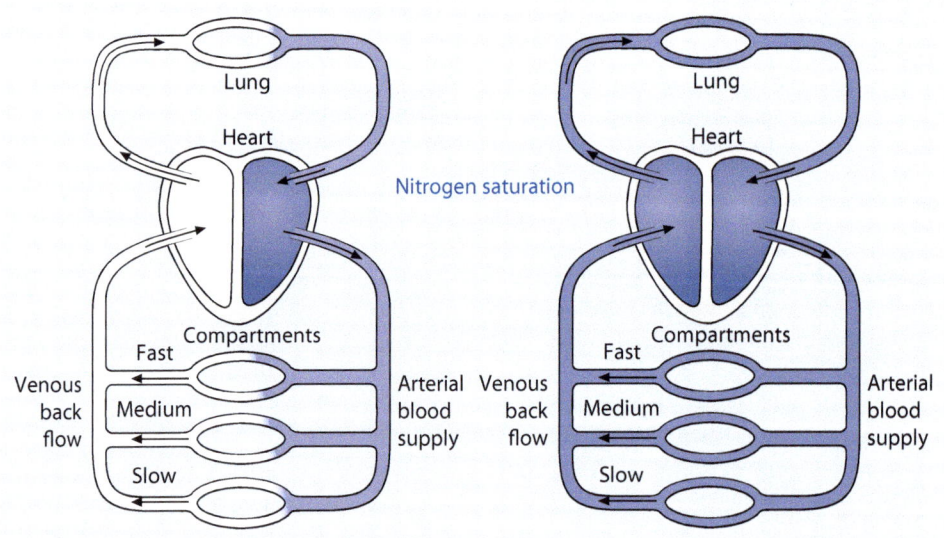

◘ **Fig. 24.4** Nitrogen saturation of the tissue compartments (With kind permission of Ecomed)

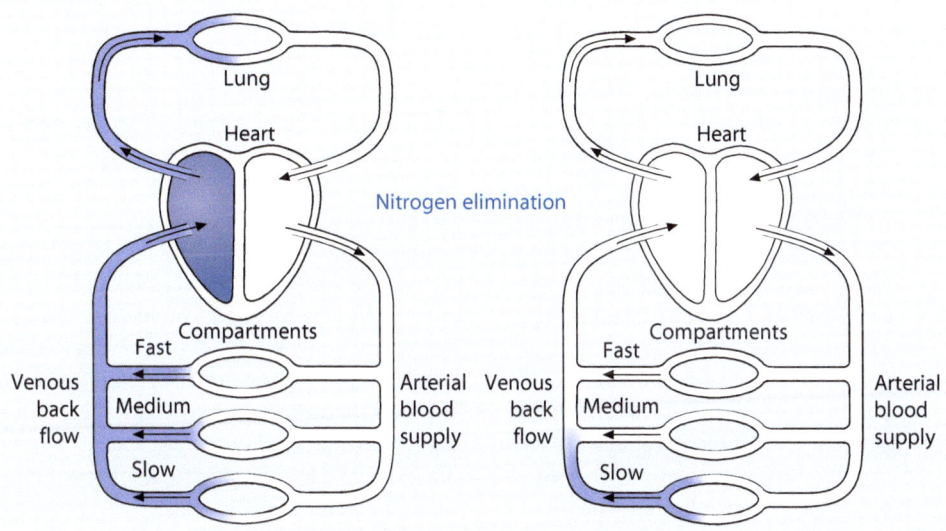

■ **Fig. 24.5**   Nitrogen elimination of the tissue compartments (With kind permission of Ecomed)

sing. During decompression ambient pressure drops, which leads to supersaturation of nitrogen in body tissues and blood, as the body can no longer sufficiently eliminate the nitrogen through exhalation. The elimination process is also called outgassing. The excess gas is either in a dissolved or free phase. During decompression microbubbles increase in size and accumulate by merging to bigger bubbles. The main locations, where bubbles are assumed to form in decompression sickness, can be subdivided:

- *Intracellular space*: Nitrogen in fatty cells, such as the myelin sheaths of nerve cells, form bubbles due to rapid decompression or interrupted perfusion. Tissue can be damaged by this. By destruction of fat tissue, tissue fragments may enter the circulation and cause fat embolisms. Gas bubbles can also enter blood vessels from the intercellular space and cause gas embolisms. This is a rather rare event. However, if perfusion is interrupted, tissue bubbles may occur.
- *Interstitial space*: Gas bubbles, formed between cells, lead to an expansion and push cells apart. The surrounding perfu-

sion might be reduced by this. Gas bubbles can also enter blood vessels from there and cause embolisms. Gas bubbles can even arise within the synaptic gap, which sometimes cause a permanent damage on the synapses. In general, the interstitial space has a slight negative pressure of approximately -0.0007 bar (-0.7 mbar) [20]. Negative tension needs to be at least 0.1 bar (100 mbar) to support bubble formation [49]; hence these values seem to be too small for being a direct reason for tribonucleation but might be a contributing factor. Also friction between tissues might support bubble formation due to tribonucleation as it might increase the negative pressure briefly.

- *Intravascular space*: Gas bubbles in arterial vessels can cause embolic events in the heart, brain and spinal cord. Embolism in arterial vessels of the lungs can lead to impairment in lung perfusion. Gas bubbles in the venous vessels can cause a pulmonary embolism or reduced blood flow. The development directly in the arterial bloodstream seems to be unlikely in diving as it requires rapid decompression. Moreover, blood seems to have a certain resistance to bubble formation in comparison to other fluids. In general, gas bubbles are mainly found in the venous system. There might be various explanations for that:

— Due to the increased partial pressure in tissues compared to venous blood, gas enters the venous system directly.
— The venous system is the elimination systems of compartments, which are storing the vast amount of nitrogen (e.g. muscles and fat).
— A relatively slow blood flow in the venous system delays nitrogen elimination and leads bubble propagation and accumulation. However, the slowest blood flow is in capillaries, which are preceding the venous system.
— Compared to arteries (430 mL) and capillaries (300 mL), the venous system (1750 mL) has a larger blood volume and hence constitutes the biggest blood pool.

In DCI a distinction between primary and a secondary development of gas bubbles has to be made. Gas bubbles may occur in veins and arteries. They predominate in veins. Gas bubbles in the arteries may develop in the arteries themselves, are released from the adjacent tissues or get redirected via shunts from the venous system. Venous gas bubbles arise from the surrounding tissue via the capillaries or within the veins themselves. Veins have a thinner and more porous wall. Therefore, they seem to be more permeable for gas than arteries. In addition to that the venous system has a lower resistance than the arterial system and a larger diameter, which slows down the blood flow. This favours gas bubble formation. The *primary* development of gas bubbles is the formation directly in the bloodstream or tissue. It only occurs with rapid pressure reduction and large pressure difference or if gas bubbles caught in tissues are unable to be eliminated via the bloodstream. Arterial as well as venous vessels can be equally affected by this. However, rapid decompression is unlikely in diving. By *secondary* development of gas bubbles, nitrogen passes from tissues into the bloodstream and accumulates there to form bigger gas bubbles. For recreational divers, most likely secondary development of gas bubbles seems to be the cause of DCI.

The shape of gas bubbles in blood vessels is slightly different than under in vitro conditions. Their shape is usually oval and club-, sickle- or cup-shaped, not spherical, and changes are highly dynamic. The initial small amount of gas enters the bloodstream. Gas bubbles may merge, accumulate and grow in their radius. At the beginning gas bubbles are growing concentric. From a certain radius on, the round shape gets distorted into an oval and club-shaped, cup-shaped or sickle-shaped gas bubbles. If they can't pass through vessels, they accumulate and cause gas arterial embolisms (AGEs). Additionally to bubble occlusion itself, blood flow is affected. Bigger bubbles might interfere significantly with blood flow and interrupt perfusion. Bubbles above a certain size might break into smaller pieces (◘ Fig. 24.6).

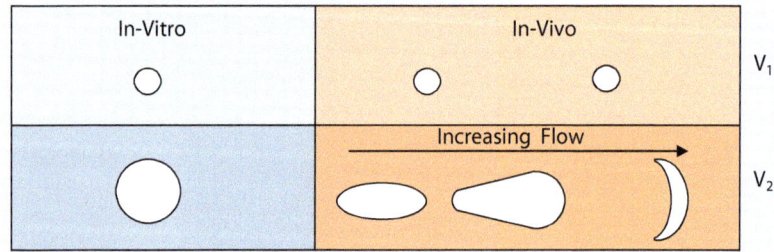

◘ **Fig. 24.6**   Shape and size of gas bubbles in correlation to the volume in vivo and in the bloodstream with various flows and volumes (V1 and V2)

◘ **Table 24.3** Quantity of gas bubbles in blood vessels
The Spencer scale
0   No bubbles
I   Occasional bubbles; the majority of the cardiac period is bubble-free
II   Bubbles in less than the half of the cardiac period
III   Continuous bubbles in the cardiac period without overriding the normal cardiac motion signals
IV   Continuous bubbles in the cardiac period with overriding the normal cardiac motion signals

(Spencer, 1974 [38])
Stage 0–II occasional DCI; Stage III–IV high likelihood of DCI

◘ **Table 24.4** Quantity of gas bubbles in blood vessels
The Eftedal-Brubakk scale
0   No observable bubbles
I   Occasional bubbles
II   At least one bubble in every four heart cycles
III   At least one bubble in every heart cycle
IV   At least one bubble per cm² in every image
V   "White-out", single bubbles cannot be discriminated

(Eftedal and Brubakk 1997 [13])

If the radius of gas bubbles is about greater than 20–30 μm [31], it seems that they can be detected via Doppler. However, several gas bubbles must have this size simultaneously to be detectable. Individual gas bubbles need a radius of 150 μm to be detected via Doppler. Spencer, Eftedal and Brubakk described different stages in Doppler detection (◘ Tables 24.3 and 24.4).

Oxygen with its increased partial pressure during diving may cause vasoconstriction. In the lungs however it causes vasodilatation. Nitric oxide (NO) is a strong vasodilator and seems to counteract this. Hyperbaric oxygen and exercise, mediated by the endothelial NO-synthase (eNOS), increase NO-synthesis. NO inhibits blood cell aggregation and possibly reduces the number of gas nuclei in caveolae of the endothelium. A reason for that might be a reduction in the hydrophobic properties of the endothelium and therefore a reduction in adherence of existing gas bubbles. Studies with NO-releasing medications (isosorbide mononitrate) in humans showed a reduction of the amount of venous gas bubbles [29, 43].

Gas bubbles don't seem to enter the venous system evenly. They seem to prefer certain structures like cavities in intracellular components of the endothelium, caveolae or points of cellular contact as well as impurities in the bloodstream with their various particles [5, 43]. The reason for that is not completely understood. It might be that tissues have some slightly increased diffusion areas for gases. It seems too that their physical property allows gas bubbles extend easier beyond a critical radius, promoting bubble growth, as they can accommodate more gas volume in their cavity compared to a flat surface. Cavities seem to be a niche, where gas nuclei rest and actually absorb more gas from supersaturated tissues. In cavities gas nuclei can exceed their critical radius still being attached, instead of being detached and freely flowing in the bloodstream. The absorption of gas from the tissue might be promoted as the flow becomes more turbulent and slower closer to the endothelium and in crevices. Hence, gas has more time to diffuse into the gas nuclei before they get washed away. Friction and tribonucleation might also contribute to this in these areas. Elliptical clefts in the endothelium created by intracellular contact points might be also exit points for gas to escape from the intracellular space (◘ Fig. 24.7).

24

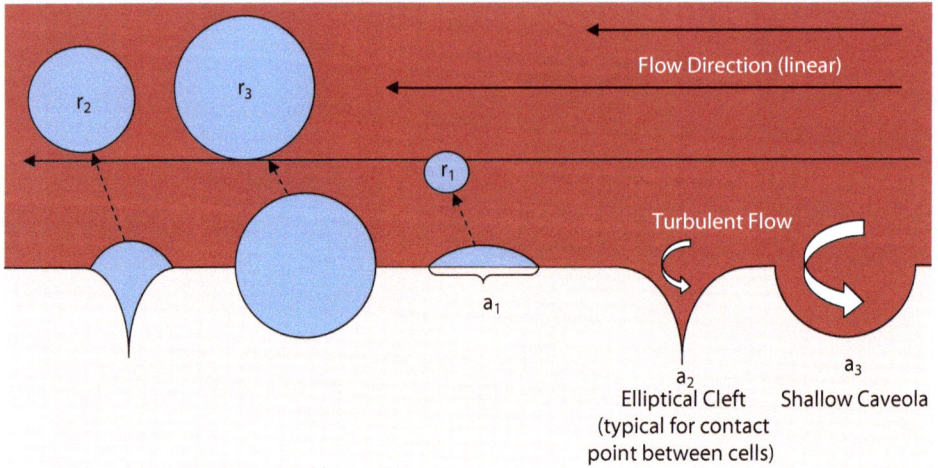

❏ **Fig. 24.7** Bubble formation arising from the endothelium: comparison from flat surface and crevices; diffusion area a_x, a_1 (flat surface) $< a_2$ (elliptical crevices) $< a_3$ (flat crevices); r = radius of gas bubble ($r_1 < r_2 < r_3$)

The development of gas bubbles from micronuclei is described in detail in the ▶ Chap. 9. The development of gas bubbles in the body is a complex process. Major factors for their development are supersaturation of nitrogen, perfusion, diffusion, elimination, dive profile, physical training of the diver and adaptation to diving. Gas bubbles develop micronuclei in blood or tissue. Gas can enter the bloodstream directly from the tissue surface or via diffusion. Smaller gas bubbles eventually grow to bigger ones. As the blood accounts only for 8% of the body, other structures of the body mainly "store" gas. The blood is the transport medium for inert gas elimination. The majority of gas bubbles in blood vessels are in the venous system, which leads to the conclusions that DCI may not only be caused by embolism but also by direct effects on tissue structures. Observation showed that trained divers develop fewer DCI than untrained person. There seems to be also a certain physiological or physical adaptation.

Gas embolisms mainly affect arterioles and capillaries. Larger gas embolism can also affect larger vessels. The larger the affected vessel, the greater is the tissue damage due to AGE. Embolic occlusions interrupt tissue perfusion. Blood flow is necessary for oxygen supply. An embolism causes a temporary oxygen deficit of affected tissues. This is to a certain extend a reversible process. Significant symptoms, particularly neurological ones, may disappear completely under HBOT. If an artery is blocked for a prolonged time, irreversible tissue damage (necrosis) develops due to a lack of perfusion and oxygen supply.

Gas embolisms probably have a similar effect on nervous tissue as strokes. The initial electrolyte shift provokes swelling of cells (cytotoxic oedema) in the affected area of the embolic event. The sodium-, chloride- and calcium-ions influx causes a fluid shift to the inside of cells. The extra calcium in the cells consumes additionally the already reduced energy carrier ATP. This results in release of lipolytic as well as protolytic enzymes and increase of the mtROS, which are causing cell death (see chapter "ppBT/AGE"). Vasogenic oedema follows the cytotoxic oedema. This is accompanied by plasma loss into the intracellular space, oedema around blood vessels (perivascular oedema), as well as paralysis of

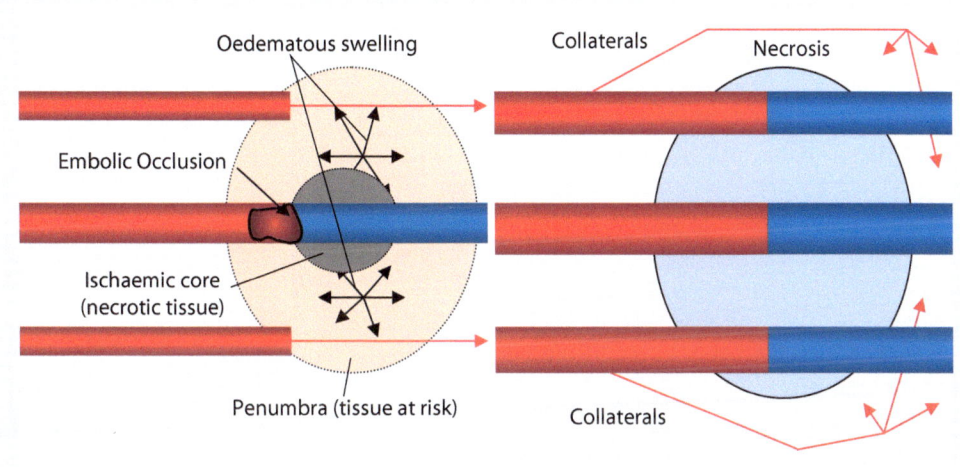

◼ Fig. 24.8 Development of a necrosis after embolic occlusion: red, intact blood vessels; bright blue, occluded blood vessels; pink, oedema; dark blue, necrotic tissue

blood vessels due to vascular active substances. This leads to further increase of the already reduced oxygen supply of already hypoxic tissues. Additionally, elimination of N_2 and CO_2 is decreased due to the obstructed blood flow at a DCI. Inert gases can further accumulate and further inert gas bubbles enhance the already persisting embolic process. Furthermore, tissues in the embolic area are acidified due to CO_2 and therefore disrupt other important metabolic cell processes (◼ Fig. 24.8).

The flow profile in the blood vessels is worsened by intravascular gas bubble formation (see ▶ Chap. 10). Secondary haematological effects may develop.

Secondary haematological effects of gas bubbles:

— Blood aggregation and consolidation of the gas bubbles (platelet aggregation, denaturation of proteins) [4, 33–35]
— Activation of the immune system (complement system) [3, 21, 22, 48]
— Leukocyte activation and adherence [1, 46]
— Endothelium damage [5, 50]
— Activation of inflammatory substances (kinin activation) [45]
— Activation of substances that initiate clotting (Hageman factor = factor XII) [4, 45]

Bubbles seem to activate the Hageman factor (factor XII), which promotes coagulation and thrombocytes aggregation. They also seem to denaturate lipoproteins, which consequently release large quantities of lipids. Solidifying lipid and protein layers around the gas bubbles may develop. Studies from Ward (1967) and Bergh et al. (1993) showed evidence of complement activation [3]. There seems to be an individual disposition that some people are sensitive and some non-sensitive to that. In particular the C5a and the C5a receptors seem to be affected. The complement activation triggers the activation of neutrophils and the formation of multiple membrane attack complexes (MAC), which lead to cell destruction and endothelium dysfunction. HBOT shows to have an effect on neutrophils and their endothelium adherence [24, 50]. Gas bubbles promote adhesion molecules of the endothelium. Some studies supporting the effects on neutrophils as neutropenic rats seemed to show less signs of a DCI [27].

Some of the secondary haematological effects either increase the probability of an embolism or reinforce already existing embolic events. Gas bubbles in blood vessels and secondary haematological effects together increase blood viscosity.

24

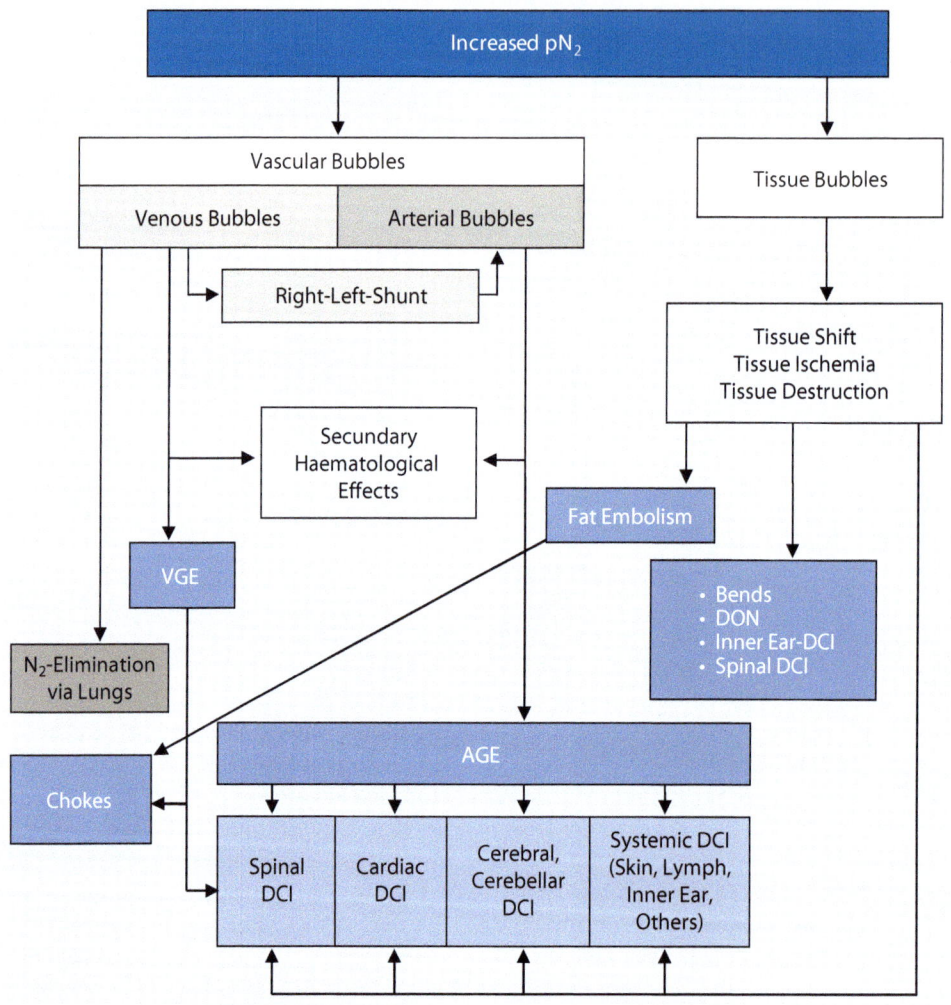

☐ **Fig. 24.9**   Effects of increased nitrogen partial pressure (pN_2) to the body

Compared to pulmonary barotraumas with its almost instant symptoms, symptoms of a DCI often occur with a timely delay after reaching the surface. It can be up to a few minutes to 12 h or more that symptoms occur. Forty-two percent of the DCI occur within 1 h, 60% within 3 h, 83% within and 98% within 24 h after reaching the surface [44] (☐ Figs. 24.9 and 24.10).

Usually cerebral manifestations of decompression sickness appear first.

24.1.1 Classifications of DCI

The decompression sickness conventionally was divided into three different types according to their severity.

In theory, DCS and AGE need to be distinguished. However, in diving accidents, often a combination of both is found, and there is of a mixture of localised and neurological symptoms. Therefore, Francis and Smith proposed a purely descriptive classification,

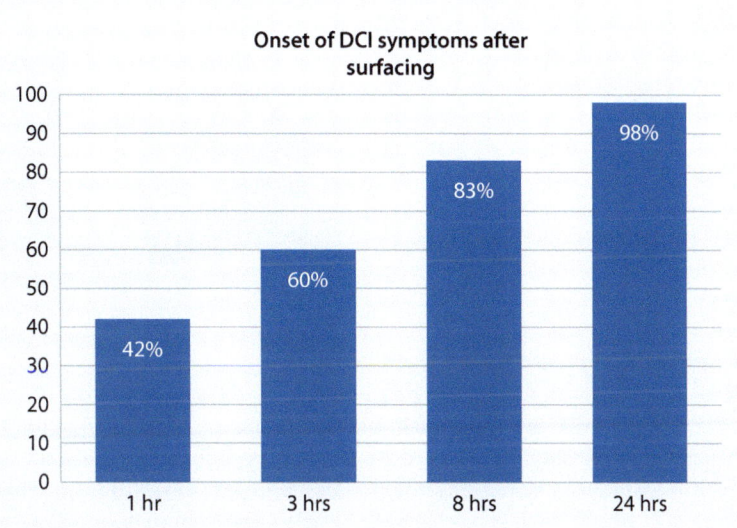

Fig. 24.10 Onset of decompression sickness symptoms after surfacing

Table 24.5 Types of dysbaric illness (modified Golding classification)

I	Mild	Mild symptoms like myalgia and arthralgia, skin eruptions other than cutis marmorata, lymphatic symptoms
II	Moderate	Neurological and symptoms of other organs (cardiovascular, inner ear and CNS-symptomatic)
III	Severe	Severe DCS in combination with AGE (combination of DCI II and AGE)
AGE		

■ **Descriptive Classification of Acute Diving Accidents (Francis and Smith)**

Progress of the symptoms
- Progressive (rapidly increasing)
- Static (symptoms unchanged)
- Spontaneous remitting
- Relapsing

Manifestations
- Musculoskeletal (muscles and ligaments)
- Neurological (cerebral, cerebellar, spinal, peripheral and autonomic nervous system)
- Pulmonary (lung)
- Cutaneous (skin)
- Lymphatic (lymphatic system)
- Audio-vestibular (hearing and balance)
- Others

as it makes no difference for treatment, if symptoms are caused by DCS or AGE. DCI seem to be also a very dynamic process, and the level of severity can rapidly change either way. This leads to confusion with the old classification of DCS types I, II and III in regard to their management and treatment (■ Table 24.5).

DCI symptoms appear often in the order of the manifestations above. However, order and combination are variable. While there is a certain correlation between initial neurological symptoms and reversibility, there is no definite answer about the recovery from a DCI.

A further category used by the US Navy but also DAN addresses the category of urgency of actions to be taken in regard to the management and treatment.

- **US Navy and DAN Categories of Diving Accidents**
  - *Category A*: Emergency
  - *Category B*: Urgent
  - *Category C*: Timely

Category A represents obviously sick divers, who develop symptoms within an hour of surfacing or symptoms are progressing. Unconsciousness and neurological and cardiovascular as well as respiratory symptoms might occur. In *category B*, pain, which is unchanged or only slightly progressed during the past few hours, is the only criterion. *Category C* combines minor non-obvious symptoms, which are not progressing or slightly progressing over several days. The symptoms are mainly mild disturbance in sensation or vague complaints about pain, which lack of evidence of injury or other causes.

24.2 Symptoms

24.2.1 Spinal Decompression Illness

Sixty-seven percent of all DCI manifestations have CNS symptoms, 24% present with pain and 9% have other symptomatic (skin, lymphatic and cardiovascular or pulmonary symptoms) [44]. Initial presentations of DCI have slightly less CNS symptoms compared to the total manifestations of DCI (CNS 57%, pain 37% and others 6%) [44]. In contrast to the AGE, the spinal cord is more frequently affected than the brain by DCI (◘ Fig. 24.11).

There are several hypotheses about the development of spinal DCI, e.g. arterial, venous, and tissue bubble (autochthonous) formation [16–18, 23]. However, the most likely explanation of the spinal DCI is rather a nitrogen bubble accumulation of

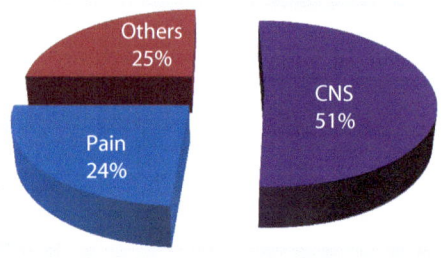

◘ **Fig. 24.11**   Manifestation of all DCI in recreational divers

the venous system in the epidural space followed by ischaemia or direct tissue damage, tissue expansion in the spinal cord, compromising the venous blood flow or a combination of both. Once perfusion is significantly reduced or halted, intra- and extravascular bubble formation is likely, resulting in direct tissue damage. Spinal DCI often occur in combination with pulmonary gas embolisms ("cokes"). The result of pulmonary gas embolisms is an outflow obstruction followed by pulmonary hypertension with increased venous pressure in the upper superior vena cava. Consequently the veins of the spinal cord (lumbar veins, ascending lumbar veins, hemiazygos vein, azygos vein, superior vena cava) are also affected in their venous return. Hence, the venous flow rate is reduced in spinal veins. Distension of the surrounding extravascular tissue by gas bubbles may reduce the venous blood flow additionally. This process promotes ischaemia and the formation of thrombosis through subsequent coagulation activation and distension. In the affected areas of the spinal cord, caused by oxygen deficiency, oedematous swelling and infarction of spinal cord tissue occurs (ischaemic myelopathy). Spinal ischaemia has a similar cascade in ischaemic tissue damage than the brain. Autopsies of divers with fatal DCI showed punctuate haemorrhages, axonal swelling, early demyelization and lacunae within the white matter [25].

The involvement of the spinal cord in DCI causes neurological deficits of the affected areas. The characteristic symptoms are similar to paraplegia, tetraplegia or a segmental neurological deficit. Ischaemia of the spinal cord often begins with severe segmental back pain, which quickly resolves. Most commonly the lower thoracic region is affected, followed by the lumbar and cervical region. Main features are motor and sensitivity dysfunction below the spinal cord lesion. Ischaemia of the anterior spinal artery causes contralateral loss of temperature sensation and pain perception and ipsilateral paralysis in accordance to the segmental level. In case of ischaemia in the area of the posterior spinal arteries, an ipsilateral disturbance of proprioception is to be expected. Paralysis is initially flaccid and then becomes spastic. The symptoms may occur on one side or on both sides. In unilateral attacks the motor function and proprioception are affected on the same side; on the opposite side, there is a reduction in pain and temperature sensation. Commonly, touch sensation is bilaterally intact. If the spine is affected bilaterally, symptoms occur on both sides. Often, bladder, bowel and sexual dysfunction develop. Usually, spinal DCI symptoms develop within a short time up to hours after surfacing. A typical accompanying complication is urinary retention. There is a risk of developing spinal shock.

The spinal cord injury can be complete and incomplete. The complete spinal cord injury has the absence of sensory and motor function in the lowest sacral segments S4–S5. The incomplete spinal cord injury has a preservation of sensory and motor functions below the level of injury, including the lowest sacral segments.

- **Symptoms of a Spinal Cord Injury**
- Initially segmental back pain
- Paraplegia and tetraplegia, below the lesion of the spinal cord (usually at thoracic level):
  - Flaccid palsy of limb according to the lesion in the spinal cord
  - Disturbance of bladder, bowel and sexual function
  - Sensitivity loss (sensation, temperature and proprioception)

- Brown-Sèquard syndrome (ipsilateral paralysis and disturbance of the deep proprioception, contralateral disturbance of temperature and pain perception)

24.2.2 Cerebral Decompression Illness

Gas embolisms can occlude arterial vessels of the *brain* (*cerebral symptoms*). The clinical manifestation is depended on the occluded artery and its supplied area. In general, the middle cerebral artery and vertebrobasilar arteries seem to be most commonly affected in cerebral-vascular events. Sensory and motor disturbances are manifested in partial or complete loss of functions (paresthesia, paralysis of single muscle groups or entire limbs, motor speech disorders, dysphasia). Almost all DCI with CNS involvement occur with pronounced symptoms. The main symptom is an altered level of consciousness. The other symptoms manifest depending on the localization of ischaemic brain tissue. The first signs of an acute hypoxia of the brain might be dizziness, nausea, inability to speak (dysphasia), coordination disturbance (apraxia), inability to recognise things and to name them (agnosia), sensory disturbances, confusion, disorientation and slowing of thought processes. Initially, unconsciousness with subsequent generalised or focal seizures and a temporary syndrome with reversible psychotic features may develop. Cerebral DCI symptoms can have a latency period of a few minutes up to several hours but no more than 12 h. The symptoms can persist or dissolve spontaneously. It depends on the extent and duration of vascular occlusion, whether the tissue is damaged and when or whether HBOT is performed. A transient ischaemic attack (TIA) lasts less than 24 h. The symptoms of a prolonged reversible ischaemic neurological deficit (PRIND) disappear within 3 weeks. In a major stroke, the symptoms remain totally or partially. As the DCI is readily treatable, symptoms are expected to partially or completely resolve with appropriate treatment, and long-term damage can be prevented.

■ **Cerebral Symptoms (See Also Hyperbaric Pulmonary Barotrauma/AGE)**
– Dizziness, nausea and vomiting
  – Disorientation, altered level of consciousness and unconsciousness
  – Sensorimotor disturbances (aphasia, dysphasia, apraxia, agnosia, paresthesia, paralysis of single muscle groups or whole limbs)
– Convulsions

24.2.3 Cerebellar Decompression Illness

The involvement of the *cerebellum* leads to disturbance in movements (ataxia), inability to perform contrasting movements in rapid sequence (dysdiadochokinesia), staccato dysphasia, tremor, asynergia with dysmetria (abnormal undershooting or overshooting movements), ocular motor disturbance, vertigo and nystagmus.

■ **Cerebellar Symptoms**
– Asynergia, ataxia and dysmetria
– Tremor
– Dysdiadochokinesia
– Nystagmus
– Vertigo
– Staccato dysphasia
– Disturbance of the fine motor skills

24.2.4 Chokes

Chokes are a severe form of DCI involving the lung. It is caused by gas bubble accumulation or fat embolism in the pulmonary bloodstream. Venous gas bubbles develop due to fast decompression either directly in the venous system or by diffusion of nitrogen from the body tissues. A direct development of gas bubbles however in the venous system is a rather unlikely event and only possible with explosive decompression, which almost never happens in diving. Fat embolism caused by destruction of fatty tissues can be a result or additional effect of cutaneous DCI

■ **Table 24.6** Severity stages of a pulmonary embolism. (Schulte, 1987)

I	Small embolism (< 25%), normal blood gas, dyspnoea
II	Moderate embolism (25–50%), pCO_2 < 35 mmHg, increased respiratory rate
III	Moderate to severe embolism (50–80%), pCO_2 < 30 mmHg, pO_2 < 65 mmHg, cyanosis, tachycardia, cardiogenic shock
IV	Severe embolism (> 80%), cardiorespiratory arrest, pO_2 < 50 mmHg

or severe DCI. Gas bubbles or fat components are transported via the venous system to the right heart from where they enter the pulmonary circulation. Pulmonary vessels are filtering gas bubbles or solid particles. Depending on the size and number of gas bubbles, an occlusion in the venous pulmonary system (*venous gas embolism* = *VGE*) can develop (■ Table 24.6). Gas bubbles may occlude some pulmonary vessels for an hour or two after diving without causing symptoms. If more than 25% of the pulmonary vessels are involved, chokes are likely. A severe complication of chokes is ARDS (adult respiratory distress syndrome). Like all other severe forms of DCI, shock may occur. Chokes may lead to pulmonary hypertension. With elevated pulmonary blood pressure, the likelihood of an arteriovenous shunt via anastomosis or septal defects (VSD, ASD, PFO, PDA) with the risk of a paradoxical AGE increases.

■ **Typical Signs of Pulmonary Embolism Are**
– Increasing shortness of breath
– High respiratory rate
– Sudden pleuritic retrosternal pain
– Dry cough with haemoptysis
– Right heart failure and refractory tachycardia
– Arrhythmias (e.g. atrial fibrillation)
– Sudden loss of consciousness

24.2.5 "Skin Bends" Cutaneous DCI (CDCI)

Skin bends are subcutaneous microembolism. It causes more or less a well-demarcated macular erythema associated with pruritus and symptoms similar to sunburn. The rash is usually not raised. Sometimes pruritus is the only symptom. More severe forms can cause papules and plaques or even cutaneous blistering and bruising. Coughing or performing a Valsalva manoeuvre will accentuate the venous markings (Mellinghoff's sign). They are painful but commonly not tender to touch. The torso, the back, the shoulders and adipose areas of the body, like thighs, triceps and, in women, the breast, most commonly are affected. Usually, a mild form disappears after few hours spontaneously. Approximately 20% of divers with skin bends have accompanying neurological symptoms. If large areas are affected, it may cause a fluid shift into the extravascular space, which might cause a relative hypovolaemia. As a result, the skin perfusion and thus the elimination of nitrogen are reduced, which can lead to a worsening of the DCI. Cutis marmorata ("marbled skin"), however, represents a serious symptom of a severe DCI. The affected area appears cyanotic and mottled and might or might not spread. During recompression skin changes are visibly disappearing completely. However, 4–6 h after HBOT the skin can become painful and tender to touch again. These symptoms can increase over the next 24–36 h. During this time the skin usually remains unchanged in colour throughout this time, except for occasional erythema. After 2–3 days, these symptoms disappear again.

24.2.6 "Lymphatic Bends" Lymphatic DCI (LDCI)

Gas bubbles can occur in the lymphatic system and prevent lymphatic flow. The rare lymphatic involvement results in lymphatic oedematous swelling in the area of the chest, trunk, face and limbs along the lymphatic pathway. Likewise, it might result in localised swelling of lymph nodes.

24.2.7 Contact Lenses and Decompression

Gas bubbles can be formed under hard contact lenses. The gas bubbles can't escape during the dive. Usually, this doesn't cause any damage to the eye, but the gas bubbles lying above the cornea may decrease the visual acuity. Soft contact lenses aren't affected by this. By using contact lenses under water, it needs to be taken in consideration that if the contact lens is lost, the diver might no longer be able to read diving instruments or identify dangers of the environment. If the diver has a poor visual acuity, it is best to correct this with optical glasses in the diving mask.

24.2.8 "Bends" Acute Dysbaric Osteo-arthralgia (ADOA)

Large joints of the shoulder (~5%) and hip (~18%) but mainly the knees (~72%) are primarily affected by ADOA. Occasionally, also elbow (~4%) and ankle joints are affected [7]. In recreational divers mainly knee joints and in professional divers with deep saturation dives shoulder joints are affected. The discomfort is caused by poor perfusion of the nutritional vessels or by extravascular gas bubbles. Expansion of extravascular gas bubbles in this non-elastic tissue causes pain. The dull pain, localised in the joint, radiates to the adjacent muscles and is often accompanied by abnormal sensations (paraesthesia), restriction of movement, muscle weakness and numbness. Sometimes the pain shifts by massaging the area. Bends can easily be confused with muscle soreness. Bends only occur after long and repetitive dives and are usually accompanied by "feeling off". Application of local pressure, e.g. by inflating a pressure cuff, can cause easing of the symptoms. Mild cases usually last only a few hours. More serious cases have increasing symptoms within the next 12–24 h and continue to persist as a dull ache, if they are left untreated. Bends usually occur only on one side and are asymmetrical.

24.2.9 Inner Ear Decompression Illness (IEDCI)

There are various hypotheses of *IEDCI*:

- *Different gas tensions* in different compartments of the inner ear support bubble formation.
- *Development of gas bubbles in osteoclasts*, where they may get trapped. This may result in destruction of adjacent bones (temporal bone) in proximity of cochlea or vestibular. These can lead to bleeding and exudation into the cochlear and vestibular system.
- *Increase of the perilymph pressure* as a consequence of gas bubble formation in the inner ear.
- *Perfusion difference* of the left and right inner ear in severe DCI.
- *Different partial pressures between endolymph* (gas exchange with the blood) *and perilymph* (gas exchange with the middle ear). Gas bubbles in the endolymph on the side of the membrane of the round and oval window may lead to its destruction or disruption of the inner ear function.
- *Vascular embolism* of the inner ear.
- *Tissue destruction* of the inner ear.
- *Helium passes via diffusion through the oval and round window into the inner ear* during saturation dives using heliox or trimix. Helium quickly saturates. Oversaturation and formation of helium gas bubbles of the perilymph during the decompression phase lead to the destruction of the fine structures of the inner ear. Helium still remains in the extracellular space, even though helium gas mixture is changed to normal air. Due to the

different solubility of the gases, it is probably a summation of mainly helium and nitrogen due to isobaric counterdiffusion causing an increased gas bubble formation.

- **The Symptoms of the Inner Ear Decompression Illness According to Origin**
- Cochlear origin
  - Tinnitus ("ear ringing")
  - Sensorineural hearing loss
- Vestibular origin
  - Vertigo, dizziness and gait instability (often permanent with fluctuation)
  - Nausea
  - Vomiting
  - Loss of consciousness

The symptoms appear suddenly, usually after reaching the surface. However, isolated inner ear involvement in a DCI is relatively rare. During heliox/trimix dives, the symptoms may also occur after changing from heliox/trimix to normal air during the decompression phase. HBOT should be performed preferably after ENT consultation. IEBT or perilymphatic fistula however has to be ruled out prior to commencement of HBOT. Any increase of symptoms during HBOT points out to IEBT or a perilymphatic fistula, and the session should be discontinued.

24.2.10 Long-Term Damage of Hyperbaric Exposure

Long-term damage of diving may occur without previous acute DCI. It rather needs to be seen as a summation of prolonged or frequent repetitive dives. Professional divers, who often stay extensive times under water, are particularly at risk. This includes also diving instructors and dive guides, which often have multiple dives a day. In these professions diving should be interrupted every 3 days for a day, to eliminate residual nitrogen from the body. Because the recreational diving industry is still very young, no studies exist for long-term damages. Data often rely only on the experience with professional divers and military divers. Previous decompression traumas can result in irreversible tissue destruction. Causes for the long-term damages are short decompression times, rapid ascent rates, long exposure times and deep dives.

24.2.10.1 Dysbaric Osteonecrosis (DON)

Osteonecrosis is caused by bone ischaemia, which leads to bone necrosis. It is an irreversible process. As mentioned above, complications can arise with long-term hyperbaric exposure. The occurrence of late damages could be reduced by adhering to dive tables, avoidance of deep diving, minimising long-term exposure and treatment of any DCI, even minor ones, with 100% oxygen and HBOT.

There are various theories for the development of dysbaric osteonecrosis (DON). Dysbaric osteonecrosis is a non-infectious destruction of bone tissue mainly of the fatty marrow-containing shaft of long bones and ball socket joints of hips (~10%) and shoulders (~42%) as well as knees (~48%) [7]. It only affects the white and not the red bone marrow. The bone marrow is enclosed in the rigid bone, and hence there is no scope of expansion within the bone marrow. As intramedullary veins only operate on a low pressure of 3–5 mmHg, little intramedullary pressure changes could affect blood flow. Small volume changes caused by gas bubble increase the pressure in the bone marrow (intramedullary) quickly. Blood supply enters the bone marrow before it reaches the bone itself. Hence, blood supply of the bone can be cut off when intramedullary pressure increases. Two-thirds of the blood supply of the inner cortex as well as the metaphysis is received from the nutrient artery, which enters the shaft and splits into ascending and descending branches. The periosteal arteries supply the outer 1/3 of the cortical blood supply. The meta- and epiphysis have their own blood supply (◘ Figs. 24.12 and 24.13).

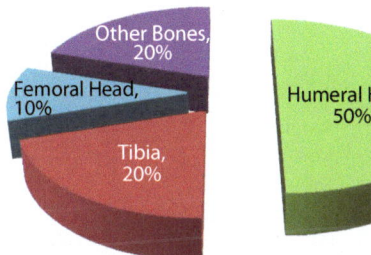

◘ **Fig. 24.12** Distribution of DON in the skeletal system

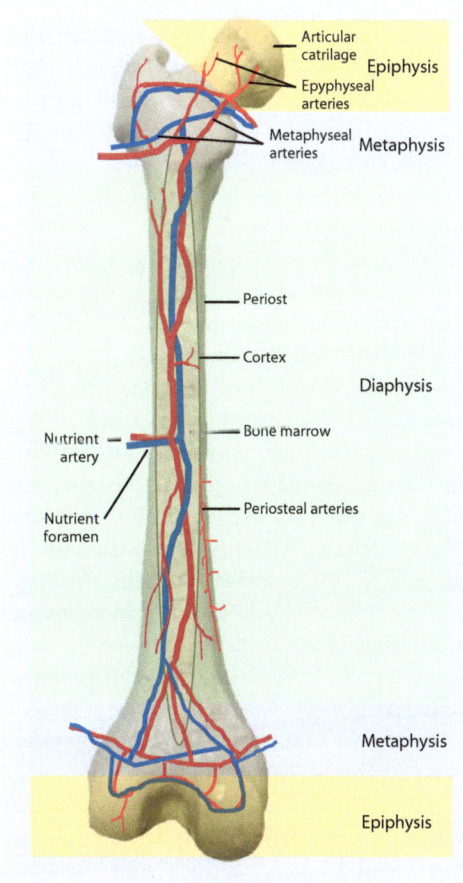

◘ **Fig. 24.13** Blood supply of the bone

24

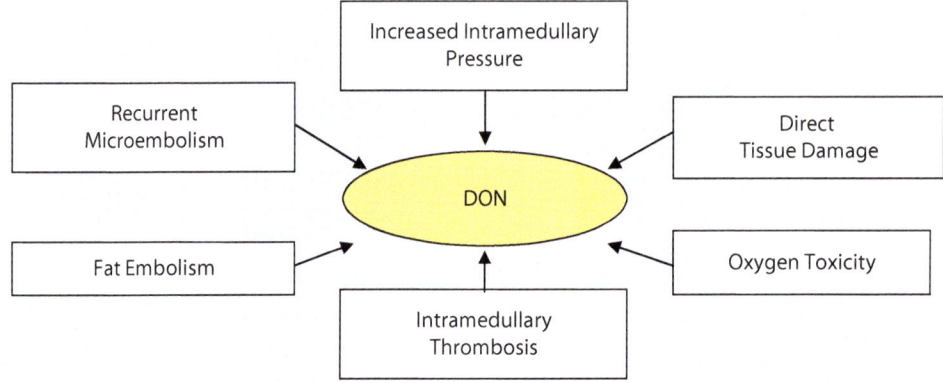

■ **Fig. 24.14**   Causes of dysbaric osteonecrosis

Gas bubbles may decrease arterial perfusion by intramedullary venous stasis. Decreased blood flow favours development of thrombi. Unnoticed, recurrent microembolism in blood vessels of the bone can lead to skeletal damage. On the other hand, gas bubbles themselves can destroy bone tissue. For this kind of damage, long hyperbaric exposures must have preceded, as bones belong to the slow tissue compartments. Gas bubbles outside blood vessels can cause fat embolisms or compress directly blood vessels of the bone. Circulating fatty constituents can then get stuck in small vessels of the bone. Another cause could be an increase of oxygen partial pressure. High oxygen partial pressure itself causes intramedullary swelling. This together with only few gas bubbles might cause sufficient swelling of intramedullary fat cells and lead to an increase in intramedullary pressure, enough to reduce blood flow. But also, rapid compression during diving reduces the venous drainage of the bone marrow and initiates intramedullary venous stasis (■ Fig. 24.14).

In mild cases small bone infarcts develop, which in most cases resolve by itself. Severe cases lead to calcifications and periosteal reactions. Commonly affected structures are the dia- and metaphysis. The epiphy-

sis is hereby spared. These skeletal changes are usually not symptomatic but can be seen on XR (■ Tables 24.7 and 24.8). Late signs of damages might even occur as late as 5–7 years after the initial damage in the absence of a noticeable DCI. After severe DCI however, DON can manifest after months. Hips, shoulders and knees are most commonly affected in decompression divers. Professional divers should get screened for DON on their initial examination. Further screening is not required unless issues arise. The preferred investigations are plain XR, MRI and bone scan. MRIs pick up changes after 2 weeks but aren't able to detect necrosis at this stage. They have good sensitivity and specificity. Bone scan also detect changes within weeks. They have good sensitivity but a poor specificity. CTs have poor sensitivity and average specificity. Additionally, they cause high radiation. Therefore, CTs aren't the preferred investigation method. Plain XRs are still a good screening method for established DON.

As during childhood and puberty bones are still growing, they are more prone for structural damages cause by hyperbaric exposure. Therefore, dive time and depth should be limited for adolescents.

- ## Radiological Changes of DON

■ **Table 24.7**   Ohta Matsunaga

Type A lesion (juxta-articular)	Type B lesion (head, neck and shaft)
A1 Normal articular cortex with possible radiopaque areas	B1 radiopaque areas
A2 Spherical opacities	B2 Irregular sclerotic, calcified areas
A3 Linear opacities	B3 Translucent and/or cystic areas
A4 Juxta-articular structural damage 1. Crescent sign 2. Cortical collapse 3. Sequestration of the cortex	
A5 Secondary, degenerative articular changes	

■ **Table 24.8**   FICAT

0	XR and MRI normal, no symptoms
I	XR: normal or minor osteopenia MRI: oedema Bone scan: increased uptake Symptoms: pain may be present
II	XR: mixed osteopenia and/or sclerosis and/or subchondral cysts, without subchondral lucency MRI: geographic defect Bone scan: increased uptake Symptoms: pain and stiffness
III	XR: crescent sign (subchondral lucency) and eventual cortical collapse MRI: same as plain film Symptoms: pain and stiffness
IV	XR: end stage with evidence of secondary degenerative changes MRI: same as plain film Symptoms: pain and limp

24.2.10.2 CNS Damages

Even without symptomatic DCI, microembolisms can cause damage to spinal cord, discs and brain. There seems to be an increased incidence of cerebral and spinal microembolism in scuba and also apnoea [14, 37, 40]. These microembolisms don't necessarily cause clinical symptoms. But if sensitive areas are affected, symptoms may arise. There is very little evidence of long-term neurological damage or neuropsychological changes.

24

24.2.10.3 Permanent Inner Ear Damage

Damages to the vestibular part of the vestibulocochlear nerve cause nystagmus and ataxia. Divers with previous head trauma are two times more affected. Diving with mixed gases imposes a higher risk. Damages to the cochlear part of the vestibulocochlear nerve rarely cause acute symptoms. They usually present after months and years. It results in sensorineural hearing loss, affecting higher frequencies, similar to noise trauma. The left ear seems to be more affected than the right. The explanation therefore seems to be that the left sigmoid sinus is longer and has lesser drainage through the smaller left jugular foramen compared to the right one.

24.3 Treatment of DCI and Hyperbaric Oxygenation Therapy (HBOT)

24.3.1 Initial Assessment and Treatment

Therapeutic action is always needed in any case of DCI. The problem is that even experienced divers often ignore minor signs of DCI and subsequently fail to be treated. It needs to be distinguished between the initial emergency treatment and the follow-up treatment with hyperbaric oxygen treatment (HBOT). Emergency care can be performed by anyone until the medical team arrives to take over. HBOT should only be performed by specifically trained medical professionals. Recognition of signs of a decompression sickness as well as of imminent life-threatening conditions is important. If stroke symptoms are present, the NIHHS scale could be used to determine the severity of the stroke. In case of a spinal DCI, the ASIA classification is a useful tool to document spinal symptoms and their progress after the accident and after the treatment. As DCI is most often a combination of DCS and AGE, both may be used at least on the initial examination.

- **Important Data Should Be Obtained on the Spot**
  - Information about the person (name, place of residence, age, contact details, next of kin)
  - Details of the diving partner
  - Details of the dive profile (diving depth, dive time, bottom time, repetitive dive, information on the previous dive, height above sea level)
  - Information about the development of the symptoms (gradual, suddenly, increasing, unchanged)
  - Time interval of becoming symptomatic after surfacing or commencement of resuscitation
  - Pre-existing conditions
  - Allergies
  - Medication

- **All Diving Accidents Require Checking and Recording of**
  - *Orientation*
    - Questions to person (name, age, address)
    - Questions about place and date
  - *Eyes*
    - Movement in all directions; symmetry; nystagmus
    - Vision
    - Pupils; papillary light response
    - Diplopia
  - *Face*
    - Facial muscles (whistling, frowning, showing their teeth)
    - Paraesthesia and sensory disturbances
    - Symmetry of facial expressions and of the soft palate, sensitivity and paraesthesia
  - *Swallowing reflex*
  - *Tongue movement (symmetry)*
  - *Skin*
    - Cutis marmorata
    - Sensitivity

- *Ears*
  - Hearing loss
  - Tinnitus
  - Vertigo
- *Shoulder*
  - Lifting resistance (strength and symmetry)
  - Paraesthesia and sensory disturbances
- *Arms, hands and legs*
  - Lifting resistance (strength and symmetry)
  - Paraesthesia and sensory disturbances
  - Reflexes
  - Grip, spreading and extending of fingers
  - Standing on the toes and lifting toes (if possible)
- *Coordination*
  - Heel-to-toe test ("drunken driver" test)
  - Finger-to-nose test
  - Heel-shin slide test
  - Romberg test
  - Rapid alternating movement tests (dysdiadochokinesia – fine motor skills)
- *Anal tone and sensation (only in case of a spinal DCI)*
- *Glasgow Coma Scale (◘ Table 24.9)*
- *Modified 5-Min neuro check, based on DAN guidelines (any diving accident) (◘ Fig. 24.15)*

NIHHS (*National Institutes of Health Stroke Scale*) if AGE suspected (◘ Fig. 24.16)
*1. The patient has to do the following tasks: description of a painting, object description and reading of sentences.
   - Examples of sentences:
     - You know how.
     - Down to earth.
     - I got home from work.
     - Near the table in the dining room.
     - They heard him speak on the radio last night.
*2. The patient has to do the following task: reading or repeating words.
   - Examples of words:
     - Mama
     - Tip-top

◘ **Table 24.9**   Glasgow Coma Scale

Eyes	
Open spontaneously	4
Open to speech	3
Open to painful stimuli	2
No response	1
Speech	
Responds sensibly to questions	5
Seems confused	4
Uses inappropriate words	3
Makes incomprehensible sounds	2
No response	1
Movement	
Obeys commands	6
Points to pain	5
Withdraws from pain	4
Bends limbs in response to pain	3
Straightens limbs in response to pain	2
No response	1
Total	15

- Fifty-five
- Thanks
- Huckleberry
- Baseball player
- *ASIA classification (standard neurological classification of spinal cord) (◘ Fig. 24.17)*
  - *Impairment Scale*
    1. No motor or sensory function in the sacral segments S4–S5.
    2. Sensory but not motor function is preserved below neurological level up to the sacral segments S4–S5.
    3. Motor function preserved below neurological level; more than half of the key muscles below that level have muscle grade < 3.

24

a

Name:	DOB:		Location:				Time :		Date:							
	Time															
Orientation*																
Age, Name	Yes															
	No															
Location	Yes															
	No															
Time, Date	Yes															
	No															
Eyes (? Symmetry)																
Diolplia (double vison; focusing of both eyes together on Fingers in 4 different positions, up, down and both sides)	Yes															
	No															
Object Identification (counting of Fingers in 2–3 different positions, seperately and both eyes together; identify objects)	Yes															
	No															
Eye Movement in all Directions with Fixed Head Position (distance from finger to face approx. 50 cm)	Yes															
	No															
Light Reactivity of Pupils	Yes															
	No															
Face (? Symmetry)																
Wisteling	Yes															
	No															
Show Teeth	Yes															
	No															
Rise eyebrow	Yes															
	No															
Equal Sensitivity on Both Sides with Closed Eyes (forhead and face)	Yes															
	No															
Hearing																
Both Sides Equal (RubbingThumbs Starting from 0.5 m Distance MovingTowards the Ear)	Yes															
	No															
Swollowing																
Visible Movement "Adam's Apple" whilst Swollowing	Yes															
	No															
Tongue and soft palate																
Symmetry when poking out	Yes															
	No															
Muscular Strength (? Symmetry, testing performed against resistance)*																
Lift Shoulders Comment:	Yes															
	No															
Upper Arm Flexation in Elbow Comment:	Yes															
	No															
Fingers and Hands (Extension and Spreading, Grip) Comment:	Yes															
	No															
Hips (Flexation) Comment:	Yes															
	No															
Knee (Extension) Comment:	Yes															
	No															
Ankle (Extension "Tiptoes") and Elevation of Toes Comment:	Yes															
	No															

Fig. 24.15   a, b Modified 5-min neuro check, based on DAN guidelines

b

Sensory Perception (? Symmetry, Starting from Top to Bottom)		
Upper Extremity Comment:	Yes	
	No	
Torso Comment:	Yes	
	No	
Lower Extremity Comment:	Yes	
	No	
Able to Squeeze Anus and Subjective Normal Sensation in Anal Area Comment:	Yes	
	No	
Balance and Motor Coordination (? Symmetry)*		
Heel-to-Toe "Drunken Driver Test" (Ataxia)	Yes	
	No	
Romberg Test (Standing with Closed Eyes and Outstreched Arms) Catch Person when Falling!	Yes	
	No	
Finger and Hand Coordination (Rapid Alternating Touching of Palm and Back of the Hand on Each Side)	Yes	
	No	
Finger-Nose-Test (Touching Nose with Fingers and Closed Eyes on Each Side)	Yes	
	No	
Knee-Heel Test (Sliding of Heel Along Shin Towards Feet with Closed Eyes)	Yes	
	No	
Other Comments or Observations:		
Examiner:		
* These examinations should be given priority, if not all can performed.		

◼ **Fig. 24.15** (continued)

4. Motor function preserved below neurological level; more than half of the key muscles below that level have muscle grade > 3.
5. Motor and sensory functions are normal.

— *Sensory scoring (light touch or pinprick)*
   - 0: Absent; no differentiation between of sharp pin and dull edge
   - 1: Impaired or hyperaesthesia
   - 2: Intact

— *Motor strength testing*
   - 0: No contraction or movement
   - 1: Minimal movement, palpable or visible contractions
   - 2: Active movement but not against gravity
   - 3: Active movement against gravity
   - 4: Active movement against resistance
   - 5: Active movement against full resistance

— *Key muscles to establish neurologic level*
   - C5: Elbow flexors (biceps, brachialis)
   - C6: Writs extensors (extensor carpi radialis longus and brevis)
   - C7: Elbow extensors (triceps)
   - C8: Long fingers flexors (flexor digitorum profundus)
   - T1: Small fingers abductors (abductor digiti minimi)
   - L2: Hip flexor (iliopsoas)
   - L3: Knee extensors (quadriceps)
   - L4: Ankle dorsiflex (tibialis anterior)
   - L5: Long toe extensors (extensor hallucis longus)
   - S1: Ankle plantar flexors (gastrocnemius soleus)

24

a

Score	Test Result	Date, Time, Examiner and Score					
LOC Responsiveness							
0	Alert; keenly responsive						
1	Arouses to minor stimulation						
2	Requires repeated stimulation to arouse; movement to pain stimulus						
3	Postures or unresponsive						
Ask month and age							
0	Both questions right						
1	1 question right; dysarthric/intubated/trauma/language barrier						
2	0 question right/aphasic						
Blink eyes & squeeze hands							
0	Performs both tasks						
1	Performs 1 task						
2	Performs 0 task						
Test horizontal extraocular movements							
0	Normal						
1	Partial gaze palsy: can be overcome; partial gaze palsy: corrects with occulocephalic reflex						
2	Forced gaze palsy: can not be overcome						
Test visual fields							
0	No visual loss						
1	Partial hemianopia						
2	Complete hemianopia						
3	Patient is bilaterally blind; bilateral hemianopia						
Testfacialpalsy							
0	Normal symmetry						
1	Minor paralysis (flat nasolabial fold, smile asymmetry)						
2	Partial paralysis (lower face)						
3	Unilateral or bilateral complete paralysis (upper/lower face)						
Test left arm motor drift (90° elevation when sitting, 45° elevation when laying)							
0	No drift for 10 seconds; amputation/joint stiffness						
1	Drift, but doesn't hit bed						
2	Drift, hits bed; some effort against gravity						
3	No effort against gravity						
4	No movement						
Test right arm motor drift (90° elevation when sitting, 45° elevation when laying)							
0	No drift for 10 seconds; amputation/joint stiffness						
1	Drift, but doesn't hit bed						
2	Drift, hits bed; some effort against gravity						
3	No effort against gravity						
4	No movement						
Test left leg motor drift (30° elevation when laying)							
0	No drift for 5 seconds; amputation/joint stiffness						
1	Drift, but doesn't hit bed						
2	Drift, hits bed; some effort against gravity						
3	No effort against gravity						
4	No movement						
Test right leg motor drift (30° elevation when laying)							
0	No drift for 5 seconds; amputation/joint stiffness						
1	Drift, but doesn't hit bed						
2	Drift, hits bed; some effort against gravity						
3	No effort against gravity						
4	No movement						

Fig. 24.16   **a**, **b** NIHSS (National Institutes of Health Stroke Scale)

b

Limb ataxia (FNF/Heel-Shin)						
0	No ataxia; amputation/joint effusion; does not understand; paralysed					
1	Ataxia in 1 limb					
2	Ataxia in 2 limbs					
Test sensation						
0	Normal; no sensory loss					
1	Mild-moderate loss: less sharp/more dull; mild - moderate loss: can sense being touched					
2	Complete loss; no response and quadriplegic; coma/unresponsive					
Test language/aphasia (Describe scene; name the objects; read the sentance *1.)						
0	Normal; no aphasia					
1	Mild-moderate aphasia: some obvious changes, without signifi cant limitation					
2	Severe aphasia: fragmentary expression, inference needed, cannot identify materials					
3	Mute/global aphasia: no usable speach/auditory comprehension; coma/unresponsive					
Test Dysarthria (read or repeat words *2.)						
0	Normal; intubated/unable to test					
1	Mild-moderate dysarthria: slurring but can be understood					
2	Severe dysarthria: unintelligible slurring or out of proportion dysarthria; mute/anarthric					
Test extinction/inattention						
0	No abnormality					
1	Extinction to bilateral simultaneous stimulation; visual/tactile/auditory/spatal/ personal inattention					
2	Profound hemi-inattention (e.g. does not recognize own hand); extinction to >1 modality					

Severity						
0	No stroke					
0–4	Minor CVA					
5–15	Moderate CVA					
16–20	Moderate to severe CVA					
21–42	Severe CVA					

◘ **Fig. 24.16** (continued)

All severe diving accidents with DCI and AGE require a thorough neurological examination of cranial nerves but also of motor and sensory functions. The examination should be commenced systematically starting with the head and ending with the toes including the lowest segment S4–S5 (rectal tone, perianal sensation, urinary retention or incontinence and priapism).

Overview of the examination scheme in a diving accident:

– *Initially*
  – At the scene of the diving accident:
    – Check vital signs
    – Start 5-min neuro check (can be done by anyone)
  – Continue 5-min neuro check from there on every 30–60 min.

– After stabilisation of the patient, a thorough examination of the first medical trained person (paramedic or doctor) should be done, including:
  – ASIA
  – NIHSS
  – General examination (skin, chest, cardiac, BP, pulse, SaO2, ECG)
– On suspicion of a pneumothorax or compromised gas exchange (ultrasound, CXR or CT chest).
– Chest drain, if necessary.
– *Immediately before HBOT*:
  – General observation (BP, pulse, SaO2, temperature).
  – Chest, cardiac and ear examination.
  – 5-min neuro check.

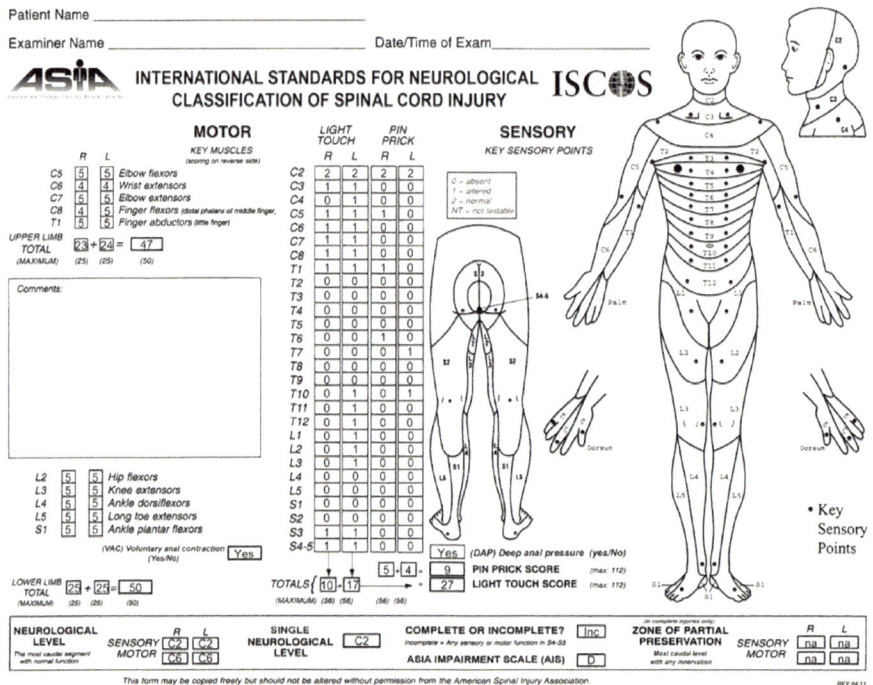

◼ Fig. 24.17 American Spinal Injury Association (ASIA) impairment scale: International Standards for Neurological Classification of Spinal Cord Injuries (updated 2015)

- Specific neurological examination according to the symptoms.
- If the patient is intubated, replace air of the cuff with fluid and check and record position of tubus.
- Paracentesis in anterior-inferior or posterior-inferior quadrant, if equalising is not possible or the patient is unconscious.
- IDC in patients with altered level of consciousness.
- *During HBOT*
  - Chest and cardiac (including JVP and trachea) examination after reaching the treatment depth and every 10–20 min; check for equal air entry.
  - General observation 10 min or more often, in particular in severe cases.
  - 5-min neuro check (in air breaks).
  - Specific neurological examination according to the symptoms (in the O2-free interval).
  - Checking of tube (cuff and position), infusion (water level in drip) and chest

drain before every pressure change and during pressure change.
- *After HOBT:*
  - Neurologist follows up and considers MRI.

A diver suffering from *DCI* should receive initially *100% normobaric oxygen* via mask to avoid progression of the symptoms. Non-Rebreather masks with 10 L / min or and on demand valves are the only efficient form of ventilation with normobaric oxygen other than intubation. Ventilation via a nasal prongs is inadequate.

◼ The Effects of Normobaric Oxygen
- Prevention of DCI progression
- Better oxygen supply to oxygen-deprived tissues
- Relapse prevention
- Extension of "oxygen window"
- Reduction of gas bubbles (size and number) through increased inert gas elimination
- Increased elimination of inert gases
- Prevention of additional venous gas embolism

The treatment with normobaric oxygen should be continued for several hours, even if symptoms resolve. Subsequent HBOT still is recommended, even if symptoms are resolved with normobaric oxygen as re-occurrence of DCI symptoms is more than likely. Equally important is to ensure that the patient has *increased fluid intake* (0.5–1 L/hrs). Urinary output in the range of 0.5 mL/kg/hour [44] is regarded as evidence of adequate intravascular volume. This leads to increased blood volume and thus to vascular dilation and reduced blood viscosity. This is important particular as after diving a certain degree of dehydration is expected (see dehydration) due to the intravascular blood shift caused by elimination of orthostatic forces under water. The fluid substitution can be either achieved by oral or intravenous intake. An unconscious or severely compromised diver should receive the fluid intravenously. The diver should be kept calm. Regardless of the person's condition even with minor or resolving symptoms, an observation period for the next 6–12 h is required. If the diver has no symptoms of DCI but it might be a possibility to develop them later, a transport in the vicinity of a recompression chamber should be considered.

Regardless of the severity, DCI has to be treated with *HBOT*! Transport to the next HBOT chamber should be sought within 4 h. There are no clear data about the maximum delay of treatment. The earlier HBOT commences, the better the outcome is to be expected. HBOT within 4 h of onset seem to result in symptom resolution of about 75–94%. Transport should be performed by trained medical professionals and with adequate means as sudden deterioration of the condition might occur. During transport, it is important to secure vital functions. Extreme heat and cold or violent vibrations should be avoided. The transport by plane or helicopter should be performed as low as possible, maximum 300 m (1000 feet) above ground. Single-patient hyperbaric chambers are no longer used since there is no way to intervene when complications arise. The "wet recompression" with 100% oxygen is not recommended either as it is not regarded safe as a medical treatment. However, in remote areas this might be the only available treatment option. Usually the transport to the hyperbaric chamber is carried out under isobaric pressure. General observation should be frequently taken.

24.3.2 Advanced Treatment: HBOT

■ **First Response**
- Stabilisation of the vital functions.
- Positioning (immobilisation; recovery positioning, if patient has an altered level of consciousness; no head-lowering positioning).
- 100% oxygen by mask (face mask 5–8 L/min; non-rebreather 10 L/min).
- For rehydration, use oral fluid intake 0.5–1 litre or intravenous access and isotonic sodium chloride solution, if patient has an altered level of consciousness or a severe DCI. Target: urine output 0.5 ml/kgbw/h. Caution needs to be applied to patients with pulmonary DCI (chokes) as they can suffer from a volume overload with aggressive fluid administration.
- Monitor blood pressure, pulse and, where appropriate, pulse oximetry, 5-min neuro checks.
- Immediate transport to the nearest recompression chamber.
- Linocaine could be considered in the treatment of AGE but not of DCI [28]. Evidence suggests to attain a serum concentration for an antiarrhythmic effect. This can be achieved by either an intravenous administration of 1 mg/kg bonus dose followed by 2–4 mg/minute continuous infusion or 0.5 mg/kg every 10 min. If no intravenous access is established, an intramuscular dose of 4–5 mg/kg (lasting for approx 10 min) will produce a therapeutic plasma concentration (Type 2 recommendation and Level C evidence for DCI, Type 2 recommendation and Level B evidence for AGE).

- VTE prophylaxis with heparin or enoxaparin only in immobilised patients after the HBOT.
- Consideration of tenoxicam or similar NSAID (Type 2 recommendation and Level C evidence for DCI, Type 3 recommendation and Level C evidence for AGE) [28].
- Consideration of aspirin for isolated AGE (Type 3 recommendation, Level C evidence) [28].

At least one qualified doctor, one nurse and a technical operator are expected for HBOT. During treatment, doctors and nursing staff are usually inside the pressure chamber. During non-emergency treatments, only a nurse may be required inside the pressure chamber with the doctor being outside on standby. The technical operator controls the settings from the outside. Inside the pressure chambers, connections for masks or hoods to supply oxygen to patients and monitoring are available. Ventilators for intubated patients can be either fitted inside the pressure chamber or being operated from the outside, depending on the chamber facilities. If patients need to be intubated, tubus cuff has to be emptied with air and replaced with fluid (normal saline solution) prior HBOT. Otherwise, the volume of the cuff would reduce with increasing pressure during compression, and the tube would start leaking. For dive accidents treatment tables and medical support inside the chamber have to be adjusted according to the severity of the dive accident. Patients with minor symptoms might only require a nurse as an attendant. However, as a guideline, every HBOT with patients who need to be treated with USN TT 6 or above (USN TT6a or Comex 30) should be accompanied with a doctor. During HBOT for diving accidents, vital signs should be regularly checked and neurological checks performed as outline above. Vital signs should be checked after each change of pressure and every 5 min at the beginning of the treatment to ensure that there is no change in the patient's condition. This can be adjusted later according to the patient's condition. Usually air breaks are a good opportunity to review patients. Treatment of severe DCI and AGE is about the same. The purpose of the treatment is primarily to eliminate gas bubbles, supply ischaemic tissue with high amounts of oxygen and avoid consequential damages. All signs of moderate to severe DCI constitute a medical emergency. They require immediate medical treatment. For DCI and AGE, *hyperbaric oxygen therapy (HBOT) in a pressure chamber* is the only treatment of choice, with the exception of an accompanied untreated pneumothorax (◘ Table 24.10). If a pneumothorax or an AGE is suspected, an ultrasound or a CXR should be performed before HBOT. Pneumothorax can be treated with thoracostomy and chest drain prior pressure chamber treatment. HBOT should be initiated as early as possible. However, if there is a delay, HBOT can be even started a few days or even weeks later. But the later HBOT commences, the lower the chances of success are. During HBOT 100% oxygen is applied under increasing ambient pressure. The aim of HBOT is to reduce gas bubbles in their radius, dissolve existing gas embolisms and thus improve perfusion. In addition, body tissues are better saturated with oxygen, and nitrogen can be eliminated at increasing rate. The administration of oxygen is applied intermittently to reduce the risk of oxygen toxicity. A treatment cycle with 100% oxygen is dependent on the HBOT scheme with 20, 30 or 60 min, with air breaks of subsequent breathing of normal air for 5, 10 or 15 min. The oxygen cycles are also referred to as BIBS (built-in breathing sessions).

- **HBOT Cycle** [44]
  - *USN TT 5*: 20 min 100% oxygen with 5-min break on normal air at 18 msw (280 kPa/2.8 bar)$_{abs}$ and 9 msw (190 kPa/1.9 bar)$_{abs}$.
  - *USN TT 6*: 20 min 100% oxygen with 5-min break on normal air at 18 msw (280 kPa/2.8 bar)$_{abs}$ and 60 min 100% oxygen with 15-min break on normal air at 9 msw (190 kPa/1.9 bar)$_{abs}$; based on the modified Table 6, up to 2 HBOT units at 18 msw (280 kPa/2.8 bar)$_{abs}$

■ **Table 24.10** Treatment options (initial HBOT aimed to commence within 4 h)

USN TT 5 (■ Fig. 24.19)	Mild DCI (with exemption of cutis marmorata)
	Asymptomatic DCI with high likelihood of developing symptoms (missed deco stops)
	Follow-up treatment for residual symptoms
USN TT 6 (■ Fig. 24.20)	AGE
	Moderate DCI and severe DCI
	Mild DCI, or if symptoms are not responding to HBOT – TT 5 (symptoms persisting more than 10 min despite HBOT)
	Cutis marmorata
	Symptomatic uncontrolled ascent
	Recurrence of symptoms at less than 18 msw
USN TT 9 (■ Fig. 24.23)	Could be considered as follow-up treatment, or if there is no complete remission of symptoms after HBOT – Table 6 within the next 24 h (no more than 2 HBOT within 24 h)
USN TT 6a or Comex 30 (■ Figs. 24.21 and 24.24)	Moderate and severe DCI, if symptoms are not easing off despite HBOT – TT 6 (symptoms persisting more than 10 min)
USN TT 4 (■ Fig. 24.18)	If symptoms are not improving after more than 30 min on 5.5 bar with USN TT 6, switch to USN TT 4
USN TT 7 (■ Fig. 24.22)	If symptoms are not improving after more than 6 h on 2.8 bar with USN TT 4, switch to USN TT 7
	Severe AGE or life-threatening DCI non-responding to treatment

Continuing treatment

USN TT 5 or 9 (■ Figs. 24.19 and 24.23)	Continuing treatment (first 5–10 days once to twice daily and then one treatment daily till the symptoms are resolved or no further improvement is expected)

and up to 6 HBOT units at 9 msw (190 kPa/1.9 bar)$_{abs}$ are added.

- *USN TT 6a*: 25 min with 5-min breaks on normal air at 50 msw (600 kPa/6 bar)$_{abs}$ and during the decompression to 18msw (280 kPa/2.8 bar)$_{abs}$ for 35 min with mixed gas composed of 50% oxygen and 50% helium or nitrogen; after that, treatment will be continued as Table 6.
- *USN TT 9*: 30 min 100% oxygen with 5-min break on normal air at 14 msw (240 kPa/2.4 bar)$_{abs}$ (oxygen cycle may vary depending on the country).
- *USN TT 4*: 25 min 100% oxygen with 5-min breaks on normal air at 18 msw (280 kPa/2.8 bar)$_{abs}$. After 4 units

oxygen breathing is adjusted to the patient's condition; 20 min 100% oxygen with 5-min break on normal air at 18 msw (280 kPa/2.8 bar)$_{abs}$, 100% oxygen 120 min prior ascent from 9 msw (190 kPa/1.9 bar)$_{abs}$ and during rest of the remaining treatment (no air breaks required).

- *USN TT 7*: 25 min 100% oxygen with 5-min break on normal air at 18 msw (280 kPa/2.8 bar)$_{abs}$. After 4 cycles follows a break on normal breathing air for 2 h. This cycle could be continued, if the patient tolerates the oxygen breathing and/or symptoms are expected to improve with oxygen breathing. In unconscious patients, oxygen breathing should be ceased after 24 cycles.

24

In general, during compression patients have to breathe normal air without mask to enable equalising. During the final decompression phase of the HBOT, 100% oxygen is supplied till 3 msw. From 3 msw (130 kPa / 1.3 bar)$_{abs}$, normal air has to be used, as technically breathing via a mask in a pressure chamber is not permitted below that pressure. To eliminate excess nitrogen, the tender requires 100% oxygen only at the end of the HBOT to minimise the risk of oxygen toxicity.

Oxygen breathing cycles with intermittent 100% oxygen for the patient [44]:

- *USN TT 5:* Time on oxygen begins on 14 msw/60 fsw (240 kPa/2.4 bar)$_{abs}$ and during ascend till 3 msw (130 kPa/1.3 bar)$_{abs}$ and during decompression from 18 msw (280 kPa/2.8 bar)$_{abs}$ to 9 msw (190 kPa/1.9 bar)$_{abs}$ for 30 min.
- *USN TT 6:* Time on oxygen begins on 18 msw/60 fsw (280 kPa/2.8 bar)$_{abs}$ and during ascend till 3 msw (130 kPa/1.3 bar)$_{abs}$ and during decompression from 18 msw (280 kPa/2.8 bar)$_{abs}$ to 9 msw (190 kPa/1.9 bar)$_{abs}$ for 30 min.
- *USN TT 6a:* Time on oxygen begins on 18 msw/60 fsw (280 kPa/2.8 bar)$_{abs}$ after the ascent from 50 msw (600 kPa/6 bar)$_{abs}$ and during ascend till 3 msw (130 kPa/1.3 bar)$_{abs}$.
- *USN TT 4:* Upon arrival at 18 msw/60 fsw (280 kPa/2.8 bar)$_{abs}$ after ascending from 50 msw/165 fsw (600 kPa) for at least 4 cycles. After that oxygen breathing is dependent on the patient's condition; time of oxygen begins 120 min prior and during the ascent from 9 msw/30 fsw (190 kPa/1.9 bar)$_{abs}$ ascend till 3 msw (130 kPa/1.3 bar)$_{abs}$.
- *USN TT 7:* 25 min 100% oxygen with 5-min break on normal air at 18 msw (280 kPa/2.8 bar)$_{abs}$. After 4 cycles follows a break on normal breathing air for 2 h. This cycle could be continued, if the patient tolerates the oxygen breathing and/ or symptoms are expected to improve with oxygen breathing. In an unconscious

patient, oxygen breathing should be ceased after 24 cycles. Breathing of normal air from 3 msw (130 kPa/1.3 bar)$_{abs}$.
- *USN TT 9:* Time on oxygen begins on 14 msw/60 fsw (240 kPa/2.4 bar)$_{abs}$ and during ascend till 3 msw (130 kPa/1.3 bar)$_{abs}$.

The tender requires intermittent 100% oxygen breathing as below [44]:

- *USN TT 5:* Time of oxygen begins starting with ascent from 9 msw/30 fsw (190 kPa/1.9 bar)$_{abs}$ to 3 msw (130 kPa/1.3 bar)$_{abs}$. If the tender had a previous hyperbaric exposure in the previous 18 h, an additional 20 min of oxygen breathing is required prior the ascent.
- *USN TT 6:* Time of oxygen begins 30 min (60 min with more than one extension) prior and during ascent from 9 msw/30 fsw (190 kPa/1.9 bar)$_{abs}$ ascend till 3 msw (130 kPa/1.3 bar)$_{abs}$. If the tender had a previous hyperbaric exposure in the previous 18 h, an additional 60 min of oxygen breathing is required prior ascent.
- *USN TT 6a:* Time of oxygen begins 60 min (90 min with more than one extension) prior and during ascent from 9 msw/30 fsw (190 kPa/1.9 bar)$_{abs}$ ascend till 3 msw (130 kPa/1.3 bar)$_{abs}$. If the tender had a previous hyperbaric exposure in the previous 18 h, an additional 120 min of oxygen breathing is required prior ascent.
- *USN TT 4:* Time of oxygen begins 120 min prior and during ascent from 9 msw/30 fsw (190 kPa/1.9 bar)$_{abs}$ ascend till 3 msw (130 kPa/1.3 bar)$_{abs}$.
- *USN TT 7:* No oxygen breathing is required.
- *USN TT 9:* Time of oxygen begins 15 min prior and during ascent from 14 msw/45 fsw (240 kPa/2.4 bar)$_{abs}$ ascend till 3 msw (130 kPa/1.3 bar)$_{abs}$. If the tender had a previous hyperbaric exposure in the previous 18 h, an additional 60 min of oxygen breathing is required prior ascent.

◻ **Table 24.11** Recommended oxygen fraction corresponding to the treatment depth

Depth (fsw)	Depth (msw)	Gas mix oxygen/ nitrogen or helium	pO_2 [bar]
0–60	0–18	100/0	1–2.82
61–165	18–50	50/50	1.42–3
166–225	50–68	36/64 (helium only)	2.17–2.81

NOAA [30]

USN Treatment Table 6 (USN TT 6) is usually the most common treatment in DCI. DCI and AGE are strongly recommended for HBOT (Type 1 recomnendation). HBOT for these indications have however a low level of evidence (Level C). Oxygen treatment with 100% oxygen starts at 2.8 bar absolute pressure corresponding to 18 m of sea water (msw). If the symptoms are unchanged after initial improvement, the *modified Treatment Table 6 (modified USN TT 6)* can be used. The modified USN TT 6 uses additionally up to 2 treatment phases with 20 min at 2.8 bar_{abs} each and/or 2 treatment phases with 60 min at 1.9 bar_{abs} each. After HBOT patients need to be monitored closely for the next 6 h and remain in the close proximity of the HBOT facility (< 30 min travel time). Regardless of that, every patient treated for DCI should stay within 60 min travel time to the HBOT facility for the next 24 h. For serious, life-threatening DCI *USN Treatment Table 6a (USN TT 6a)* can be used, which starts at 6 bar_{abs} (equivalent to 50 msw) with normal air or with a mixture of oxygen and nitrogen or helium with the ratio of 50/50 (or 40/60) (◻ Table 24.11). Alternatively *Comex 30* can be used instead of the USN TT 6a. If symptoms resolve or improve significantly during compression on USN TT 6a, the maximum treatment depth can be less than 50 msw. However, the remaining table regime stays unchanged. If symptoms remain unchanged on 50 msw for more than 30 min, USN TT 6a can be switched to *Treatment Table 4 (USN TT 4)*, which will initially continue at 50 msw. If there is no improvement on Table 4, the treatment can be switched to *Treatment Table 7 (USN TT 7)* at 18 msw. Here, the minimum duration at 18 msw is 12 h, before further decompression can be commenced. Even if the symptoms increase, the treatment depth shouldn't be changed. If there is no improvement after 12 h, decompression can commence. Other indications for the USN TT 7 are severe AGE or life-threatening DCI, non-responding to treatment. USN TT 7 is an extension of Table 6, 6a and 4. A long-term HBOT of DCI or AGE is commonly followed with the *Treatment Table 9 (USN TT 9)*, *Treatment Table 5 (USN TT 5)* or occasionally *Treatment Table 6* over the following days. Long-term HBOTs are performed initially up to two times daily or in case of USN TT six once daily only for the first 5–10 days. After 5 days, a break of 1 day should follow. Treatment continues until there is no further improvement in symptoms for at least 2–3 treatments. If no improvement is achieved for 3–5 days, HBOT can be ceased. The usual duration is approximately 5–10 treatments. For long-term HBOT pulmonary oxygen toxicity needs to be taken in consideration. In particular USN TT 6a with extensions, USN TT 4 and USN TT 7 bear a risk for pulmonary oxygen intoxication. USN TT 4 and USN TT 7 hardly get used nowadays, and it needs to be noted that during the USN TT 4, 20% of tenders suffered from a DCI. Both USN TT 4 and 7 also carry a risk of oxygen toxicity mainly manifested in the lungs. Even not commonly used, the Hawaiian Deep Tables seem to have good properties for treating especially severe DCI. They generally start at a greater

24

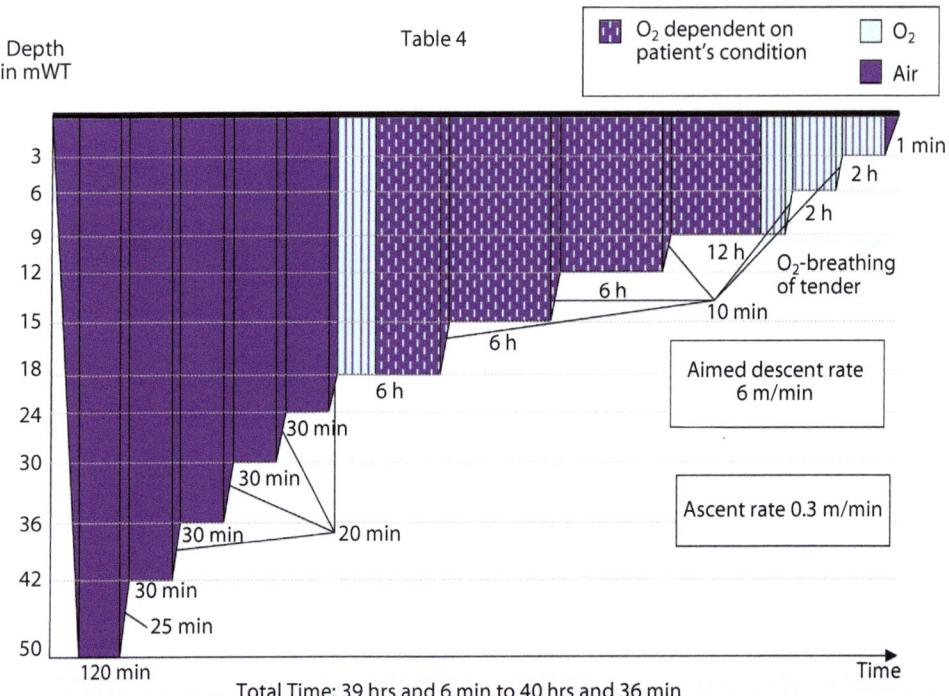

Fig. 24.18   USN Hyperbaric Oxygen Treatment Table 4 (USN TT 4)

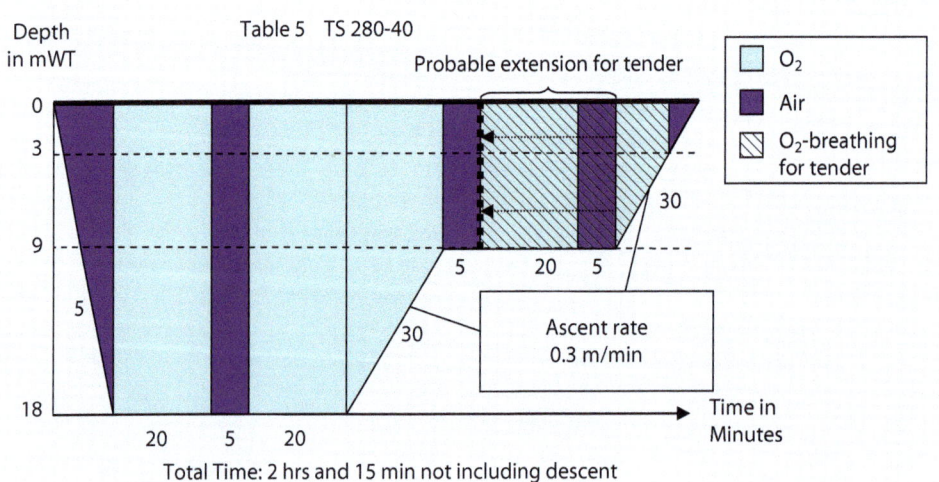

Fig. 24.19   USN Hyperbaric Oxygen Treatment Table 5 (USN TT 5)

depth varying from 49 m to 85 m (160 f to 280 f), with a following staged decompression (■ Figs. 24.18, 24.19, 24.20, 24.21, 24.22, 24.23, 24.24, 24.25 and 24.26).

■ **Complications of HBOT**
– Barotrauma of the ear and sinuses
– Myopia (during prolonged treatment, but commonly resolves spontaneously)

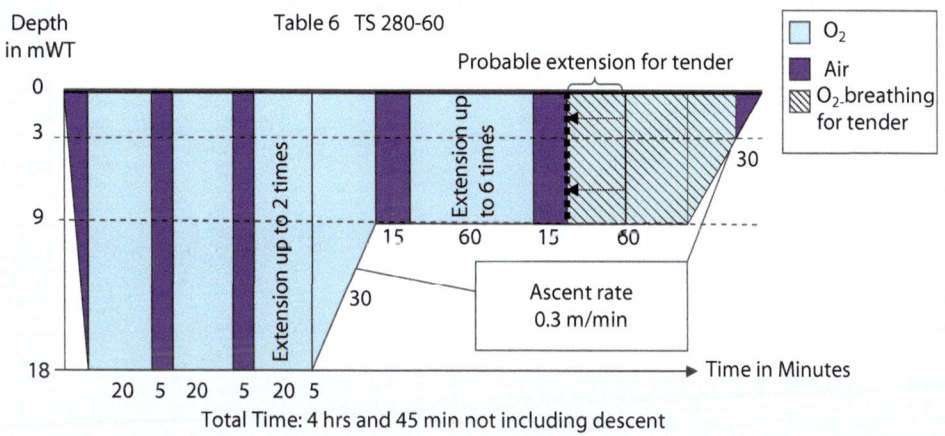

Fig. 24.20   USN Hyperbaric Oxygen Treatment Table 6 (USN TT 6)

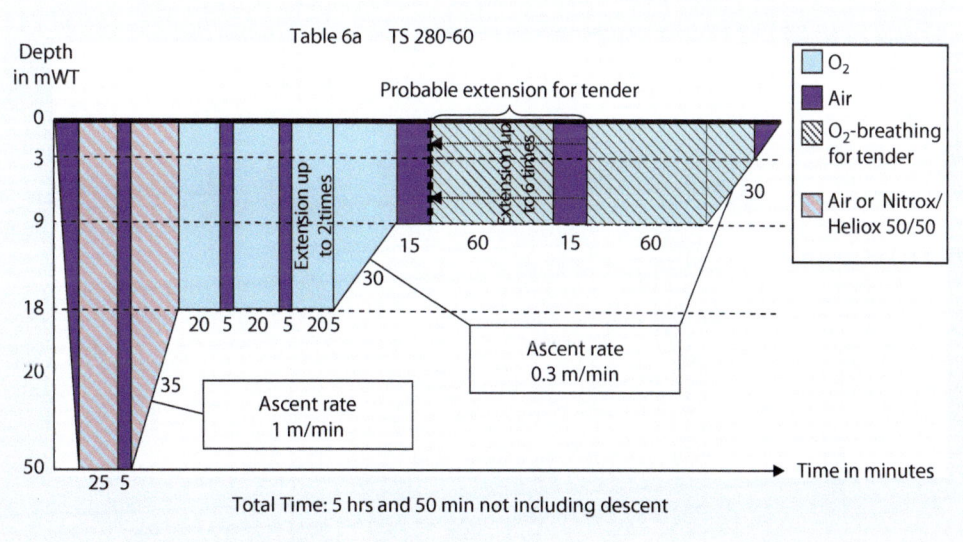

Fig. 24.21   USN Hyperbaric Oxygen Treatment Table 6a (USN TT 6a)

- Cataract (only >100 HBOT)
- Pulmonary barotrauma
- CNS oxygen toxicity with seizures, incidence 1:10000
- Pulmonary oxygen intoxication with interstitial pulmonary fibroses and rarely ARDS
- Claustrophobia

■ **Contraindications for HBOT**
- Absolute
  - Pneumothorax
  - Medications: bleomycin (for extended time), cisplatin, disulfiram, doxorubicin, sulfamylon
- Relative
  - Asthma

24

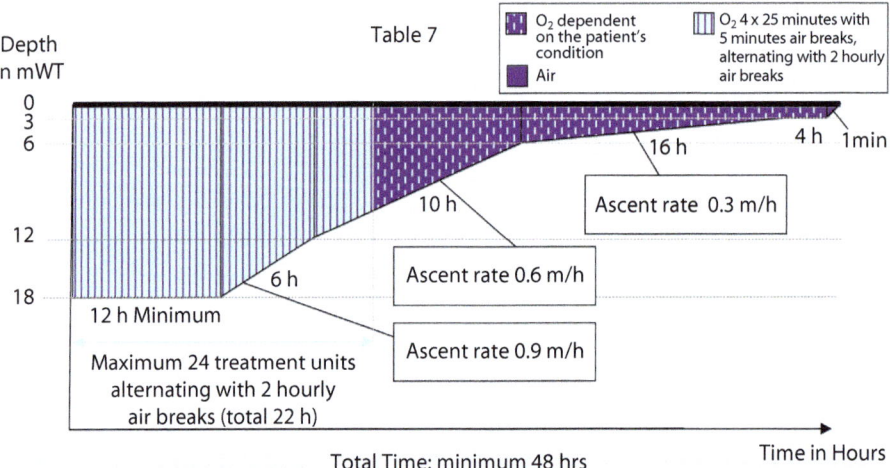

□ Fig. 24.22   USN Hyperbaric Oxygen Treatment Table 7 (USN TT 7)

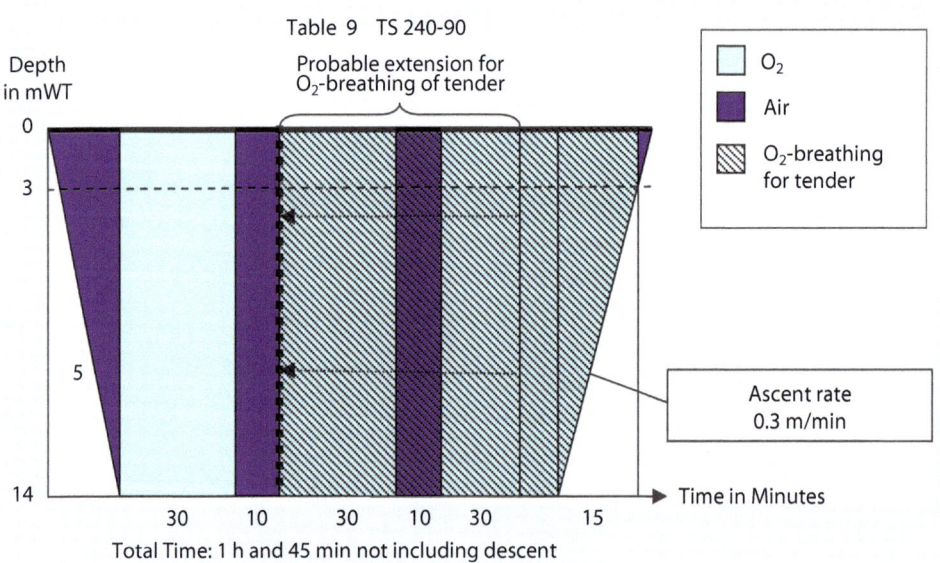

□ Fig. 24.23   USN Hyperbaric Oxygen Treatment Table 9 (USN TT 9)

COPD   High fever
Claustrongenital spherocytosis   Pregnancy
Eustachian tube dysfunction   Seizures
Pacemaker   Upper and lower respiratory infections

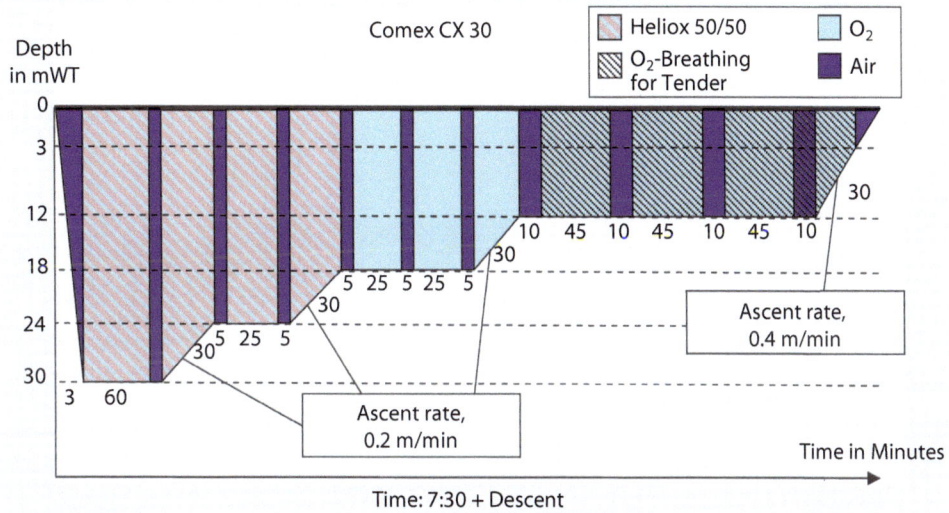

■ Fig. 24.24 Comex 30

■ Fig. 24.25 Mild DCI treatment schema

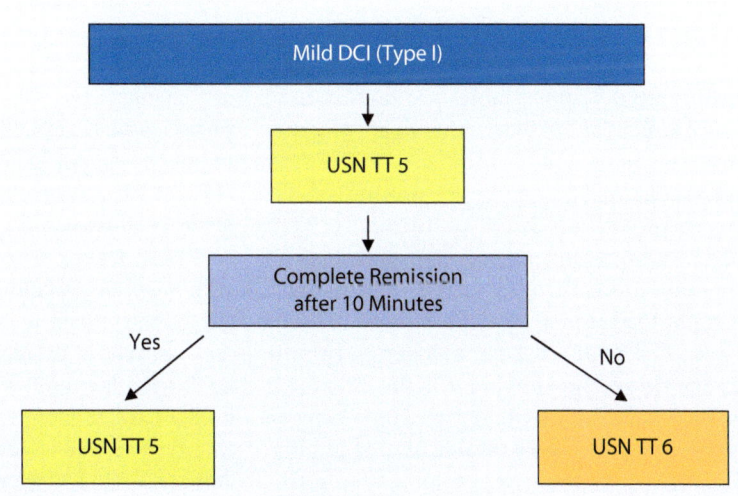

The compression or descent rate is usually 6 m/minute (20 ft/minute). If complications occur during this time, the compression can be halted or commenced with a reduced compression rate. The decompression and ascent rates vary according to treatment tables and depth. Various tables are also referred to the TS classification. "TS" stands for therapeutic schema. The first number describes the treatment depth in [kPa], e.g. 280 kPa, which corresponds to 18 msw. The second number stands for the treatment time on the treatment depth. The treatment time or the depth of treatment involves only the total oxygen time and not the compression or neither decompression time nor the oxygen breaks with normal breathing air.

Besides the above-mentioned USN HBOT Tables, other tables from Comex

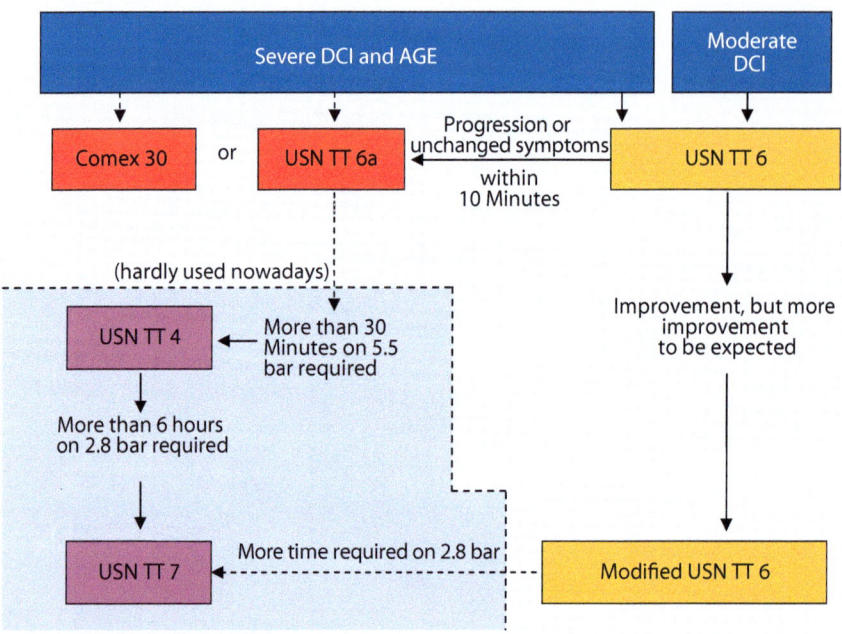

■ **Fig. 24.26**   AGE and severe DCI treatment schema

can be used. Comex tables are mainly used in commercial offshore and deep sea diving. The most common table is the Comex table 30 (Cx30). At the beginning of the treatment, heliox 50/50 or nitrox 50/50 is used as breathing gases. The advantage of the helium or nitrogen mix is that the total oxygen load under hyperbaric conditions is lowered. The pO_2 is 2 bar at 4 bar$_{abs}$ with the Cx30, decreasing further till the breathing gas eventually is switched to 100% oxygen at 2.8 bar$_{abs}$, which equals a pO_2 of 2.8 bar. Helium is lighter and less soluble than nitrogen. Hence, diffusion of helium is easier and doesn't get dissolved as much in blood and tissue. Another advantage of helium is the lower density which eases the respiratory flow and consequently the ventilation. As not all HBOT centres have the facility to treat with mixed gases, Comex tables are not always used (■ Fig. 24.24).

HBOT addresses the reduction of gas bubbles and supersaturation as well as oxygenation of ischaemic tissue and reversion of second-

ary changes. HBOT can be divided into two phases, which are addressing different targets in the treatment of DCI. Enhanced oxygenation of tissues and elimination of nitrogen are given in all phases to various degrees.

Phase I aims to restore perfusion and to eliminate DCI symptoms. This means inert gas bubbles need to be reduced in their size and numbers. Bubble reduction is driven by Boyle's law and diffusion. The bigger gas bubbles are, the longer it takes to reduce them in size. For example, microbubbles of 10 μm collapse within 6 sec due to their constrictive surface tension. Bigger bubbles take far longer to reduce their size. This is due to the Laplace's law but also to the effects on diffusion. Smaller bubbles are mainly influenced by Boyle's law and bigger bubbles mainly to diffusion. Bigger bubbles have additionally a surface-volume mismatch, which makes them more unfavourable in diffusion compared to smaller ones. Diffusion always requires a gradient. In case of a gas bubble, diffusion is driven by the diffusion area and the pressure difference. If the gas

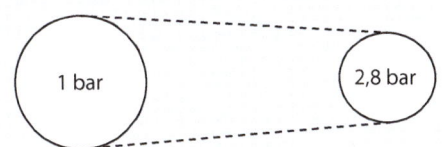

☐ **Fig. 24.27** Bubble size change under different pressures

bubble is stabilised by impurities or blood contents, diffusion distance might even increase, and diffusion is more or less slowed down. The mainstream treatment of DCI is USN TT 6. In severe cases Comex 30 or USN TT 6a are used. During HBOT (USN TT 6) at 2.8 bar, the theoretical bubble volume is reduced by 64% and however the diameter only by 29%. HBOT (Comex 30) at 4 bar reduces the volume by 75% and its diameter by 37%. HBOT (USN TT 6a) at 6 bar reduces the volume by 83% and its diameter by 45%. Before gas bubbles reduce their diameter, they have to have a spherical shape. Most bubbles in the bloodstream are however club- or sickle-shaped. HBOT reduces their length before their diameter is changed. Regardless of shape, passage of gas bubbles is eased by volume reduction. The smaller the gas bubble the quicker they pass through capillaries. It needs to be mentioned that elevated oxygen partial pressure initially increases the bubble size and decreases bubble elimination before it eventually decreases [14, 53]. This is best explained by ICD and the fact that individual gases diffuse individually depending on their partial pressure regardless of the partial pressures of other gases, which may be present. This may counteract the volume lowering effect of HBOT in Phase I (☐ Fig. 24.27).

Diffusion enhances the bubble size reduction by pressure increase. According to Fick's law, diffusion is driven by its partial pressure difference, exchange surface, diffusion distance and solubility. Increasing pressure leads to smaller supersaturation gradients of tissue and blood. This inhibits new bubble formation but doesn't reduce existing bubbles. The reversal of supersaturation by pressure changes by itself

has little effect on existing gas bubbles. In DCI gas bubbles are assumed to have almost the same partial pressure as their surroundings. Additionally, gas bubbles contain water vapour. In general, that means tissue and blood have approximately the same partial pressures as gas bubbles, even with changing pressure. Hence, there is no or little gradient and no diffusion out of gas bubbles to be expected. Gas transfer is driven by gradients of individual gases not by gases in total. That means each individual gas follows its own gradient. Bubbles reduce their volume by diffusion, only if a gradient is present. This can be found in the lungs, but also tissues or fluids, which are undersaturated by specific gases like nitrogen. In Phase I of HBOT, a drastic elimination of nitrogen in the fast compartments is achieved. Inert gas is kept in the dissolved phase and can be eliminated via the lungs. As 100% oxygen is administered, only little inert gas is in the alveolar air. Hence, a large inert gas gradient between pulmonary capillary and lungs leads to a relative quick off-gassing. By breathing an inert gas-free mix, the arterial blood is also assumed to be relatively inert gas-free. A gradient between gas bubble and blood/tissue develops, and gas can diffuse from bubble to blood or tissue. Inert gas, which is released from bubbles, can be eliminated via the blood in a dissolved phase. However, it applies only to areas where perfusion is possible. In areas where perfusion is cut off, the gas composition of blood and tissue is expected to remain almost unchanged. In case of a DCI, this produces an unfavourable cascade. As tissue continues to off-gas and inert gas isn't eliminated, swelling of the affected area increases due to ischaemia and gas bubbles. This further reduces perfusion. The only way to interrupt this cascade is to shrink bubbles with increased pressure according to Boyle's law. This is only achieved by high pressure, but not by changing gradients on its own.

Phase II aims to reduce the remaining inert gas load of compartments with their different M-values (☐ Fig. 24.28). As inert gas of the fast compartments is almost removed, only slower compartments are targeted in this phase. As slow compartments release excess

24

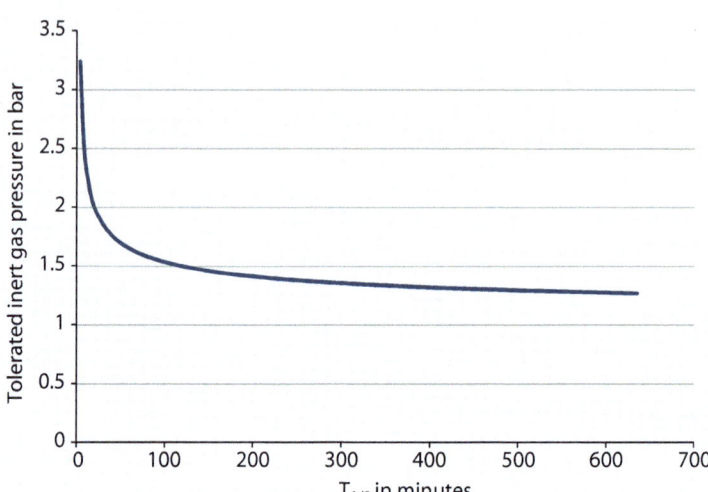

◻ Fig. 24.28
Tolerated inert gas
pressure in relation to
compartments with
different half times.
(From Bühlmann
1984 [6])

inert gas slowly, high peaks of inert gases are not expected. Hence, not treatment depth but treatment time has priority. Slower compartments begin off-gassing from the commencement of HBOT on. Nitrogen half times of muscles, for example, are about 100–240 min. In comparison, the total oxygen cycles of USN TT 6 combined take 230 min. Phase II requires enough capacity to reduce supersaturation to a safe level, so no total elimination is required. Current treatments have either 9 msw allocated for Phase II. The oxygen window HBOT at 1.9 bar_{abs} is 811 mmHg, supersaturation reduction by pressure of 633 mmHg, totalling to 1444 mmHg (approx. 2 bar).

During HBOT, but also during normobaric oxygen therapy, the oxygen window (OW) increases. The increased oxygen window offers a greater capacity to absorb inert gases from highly saturated tissues. As alveolar air has only little inert gas during HBOT, only little inert gas enters the pulmonary capillary. However, some nitrogen will still enter the arterial system via shunting depending on the extent of the intrapulmonary shunt. The intrapulmonary shunt is influenced by occluded pulmonary capillaries due to VGE. An almost complete inert gas elimination of fast compartments like blood and CNS tissue is achieved within approx.

100–120 min (5–6 x $T_{1/2}$). As long as a gradient exists, treatment time is more important than treatment depth, as elimination is rather driven by perfusion than diffusion.

All HBOT outlined below show a sufficient reduction in supersaturation to various degrees. In all HBOT the oxygen window alone can absorb nitrogen supersaturation by more than 1 bar. The total supersaturation reduction is a combination of OW and pressure increase. The lowest total theoretical reduction in supersaturation is 2.6 bar (1959 mmHg), and the highest is 5.8 bar (4334 mmHg) of the current treatment tables. 3.2–3.5 bar (2400–2625 mmHg) is the maximum tolerated inert gas pressure in fast compartments and 1.27 mmHg (952 mmHg) in the slowest compartment [6] (◻ Table 24.12).

Recreational diving rarely exceeds 70 m depth. The nitrogen partial pressure is there approximal 6.2 bar. Taking both, tolerated inert gas pressures of slow and fast compartment in consideration with the supersaturation are independent from exposure time something between 3 and 5 bar (2250 and 3750 mmHg). There is no clear limit to which extent the bubble sizes should be reduced. At 6 bar the bubble size is almost half of the original size and at 2.8 bar only about 1/3.

□ **Table 24.12** HBOT effects at maximum treatment depths

HBOT	100% oxygen				Heliox 50/50			
	1.5 bar[a]	1.9 bar	2.2 bar	USN TT 6 (2.8 bar)	Comex 30 (4 bar)	4.5 bar[a]	5 bar[a]	USN TT 6a (6 bar)
Reduction in volume	34%	47%	55%	64%	75%	78%	80%	83%
Reduction in diameter	13%	19%	23%	29%	37%	40%	42%	45%
P_{SS} reduction by pressure [mmHg]	348	633	842	1274	2129	2485	2842	3554
P_{SS} reduction by OW [mmHg][b]	801	811	812	809	781	779	783	780
Total P_{SS} reduction [mmHg][b]	1150	1444	1695	1959	2910	3265	3625	4334
Alveolar pO_2 [mmHg][b]	1006	1287	1498	1919	1286	1449	1613	1940

[a]Not included in current treatment tables
[b]Approximate theoretical values
P_{SS} = supersaturation

In summary, USN TT 6 is a good treatment option for most DCI patients and hence is regarded as the streamline treatment for DCI. It provides good oxygenation as well as bubble and supersaturation reduction. For severe DCI, where initial bubble reduction has priority for the reinstitution of perfusion, USN TT 6a performs best. However, the possibility of IGN for the attendant might significantly interfere with clinical judgement and performance. Phase II of USN Table 6 and 6a is at 9 msw. There is still a minimal risk of CNS oxygen intoxication for the tender at this depth. Additionally, the OTU for patients still increases.

■ **Effects of HBOT**
— *Reduction of nitrogen supersaturation by increased partial pressure gradient.* The mixture of gases in gas bubbles is similar to the mixture of the gases in its surroundings. Therefore, just pressure reduction doesn't enhance diffusion of gases out of the bubble into blood and tissue. As almost no nitrogen is in the arterial system, a large gradient exists between the arterial blood and tissue. Hence, only nitrogen of tissues adds to the venous nitrogen partial pressure. Under normobaric conditions oxygen partial pressure is 0.21 bar. During the HBOT the ambient pressure increases to approx. 2.8 bar when breathing 100% oxygen, which increases the blood oxygen partial pressure by almost 20-fold. Breathing 100% oxygen reduces dramatically arterial and venous nitrogen partial pressures. Additionally, the oxygen window increases with HBOT and allows more nitrogen to be carried in the blood before reaching supersaturation.

24

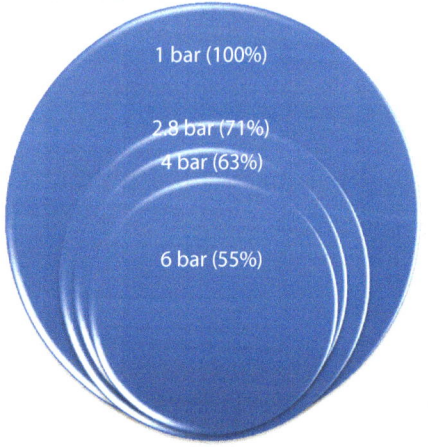

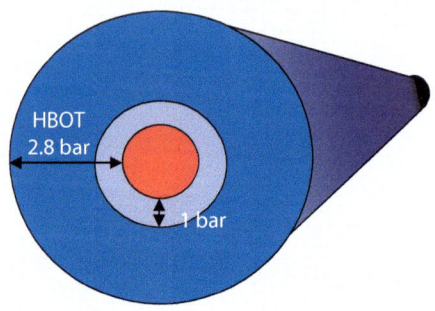

Fig. 24.30 Krogh cylinder model. 4-fold radius of the oxygen diffusion distance during HBOT (2.8 bar) in comparison to normobaric conditions (1 bar)

Fig. 24.29 Decrease of gas volume during HBOT

– *Reversing the supersaturation gradient.* With increasing pressure the supersaturation gradient is reduced. New bubble formation is therefore reduced or inhibited.
– *Mechanical reduction of gas bubbles.* At treatment pressure of 2.8 bar_{abs}, a theoretical reduction of the gas bubble volume by 64% is achieved. However, the diameter reduces only by 29%. HBOT with Comex 30 at 4 bar_{abs} reduces the volume by 75% and its diameter by 37%. HBOT with USN Table 6a at 6 bar_{abs} reduces the volume by 83% and its diameter by 45%. Additionally, it needs to be taken into consideration that gas bubbles in the bloodstream first change their shape from club-shaped to spherical before they change their diameter. Hence the real diameter reduction in vivo might be even less (Fig. 24.29).
– Approx. 15–20-fold *increased oxygen partial pressure* in blood (the oxygen partial pressure change in tissues is only minimal).
– *Increased penetration of oxygen* into the hypoxic tissue. Due to the increased oxygen partial pressure gradient, there is up to 4-fold radius of oxygen saturation around the blood vessels with 100% oxygen at 2.8 bar_{abs}. Additionally, hypoxic tissue

is less affected by the HBOT-produced vasoconstriction. Hence, there is a relative shift of blood flow into hypoxic tissues (Fig. 24.30).
– *Vasoconstriction* (with exemption of the pulmonary arteries).
– *Oedema reduction* due to vasoconstriction but also an approx. 8.5% increase of the oncotic pressure by oxygen itself. Anti-inflammatory effects may also contribute to the oedema reduction. This causes CNS reduction of penumbra and intracranial pressure. During HBOT oxygen remains mainly in blood vessels and not in tissues.
– *Oxygenation of hypoxic marginal tissues.*
– Hyperbaric oxygen stimulates *angiogenesis* [19, 41]. Neovascularisation is significantly increased in HBOT.
– *Impeded neutrophil activation* results in anti-inflammatory effects [24].
– *Reduction of lipid peroxidase* resulting in reduction of cytotoxic effects of ischaemia [42].
– *Reduction of leukocyte adhesion.* Decreased interaction of the immune system and endothelium (NO and inhibition of β-2 integrin with subsequent reduced ICAM-1-activation) [24]. Bubble-induced hypoxia provokes perivascular stress and NO increase and leads to leukocyte activation and adhesion to the endothelium. The adhesion takes place in two phases.

The initial phase is unsteady and mediated by selectins. The second phase is stable due to β-2 integrins activation. Hence, by inhibition of β-2 integrins, HBOT prevents the occurrence of subsequent processes causing cellular damage. HBOT doesn't seem to increase ROS in ischaemic tissue and ischaemia-reperfusion injury. It rather seems to increase antioxidant expression and decreases prooxidant expression (iNOS and gp91-phox) in ischaemic tissue [52].

Patients should be positioned horizontally without elevation or lowering of the head. Lowering of the head should be avoided, since it increases the risk of cerebral oedema. On the other hand, an elevation of the head seems to favour cerebral or cerebellar gas embolism, as gas travels up even against the flow. Unconscious patients should be initially positioned in a stable side position on the left (with the exception of right-side pneumothorax). If the GCS is less than 8, the patient might need to be intubated. 100% oxygen should be applied. A slightly increased respiration (*moderate hyperventilation*) is effective to reduce the intracerebral pressure (ICP). However, an excessive hyperventilation should be avoided. The desired pCO_2 is 20–35 mmHg. Euvolaemia or a mild hypovolaemia is useful to reduce intracranial pressure and to avoid brain oedema. The CPP (cerebral perfusion pressure) should be 50–70 mmHg. The CPP can be estimated by

$$CPP = MAP - ICP \text{ or } MAP - CVP$$

- CPP = cerebral perfusion pressure
- MAP = mean arterial pressure
- ICP = intracranial pressure
- CVP = central venous pressure.

Treatment with PEEP worsens the potentially damaged lung tissue and should be therefore avoided.

Cerebral oedema occurs usually 2–5 days after embolic occlusions. Considered treatment for increased intracranial pressure may be osmotic therapy with a bolus of mannitol (0.25–1.5 g/kg bw). To compensate increased blood viscosity, Ringer's lactate solution with 5% albumin can be administered. Otherwise, in the absence of brain oedema, parenteral hydration (e.g. isotonic sodium chloride solution) can be started immediately after a decompression accident. However, if chokes are present, fluids need be administered carefully. Parenteral fluid administration with pulmonary DCI (chokes) can lead to right heart failure. Hence, parenteral fluid administration with chokes requires fluid balance and is usually not exceeding 700–1000 mL/day till recovery.

The use of enoxaparin 40 mg SC per day or heparin 5000 IU SC 2–3 times per day and compression stockings are only indicated for the bed-ridden patients for VTE prophylaxis after the commencement of HBOT. Steroids are not recommended to reduce cerebral oedema. Administering cortisone leads to a quantitative transfer glucose from the interior of the cell into the blood (reactive hyperglycaemia) and leads to a deterioration of the metabolic balance of the brain.

Acute ischaemic cerebral events can increase cerebral blood pressure. Reactively, blood pressure in the entire body increases. Due to the increase of the blood pressure in the body, in the cerebral blood pressure increases again. The result is a fatal cycle. The increased blood pressure normalises after approximately 2 days. A blood pressure above 220/150 mmHg should be treated (e.g. labetalol IV or oral, lisinopril oral) in ischaemic strokes with suspicion of increased intracranial pressure. The initial lowering of the blood pressure shouldn't be more than 25% in the first 2 h. Aggressive lowering of blood pressure with nitrates should be avoided. Vasodilator drugs increase oxygen deficiency in affected areas. Vasodilatation of the penumbra "steals" the blood from the already underperfused tissue in the stroke area. The target blood pressure is at 160/95 mmHg. Blood pressure under 120 mmHg is equally unfavourable, as it reduces the cerebral blood flow. To increase blood pressure, Ringer's solution is recommended.

The use of drugs that inhibit platelet aggregation, such as aspirin, for example, in DCI is controversial. Currently, it is believed that acetylsalicylic acid (Aspirin®) should be omitted, since it may cause spinal or inner ear bleeding, if used as treatment of DCI. However, Aspirin for isolated AGE might be a reasonable treatment option.

Dysbaric osteonecrosis is treated with HBOT (approximately 30 treatments with USN Table 9). The affected area may be surgically treated as well. The success rate in the treatment of a dysbaric osteonecrosis is however moderate. Next beside diving related injuries, HBOT is used to treat other medical conditions (◘ Table 24.13)

■ Prophylaxis

There are different ways to reduce the probability of suffering from DCI. Dive tables have been developed over the years to minimise risks. Diving tables from different providers have only minor differences in details such as surface intervals and diving groups at various dive times and depths. There are also tables (wheel), which allow the calculation of dive profiles with different depths during a single dive. In normal diving tables, only the maximum depth and the bottom time are included. Theoretical calculations of these tables are based on *dive time*, *depth*, *surface intervals and ascent rate* after Hampleman, Bassett, Haldane, Hills and Bühlmann, verified by practical comparison. The calculations are quite similar for diving computers. The advantage of diving computers is that they involve each change of the diving profile (dive time and depth as well as ascent rate and surface intervals) in their calculations. Failure to comply with deco stops and bottom time and exceeding the ascent rate result in a visually or acoustically warning of the dive computer (◘ Fig. 24.31).

In general the maximum diving depth should be at the beginning of the dive. Yo-yo dives with frequent changes in depth, and frequent surface contacts increase the risk of DCI and should be therefore avoided. For diving deeper than 18 m, safety stops in 5 m for at least 3 min are recommended. The old rule of 5 min at 3 m is less favourable, since the short distance of only 3 m to the surface often can't be always met (e.g. when there are waves) and poses a risk of accidental surface contact. However, due to the greater pressure difference between underwater and surface at altitude dives, safety stops for altitude dives are at 2-m depth for 5 min. Dives below 40 m deep shouldn't be performed in recreational scuba diving. In general, deep stops at half of the maximum depth for 2.5 min for recreational diving are recommended (Bennett and Maronni [2]). For example, in a 40-m dive, a deep deco stop at 20 m for 2.5 min should be included. This significantly reduces the formation of microbubbles by reducing the inert gas amount in the dissolved phase and thus the risk of DCI. This is usually not displayed in diving computers but should be implemented in the diving profile. Despite adherence to all safety rules, DCI still can occur. About 1/3 of all DCI divers complied with diving tables or computers. That suggests that other factors and then the diving profile only may play a role in DCI development. These might be personal disposition, external influences and diving habits.

■ Personal Dispositions that May Pose an Increased DCI Risk

− Because nitrogen is highly soluble in lipid, inert gas may accumulate more in *obese* people. Additionally, comorbidities and reduced physical fitness are often associated with obesity. Therefore, it can be assumed that obese people are exposed to a higher DCI risk. The BMI seems to be a good guidance in the assessment of obesity.

− Some studies in the past suggested that women are more often affected by decompression accidents than men. The explanation of this supposed to be the difference in *gender*. Women have physiologically approximately twice as much body fat compared to men, and their perfusion of muscles and skin is also higher. In addition, the water content in their bodies is lower than in men. The different hormonal

◼ **Table 24.13** Other indications for HBOT [44]

Indication	USN TT	Minimum treatment	Maximum treatment
CO intoxication[1B]	USN TT 5 or 6	1	5
Clostridial myositis and myonecrosis[1B]	USN TT 5: first day 3x/day, followed by 2x/day	5	10
Crush injury, compartment syndrome and other acute traumatic ischaemias[1B]	USN TT 9 depending on symptoms: 3x/day, 2x/day or 1x/day	3	12
Poor wound healing caused by poor perfusion (DM, venous and arterial ulcerations, pressure ulcers)[2B]	USN TT 9: 2x/day or 1x/day	10	60
Necrotising soft tissue infection[1C]	USN TT 9: initially 2x/day and then 1x/day	5	30
Refractory osteomyelitis[2C]	USN TT 9	20	60
Delayed radiation injury (soft tissue)[1B]	USN TT 9	20	60
Osteoradionecrosis[1B] (mandible),[2C] (other than mandible)	USN TT 9	20	60
Compromised skin grafts and skin flaps[2C]	USN TT 9	6	40
Acute thermal burn injury (second-degree burn >20% body surface area, with burns to face, neck, hands and fingers and perineum)[2C]	USN TT 9: initially 3x/day and then 2x/day	5	45
Intracranial abscess (multiple abscesses, abscess in a deep or dominant location, compromised host, contraindication to surgery, lack of response in spite of standard treatment)[1C]	USN TT 9: 1–2/day		As needed
Central retinal artery occlusion[2C] <24 h If normobaric high-flow oxygen is not sufficient (> 5 min) Corrected vision acuity 20/200 or worse Age > 40 No recent eye surgery of trauma No acute onset of flashes or floater prior vision loss	Start with 100% oxygen at normobaric (90 min); if there is no improvement after 5 min, start USN TT 5 If there is no improvement after 20 min with USN TT 5, change to USN TT 6 2x/day		Until resulting in 3 days without further improvement
Severe anaemia	US NTT 9 or USN TT 5 Up to 3–4x/day		As needed
Idiopathic sudden sensorineural hearing loss (within 2 weeks of onset)[1B]	USN TT 9	10	20

1 = Type 1 recommendation (recommended treatment option), 2 = Type 2 recommendation (suggested treatment option), 3 = Type 3 recommendation (reasonable treatment option); level of evidence: A = high level of evidence, B = moderate level of evidence, C = low level of evidence, D = very low level of evidence [28]

24

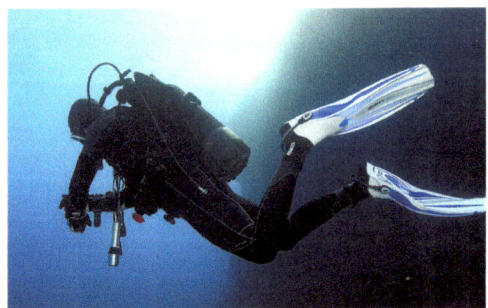

■ **Fig. 24.31** Adherence to deco and safety stops. (With kind permission of Mares, Photo Bernd Humberg)

system or its secondary effects on the cardiovascular system possibly might influence the development of DCI as well. During menstruation and by using contraceptives, the susceptibility of decompression accidents was deemed to be higher. The use of contraceptives as a sole factor seemed to play a minor role. The likelihood of clots formation with female smokers on oral contraceptives may increase the DCI risk as well. However, there is no support in studies to show an increased risk in female developing DCI. Moreover, as males tend to choose riskier diving profiles and perform often physically more demanding dives, some studies suggested a higher incidence of DCI in males.

- The increased occurrence of DCI at *higher age* is most likely due to reduced perfusion of the different tissues, multi-morbidity, reduced body responsiveness on environmental factors, lack of fitness, changes of the cardiovascular system and respiratory changes.
- *Poor training or physical fitness* (e.g. after illness) making divers more susceptible to DCI.
- *Dehydration* may reduce the blood volume and thus the diameter of the blood vessels, which encourages the formation of gas embolism. The blood may be more concentrated and hence may have increased viscosity.

- *Pathological changes* of the cardiovascular system (e.g. PFO), of the nervous system, of the haematological system and of the pulmonary system promote the occurrence of DCI.
- *Alcohol and drugs* may lead to inappropriate behaviour underwater and to misjudgement and neglecting basic diving rules. Alcohol itself is a causative factor for dehydration, bradycardia and respiratory depression. Reduced perfusion minimizes off-gassing of nitrogen, which can lead to its accumulation. Other drugs such as amphetamines and cocaine cause vasoconstriction.
- *Medication*, which acts on the cardiovascular system and blood, may increase the risk of DCI.
- *Smoking* with its increased carbon monoxide content reduces the oxygenation of blood and hence oxygen supply to tissue. Smoking causes an increased thrombocytes aggregation and therefore increased coagulation. Additionally, it causes endothelial stress.
- *Poor acclimatisation* leads to an increased cardiovascular stress and dehydration with an increased risk of decompression accidents.
- *Poor adaptation* to diving increases the risk of DCI. The adaptation to diving itself seems to have a protective factor against DCI. Frequent diving seems to lower the risk of DCI [47], which may be due to either physical or physiological adaption of the diver. Hence, recreational divers, in particular at the beginning of their holiday, are at risk. A slow start with shallow dives is recommended.
- *Strenuous physical exercise* before, during and after diving seems to increase the risk of decompression accidents. However, mild to moderate exercise before diving and during decompression seems to lower the risk of a DCI [9–12].
- *Previous DCI*.

■ **External Influences and Diving Behaviour**
- *Rapid ascent rates* promote gas bubble formation.
- With the number of *repetitive dives* the risk of decompression accidents increases. Inert gas in the body accumulates through repetitive dives. This causes particularly inert gases in slow compartments with long half-lives to rise. That's why it is recommended to take 1 day of diving with more than 3 consecutive days of repetitive dives. In general it is recommended not to exceed two dives per day.
- Due to low *temperatures*, oxygen turnover, respiration and hence inert gas intake are increased. The narrowing of skin capillaries causes a shift of the blood volume centrally. The nitrogen solubility depends on temperature as well. The solubility increases with decreasing temperature. During diving the temperature in the body core is higher than in the periphery, which is exposed to cold ambient temperatures. This means that, due to the lower temperatures in the body periphery, the gas is better resolved than in the core of the body. This leads to increased nitrogen saturation in peripheral tissues but also release of nitrogen into the free phase in central body parts. These two factors might promote the occurrence of subcutaneous embolism and bends. If nitrogen-rich cool blood of the body periphery enters the core of the body and warms up, the solubility of nitrogen decreases and increases the risk of forming gas bubbles, which in turn increases the risk of air embolism. Strong exposure to the sun and hot showers or baths after the dive should be avoided, because it increases skin perfusion, reduces gas solubility and thus increases gas bubbles formation (■ Fig. 24.32).
- *Dive profiles* with the maximum depth at the end of the dive, frequent change

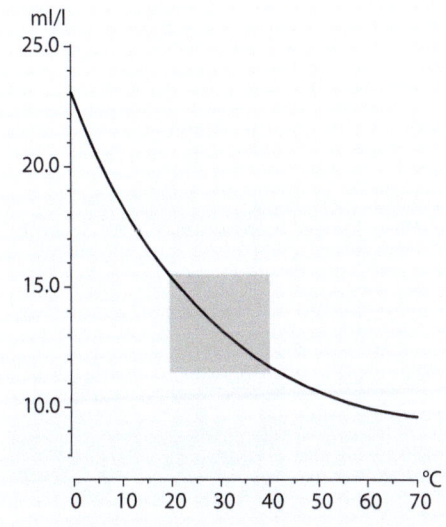

■ **Fig. 24.32** Exponential increase of N_2 solubility in water with decreasing ambient temperature at 1.0 bar. (From Bühlmann 2002 [7])

of depth (yo-yo dives), frequent surfacing, neglecting of decompression times, emergency ascents, strong physical stress during deep dives and long stays in great depth promote the occurrence of decompression accidents (■ Fig. 24.33).
- *Short surface intervals* increase the risk of DCI. The surface interval should be at least 90 min. The RGBM proposes that the surface intervals should be prolonged to reduce inert gas loading between dives.
- *Altitude changes above sea level after diving* can trigger DCI. Altitude diving requires other tables. Ambient pressure decreases approximately by 0.1 bar per 1000 m (1 hPa per 30 ft). The difference of underwater and surface pressure increases as the ambient pressure above water is lower in altitude compared to the one at sea level, but pressure changes below the surface are unchanged. For example, at 2000 m above water, the ambient pressure is 0.8 bar compared to 1 bar at sea level. Pressure

24

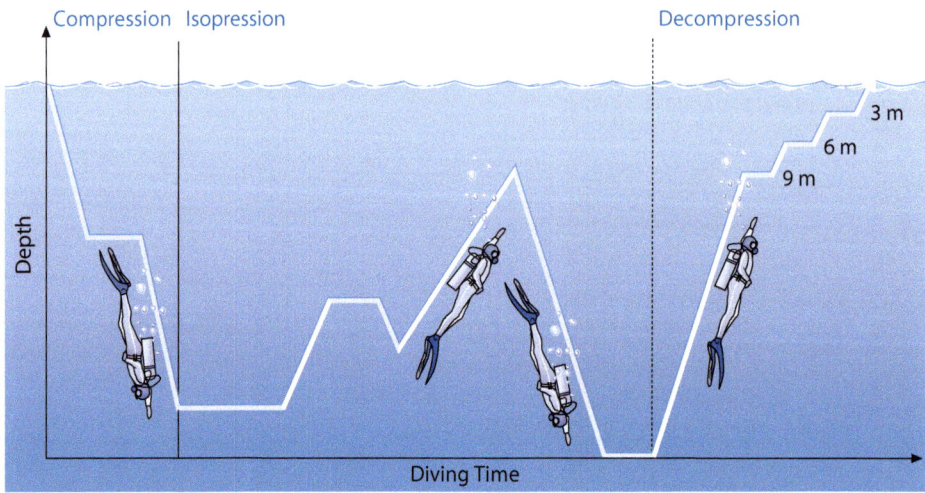

■ **Fig. 24.33** Risky dive profile with frequent changes of depth, dive requiring deco stops, fast ascent to surface and maximum depth at the end of the dive (Ecomed)

changes underwater are not affected by the ambient pressure above water as they are related to the water column. The water column is the main driver for the pressure increase underwater. Hence, the inert gas uptake is similar in altitude and normal diving. However, divers are exposed to lower ambient pressure at altitude diving on exiting the water, and hence gradients are bigger. Dive computers have the ability to switch to altitude diving to adjust calculations. Travel along ridges or flights should be avoided for at least 12 h after diving, as ambient pressure is decreased. Emergency ascents require a waiting period of 24 h before flying or travelling at greater heights and of at least 48 h after decompression accidents with a complete remission of symptoms.

— The use of *different gas mixtures* (nitrox, heliox) with different densities can cause DCI when changing to normal breathing air. When switching from a helium mix to air, helium leaves the tissue faster than nitrogen. As gas bubbles contain mainly helium from the helium mixture and only little nitrogen,

nitrogen diffuses into gas bubbles at a fast rate and add onto bubble volume additionally to the existing helium (*ICD* = isobaric counterdiffusion). Switching from normal air to a helium mix is even worse (see ▶ Chap. 5). Remember that diffusion of gases happens separately according to each individual gas and not as a sum of all gases. The symptoms appear almost immediately after switching the gas mixture. The change of gases may trigger gas bubble formation, mainly manifesting as IEDCI. Recently there are alternative suggestions that vestibular symptoms could be also related to damages to the cerebellum. Vestibular and cerebellar symptoms can be quite similar and can be easily confused.

— Vertical *body positions* compared to horizontal may decrease inert gas elimination. In horizontal position inert gas bubbles seem to be better distributed through the body, accumulate less and hence can be eliminated easier via the lung. Immersion in *horizontal position and slight movement* may therefore promote inert gas elimination. The reduction of V/Q mismatch in horizontal position increases the overall gas exchange and hence inert gas elimination. In horizontal positions, the pressure difference within the body between the least and the greatest is smaller depth compared to upright positions. This is particularly pronounced at shallow depth, where pressure differences are bigger. For example, a change of 1.8 m (size of a diver) in 3 m depth creates a significant pressure difference in the body. In 30 m the same change would be negligible. Moreover, bigger gas bubbles also find their way up, even against the bloodstream in the venous system [36] and hence potentially increase the risk of ceAGE.

- During *flights*, cabin pressure decreases up to approx. 0.7 bar. This increases the risk of DCI. To reduce risks, time intervals between last dive and flight of 12 h after a single dive, 24 h after repetitive dives and 24–48 h after diving requiring deco stops should be kept. Patients treated for DCI or AGE should not fly for a minimum of 72 h. Tender who had been with a patient in USN TT 5, 6, 6A, 1A, 2A or 3 should not fly for 24 h, and tenders who had been with a patient treated with USN TT 4 or 7 should not fly for a minimum of 72 h.

In general, DCI is caused by a summation of several factors. Health, fitness, diving experience, adaptation and acclimatization, as well as adjustments to the conditions of the diving spot, can reduce the risk of DCI.

References

1. Benestad HB, Hersleth IB, Hardersen H, Molvaer OI. Functional capacity of neutrophil granulocytes in deep-sea divers. Scand J Clin Lab Invest. 1990;50:9–18.
2. Bennett PB, Marroni A, Cronje FJ, Cali-Corleo R, Germonpre P, Pieri M, et al. Effect of varying deep stop times and shallow stop times on precordial bubbles after dives to 25 msw (82 fsw). Undersea Hyperb Med. 2007;34(6):399–406.
3. Bergh K, Hjelde A, Iversen OJ, Brubakk AO. Variability over time of complement activation induced by air bubbles in human and rabbit sera. J Appl Physiol. 1993;74:1811–5.
4. Boussuges A, Succo E, Juhan-Vague I, Sainty JM. Activation of coagulation in decompression illness. Aviat Space Environ Med. 1998;69(2):129–32.
5. Brubakk AO. Endothelium and bubble injury. The role of endothelium in decompression illness; 30th annual scientific meeting of the European Underwater Baromedical Society, Ajaccio, Corsica, France EUBS; 2004
6. Bühlmann AA. Decompression/decompression sickness. Berlin: Springer; 1984.
7. Bühlmann AA, Völlm EB, Nussberger P. Tauchmedizin, barotrauma, Gasembolie, Dekompensation, Dekompensationskrankheit. 5th ed. Berlin: Springer; 2002.
8. Butler BD, Hills BA. The lung as a filter for microbubbles. J Appl Physiol Respir Environ Exerc Physiol. 1979;47(3):537–43.
9. Dujic Z, Duplancic D, Marinovic-Terzic I, Bakovic D, Ivancev V, Valic Z, et al. Aerobic exercise before diving reduces venous gas bubble formation in humans. J Physiol. 2004;555(Pt 3):637–42.
10. Dujic Z, Obad A, Palada I, Ivancev V, Valic Z. Venous bubble count declines during strenuous exercise after an open sea dive to 30 m. Aviat Space Environ Med. 2006;77(6):592–6.
11. Dujic Z, Palada I, Obad A, Duplancic D, Bakovic D, Valic Z. Exercise during a 3-min decompression stop reduces postdive venous gas bubbles. Med Sci Sports Exerc. 2005;37(8):1319–23.
12. Dujic Z, Valic Z, Brubakk AO. Beneficial role of exercise on scuba diving. Exerc Sport Sci Rev. 2008;36(1):38–42.
13. Eftedal OS, Lydersen S, Brubakk AO. The relationship between venous gas bubbles and adverse effects of decompression after air dives. Undersea Hyperb Med Soc UHM. 2007;35(2)
14. Erdem I, Yildiz S, Uzun G, Sonmez G, Senol MG, Mutluoglu M, Mutlu H, Oner B. Cerebral whitematter lesions in asymptomatic military divers. Aviat Space Environ Med. 2009;80:2–4.
15. Erdmann. Klinische Kardiologie – Krankeiten des Herzens, des Kreislaufs und der herznahen Gefäße. 6th ed: Springer; 2006.
16. Francis TJR. The pathophysiology of decompression sickness. In: Bennett PB, Moon RE, editors. Diving accident management. North Palm Beach: UHMS; 1990. p. 38–56.
17. Francis TJ, Dutka AJ, Flynn ET. Experimental determination of latency, severity, and outcome in CNS decompression sickness. Undersea Biomed Res. 1988;15(6):419–27. 83
18. Francis TJ, Pezeshkpour GH, Dutka AJ, Hallenbeck JM, Flynn ET. Is there a role for the autochthonous bubble in the pathogenesis of spinal cord decompression sickness? J Neuropathol Exp Neurol. 1988;47(4):475–87.

24

19. Grassmann JP, Schneppendahl J, Hakimi AR, Herten M, Betsch M, Lögters TT, Thelen S, Sager M, Wild M, Windolf J, Jungbluth P, Hakimi M. Hyperbaric oxygen therapy improves angiogenesis and bone formation in critical sized diaphyseal defects. J Orthop Res. 2015;33(4):513–20. https://doi.org/10.1002/jor.22805.

20. Guyton AC. A concept of negative interstitial pressure based on pressure in implanted capsules. Circ Res. 1963;XII

21. Hjelde A, Bergh K, Brubakk AO, Iversen OJ. Complement activation in divers after repeated air/heliox dives and its possible relevance to DCS. J Appl Physiol. 1995;78(3):1140–4.

22. Huang KL, Lin YC. Activation of complement and neutrophils increases vascular permeability during air embolism. Aviat Space Environ Med. 1997; 68(4):300–5.

23. Jain KK. Oxygen toxicity. In: Textbook of hyperbaric medicine. Cham: Springer; 2017. p. 49–60.

24. Kalns J, Lane J, Delgado A, Scruggs J, Ayala E, Gutierrez E, et al. Hyperbaric oxygen exposure temporarily reduces mac-1 mediated functions of human neutrophils. Immunol Lett. 2002;83(2):125–31. 12067761

25. Kitano M, Hayashi K, Kawashima M. Three autopsy cases of acute decompression sickness consideration of pathogenesis about spinal cord damage in decompression sickness. Jpn Orthop Traum. 1977;26:402.

26. Loset A Jr, Mollerlokken A, Berge V, Wisloff U, Brubakk AO. Post-dive bubble formation in rats: effects of exercise 24 h ahead repeated 30min before the dive. Aviat Space Environ Med. 2006;77(9):905–8.

27. Madden LA, Laden G. Gas bubbles may not be the underlying cause of decompression illness - the at-depth endothelia dysfunction hypothesis. Med Hypothesis. 2009;72:389–92.

28. Mathieu D, Marroni A, Kot J. Consensus conference of hyperbaric medicine. Diving Hyperb Med. 2017;47(1):24–32.

29. Mollerlokken A, Berge VJ, Jorgensen A, Wisloff U, Brubakk AO. Effect of a short-acting NO donor on bubble formation from a saturation dive in pigs. J Appl Physiol. 2006;101(6):1541–5.

30. National Oceanic and Atmospheric Administration. NOAA diving manual: Diving for science and technology. 6th ed. revised. Washington: DC; 2017.

31. Papadopoulou V, Tang M, Belestra C, Thodoris RJE, Karapantsios TD. Circulatory bubble dynamics: from physical to biological aspects. Adv Colloid Interface Sci Elsevier. 2014;206:239–49.

32. Patra M. Laterall-Pressure Profiles in Cholesterol-DPPC Bilayers, arXiv:cond-mat/0504101v1 [cond-mat.soft] 5 April 2005.

33. Philp RB, Freeman D, Francey I, Bishop B. Hematology and blood chemistry in saturation diving:

I. Antiplatelet drugs, aspirin, and VK744. Undersea Biomed Res. 1975;2(4):233–49.

34. Pontier JM, Blatteau JE, Vallée N. Blood platelet count and severity of decompression sickness in rats after a provocative dive. Aviat Space Environ Med. 2008;79(8):761–4.

35. Pontier JM, Jimenez C, Blatteau JE. Blood platelet count and bubble formation after a dive to 30 msw for 30 min. Aviat Space Environ Med. 2008;79(12): 1096–9.

36. Schlimp CJ, Bothma PA, Brodbeck AE. Cerebral venous air embolism: what is it and do we know how to deal with it properly? JAMA Neurol. 2014;71(2):243. https://doi.org/10.1001/jamaneurol.2013.5414.

37. Sparacia G, Banco A, Sparacia B, Midiri M, Brancatelli G, Accardi M, et al. Magnetic resonance findings in scuba diving-related spinal cord decompression sickness. MAGMA. 1997;5(2):111–5.

38. Spencer MP, Johanson DC. Investigation of new principles for human decompression schedules using the Doppler ultrasonic blood detector. Tech report to ONR on contract N00014–73-C-0094. Seattle, Washington: Institute for Environmental Medicine and Physiology; 1974.

39. Stickland MK, Lovering AT. Exercise-induced intra pulmonary arteriovenous shunting and pulmonary gas exchange. Exerc Sport Sci Rev. 2006; 34(3):99–106.

40. Tetzlaff K, Friege L, Hutzelmann A, Reuter M, Holl D, Leplow B. Magnetic resonance signal abnormalities and neuropsychological deficits in elderly compressed-air divers. Eur Neurol. 1999;42(4):194–9.

41. Thom SR. Hyperbaric oxygen: its mechanisms and efficacy. Plast Reconstr Surg. 2011;127:131S–41S. https://doi.org/10.1097/PRS.0b013e3181fbe2bf.

42. Thom SR, Elbuken ME. Oxygen-dependent antagonism of lipid peroxidation. Free Radic Biol Med. 1991;10:413–26.

43. Tikuisis P. Modeling the observations of in vivo bubble formation with hydrophobic crevices. Undersea Biomed Res. 1986;13(2):165–80.

44. US Navy Diving Manual: www.uhms/images/DCS-and-AGE-Journal-Watch/recompression_therapy_usn_di.pdf. Accessed 04.10.2015.

45. Van Poucke S, Jorens P, Beaucourt L. Chapter 1.7 Physiologic effects of hyperbaric oxygen on ischemia-reperfusion phenomenon. In: Mathieu D, editor. Handbook on hyperbaric medicine: Springer; 2006.

46. Walder DN. Prevention of DCS in compressed air workers. In: Bennett PB, Elliott DH, editors. The physiology and medicine of diving and compressed air work. 1st ed. London: Bailliére Tindall and Cassell; 1969. p. 437–50.

47. Walder DN. Adaptation to decompression sickness in caisson work. Biometeor. 1968;11:350–9.

48. Ward CA, McCullough D, Fraser WD. Relation between complement activation and susceptibility to decompression sickness. J Appl Physiol. 1987; 62:1160–6.

49. Wienke BR. Diving decompression models and bubble metrics: modern computer synthesis. Comput Biol Med. 2009;39(2009):309–31.

50. Yu X, Xu J, Huang G, Zhang K, Qing L, Liu W, et al. Bubble-induced endothelial microparticles promote endothelial dysfunction. PLoS One. 2017; 12(1):e0168881. https://doi.org/10.1371/journal.pone.0168881.

51. Yusupov M, Wende K, Kupsch S, Neyts EC, Reuter S, Bogaerts A. Effect of head group and lipid tail oxidation in the cell membrane revealed through integrated simulations and experiments, Scientific Reports 7, Article number: 5761(2017) https://doi.org/10.1038/s41598-017-06412-8.

52. Zhang K, et al. Endothelial dysfunction correlates with decompression bubbles in rats. Sci Rep. 2016;6:33390. https://doi.org/10.1038/srep33390.

53. Zhu J, Hullett JB, Somera L, Barbee RW, Ward KR, Berger BE, et al. Intravenous perfluorocarbon emulsion increases nitrogen washout after venous gas emboli in rabbits. Undersea Hyperb Med. 2007;34(1):7–20.

Suggested Reading

Aksoy FG. MR imaging of subclinical cerebral decompression sickness. A case report. Acta Radiol. 2003;44(1):108–10.

Anaesthesia UK; spinal cord; www.frca.co.uk/article.aspx?articleid=100360. Accessed 30.01.2016.

Antonelli C, Franchi F, Della Marta ME, Carinci A, Sbrana G, Tanasi P, De Fina L, Brauzzi M. Guiding principles in choosing a therapeutic table for DCI hyperbaric therapy. Minerva Anaestesiol. 2009;75(3):151–61.

Arness MK. Scuba decompression illness and diving fatalities in an overseas military community. Aviat Space Environ Med. 1997;68(4):325–33.

Aslam F, Shirani J, Haque AA. Patent foramen ovale: assessment, clinical significance and therapeutic options. South Med J. 2006;99(12):1367–72.

Assessing Fitness to Return to Diving After Decompression Illness: DMAC 13 Rev. 1 – October 1994.

Auten JD, Kuhne MA, Walker HM, Porter HO. Neurologic decompression sickness following cabin pressure fluctuations at high altitude. Aviat Space Environ Med. 2010;81(4):427–30.

Barratt DM, Van Meter K. Decompression sickness in Miskito Indian lobster divers: review of 229 cases. Aviat Space Environ Med. 2004;75(4):350–3.

Bennett MH, Lehm JP, Mitchell SJ, Wasiak J. Recompression and adjunctive therapy for decompression illness. Cochrane Database Syst Rev. 2012;5: CD005277.

Bennett PB, Elliott DH. The physiology and medicine of diving and compressed air work. 2nd ed. Baltimore: Lippincott William & Wilkins; 1975.

Marroni A, Bennett PB, Cronje FJ, Carli-Corleo R, Germonpre P, Pieri M, Bonuccelli C, Balestra B. A deep stop during decompression from 82 few (25 m) significantly reduces bubbles and fast tissue gas tension. UHM. 2004;31(2):233–43.

Goldman S. A new class of biophysical models for predicting the probability of decompression sickness in scuba diving. J Appl Physiol. 2007;103: 484–93.

Berge VJ, Jørgensen A, Løset A, Wisløff U, Brubakk AO. Exercise ending 30 min pre-dive has no effect on bubble formation in the rat. Aviat Space Environ Med. 2005;76(4):326–8.

Bessereau J, Coulange M, Genotelle N, Barthélémy A, Michelet P, Bruguerolle B, et al. Aspirin in decompression sickness. Therapie. 2008;63(6):419–23.

Bhardwaj A, Ulatowski JA. Cerebral edema: hypertonic saline solutions. Curr Treat Options Neurol. 1999;1:179–88.

Blatteau JE, Boussuges A, Gempp E, Pontier JM, Castagna O, Robinet C, et al. Haemodynamic changes induced by submaximal exercise before a dive and its consequences on bubble formation. Br J Sports Med. 2007;41(6):375–9.

Blatteau JE, Gempp E, Balestra C, Mets T, Germonpre P. Predive sauna and venous gas bubbles upon decompression from 400 kPa. Aviat Space Environ Med. 2008;79(12):1100–5.

Blatteau JE, Gempp E, Simon O, Coulange M, Delafosse B, Souday V, et al. Prognostic factors of spinal cord decompression sickness in recreational diving: retrospective and multicentric analysis of 279 cases. Neurocrit Care. 2011;15(1):120–7.

Blatteau JE, Jean F, Pontier JM, Blanche E, Bompar JM, Meaudre E. Decompression sickness accident management in remote areas. Use of immediate in-water recompression therapy. Review and elaboration of a new protocol targeted for a mission at Clipperton atoll. Ann Fr Anesth Reanim. 2006;25(8):874–83.

Blatteau JE, Brubakk AO, Gempp E, Castagna O, Risso JJ, Vallee N. Sildenafil pre-treatment promotes decompression sickness in rats. PLoS One. 2013;8:e60639.

Blogg SL, Loveman GA, Seddon FM, Woodger N, Koch A, Reuter M, et al. Magnetic resonance imaging and neuropathology findings in the goat nervous system following hyperbaric exposures. Eur Neurol. 2004;52(1):18–28.

Bove AA. Risk of decompression sickness with patent foramen ovale. Undersea Hyperb Med. 1998; 25(3):175–8.

Brain Trauma Foundation. American Association of Neurological Surgeons, joint section on Neurotrauma and critical care: guidelines for cerebral perfusion pressure. J Neurotrauma. 2000;17:507–11.

Brodsky SV, Zhang F, Nasjletti A, Goligorsky MS. Endothelium-derived microparticles impair endothelial function in vitro. Am J Physiol. 2004;286:H1910–5.

Brott TG. NIH Stroke/Score (NIHSS), http://www.mdcal.com/nih-stroke-scale-score-nihss/#how-to-use. Accessed 07.10.2015.

Brubakk AO, Arntzen AJ, Wienke BR, Koteng S. Decompression profile and bubble formation after dives with surface decompression: experimental support for a dual phase model of decompression. Undersea Hyperb Med. 2003;30:181–93.

Brubakk AO, Neuman TS, editors. Bennett and Elliott's physiology and medicine of diving. 5th ed. London: Saunders; 2003.

Bruno A, Williams LS, Kent TA. How important is hyperglycemia during acute brain infarction? Neurologist. 2004;10:195–200.

Buch DA, El Moalem H, Dovenbarger JA, Uguccioni DM, Cigarette MRE. Smoking and decompression illness severity: a retrospective study in recreational divers. Aviat Space Environ Med. 2003;74(12):1271–4.

Butler BD, Little T, Cogan V, Powell M. Hyperbaric oxygen pre-breathe modifies the outcome of decompression sickness. Undersea Hyperb Med. 2006;33(6):407–17.

Camporesi EM. Diving and pregnancy. Semin Perinatol. 1996;20(4):292–302.

Candito M, Candito E, Chatel M, van Obberghen E, Dunac A. Homocysteinemia and thrombophilic factors in unexplained decompression sickness. Rev Neurol (Paris). 2006;162(8–9):840–4.

Candito M, Chatel M, Candito E, Lapoussiere M, Mengual R, Van Obberghen E, et al. Thrombophilic factors in divers with undeserved decompression sickness. Pathol Biol (Paris). 2006;54(3):155–8.

Cartoni D, De Castro S, Valente G, Costanzo C, Pelliccia A, Beni S, et al. Identification of professional scuba divers with patent foramen ovale at risk for decompression illness. Am J Cardiol. 2004;94(2):270–3.

Carturan D, Boussuges A, Burnet H, Fondarai J, Vanuxem P, Gardette B. Circulating venous bubbles in recreational diving: relationships with age, weight, maximal oxygen uptake and body fat percentage. Int J Sports Med. 1999;20(6):410–4.

Chang Y, Chen TY, Chen CH, Crain BJ, Toung TJ, Bhardwaj A. Plasma arginine-vasopressin following experimental stroke: effect of osmotherapy. J Appl Physiol. 2006;100:1445–51.

Chappell M. Modelling and measurement of bubbles in decompression sickness, University of Oxford; 2006. https://users.fmrib.ox.ac.uk/~Chappell/papers/m_chappell_thesis.pdf. (Accessed 16 Oct 2016).

Cheshire WP. Headache and facial pain in scuba divers. Curr Pain Headache Rep. 2004;8:315–20.

Chryssanthou C. Animal model of human disease: dysbaric osteonecrosis. AM J Pathol. 1981;103(2):334–6.

Cimsit M, Ilgezdi S, Cimsit C, Uzun G. Dysbaric osteonecrosis in experienced dive masters and instructors. Aviat Space Environ Med. 2007;78(12):1150.

Clenney TL, Lassen LF. Recreational scuba diving injuries. Am Fam Physician. 1996;53:1761–6.

Dainer H, Nelson J, Brass K, Montcalm-Smith E, Mahon R. Short oxygen prebreathing and intravenous perfluorocarbon emulsion reduces morbidity and mortality in a swine saturation model of decompression sickness. J Appl Physiol. 2007;102(3):1099–104.

de Watteville G. A critical assessment of Trendelenburg's position in the acute phase after a diving accident. Schweiz Z Sportmed. 1993;41(3):123–5.

Dietrich A. U. S. navy diving Manual: air diving: 1. New York: Diane Pub Co; 1999.

Diringer MN, Zazulia AR. Osmotic therapy: fact or fiction. Neurocrit Care. 2004;1:219–34.

Divers Alert Network, de Lisle Dear G. Asthma and diving. Available at: http://www.diversalertnetwork.org/medical/articles/article.asp?articleid=22. Accessed 02.03.2015.

Divers Alert Network. Annual diving report 2006 edition. Durham, North Carolina, US: Divers Alert Network; Oct 11, 2006.

Divers Alert Network. Report on decompression illness, diving fatalities and project dive exploration 2005 edition. Durham, North Carolina: Divers Alert Network; 2005.

Doolette DJ, Mitchell SJ. Biophysical basis for inner ear decompression sickness. J Appl Physiol. 2003;94:2145–50.

Drighil A, El Mosalami H, Elbadaoui N, Chraibi S, Bennis A. Patent foramen ovale: a new disease? Int J Cardiol. 2007;122(1):1–9.

Dromsky DM, Spiess BD, Treatment FA. Of decompression sickness in swine with intravenous perfluorocarbon emulsion. Aviat Space Environ Med. 2004;75(4):301–5.

Duggan C, Fontaine O, Pierce NF, et al. Scientific rationale for a change in the composition of oral rehydration solution. JAMA. 2004;291(21):2628–31.

Dujic Z, Palada I, Obad A, Duplancic D, Brubakk AO, Valic Z. Exercise-induced intrapulmonary shunting of venous gas emboli does not occur after open-sea diving. J Appl Physiol. 2005;99(3):944–9.

Dujic Z, Palada I, Valic Z, Duplancic D, Obad A, Wisløff U. Exogenous nitric oxide and bubble formation in divers. Med Sci Sports Exerc. 2006;38(8):1432–5.

Dunford RG, Vann RD, Gerth WA, Pieper CF, Huggins K, Wacholtz C, et al. The incidence of venous gas emboli in recreational diving. Undersea Hyperb Med. 2002;29(4):247–59.

Eccher M, Suarez JI. Cerebral edema and intracranial pressure. Monitoring and intracranial dynamics. In: Suarez JI, editor. Critical care neurology and neurosurgery. Totowa: Humana Press; 2004. p. 47–100.

Edmonds CW, Lowry C, Pennefather JW. Diving and subaquatic medicine. 4th ed. London: Edward Arnold; 2005.

Ehm OF. Tauchen - noch sicherer!. 5. Auflage. Zürich: Müller Rueschlikon; 1991.

Endres M, Dirnagl U, Moskowitz MA. The ischemic cascade and mediators of ischemic injury, stroke, part I, chapter 2. In: Handbook of clinical neurology, vol. 92. Philadelphia: Elsevier; 2009. p. 31–41.

Fahlman. On the physiology of hydrogen diving and its implication for hydrogen biochemical Dekompression;B.Sc. Hawaii Pacific University; 1996.

Fahlman A, Dromsky DM. Dehydration effects on the risk of severe decompression sickness in a swine model. Aviat Space Environ Med. 2006;77(2): 102–6.

Francis A, Baynosa R. Ischaemia-reperfusion injury and hyperbaric oxygen pathways: a review of cellular mechanisms. Diving Hyperb Med SPUMS. 2017;47(2):110.

Frank JI. Management of intracranial hypertension. Med Clin North Am. 1993;77:61–76.

Fremont-Smith F, Forbes HS. Intravascular and intracranial pressure: an experimental study. Arch Neurol Psychiatr. 1927;18:550–64.

Fyneface-Ogan S. Epidural analgesia - current views and approaches. London: InTech; 2010.

Gao GK, Wu D, Yang Y, Yu T, Xue J, Wang X, et al. Cerebral magnetic resonance imaging of compressed air divers in diving accidents. Undersea Hyperb Med. 2009;36(1):33–41.

Gemma M, Cozzi S, Poccoli C, Magrin S, De Vitis A, Cenzato M. Hypertonic saline fluid therapy following brain stem trauma. J Neurosurg Anesthesiol. 1996;8:137–41.

Gemma M, Cozzi S, Tommasino C, Mungo M, Calvi MR, Capriani A, et al. 7.5% hypertonic saline versus 20% mannitol during elective neurosurgical supratentorial procedures. J Neurosurg Anesthesiol. 1997;9: 329–34.

Gempp E, Blatteau JE, Pontier JM, Balestra C, Louge P. Preventive effect of pre-dive hydration on bubble formation in divers. Br J Sports Med. 2009;43(3):224–8.

Gempp E, Blatteau JE. Neurological disorders after repetitive breath-hold diving. Aviat Space Environ Med. 2006;77(9):971–3.

Gempp E, Blatteau JE. Preconditioning methods and mechanisms for preventing the risk of decompression sickness in scuba divers: a review. Res Sports Med. 2010;18(3):205–18.

Gempp E, Blatteau JE, Stephant E, Pontier JM, Constantin P, Peny C. MRI findings and clinical outcome in 45 divers with spinal cord decompression sickness. Aviat Space Environ Med. 2008;79(12):1112–6.

Germonpre P, Dendale P, Unger P, Balestra C. Patent foramen ovale and decompression sickness in sports divers. J Appl Physiol. 1998;84(5):1622–6.

Gil A, Shupak A, Lavon H, Adir Y. Decompression sickness in divers treated at the Israel Naval Medical Institute between the years 1992 to 1997. Harefuah. 2000;138(9):751–4. 806

Gold D, Geater A, Aiyarak S, Juengprasert W, Chuchaisangrat B, Samakkaran A. The indigenous fisherman divers of Thailand: in-water recompression. Int Marit Health. 1999;50(1–4):39–48.

Goldenberg I, Shupak A, Oxy-helium SO. Treatment for refractory neurological decompression sickness: a case report. Aviat Space Environ Med. 1996;67(1):57–60.

Goldhahn RT Jr. Scuba diving deaths: a review and approach for the pathologist. Leg Med Annu. 1976;1977:109–32.

Goplen FK, Grønning M, Irgens A, Sundal E, Nordahl SH. Vestibular symptoms and otoneurological findings in retired offshore divers. Aviat Space Environ Med. 2007;78(4):414–9.

Gorman D, Sames C, Drewry A, Bodicoat S. A case of type 3 DCS with a radiologically normal spinal cord. Intern Med J. 2006;36(3):193–6.

Gutvik CR, Brubakk AO. A dynamic 2-phase model for vascular bubble formation during decompression of divers, TBME-00076-2008.

Hajat C, Hajat S, Sharma P. Effect of poststroke pyrexia on stroke outcome. A meta-analysis of studies in patients. Stroke. 2000;31:410–4.

Hampson NB, Dunford RG, Kramer CC, Norkool DM. Selection criteria utilized for hyperbaric oxygen treatment of carbon monoxide poisoning. J Emerg Med. 1995;13(2):227–31.

Hardy KR. Diving-related emergencies. Emerg Med Clin North Am. 1997;15(1):223–40.

Hart AJ, White SA, Conboy PJ, Bodiwala G, Quinton D. Open water scuba diving accidents at Leicester: five years' experience. J Accid Emerg Med. 1999;16(3):198–200.

Harukuni I, Kirsch J, Bhardwaj A. Cerebral resuscitation: role of osmotherapy. J Anesth. 2002;16:229–37.

Helps SC, Gorman DF. Air embolism of the brain in rabbits pretreated with mechlorethamine. Stroke. 1991;22:351–4.

Hennessy TR, Hempleman HV. An examination of the critical released gas concept in decompression sickness. Proc R Soc London B. 1977;197:299–313.

Holzer M, Bernard SA, Hachimi-Idrissi S, Roine RO, Sterz F, Mullner M, et al. Hypothermia for neuroprotection after cardiac arrest: systematic review and individual patient data meta-analysis. Crit Care Med. 2005;33:414–8.

Honek T, Veselka J, Tomek A, Srámek M, Janugka J, Sefc L, et al. Paradoxical embolization and patent foramen ovale in scuba divers: screening possibilities. Vnitr Lek. 2007;53(2):143–6.

Hughes JT. Venous infarction of the spinal cord. Neurology. 1971;21(8):794–800. 82.

Hutter CD. Dysbaric osteonecrosis: a reassessment and hypothesis. Med Hypotheses. 2000;54(4):585–90.

Hyldegaard O, Jensen T. Effect of heliox, oxygen and air breathing on helium bubbles after heliox diving. Undersea Hyperb Med. 2007;34(2):107–22.

James HE, Langfitt TW, Kumar VS, Ghostine SY. Treatment of intracranial hypertension. Analysis of 105 consecutive, continuous recordings of intracranial pressure. Acta Neurochir. 1977;36:189–200.

James PB. Hyperbaric oxygenation in fluid microembolism. Neurol Res. 2007;29(2):156–61.

Jankowski LW, Tikuisis P, Nishi RY. Exercise effects during diving and decompression on post-dive venous gas emboli. Aviat Space Environ Med. 2004;75(6):489–95.

Jauch EC. Acute management of stroke, http://emedicine.medscape.com/article/1159752-overview. Accessed 12.7.2015.

Jauch EC. Ischemic Stroke, http://emedicine.medscape.com/article/1916852-overview. Accessed 10.7.2015.

Jerrard DA. Diving medicine. Emerg Med Clin North Am. 1992;10(2):329–38.

Keller H, Buhlmann AA. Deep diving and short decompression by breathing mixed gases. J Appl Physiol. 1965;20:1267.

Kizer KW. Dysbarism. In: Rosen R, Barken RM, Brean CR, et al., editors. Emergency medicine: concepts and clinical practice: St Louis Mosby; 1992. p. 881–8.

Klingman C, Tetzlaff K. Moderne Tauchmedizin. 2 Auflage ed. Stuttgart: Gentner Verlag; 2012.

Klingmann C, Praetorius M, Baumann I, Plinkert PK. Barotrauma and decompression illness of the inner ear: 46 cases during treatment and follow up. Otol Neurotol. 2007;28:447–54.

Koch AE, Kirsch H, Reuter M, Warninghoff V, Rieckert H, Deuschl G. Prevalence of patent foramen ovale (PFO) and MRI-lesions in mild neurological decompression sickness (type B-DCS/AGE). Undersea Hyperb Med. 2008;35(3):197–205.

Koch AE, Wegner-Bröse H, Warninghoff V, Deuschl G. Viewpoint: the type A- and the type B-variants of decompression sickness. Undersea Hyperb Med. 2008;35(2):91–7.

Korenkov AI, Pahnke J, Frei K, Warzok R, Schroeder HW, Frick R, et al. Treatment with nimodipine or mannitol reduces programmed cell death and infarct size following focal cerebral ischemia. Neurosurg Rev. 2000;23:145–50.

Kot J, Sicko Z, Michalkiewicz M, Lizak E, Góralczyk P. Recompression treatment for decompression illness: 5-year report (2003-2007) from National Centre for hyperbaric medicine in Poland. Int Marit Health. 2008;59(1–4):69–80.

Kunkle TD, Beckman EL. Bubble dissolution physics and the treatment of decompression sickness. Med Phys. 1983;10:184–90.

Lafay V. The heart and underwater diving. Arch Mal Coeur Vaiss. 2006;99(11):1115–9.

Lambertson CJ. Effects of excessive pressures of oxygen, nitrogen, helium, carbon dioxide, and carbon monoxide. In: Mountcastle VB, editor. Medical physiology. Missouri: CV Mosby Co.; 1980. p. 1901–46.

Lang EW, Chestnut RM. Intracranial pressure: monitoring and management. Neurosurg Clin N Am. 1994;5:573–605.

Lang MA, Brubakk AO. The future of diving: 100 years of Haldane and beyond. Washington, DC: Smithsonian Institution Scholaryly Press; 2009.

Landsberg PG. South African underwater diving accidents, 1969-1976. S Afr Med J. 1976;50(55):2155–9.

Leffler CT, White JC. Recompression treatments during the recovery of TWA flight 800. Undersea Hyperb Med. 1997;24(4):301–8.

Lemaitre F, Carturan D, Tourney-Chollet C, Gardette B. Circulating venous bubbles in children after diving. Pediatr Exerc Sci. 2009;21(1):77–85.

Longphre JM, Denoble PJ, Moon RE, Vann RD, Freiberger JJ. First aid normobaric oxygen for the treatment of recreational diving injuries. Undersea Hyperb Med. 2007;34(1):43–9.

MacDonald RD, O'Donnell C, Allan GM, Breeck K, Chow Y, DeMajo W. Interfacility transport of patients with decompression illness: literature review and consensus statement. Prehosp Emerg Care. 2006;10(4):482–7.

Magnaes B. Body position and cerebrospinal fluid pressure. Part I: clinical studies on the effect of rapid postural changes. J Neurosurg. 1976;44:687–97.

Manabe Y, Sakai K, Kashihara K, Shohmori T. Presumed venous infarction in spinal decompression sickness. AJNR Am J Neuroradiol. 1998;19(8):1578–80.

Marabotti C, Chiesa F, Scalzini A, Antonelli F, Lari R, Franchini C, et al. Cardiac and humoral changes induced by recreational scuba diving. Undersea Hyperb Med. 1999;26(3):151–8.

Marroni A, et al. Chapter 2.2.1 Dysbaric illness. In: Mathieu D, editor. Handbook of hyperbaric medicine: Springer; 2006. p. 173–216.

Mathieu D, Nolf M, Durocher A, et al. Acute carbon monoxide poisoning. Risk of late sequelae and treatment by hyperbaric oxygen. J Toxicol Clin Toxicol. 1985;23:315.

McCormac J, Mirvis SE, Cotta-Cumba C, Shanmuganathan K. Spinal myelopathy resulting from decompression sickness: MR findings in a case and review of the literature. Emerg Radiol. 2002;9(4):240–2.

McGuire G, Crossley D, Richards J, Wong D. Effects of varying levels of positive end-expiratory pressure on intracranial pressure and cerebral perfusion pressure. Crit Care Med. 1997;25:1059–62.

McManus ML, Soriano SG. Rebound swelling of astroglial cells exposed to hypertonic mannitol. Anesthesiology. 1998;88:1586–91.

Meijer LA, Leermakers FAM, Lyklema J. Self-consistent-field modeling of complex molecules with united atom detail in inhomogeneous systems. Cyclic and branched foreign molecules in dimyristoylphosphatidylcholine membranes. J Chem Phys. 1999;110(6560):6560–79.

Mekjavić B, Golden FS, Eglin M, Tipton MJ. Thermal status of saturation divers during operational dives in the North Sea. Undersea Hyperb Med. Edition 3/2001; S. 149–155.

Miller JD, Leech P. Effects of mannitol and steroid therapy on intracranial volume-pressure relationships in patients. J Neurosurg. 1975;42:274–81.

Mitchell SJ, Doolette DJ. Selective vulnerability of the inner ear to decompression sickness in divers with right-to-left shunt: the role of tissue gas supersaturation. J Appl Physiol. 2009;106(1):298–301.

Montcalm-Smith E, Caviness J, Chen Y, McCarron RM. Stress biomarkers in a rat model of decompression sickness. Aviat Space Environ Med. 2007;78(2):87–93.

Moses H. casualties in individual submarine escape, Bureau of Medicine and Surgery, Navy Department Reserch Project MR005.14–3002-4.17, Report No. 438; 1964.

Muizelaar JP, Marmarou A, Ward JD, Kontos HA, Choi SC, Becker DP, et al. Adverse effects of prolonged hyperventilation in patients with severe head injury: a randomized clinical trial. J Neurosurg. 1991;75:731–9.

Muizelaar JP, van der Poel HG, Li ZC, Kontos HA, Levasseur JE. Pial arteriolar vessel diameter and CO 2 reactivity during prolonged hyperventilation in the rabbit. J Neurosurg. 1988;69:923–7.

Neuman TS, Thom SR. Physiology and medicine of hyperbaric oxygen therapy. Philadelphia: Saunders Elsevier; 2008.

Nishi RY. Development of surface decompression tables for helium–oxygen diving to depths of 100msw. Undersea Biomed Res. 1991;18:66–7.

Nishi RY. Development of new helium–oxygen decompression tables for depths to 100 msw. Undersea Biomed Res. 1989;16:26–7.

Obad A, Palada I, Valic Z, Ivancev V, Bakovic D, Wisloff U, et al. The effects of acute oral antioxidants on diving-induced alterations in human cardiovascular function. J Physiol. 2007;578(Pt 3):859–70.

O'Connor PE. The nontechnical causes of diving accidents: can U.S. navy divers learn from other industries? Undersea Hyperb Med. 2007;34(1):51–9.

Papadopoulos MC, Saadoun S, Binder DK, Manlet GT, Krishna S, Verkman AS. Molecular mechanisms of brain tumor edema. Neuroscience. 2004;129:1011–20.

Parsons MW, Barber PA, Desmond PM, Baird TA, Darby DG, Byrnes G, et al. Acute hyperglycemia adversely affects stroke outcome: a magnetic resonance and spectroscopy study. Ann Neurol. 2002;52:20–8.

Pendergast DR, Tedesco M, Nawrocki DM, Fisher NM. Energetics of underwater swimming with SCUBA. Med Sci Sports Exerc. 1996;28:573–80.

Pontier JM, Guerrero F, Castagna O. Bubble formation and endothelial function before and after 3 months of dive training. Aviat Space Environ Med. 2009;80(1):15–9.

Pöppel E., Bullinger M. Medizinische Psychologie. VHC ed. Medizin: Weinheim; 1990.

Poungvarin N. Steroids have no role in stroke therapy. Stroke. 2004;35:229–30.

Pulley SA. Decompression Sickness, http://emedicine.medscape.com/article/769717-overview.   Access date 8.10.2015.

Qureshi AI, Suarez JI, Bhardwaj A, Mirski M, Schnitzer MS, Hanley DF, et al. Use of hypertonic (3%) saline/acetate infusion in the treatment of cerebral edema: effect on intracranial pressure and lateral displacement of the brain. Crit Care Med. 1998;26:440–6.

Qureshi AI, Suarez JI. Use of hypertonic saline solutions in treatment of cerebral edema and intracranial hypertension. Crit Care Med. 2000;28:3301–13.

Qureshi AI, Wilson DA, Traystman RJ. Treatment of elevated intracranial pressure in experimental intracerebral hemorrhage: comparison between mannitol and hypertonic saline. Neuro Surg. 1999;44:1055–64.

Rabinstein AA. Found comatose. In: Rabinstein AA, Wijdicks EFM, editors. Tough calls in acute neurology. Philadelphia: Elsevier; 2004. p. 3–18.

Rabinstein AA. Treatment of brain edema. Neurologist. 2006;12:59–73.

Reinertsen RE, Flook V, Koteng S, Brubakk AO. 1996 Effect on oxygen tension and rate of pressure reduction during decompression on central gas bubbles; http://jap.physiology.org/content/jap/84/1/351.full.pdf. Accessed 4/7/2017.

Reuter M, Tetzlaff K, Hutzelmann A, Fritsch G, Steffens JC, Bettinghausen E, et al. MR imaging of the central nervous system in diving-related decompression illness. Acta Radiol. 1997;38(6):940–4.

Reuter M, Tetzlaff K, Warninghoff V, et al. Computed tomography of the chest in diving-related pulmonary barotrauma. Br J Radiol. 1997;70(833):440–5.

Riede UN, Werner M, Freudenberg N. Basiswissen Allgemeine und Spezielle Pathologie. 2nd ed. Stuttgart: Georg Thieme Verlag; 2009

Roberts I, Yates D, Sandercock P, Farrell B, Wasserberg J, Lomas G, et al. Effect of intravenous corticosteroids on death within 14 days in 10008 adults with clinically significant head injury (MRC CRASH trial): randomised placebo controlled trial. Lancet. 2004;364:1321–8.

Rockswold GL, Ford SE, Anderson DC, Bergman TA, Sherman RE. Results of a prospective randomized trial for treatment of severely brain-injured patients with hyperbaric oxygen. J Neurosurg. 1992;76:929–34.

Ropper AH, Gress DR, Diringer MN, Green DM, Mayer SA, editors. Neurological and neurosurgical intensive care. Philadelphia: Lippincott, Williams & Wilkins; 2004. p. 26–51.

Ropper AH, O'Rourke D, Kennedy SK. Head position, intra cranial pressure, and compliance. Neurology. 1982;32:1288–91.

MJ CIB. Cerebral perfusion pressure, intracranial pressure, and head elevation. J Neurosurg. 1986;65: 636–41.

24

Sastry S, MacNab A, Daly K, Ray S, McCollum C. Transcranial Doppler detection of venous-to-arterial circulation shunts: criteria for patent foramen ovale. J Clin Ultrasound. 2009;37(5):276–80.

Schell RM, Applegate RL II, Cole DJ. Salt, starch, and water on the brain. J Neurosurg Anesthesiol. 1996;8:178–82.

Schipke JD, Gams E, Kallweit O. Decompression sickness following breath-hold diving. Res Sports Med. 2006;14(3):163–78.

Schmoker J, Zhuang J, Shackford S. Hypertonic fluid resuscitation improves cerebral oxygen delivery and reduces intracranial pressure after hemorrhagic shock. J Trauma. 1991;31:1607–13.

Schrot RJ, Muizelaar JP. Mannitol in acute traumatic brain injury. Lancet. 2002;359:1633–4.

Schwab S, Geordiadis D, Berrouschot J, Schellinger PD, Graf fag nino C, Mayer SA. Feasibility and safety of moderate hypothermia in acute ischemic stroke. Stroke. 2001;32:2033–5.

Schwarz S, Georgiadis D, Aschoff A, Schwab S. Effects of body position on intracranial pressure and cerebral perfusion in patients with large hemispheric stroke. Stroke. 2002;33:497–501.

Schwarz S, Georgiadis D, Aschoff A, Schwab S. Effects of hypertonic (10%) saline in patients with raised intracranial pressure after stroke. Stroke. 2002;33:136–40.

Schwarz S, Schwab S, Bertram M, Aschoff A, Hacke W. Effect of hypertonic saline hydroxyethyl starch solution and mannitol in patients with increased intracranial pressure after stroke. Stroke. 1998;29:1550–5.

Scubamed. Underwater medicine 2008. Dominica. January 12–19. Available at: http://www.scubamed.com/tuum_prg.htm. Accessed 15.05.2013.

Shastri KA, Logue GL, Lundgren CE, Logue CJ, Suggs DF. Diving decompression fails to activate complement. Undersea Hyperb Med. 1997;24(2):51–7.

Shupak A, Gil A, Nachum Z, Miller S, Gordon CR, Tal D. Inner ear decompression sickness and inner ear barotrauma in recreational divers: a long-term follow-up. Laryngoscope. 2003;113(12):2141–7.

Shupak A, Melamed Y, Ramon Y, Bentur Y, Abramovich A, Kol S. Helium and oxygen treatment of severe air-diving-induced neurologic decompression sickness. Arch Neurol. 1997;54(3):305–11.

Sinha S, Bastin ME, Wardlaw JM, Armitage PA, Whittle IR. Effects of dexamethasone on peritumoral oedematous brain: a DT-MRI study. J Neurol Neurosurg Psychiatry. 2004;75:1632–5.

Slivka AP, Murphy EJ. High-dose methylprednisolone treatment in experimental focal cerebral ischemia. Exp Neurol. 2001;167:166–72.

Smerz RW. Age associated risks of recreational scuba diving. Hawaii Med J. 2006;65(5):140–1. 153

Sobakin AS, Wilson MA, Lehner CE, Dueland RT, Gendron-Fitzpatrick AP. Oxygen pre-breathing decreases dysbaric diseases in UW sheep undergoing hyperbaric exposure. Undersea Hyperb Med. 2008;35(1):61–7.

Spiess BD, Zhu J, Pierce B, Weis R, Berger BE, Reses J, et al. Effects of perfluorocarbon infusion in an anesthetized swine decompression model. J Surg Res. 2009;153(1):83–94.

Spiess BD. Perfluorocarbon emulsions as a promising technology: a review of tissue and vascular gas dynamics. J Appl Physiol. 2009;106(4):1444–52.

Spira A. Diving and marine medicine review part II: diving diseases. J Travel Med. 1999;6(3):180–98.

Stringer WA, Hasso AN, Thompson JR, Hinshaw DB, Jordan KG. Hyperventilation-induced cerebral ischemia in patients with acute brain lesions: demonstration by xenon-enhanced CT. AJNR Am J Neuroradiol. 1993;14(2):475–84.

Su CL, Wu CP, Chen SY, Kang BH, Huang KL, Lin YC. Acclimatization to neurological decompression sickness in rabbits. Am J Physiol Regul Integr Comp Physiol. 2004;287(5):R1214–8.

Suarez JI, Qureshi AI, Bhardwaj A, Williams MA, Schnitzer MS, Mirski M, et al. Treatment of refractory intracranial hypertension with 23.4% saline. Crit Care Med. 1998;26:1118–22.

Taylor DM, Lippmann J, Smith D. The absence of hearing loss in otologically asymptomatic recreational scuba divers. Undersea Hyperb Med. 2006;33(2):135–41.

Tempel R, Severance HW. Proposing short-term observation units for the management of decompression illness. Undersea Hyperb Med. 2006;33(2):89–94.

Tetzlaff K, Thorsen E. Breathing at depth: physiologic and clinical aspects of diving while breathing compressed gas. Clin Chest Med. 2005;26:355–80.

Thenuwara K, Todd MM, Brian JE Jr. Effect of mannitol and furosemide on plasma osmolality and brain water. Anesthesiology. 2002;96:416–21.

Tietjen CS, Hurn PD, Ulatowski JA, Kirsch JR. Treatment modalities for hypertensive patients with intracranial pathology: options and risks. Crit Care Med. 1996;24:311–22.

Tomassoni AJ. Cardiac problems associated with dysbarism. Cardiol Clin. 1995;13(2):266–71.

Toung TJ, Chang Y, Lin J, Bhardwaj A. Increases in lung and brain water following experimental stroke: effect of mannitol and hypertonic saline. Crit Care Med. 2005;33:203–8.

Toung TJ, Chen CH, Lin C, Bhardwaj A. Osmotherapy with hypertonic saline attenuates water content in brain and extra cerebral organs. Crit Care Med. 2007;35:526–31.

Toung TJ, Hurn PD, Traystman RJ, Bhardwaj A. Global brain water increases after experimental focal cerebral ischemia: effect of hypertonic saline. Crit Care Med. 2002;30:644–9.

Trevett AJ, Sheehan C, Forbes R. Decompression illness presenting as breast pain. Undersea Hyperb Med. 2006;33(2):77–9.

Tufan K, Ademoglu A, Kurtaran E, Yildiz G, Aydin S, Egi SM. Automatic detection of bubbles in the subclavian vein using Doppler ultrasound signals. Aviat Space Environ Med. 2006;77(9):957–62.

Undersea Medical Society. Program and abstracts: undersea medical society annual scientific meeting. 11-14 June 1985, Long Beach, California. Undersea Biomed Res. 1985;12(1 Suppl):1–65.

van der Hulst GA, Buzzacott PL. Diver health survey score and probability of decompression sickness among occupational dive guides and instructors. Diving Hyperb Med. 2012;42(1):18–23.

Van Rees Vellinga TP, Verhoeven AC, Van Dijk FJ, Sterk W. Health and efficiency in trimix versus air breathing in compressed air workers. Undersea Hyperb Med. 2006;33(6):419–27.

Vann RD, Butler FK, Mitchell SJ, Moon RE. Decompression illness. Lancet. 2011;377:153–64.

Vann RD, Clark HG. Bubble growth and mechanical properties of tissue in decompression. Undersea Biomed Res. 1975;2:185–94.

Wakai A, Roberts I, Schierhout G. Mannitol for acute traumatic brain injury. Cochrane Database Syst Rev. 2007;1:CD001049.

Wang J, Corson K, Minky K, Mader J. Diver with acute abdominal pain, right leg paresthesias and weakness: a case report. Undersea Hyperb Med. 2002;29(4):242–6.

Ward CL. Scuba diving - biologic and physical aspects. Aeromed Rev. 1967;1:1–25.

Weaver LK. Monoplace hyperbaric chamber use of U.S. navy table 6: a 20-year experience. Undersea Hyperb Med. 2006;33(2):85–8.

Weisher DD. Resolution of neurological DCI after long treatment delays. Undersea Hyperb Med. 2008; 35(3):159–61.

Wienke BR. Basic decompression theory and application. Flagstaff: Best Publishing Company; 2001.

Williams ST, Prior FG, Bryson P. Hematocrit change in tropical scuba divers. Wilderness Environ Med. 2007;18(1):48–53. [Medline]

Wilmshurst PT, Nightingale S, Walsh KP, Morrison WL. Effect on migraine of closure of cardiac right-to-left shunts to prevent recurrence of decompression illness or stroke or for haemodynamic reasons. Lancet. 2000;356(9242):1648–51.

Wisløff U, Brubakk AO. Aerobic endurance training reduces bubble formation and increases survival in rats exposed to hyperbaric pressure. J Physiol. 2001;537(Pt 2):607–11.

Wisløff U, Richardson RS, Brubakk AO. Exercise and nitric oxide prevent bubble formation: a novel approach to the prevention of decompression sickness? J Physiol. 2004;555:825–9.

Wisløff U, Richardson RS, Brubakk AO. NOS inhibition increases bubble formation and reduces survival in sedentary but not exercised rats. J Physiol. 2003;546:577–82.

Wolf AL, Levi L, Marmarou A, Ward JD, Muizelaar PJ, Choi S, et al. Effect of THAM upon outcome in severe head injury: a randomized prospective clinical trial. J Neurosurg. 1993;78:54–9.

Xing C, Arai LEH. Pathophysiologic Cascade in ischemic stroke. Int J Stroke. 2012;7:378–85.

Yoshiyama M, Asamoto S, Kobayashi N, Sugiyama H, Doi H, Sakagawa H, et al. Spinal cord decompression sickness associated with scuba diving: correlation of immediate and delayed magnetic resonance imaging findings with severity of neurologic impairmentDOUBLEHYPHENa report on 3 cases. Surg Neurol. 2007;67(3):283–7.

Zhang Q, Chang Q, Cox RA, Gong X, Gould LJ. Hyperbaric oxygen attenuates apoptosis and decreases inflammation in an ischemic wound model. J Invest Dermatol. 2008;128(8):2102–12. pmid:18337831

Zhang Q, Gould LJ. Hyperbaric oxygen reduces matrix metalloproteinases in ischemic wounds through a redox-dependent mechanism. J Invest Dermatol. 2013;134:237–46.

Zhao Y, Vanhoutte PM, Leung SWS. Vascular nitric oxide: beyond eNOS. J Pharmacol Sci. 2015;129:83–94.

Oxygen Window

© Springer International Publishing AG, part of Springer Nature 2018
O. Rusoke-Dierich, *Diving Medicine*, https://doi.org/10.1007/978-3-319-73836-9_25

The oxygen window first was described by Momsen, Behnke, Thalmann, Van Liew and Sass in the mid-twentieth century. They picked up the already described phenomenon of the undersaturation of blood compared to air at ambient pressure by Krogh at the beginning of the twentieth century. Behnke originally described the oxygen window as the difference between arterial and venous oxygen pressure with its 60 mmHg [1]. Kot described the extended oxygen window (EOW) in 2015 [3]. Additionally to the gas tension difference of oxygen and carbon dioxide, he included the total carbon dioxide and water vapour to the oxygen window. In his concept, water vapour was included as it doesn't participate in the development of gas bubbles, even if it joins the contents of gas bubbles as a consequence of temperature. As carbon dioxide is highly reactive and doesn't contribute to bubble formation, he added it to the EOW as well. His estimated EOW was approximately 150 mmHg, which is close to the oxygen partial pressure of the air at ambient pressure (not to be confused with alveolar air).

During exposure of increased ambient pressure, inert gases are dissolved to a higher rate. They are stored into the different compartments. The initial five compartments of Haldane were extended during the time up to 16 compartments. The compartments are defined by their half-times. Haldane advocated 5, 10, 20, 40 and 75 min. Later, maximum elimination half-times for nitrogen were mathematically extended up to 1280 min (Miller). The physiological values seem to be somewhere between 320 and 420 min. Experiments and calculations were carried out to determine a safe decompression rate from a fully saturated state. Haldane proposed that there is a no decompression limit in dives below 10 m. However, some reports showed a 50% DCI rate after saturation with air about 8.7–9 m, 25% between 7.7 and 8 m and 16% deeper than 6 m. No DCI for saturation dives in depth shallower than 6 m had been reported. However, venous gas bubbles were detected in ultrasound even at saturation dives from 3.8 m. The EWO postulates a safe limit of 2.5 m. Behnke and Griffiths suggested even lower values of 1 and 0 m. To a certain degree, supersaturation of inert gases can be compensated by the oxygen window. Basically, the amount of inert gas can be dissolved to such amount as the value of unsaturation due to the oxygen window. With a closer review, the oxygen window needs to be broken down in two major compartments. The first reduction of pressure is due to the alveolar-arterial gradient. The second reduction is after metabolism of oxygen in the cells. All these calculations are mathematical and represent a virtual space.

25.1 Physiological Basics in Relation to Pressure

As we know, the air is a sum of various partial pressures of gases. At sea level, the ambient pressure is 100 kPa. Kilopascal [kPa] is the international unit for atmospheric pressure. In diving usually bar or PSI is used. In medical terms, usually mm Hg or Torr is used (mm Hg = Torr). For example, our blood pressure or blood gases are measured in mm Hg (◘ Table 25.1). Therefore for consistency, all units are used in mm Hg in this chapter.

Pressure adjusts to changes in ambient pressure. With its changes, partial pressures of individual gases change too. The partial pressure of a gas can be determined by multiplying the fraction (percentage) of the total gas and ambient pressure:

$$p_{gas} = f_x \times p_{amb}$$

- p_{gas} = partial pressure individual gas
- f_x = fraction of individual gas in air
- p_{amb} = ambient pressure

The different fractions apply to dry air. As we always have some saturation of water vapour in the air, the partial pressure of each individual gas will be reduced by the water vapour pressure. Water vapour is the amount of fluid, which is vaporising at a certain temperature. For example, it is 17.4 mmHg at 20 °C, 47 mmHg at 37 °C, 55.1 mmHg at 40 °C and 760 mg at 100 °C. After entering the airways,

◘ **Table 25.1** Units of pressure

	Bar	Atm	PSI	kPa	mmHg = Torr	mmWC
1 bar	1	0.987	14.7	100	750.062	10.02
1 atm	1.013	1	14.89	101.32	759.99	10.33
1 PSI	0.068	0.067	1	6.802	51.02	0.6816
1 kPa	0.01	0.099	0.147	1	7.5	0.102
1 mmHg/Torr	0.00131	0.00132	0.0195	0.133	1	0.1336
1 mmWC	0.099	0.097	1.455	0.98	7.48	1

air will be fully saturated with 47 mmHg water vapour at the level of the trachea. As vapour and fluids are hardly get affected by pressure changes, the value of water vapour remains constant within the blood and tissues:

$$P_{gas} = F_{gas} \left(P_{amb} - P_{H_2O} \right)$$

- F_{gas} = fraction
- P_{H_2O} = 47 mmHg (water vapour) at 37 °C body temperature

Air is usually described under standard temperature, ambient pressure at sea level and dry conditions (STPD), with $T = 273$ K, $P_{amb} = 760$ mmHg and $P_{H_2O} = 0$ mmHg. This doesn't apply for real conditions in the alveoli. In the alveoli, the temperature is similar to the body temperature, ambient pressure is variable and air is saturated with water vapour (BTPS). The standard temperature is defined as 273 K. The body temperature is 310 K (273 + 37 K), and the ambient pressure is variable. Hence, STPD conditions need to be transferred to BTPS conditions and vice versa for calculations. This correction factor respects the temperature (K 310 at $T = 37$ °C) and ambient pressure:

$$\frac{V_{(BTPS)}}{V_{(STPD)}} = \left(\frac{(273 + T) \times P_{amb}}{273 \times (P_{amb} - 47)} \right)$$

By respecting this, the equation for alveolar partial pressure oxygen is

$$P_{A_{O_2}} = P_{I_{O_2}} - \frac{\dot{V}_{O_2(STPD)}}{\dot{V}_{A(BTPS)}} \times \frac{310 \times P_{amb}}{273}$$

with

- $\dot{V}_{A(BTPS)}$ = 5 L/min alveolar ventilation (resting condition, might go up to 350 L/min under extreme exercise); minute volume: $V_E = V_T \times f$ (V_T = tidal volume, f = frequency)
- $\dot{V}_{O_2(STPD)}$ = 0.28 L/min O_2 absorption resting condition (it might go up to 3.5 L/min for young men and 2.3 L/min for young women under extreme exercise); men, $\dot{V}_{O_2(STPD)max} = 4.2 - (0.032 \times Age)$; women, $\dot{V}_{O_2(STPD)max} = 2.6 - (0.014 \times Age)$
- $P_{I_{O_2}}$ = partial pressure of oxygen at ambient pressure in airways on inspiration
- $P_{A_{O_2}}$ = alveolar oxygen partial pressure

Other equations for calculating the alveolar oxygen partial pressure are

$$P_{A_{O_2}} = FiO_2 \cdot \left(P_{amb} - P_{H_2O} \right) - \frac{PaCO_2 \left[1 - FiO_2 (1 - RQ) \right]}{RQ}$$

or simplified when $FiO_2 (1 - RQ) \ll 1$

$$P_{A_{O_2}} = FiO_2 \cdot \left(P_{amb} - P_{H_2O} \right) - \frac{PaCO_2}{RQ}$$

25

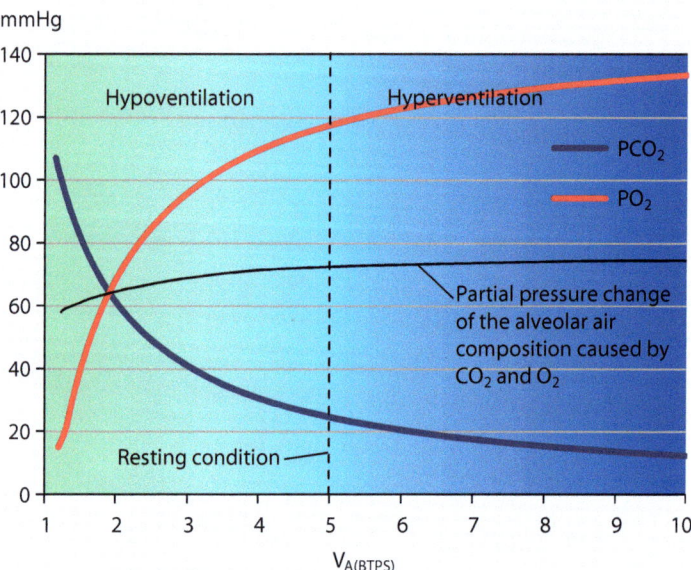

◘ Fig. 25.1 Alveolar CO_2 and O_2 in relation to ventilation

Under exertion the tidal volume and respiratory rate increases and so does the O_2 absorption. With increasing tidal volume and respiratory rate, the alveolar ventilation increases. There is however a maximum oxygen uptake (VO_{2max}) in relation to the ventilation, where no further increase of oxygen uptake is expected. The alveolar oxygen partial pressure increases at a quite similar rate as pCO_2 declines till both plateau out (◘ Fig. 25.1).

By increasing the minute volume, arterial pO_2 increases in a similar curve as the alveolar pO_2 increases. Changes in exertion also affect the nitrogen absorption and elimination as there is an increased cardiac output, exchange of alveolar ventilation and minute volume.

25.2 Respiratory Basics in Relation to the Oxygen Window

By passing through the surfactant, the endothelium of the alveoli, interstitial fluid, collagen tissue and the capillary walls, oxygen transfer is reduced, and intrapulmonary shunts redirect venous into arterial blood. All this is described as the alveolar-arterial gradient (AaG).

■ **Aa Gradient**

$$Aa = P_A O_2 - P_a O_2$$

or

$$AaG = \left(Fi_{O_2} \cdot \left(p_{amb} - pH_2O \right) \right) - \left(\frac{pCO_2}{RQ} \right)$$
$$+ \left(pCO_2 \times Fi_{O_2} \times \left(\frac{1-RQ}{RQ} \right) \right) - paO_2$$

The Aa gradient assesses the degree of shunting and V/Q mismatch. Under normal conditions, it is mainly determined by perfusion and not diffusion. It depends on age, FiO_2 and comorbidities. Important factors are alveolar ventilation, pulmonary capillary blood flow, shunting and the oxygenation of Hb. It declines in average by 4 mmHg per decade in a lifespan. According to age, an AaG can be estimated in different ways. The equations are in order from the lowest expected AaG to the highest:

$$\text{Expected AaG} = 2.5 + \left(0.21 \times \text{Age} \right) \text{ or}$$
$$= \left(\text{Age} + 10 \right) / 4, \text{ or}$$
$$= \left(\text{Age} / 4 \right) + 4$$

The AaG is believed to increase 5–7 mmHg (average 6 mmHg) for every 10% increase of FiO_2. This increase seems to be mainly due to the resulting absorption atelectasis. There are no studies available for simple hyperbaric exposure with normal air, but due to the higher pO_2 difference in the alveoli and precapillary arteries, this might have an effect during diving too. For its estimation in normobaric conditions the difference ΔFiO_2, the actual oxygen fraction $F_{iO_{2x}}$ needs to be deducted from the baseline oxygen faction of normal air ($F_{iO_{20}} = 0.20947$) and adjusted to the AaG increase per 10% (= 0.1) of ΔFiO_2:

$$c_{AaG} = \left(F_{iO_{2x}} - F_{iO_{20}} \right) \times \frac{6\,mmHg}{0.1}$$

If that also should apply to changes in ambient pressure at normal air, the given inspired oxygen partial pressure $(P_{ambO_{2x}})$ needs to be correlated to the corresponding oxygen fraction $(F_{iO_{2x}})$. At a given ambient pressure, the modified equation for the fraction would be

$$\frac{P_{ambO_{2x}}}{P_{ambO_{2Atm}} - P_{H_2O}} = F_{iO_{2x}}$$

By combining that with the above equation, the AaG correction factor (c_{AaG}) for changes in ambient pressure is

$$c_{AaG} = \left(\frac{P_{ambO_{2x}}}{713\,mmHg} - 0.20947 \right) \times \frac{6\,mmHg}{0.1}$$

The rate of transfer is described by *Fick's law*, which includes the area, the tissue thickness, the diffusion constant and the gas tension.

$$\dot{V}_{gas} = \frac{A}{T} \times D \times \Delta P$$

- $\dot{V}_{gas}$ = Rate of gas diffusion across permeable membrane
- D = Diffusion coefficient
- A = Surface area

- ΔP = Difference in partial pressure of the particular gas across the membrane
- T = Thickness

The Bunsen coefficient (STPD) and the Ostwald coefficient (temperature dependent) describe different solubilities and amount of gas, which dissolves in unit volume of a liquid at 1 atm. Gas solubility is dependent on temperature. In general, the more soluble a gas is, the more gas could get dissolved in liquid. The solubility varies in different solutes, like water, blood or fat. The n-octanol/water partition coefficient is a good guideline for fat solubility. Its unit is often described as log K_{OW}. If the log K_{OW} is resolved with log 10, the fat solubility can be determined. The lower the fat solubility is, the more hydrophobic the substance is, and the higher it is, the more hydrophilic the substance becomes. Hence, the higher the fat solubility is, the more readily the gas can diffuse via cell membranes. All factors together influence the diffusion rate relative to oxygen. Moreover, lighter and more soluble gases diffuse in general quicker (□ Table 25.2).

$$Q_{g_d} = \frac{c * f_c}{760\,mmHg}$$

- Q_{g_d} = Quantity of dissolved gas in blood in [mL/dL/mmHg]
- c = solubility coefficient in [mL/mL]
- f_c = conversion factor (for mL to dL it equals 100)

CO_2 and O_2 are involved in metabolic processes and get bound to protein structures. So they easily can have higher contents in the body with far less being dissolved. Inert gases, like He and N_2, solely in- and outgas. Hence, their partial pressures represent only the dissolved phase. If gas contents exceed the dissolved phase, tissues and blood become supersaturated and hence form a free phase (bubbles). The dissolved and the free content together represent then the total amount.

◻ Table 25.2 Specifications of different gases

Gas	MV	Solubility coefficient in blood [mL/mL/1 atm] at 310 K	Solubility coefficient in water at 310 K	Solubility coefficient in olive oil at 307 K [mL/mL]	Quantity dissolved in blood [mL/dL/mmHg] at 310 K	Partition coefficient: n-octanol/water [logK$_{OW}$]	Diffusion rate in relation to oxygen
O_2	32	0.028	0.023	0.117	0.0037	0.65	1
CO_2	44	0.47	0.545	1.105	0.062	0.83	0.852
N_2	28	0.015	0.0125	0.057	0.00197	0.67	1.068
He	4	0.0086	0.0085	0.0157	0.00113	0.28	2.825

Reaching the pulmonary capillary blood, CO_2 diffuses from the blood along the gradient with 45 mmHg into the lung with its 40 mmHg. High alveolar CO_2 contents compared to normal air are related to incomplete ventilation (relative alveolar hypoventilation). With increased minute volume, CO_2 decreases. At vigorous exercise, the pCO_2 in the blood can increase to 75 mm Hg and the alveolar CO_2 can drop as low as 10 mmHg. Increasing difference in concentration enhances the gas exchange. The CO_2 production is only minimally affected by hyperbaric condition as it is a metabolic product related to oxygen consumption. For example, CO_2 partial pressure in 80 msw increases only from 0.226 mmHg to 2.03 mmHg in the dry air inhaled from the tank, which is 1.92 mmHg on fully saturated air in the airways. The regular 40 mmHg in the alveoli exceeds that by far and no change of alveolar CO_2 would be expected. The CO_2 in the venous part of the pulmonary capillaries is 45 mmHg. CO_2 would still diffuse out in the lungs. Additionally, increased $paCO_2$ triggers an increase of minute volume, which counteracts CO_2 accumulation in the body. However, increased viscosity of the gas mixture at depth increases the alveolar pCO_2 to a certain degree.

The total alveolar contact time of pulmonary capillaries is approximately 0.75 s.

Oxygen is usually completely absorbed within 0.25 s. Nitrogen probably is absorbed even a bit faster. Even under vigorous exertion, oxygen still gets fully absorbed within the 0.75 s. O_2 diffuses from the alveoli with its approx. 101 mm Hg into the capillaries (98 mmHg) and loses its first fraction of oxygen. The following measured arterial blood is a combination of arterial and a small amount of venous blood and will be hereby further reduced to approx. 94 mmHg. The mixed arterial blood is a result of the total intrapulmonary shunt which bypasses the lungs. The shunt has two components. The physiological shunt is a redirection of blood within the pulmonary vessels. Anatomical shunt occurs by bypassing the pulmonary vessels completely. The anatomical shunt is a real shunt with approximately 2–5% of the cardiac output, via the Thebesian veins from the left ventricle and the vessels for the blood supply of the pulmonary as well as pleural tissue. The Thebesian veins enable a form of collateral circulation unique to the heart. The admixture of the poorly oxygenated blood relates to an approximately 10% of total shunt volume. Bubbles get caught in the pulmonary capillary filter, which increases shunting. With increased shunt, the arterial pO_2 gets reduced. The arterial pCO_2 in contrast only changes minimal. The intrapulmonary shunt is a ratio of the alveolar and arterial (A-a) and the arterial and venous (a-v) differences dependent on the cardiac output. In DCI pulmonary gas embolism is always in various degrees present. This increases the shunt. Shunts in general with more than 35% significantly reduce the gas exchange For example, shunts up to 30–40% can be restored with increased oxygen supply. The bigger the shunt, the more oxygen needs to be supplied. Shunts above 40–50% don't benefit from additional oxygen delivery. Blocked pulmonary vessels by pulmonary embolism redirect blood to other vessels and therefore reduce the V/Q ratio. The same can be assumed after diving when gas bubbles, blocking off pulmonary capillaries, redirect the blood flow and increase shunting and hence result in decreased inert gas elimination:

$$\frac{\dot{Q}_S}{\dot{Q}_T} = \frac{C_{c'O_2} - C_{\bar{a}O_2}}{C_{c'O_2} - C_{\bar{v}O_2}}$$

- $\dot{Q}_S$ = shunted blood flow
- $\dot{Q}_T$ = cardiac output
- $C_{c'O_2}$ = oxygen content of pulmonary end-capillary blood equally to the alveolar oxygen content
- $C_{\bar{a}O_2}$ = oxygen content of arterial blood
- $C_{\bar{v}O_2}$ = oxygen content of mixed venous blood

Next to the real shunt, the V/Q *mismatch* is an important factor determining the AaG. The V/Q ratio describes the ventilation-perfusion relationships:

$$\frac{\dot{V}_A}{Q} = p_{amb} \times \frac{310}{273} \times R \times \frac{Ca_{O_2} - Cv_{O_2}}{pA_{O_2}}$$

V/Q mismatch can occur either by factors affecting ventilation, perfusion or both. The perfect V/Q equals 1. Practically, that means that all parts of the lung have equal perfusion and ventilation. However, in reality that is not the case. Moreover, the average V/Q value doesn't reflect the real gas exchange capacity of the entire lung. The ventilation-perfusion (V/Q) ratio describes the relation between the alveolar ventilation and cardiac output. The mean V/Q ratio is ~ 0.8. The lung is also not evenly perfused and ventilated. There are three zones (West) (■ Table 25.3). From the upper zones to the lower zones [7], the hydrostatic pressure increases. That means in the upper zone I is more ventilated but less perfused. The V/Q varies there between 1.3 and 3.3. In the mid zone II, the V/Q is between 0.8 and 1.0. In the lower zone III where perfusion outweighs ventilation, the V/Q is between 0.63 and 0.73. A high V/Q contributes to alveolar dead space and a low V/Q to physiological shunt. The posture but also in water immersion with reduction of the hydrostatic pressure reduces the V/Q ratio due to the blood shift.

Any V/Q with a different value than 1 has a reduced efficiency in the gas exchange. Critical V/Q values, where gas exchange is significantly impacted, are <0.4 and >4. Under perfect conditions, a misbalance in one area of the lung would be counterbalanced in other parts. For example, during exercise, mainly the upper parts of the lung increase the perfusion and hence lower the local V/Q and enhance gas exchange. The redirection of the total blood means that the increased perfusion of the upper part reduces the average perfusion of the rest, which improves the overall V/Q. Still there will be a mismatch. During diving in horizontal position, the average V/Q is improved. After diving there is a certain amount of gas bubbles, which decrease perfusion on the one hand and increase shunt on the other hand. Additionally, the horizontal position is changed to a vertical. Both lead to an increased V/Q mismatch and reduce gas exchange.

The airways have an anatomical and physiological *dead space* (■ Table 25.4), which is not included in any gas exchange. The physiological dead space (V_D^{phys}) influences the tidal ventilation (V_T). If the dead space is deducted from the alveolar ventilation, the tidal ventilation can be calculated. The physiological dead space

◘ **Table 25.3** Lung zones after West [7]

	V_A	Q	pO_2 [mmHg]	pCO_2 [mmHg]	R	% of the total lung volume [VI]	V/Q
Apex	0.24	0.07	132	28	2	7	3.43
	0.33	0.19	121	34	1.3	8	1.74
	0.42	0.33	114	37	1.1	10	1.27
Mid	0.52	0.5	108	39	0.92	11	1.04
	0.59	0.66	102	40	0.95	12	0.89
	0.67	0.83	98	41	0.78	13	0.81
Base	0.72	0.98	95	41	0.73	13	0.73
	0.78	1.15	92	42	0.68	13	0.68
	0.82	1.29	89	42	0.65	13	0.64
Mean value	5.09	6	106	38	1.01	100	0.85/0.81[a]

[a]Adjusted to the lung volume distribution in %

◘ **Table 25.4** Factors affecting dead space

Increase for dead space ↑	Decrease of dead space ↓
Large body	Small body
Position sitting (V_D ~ 100 mL)	Position supine (V_D~145 mL)
Increased oxygen partial pressure	Hypoxia
Age	
Increased lung volume (~20 mL for each L of lung volume)	
Emphysema	

(V_D^{phys}) equals the sum of alveolar (V_D^{Alv}) and anatomical dead space (V_D^{anat}):

$$V_T = V_A - V_D^{phys}$$

with

$$V_D^{phys} = V_D^{Alv} + V_D^{anat}$$

Usually the anatomical dead (V_D^{anat}) space equals the physiological dead space with ~150 mL; hence the alveolar dead space is 0.

The expired volume (V_E) is

$$V_E = V_A + V_D^{phsy}$$

O_2 is consumed in the body and CO_2 is produced. As a baseline of all equations, the O_2 consumption needs to be calculated:

$$O_2 \text{ consumed} = O_2 \text{ in} - O_2 \text{ out}$$

or

$$\dot{V}_{O_2} = F_{I_{O_2}} \times \dot{V}_I - F_{E_{O_2}} \times \dot{V}_E$$

- $\dot{V}_{O_2}$ = Oxygen consumption
- $F_{I_{O_2}}$ = Fraction of oxygen in the inspired air
- $F_{E_{O_2}}$ = Fraction of oxygen in the exhaled air
- V_I = Quantity of the inspired gas
- V_E = Quantity of the exhaled gas

By assuming that the inhaled gas quantities equal the exhaled quantities by calling both $\dot{V}_E$. But in reality $\dot{V}_I > \dot{V}_E$:

$$\dot{V}_{O_2} = \dot{V}_E \left(F_{I_{O_2}} - F_{E_{O_2}} \right)$$

By solving to the outgoing O_2,

$$F_{E_{O_2}} = F_{I_{O_2}} - K \times \frac{\dot{V}_{O_2}}{\dot{V}_E}$$

or

$$P_{E_{O_2}} = P_{I_{O_2}} - 0.863 \frac{\dot{V}_{O_2}}{\dot{V}_E}$$

with $K = 0.836$, given that the dimension of $\dot{V}_{O_2}$ is in [mL/min].

The *Bohr equation* describes the ratio between dead space and tidal volume:

$$\frac{V_D^{phys}}{V_T} = \frac{F_{A_{CO_2}} - F_{E_{CO_2}}}{F_{A_{CO_2}}}$$

The *Enghoff modification* for partial pressure is

$$\frac{V_D^{phys}}{V_T} = \frac{P_{A_{CO_2}} - P_{E_{CO_2}}}{P_{A_{CO_2}}}$$

The normal range is 0.2–0.35, which means that the dead space is approximately 20–35% of the tidal lung volume.

For CO_2 the equation is the same, but as there is essentially no CO_2 in the inspired air, the expired CO_2 is:

$$P_{A_{CO_2}} = K \times \frac{\dot{V}_{CO_2}}{\dot{V}_E}$$

A further factor in ventilation is the respiratory quotient (R_Q) as a ratio of CO_2 production and O_2 consumption.

$$R_Q = \frac{\dot{V}_{CO_2}}{\dot{V}_{O_2}}$$

The R_Q is a ratio describing the body's burning of fuel such as glucose, fat and proteins. R_Q 1 means that as much CO_2 is produced as O_2 is consumed. If R_Q is <1, that means more O_2 is consumed than CO_2 produced, e.g. proteins have a R_Q around 0.84 and fat around 0.7. Another equation for the estimation of $P_{A_{CO_2}}$ including the R_Q is

$$P_{A_{CO_2}} = \frac{R_Q \times P_{I_{O_2}}}{\left(1 - F_{I_{O_2}}\right) \times \left(1 - R_Q\right)}$$
$$- \frac{R_Q}{\left(1 - F_{I_{O_2}}\right) \times \left(1 - R_Q\right)} \times P_{A_{O_2}}$$

25.3 Oxygen Window (OW)

Both reductions of pO_2 by gas exchange and shunt are defined as the *alveolar-arterial gradient* (AaG), which I describe as the *pulmonary oxygen window* (OW_p). The total decline in gas tension is hereby about 10 mmHg, depending on age and health. It doesn't really

25

change with exertion or ambient pressure. But it depends on various factors, like perfusion, gas exchange, ventilation, shunt, gas density, amount of haemoglobin, etc. The alveolar air is influenced by ambient pressure, gas fraction, minute volume and pulmonary oxygen uptake. During compression, nitrogen is slightly undersaturated in blood. Gas tensions are expected to adopt quite quickly and evenly. Hence, nitrogen uptake is not really affected by the pulmonary oxygen window. The Aa-gradient however might be an important factor for nitrogen elimination. It doesn't only give an idea how much nitrogen can leave during the passage of the pulmonary capillaries but also how much nitrogen will be bypassed and re-enters arteries. Ageing reduces ventilatory control, respiratory muscle strength, respiratory mechanics and gas exchange. The alveolar-arterial gradient increases with age (approx. 4 mmHg per 10 years in life) or with pulmonary dis-

eases. The V/Q inequality of the different lung zones and reduced cardiac output seem also to influence gas exchange. During diving gravity is reduced, and usually the diver is in a horizontal position. This changes the overall V/Q ratio to slightly higher values as the average Q decreases and enhances gas exchange. Out of the water, this reverses, and gas exchange is reduced compared to water immersion, which is not in favour of nitrogen elimination.

Once oxygen enters the bloodstream, it is transported to tissues. The majority is transported in haemoglobin. One haemoglobin can hold four oxygen molecules. Without this mechanism, oxygen supply wouldn't be sufficient. A smaller part of oxygen is transported dissolved in blood. Only the dissolved oxygen is measured in arterial blood gas analysis. Both together, the dissolved and the haemoglobin-bound oxygen, represent the total oxygen amount in blood (◘ Fig. 25.2).

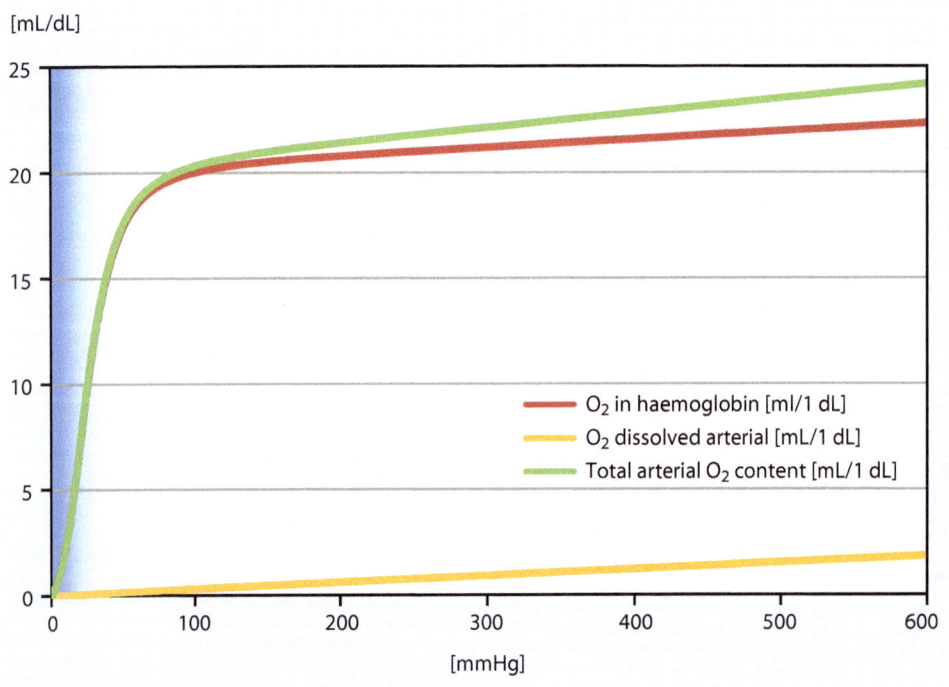

[mL/dL]

— O_2 in haemoglobin [ml/1 dL]
— O_2 dissolved arterial [mL/1 dL]
— Total arterial O_2 content [mL/1 dL]

[mmHg]

◘ **Fig. 25.2** O_2 content in relation to absolute O_2 partial pressure

The total oxygen content is a result of the combined O_2 in the haemoglobin and the dissolved O_2 in plasma:

$$\text{total oxygen content} = O_2 \text{ in Hb} + \text{dissolved } O_2 \text{ in plasma}$$

with

- **O_2 in Hb**

$$C_{haem_{O_2}} = 1.34 \times Hb \times SO_2 \times 0.01 + 0.0037 \times pO_2$$

- Hb assumed at 15 g Hb/dL
- 0.0037 = constant, which represents the amount of oxygen dissolved in plasma (mL O_2 in 1 dL plasma)
- 1.34 = Huefner's constant: amount of oxygen bound per gram of haemoglobin (varies from 1.34 to 1.36)

and

- **Dissolved O_2 in Plasma**

$$C_{diss_{O_2}} = a_{O_2} \times pO_2$$

- a_{O_2} = mL of O_2 dissolved in 1 dL plasma: 0.0037 mL/dL O_2/mmHg blood (applies also for other pressure units eg. kPa)
- pO_2 = oxygen partial pressure

- **Total cO_2**

$$cO_2 = \left(1.34 \times Hb \times SO_2 \times 0.01 + 0.0037 \times pO_2\right) + \left(a_{O_2} \times pO_2\right)$$

By knowing the arterial or venous oxygen partial pressure, the oxygen saturation of haemoglobin (SO_2) can be calculated. Venous blood is slightly more acidic, which causes a right shift of the dissociation curve. Hence, slightly higher venous oxygen partial pressures can be expected in relation to the calculated SO_2.

- **Oxygen Saturation of Haemoglobin (Severinghaus)** [5]

$$SO_2 = \left(23400 \times \left(pO_2^3 + 150 + pO_2\right)^{-1} + 1\right)^{-1}$$

and vice versa. By knowing the SO_2, the partial pressure can be calculated:

$$pO_2 = \sqrt[3]{\frac{1}{2}\left(-y_N + \sqrt{y_N^2 - h^2}\right)} + \sqrt[3]{\frac{1}{2}\left(-y_N - \sqrt{y_N^2 - h^2}\right)}$$

with

$$h^2 = 500,000$$

$$y_N = \frac{23400 \times SO_2}{1 - SO_2}$$

Alternatively the SO_2 can be calculated with the *Hill equation*:

$$SO_2 = \frac{pO_2^n}{\left(p_{50} + pO_2^n\right)}$$

- n = Hill constant (for blood 2.5–2.8)
- p50 = oxygen gas tension at 50% SO_2 (approx. 27 mmHg in arterial blood)

The more oxygen is bound to haemoglobin, the more its affinity increases. This is reflected in the beginning of the dissociation curve as it starts flat but increases continuously and flattens out again. Between 20 and 90 mmHg, the dissociation curve has a sharp increase. In this part, little changes in the SO_2 or pO_2 have great impact on the oxygen content. There is a significant reduction of oxygen from the bloodstream to the cell from about 92 mmHg in the arterial blood to 10–19 mmHg intracellular, depending on the cells. The mitochondrial pO_2 can drop to as little as 1–2 mmHg in times of demand. The capillary pO_2 varies from tissue to tissue and is dependent on its perfusion (◘ Table 25.5).

Intracellular fluid (ICF) is composed of at least 10^{13} cells. It has to be seen as a sum of tiny compartment. The extracellular fluids (ECF) are composed of different compartments. It contains plasma, interstitial fluid, dense connective tissue water, bone water and transcellular water. The plasma is a major single fluid compart-

◘ Table 25.5 capillary pO$_2$ of different tissues [2]

Tissue	pO$_2$ [mmHg]
Brain	33.8 ± 2.6
Lung	42.8
Muscle	29.2 ± 1.8
Bone marrow	48.9 ± 4.5
Superficial skin	8 ± 3.2
Skin (sub-papillary plexus)	35.2 ± 8
Skin (dermal papillae)	24 ± 6.4
Intestinal tissue	57.6 ± 6.4

ment. It basically is blood without blood components like red and white blood cells. White and red blood cells are included in the ICF. The interstitial fluid (ISF) is the fluid between body tissues. The dense connective tissue water and the bone water fluid content is quite significant as it makes 15% of the total body water. The transcellular water is a small compartment contained within epithelial lined spaces, including joint spaces, GI fluids, CSF and urine.

The partial pressure in blood seems high compared to the intracellular pressure. Blood has a volume of 5 L with 3.2 L belonging to plasma. This is included in the 42 L of the total body volume. The intracellular fluid (ICF) has 23 L and the extracellular fluid (ECF) 19 L, totalling 42 L. That means the ICF alone has a 7 times larger volume than plasma. If the interstitial fluid, which is closely linked to cells, is added it would contribute to a 10 times larger volume than plasma (◘ Table 25.6). This factor would be expected in pressure drop just by distribution from blood to cells. The expected pressure would be 1/10 of the arterial blood, equalling 9 mmHg, which comes close to the real average value. If the entire blood volume of 5 L is taken, the oxygen gas tension would be 1/6 or 15 mmHg. However, physiological gas exchange and distribution is a highly dynamic process. Tissues are differently perfused, and hence blood volume is not evenly distributed, so the individual oxygen partial pressure of cells might vary. Oxygen supply and consumption strongly depend on the metabolic rate of cells but also on perfusion rate. Intracellular carbon dioxide can be quite high with 78 mmHg on vigorous exertion. With increased exertion, more CO_2 is produced. Of the oxygen uptake, approximately 20% less CO_2 is produced. As CO_2 has a high diffusion rate, it quickly is expected to leave cells. The intracellular oxygen drops as it is rapidly consumed and the total oxygen gas tension further declines of

◘ Table 25.6 Body fluid compartments (70 kg male)

	% of body weight	% of total body water	Volume [L]
ECF (extracellular)	27	45	19
Plasma	4.5	7.5	3.2
ISF (interstitial fluid)	12	20	8.4
Dense connective tissue water	4.5	7.5	3.2
Bone water	4.5	7.5	3.2
Transcellular water	1.5	2.5	1
ICF (intracellular fluid)	33	55	23
TBW (total body water)	60	100	42

about 10–19 mmHg from arterial blood to cells. This step of partial pressure changes can be described as *tissue oxygen window* (OW$_{tis}$). An important influencing factor for the OW$_{tis}$ is the perfusion and the solubility in blood and tissue. As nitrogen and oxygen have quite similar diffusion rates, the OW$_{tis}$ could be also a good indicator for the absorption of nitrogen into cells. OW$_{tis}$ doesn't contribute itself to the total oxygen window, but it is an important influencing factor. Oxygen is utilised and has intracellular lower oxygen partial pressure compared to venous oxygen partial pressure. Therefore it doesn't leave cells.

The venous blood is only left with approximately 40–45 mmHg of oxygen partial pressure due to the oxygen consumption. The normal resting O_2 consumption is 3.1–4.0 mL/kg/min but can increase to over 40 mL/kg/min during exercise and has an individual cut-off. The average O_2 consumption is 280 mL/min in an adult at rest. At exercise it might reach 3000–4000 mL/min:

- **Oxygen Consumption**

$$\dot{V}_{O_2} = Q\left(Ca_{O_2} - Cv_{O_2}\right)$$

- $\dot{V}_{O_2}$ = oxygen consumption [mL/min]
- Ca_{O_2} = total arterial oxygen content [mL/min]
- Cv_{O_2} = total venous oxygen content [mL/min]
- Q = cardiac output [dL/min]

Hence, the venous oxygen [mL/min] content is

$$Cv_{O_2} = Ca_{O_2} - \frac{\dot{V}_{O_2}}{Q}$$

- **The Oxygen Delivery DO$_2$ [mL/min] Is with an Assumed Cardiac Output of 50 dL/min at Rest**

$$D_{O_2} = Ca_{O_2} \times Q$$

- Ca_{O_2} = total arterial oxygen content
- Q = cardiac output assumed at 50 dL/min

In venous blood, 60% of carbon dioxide is bound by HCO_3 and 30% in Hb, and only 10% is dissolved. In the arterial blood, 90% of carbon dioxide is bound by HCO_3 and 5% in Hb, and only 5% is dissolved. Again, only the dissolved CO_2 is measured in blood gas analysis. The pCO_2 is approx. 47 mmHg in the venous blood and 40 mmHg in the arterial blood. Carbon dioxide is 20 times more soluble in blood than oxygen. All this explains why the consumption of 50 mmHg in oxygen causes only a 5 mmHg increase in CO_2. CO_2 easily diffuses through cell membranes and is highly interactive in biochemical processes.

The arterial-venous difference in partial pressures is described as the classical oxygen window, which resembles the *vascular oxygen window* (OW$_v$). The total partial pressure difference between alveolar air and veins is approx. −64 mm Hg at rest. OW$_p$ and OW$_v$ together represent the *total oxygen window* (Ow$_{tot}$). The OW$_{tis}$ isn't included in the calculation of the OW$_{tot}$, but is an influencing factor of the OW$_v$. The model of the oxygen window has similarities to the two-compartment model of pharmacokinetics (◘ Figs. 25.3 and 25.4).

Gas exchange usually appears to be in a steady state. However, by changing ambient pressure, a mismatch of ingassing and outgassing can occur:

$$\left(p_i - p_a\right) + \left(p_a - p_t\right) + \left(p_t - p_v\right) + \left(p_v - p_i\right) = 0 = \Delta p$$

Supersaturation (P_{SS}) and cavitation are expected to occur, when inert gas exceeds unsaturation, determined by pO_2 and pCO_2. This can happen by decompression or by ascending during diving. The limits of pressure difference are based on the alveolar air and venous blood. As gas is usually filtered and eliminated by pulmonary capillaries, only little excess inert gas is expected to enter the arteries after diving. However, when gas emboli block off pulmonary capillaries, intrapulmonary shunt increases and blood with its inert gas bypasses the lungs. Depending on the shunt, inert gas might exceed the OW$_p$ and theoretically cause arterial gas bubbles. Tissue

25

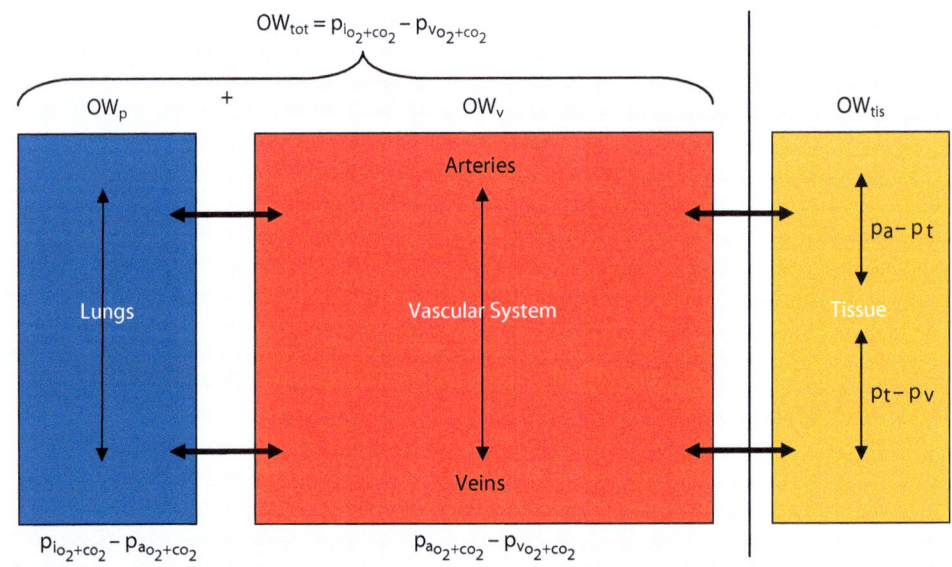

$$OW_{tot} = p_{io_2+co_2} - p_{vo_2+co_2}$$

OW_p + OW_v OW_{tis}

Arteries

$p_a - p_t$

Lungs   Vascular System   Tissue

$p_t - p_v$

Veins

$p_{io_2+co_2} - p_{ao_2+co_2}$ $p_{ao_2+co_2} - p_{vo_2+co_2}$

▫ **Fig. 25.3**   Oxygen window with its individual components

absorbs and releases inert gas during diving. Inside the cells, there is a dramatic reduction of oxygen partial pressure but also an increase of pCO_2. Depending on perfusion and oxygen supply as well as oxygen consumption, the total gas tension difference between arterial blood and tissues varies from 15 to 50 mmHg. There is a further drop of gas tensions between tissues and cells. The relative unsaturation between arterial blood and cells of approx. 70 mmHg facilitates inert gas absorption into cells. The excess venous inert gas determines the capacity of tissue holding inert gas without being supersaturated. If excess tissue inert gas exceeds the excess venous inert gas, gas bubbles are expected to form in or around cells. Together with perfusion, solubilities and metabolic rate of tissues influence the gas exchange rate. Decreased perfusion or high metabolic rate decreases the OW_v and makes the tissue more prone to develop gas bubbles. High fat contents of cells allow higher N_2 dissolution due to higher solubility. Fatty tissues can hold more N_2 contents without influencing partial pressure compared to watery solutions (con-

tent and partial pressure can't be confused). By releasing N_2 due to decreasing partial pressure from fatty tissues into watery solutions, gas bubbles may form just by the fact that water allows smaller contents in dissolution compared to fat. However, these bubbles dissolve rapidly, if unsaturation in venous blood is still present.

Bubbles form, if the excess inert gas in either veins, tissues or arteries exceeds the sum of its pressure (blood pressure or intracellular pressure) and its following OW subunit or OW unit. OW units are lungs, vascular system or tissue. The OW subunit describes the unsaturation of either the arterial or the venous system. Unsaturation is defined as the inspired partial pressure of oxygen and carbon dioxide minus either arterial or venous oxygen and carbon dioxide partial pressure. The tissue OW unit acts slightly different as it is not actually a part of the OW but a modulating factor. As such the following OW subunit is not determined by the unsaturation of the venous system as expected, but by the inert gas saturation of the venous system. The excess inert gas can be calculated, if the expected ambient inert gas tension is deducted from the actual inert gas tension.

■ **Veins**

No bubbles : $\left(p_{v(ig)} - p_{v(ig)_{amb}}\right)$

$$< \left(p_{i_{O_2+CO_2}} - p_{v_{O_2+CO_2}}\right) + BP_v$$

Bubbles : $\left(p_{v(ig)} - p_{v(ig)_{amb}}\right)$

$$> \left(p_{i_{O_2+CO_2}} - p_{v_{O_2+CO_2}}\right) + BP_v$$

■ **Tissue (Cells and Interstitial Space)**

No bubbles : $\left(p_{t(ig)} - p_{t(ig)_{amb}}\right)$

$$< \left(p_{v(ig)} - p_{v(ig)_{amb}}\right) + p_{ic}$$

Bubbles : $\left(p_{t(ig)} - p_{t(ig)_{amb}}\right)$

$$> \left(p_{v(ig)} - p_{v(ig)_{amb}}\right) + p_{ic}$$

■ **Arteries**

No bubbles : $\left(p_{a(ig)} - p_{a(ig)_{amb}}\right)$

$$< \left(p_{i_{O_2+CO_2}} - p_{a_{O_2+CO_2}}\right) + BP_a$$

Bubbles : $\left(p_{a(ig)} - p_{a(ig)_{amb}}\right)$

$$> \left(p_{i_{O_2+CO_2}} - p_{a_{O_2+CO_2}}\right) + BP_a$$

- p_i = partial pressure in the inspired air
- p_a = arterial partial pressure
- p_t = tissue partial pressure
- p_v = venous partial pressure
- BP_a = arterial blood pressure
- BP_v = venous blood pressure
- p_{ic} = intracellular pressure
- (ig) = inert gas.

According to Dalton's law, the blood pressure (BP) and intracellular pressure theoretically have some influence in extending the oxygen window. In arteries, the mean blood pressure is 100 mmHg, in veins 10 mmHg and in end pulmonary capillaries 20 mmHg and the intracellular pressure (p_{ic}) is something about

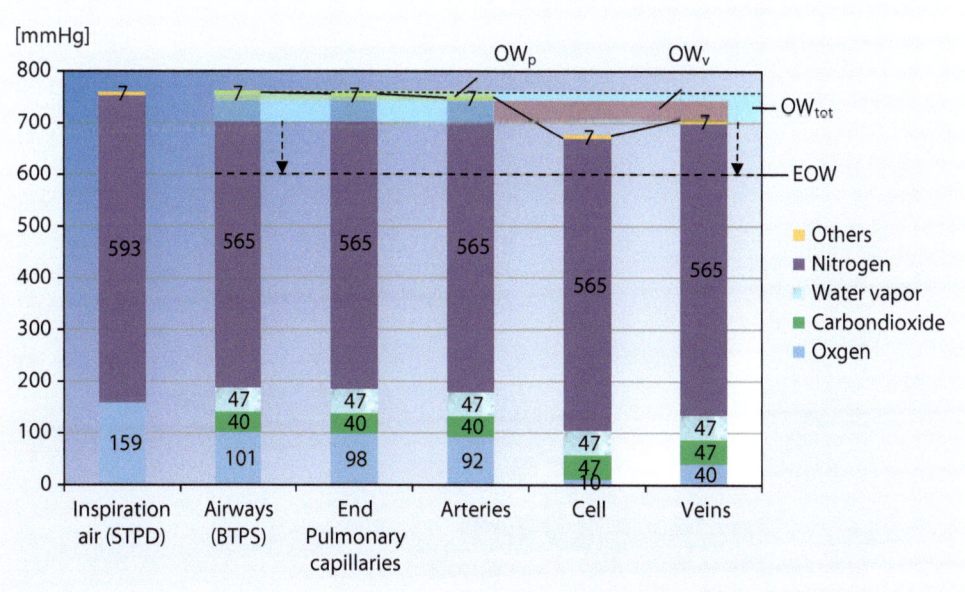

□ **Fig. 25.4** Partial pressures of gases in normal air in inspiration air (STPD), airways (BTPS), end pulmonary capillaries, arteries, cells and veins and the role of total, pulmonary, vascular and extended oxygen window

0.4–4 mmHg. That means that due to the pressure in compartments a more or less higher unsaturation than only the differences in partial pressures is expected. Due to the higher blood pressure in arteries compared to veins, it requires higher inert gas partial pressures and/or shunt to form bubbles in arteries. However, the impact in decompression algorithms seems to be negligible and is therefore not included in current calculations. Water vapour is assumed to be unchanged by pressure. It is mainly influenced by factors like temperature and properties of the gas environment. Bubble seeds contain only water vapour. Depending on the growth of the seeds to bubbles, they either contain only water vapour (fast growth) or absorb gases from the supersaturated surrounding liquid (slow growth). As water vapour doesn't participate in saturation processes in liquid, it could be discussed to be included in the OW. If water vapour would be included and blood pressure/intracellular pressure is considered in the OW, the unsaturation of arteries would

be about 156 mmHg, of veins 91 mmHg, of tissue 122–135 mmHg and of end pulmonary capillaries 70 mmHg at ambient pressure. This might be a further contributing factor that bubbles are rather found in veins compared to arteries. But it also indicates, that if arterial bubbles are present, a disastrous DCI is to be expected.

The total oxygen window increases almost at the same rate as the alveolar oxygen partial pressure at increasing ambient pressure before it plateaus out at approximately 80 msw with normal air or 1.7 bar with 100% oxygen during HBOT. There is also an upper limit for the calculation of the OW, because high oxygen levels are unrealistic as they would exceed the toxic range. There are slight age-related changes in the Aa gradient. With increasing age, the Aa gradient increases slightly and hence the OW_p increases. At the same time, the OW_v decreases accordingly. However, OW_p and OW_v together always equal the total oxygen window (◘ Figs. 25.5 and 25.6).

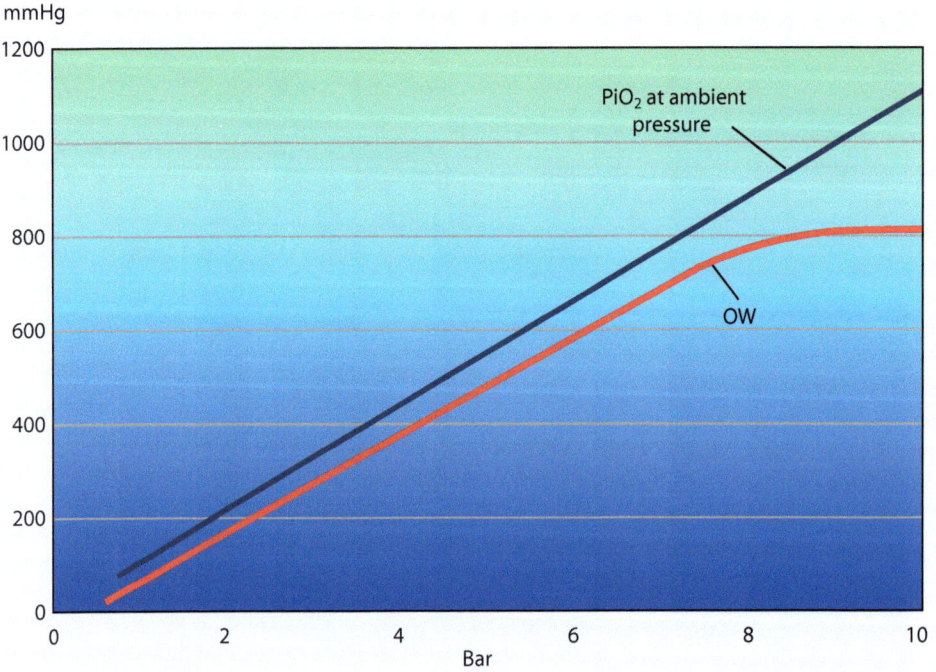

◘ **Fig. 25.5**   Inspiratory oxygen partial pressure and oxygen window in relation to increasing ambient pressure

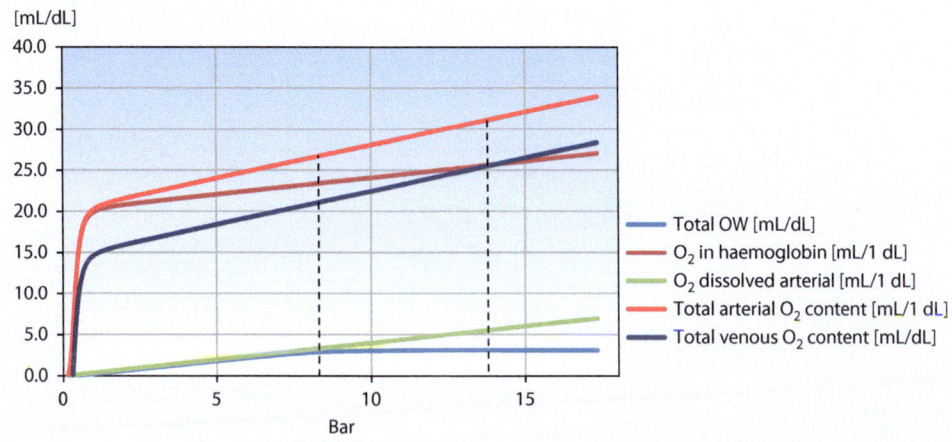

Fig. 25.6 Oxygen window when breathing normal air compared to O_2 content in haemoglobin, dissolved O_2 as well as total arterial and venous O_2 content in relation to increasing ambient pressure; plateauing out from approx. 8–9 bar and no further increase at approx. 14 bar

During exercise, oxygen is metabolised to a higher rate, and hence oxygen partial pressure decreases initially in the venous blood. At the same time, CO_2 partial pressure increases. Under vigorous exercise, CO_2 can reach 78 mm Hg. CO_2 production is determined by the O_2 consumption. Normal resting O_2 consumption is 3.1–4.0 mL/kg/min. It can increase to over 40 mL/kg/min during exercise and has an individual cut-off. The VO_2max [mL/kg/min] is a measure of the maximal oxygen uptake and varies in gender, age and physical fitness. Men at young age have a VO_2 max of approx. 40–50 mL/kg/min and at older age 30–40 mL/kg/min, compared to female 30–40 mL/kg/min at young age and 20–30 mL/kg/min at older age. In physical fit people, another 10–20 mL/kg/min can be added. Average oxygen consumption of an adult at rest is approximately 280 mL/min and increases at exercise up to 3000–4000 mL/min. Triggered by higher CO_2 levels during exercise, the minute volume increases. Contents of CO_2 can be estimated with $R = 0.8$ times the oxygen demand. At rest, it equals approximately to CO_2 of 220 mL/min.

By assuming that 10% of the CO_2 is dissolved equalling approximately 47 mmHg, the total CO_2 concentration would be 3 mL/dL in venous and 2.5 mL/dL in arterial blood. CO_2 is eliminated in the lungs and returns with about 40 mmHg arterial CO_2 partial pressure. The increase of the oxygen alveolar partial pressure during exercise is less dramatic than that of CO_2. The alveolar pO_2 reaches about 130 mm Hg during exertion. During exertion, venous oxygen partial pressure is only minimally decreased. Venous pCO_2 increases initially with a slight delay due to aerobic glycolysis but increases then initially sharply and can reach even 78 mm Hg. These initial high CO_2 levels decrease again after continuing exertion. During exercise, pCO_2 but also pO_2 are influenced by changes in minute volume.

There is no significant change of arterial pO_2 during moderate exercise, but in strenuous exercise, there is a mild increase. The venous pO_2 drops at rest by approx. 25% but can decrease at vigorous exercise by 75%.

Exercise slightly increases the OW_v (■ Fig. 25.7).

25

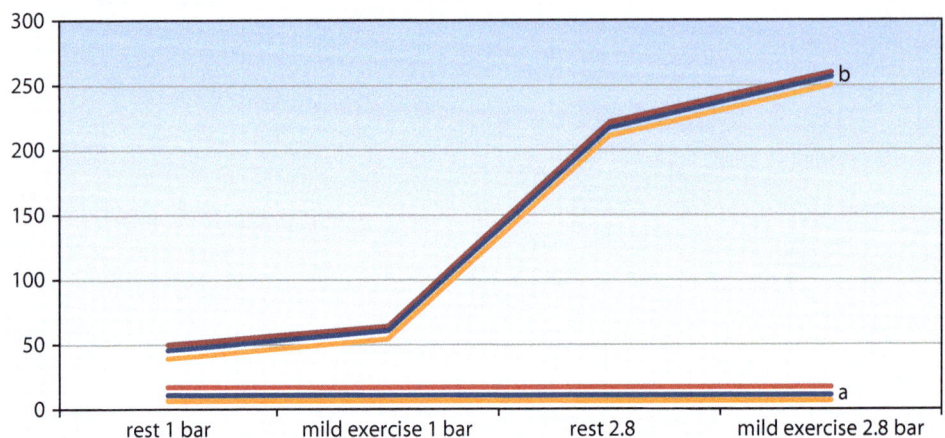

● **Fig. 25.7**   Oxygen window in relation to exercise at 1 and 2.8 bar absolute at different age groups (20/orange, 40/blue and 79/red YOA); **a** pulmonary oxygen window, **b** vascular oxygen window

25.4 Oxygen Window in HBOT

The oxygen window is an important factor in relation to the absorption and elimination pathway of inert gases. Vann and Thalmann described the linear relationship between an acceptable decompression rate (r_d) and inspired pO_2 (PiO_2). They formulated out of this quotient the K value [6].

$$K = \frac{r_d}{Pi_{O2}}$$

It seemed the higher the K value is the more likely DCI is to occur. K values of 10 were regarded as critical values for Helium decompression dives. With increasing depth, the safe K value was thought to decrease. For nitrogen mixture dives, the K values with 3.5–5 were even lower. Later studies confirmed the theory behind this. It showed good correlation in oxygen window (Kw), inspired (Ki) and arterial O_2 partial pressures (Ka). However, the inspired and arterial O_2 partial pressure seemed to have a slightly better correlation to decompression rates than the oxygen window.

The results of this study [4] were:
- Ki: correlation coefficient 0.72, $t = 5.9$; bubbles = 3.43 Ki + 0.71

- Ka: correlation coefficient 0.72, $t = 5.5$; bubbles = 2.65 Ka − 1.34
- Kw: correlation coefficient 0.65, $t = 4.6$; bubbles = 1.86 Kw + 1.75

They all display a good correlation between K value and decompression stress, but K values of the inspired O_2 partial pressure are not only slightly better but also easily obtained or calculated as it is not influenced by various factors. It is probably a good way to estimate the severity of decompression stress.

The understanding of the oxygen window is important for understanding HBOT for DCI treatment. The supersaturation of inert gas, mainly nitrogen, is the causative factor for DCI. The excess nitrogen reflects the conversion of unsaturation to supersaturation. In other words, when excess nitrogen exceeds the oxygen window, supersaturation commences. The oxygen window easily can be extended by supplying extra oxygen, even with normobaric oxygen treatment with high flow rebreather masks. That might reduce or reverse the supersaturation gradient of nitrogen to a greater extent than recompression with normal air. The calculated OW_t with 60% normobaric oxygen with a rebreather is 332 mmHg, compared to the nitrogen gas tension reversal on normal

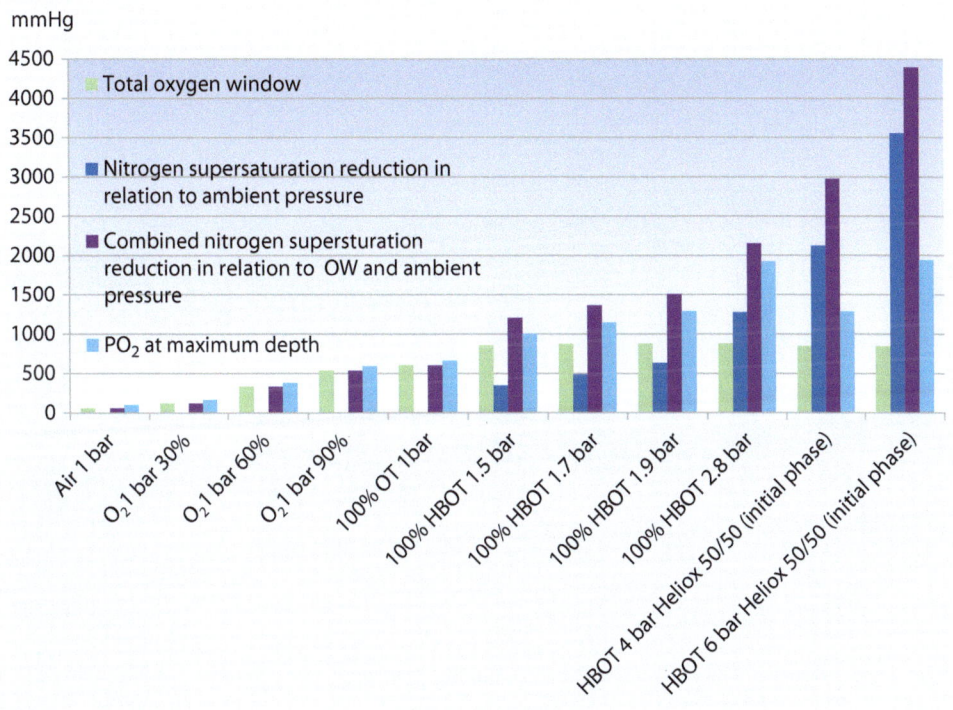

Fig. 25.8 Oxygen window, nitrogen saturation reduction, combined nitrogen reduction in relation to oxygen window and oxygen partial pressure at different oxygen fractions and ambient pressure

air at 1.7 bar air with 377 mmHg. A nitrogen supersaturation of 0.4 bar equals 300 mmHg, which can be associated with an approx. 60% chance of developing DCI. To totally reverse this supersaturation with normal air, an ambient pressure of about 1.7 bar would be needed. On the other hand, 60% normobaric oxygen would already reverse the supersaturation gradient at 1 bar just with the OW_t (Fig. 25.8).

However, as DCI is not only about bubbles, reducing supersaturation might not be enough for a sufficient treatment on its own. But it stresses that high flow oxygen should be delivered as soon as possible in DCI. HBOT is superior for DCI treatment, as it increases OW, ambient pressure but also oxygen supply to damaged and ischemic tissue. In HBOT at 2.8 bar, the venous SaO_2 is 100%. Theoretically, venous SO_2 of 98% is already reached with HBOT at 1.35 bar. 100% oxygen supply at 1 bar

theoretically should achieve a venous SO_2 of 91%. That means tissues are highly saturated, and even after intracellular oxygen consumption, it leaves enough oxygen to saturate haemoglobin in the venous blood to high levels. In HBOT the OW start to plateau out at approx. 1.7 bar, with normal air at 8 bar, when the venous SO_2 is close to 100% (Fig. 25.9).

HBOT increases the oxygen window. It supplies tissue with high O_2 partial pressure and minimised ischemic damage but also reverses the supersaturation gradient. Existing gas bubbles only reduce to some degree their diameter under hyperbaric conditions, and their volume reduction according to Boyle's law is minimal with regular HBOT for DCI. However, gas bubbles get relatively quickly eliminated via the lung, and reversion of the supersaturation gradient forces gas from the free phase into the dissolved phase. By reducing or reversing the

25

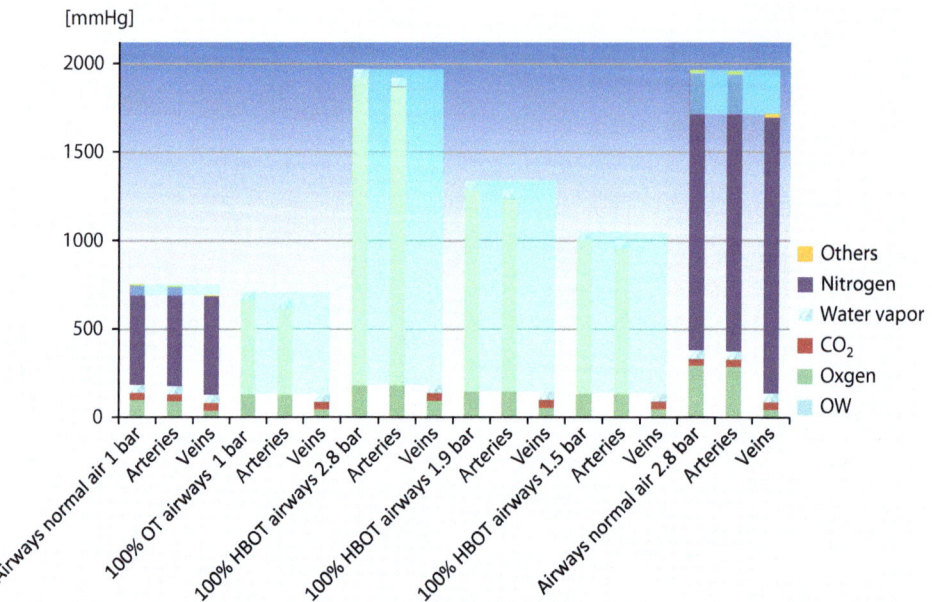

□ Fig. 25.9   Proportion of the oxygen window to gas partial pressures in airways, arteries and veins with different gas composition and ambient pressure

supersaturation gradient, new bubble formation is reduced or stopped completely. With HBOT the fast compartments are expected to empty within a short time. In severe DCI, deeper recompression might be helpful to empty these compartments, reduce their high bubble load and reduce the size of existing bubbles. Phase 1 of HBOT is an important part of reducing the free phase and emptying fast compartments. Theoretically, compartments like nerve cells with their $t_{1/2}$ of 10–20 min will be emptied completely within 60–120 min. For slower compartments, treatment duration is more important than depth. As DCI is often a result of repetitive dives, slower compartments fill up too. These require longer elimination times, which can't be accomplished in a single treatment session.

Hyperbaric and normobaric oxygen treatment can be adjusted in various ways. However, the risk and benefits need to be carefully considered. The OW of high flow normobaric oxygen is quite significant, particularly in the elimination of nitrogen from slow compartments. A simple face mask delivers FiO_2 40–60% at 5–10 L/min and a non-rebreather with tight sitting mask with reservoir up to FiO_2 90% at 15 L/min.

25.5   Extended Oxygen Window (EOW)

The extended oxygen window (EOW) was suggested by Kot in 2015 [3]. In addition to oxygen, carbon dioxide and water vapour were included. This extended the classical oxygen window from 60 mmHg to approximately 150 mmHg (oxygen 60 mmHg + water vapour 47 mmHg + carbon dioxide 45 mmHg). The value of the EOW comes close to inspired oxygen partial pressure outside the airways. Water vapour was included as it doesn't participate in the creation of gas bubbles. In the classical oxygen window, water vapour is included in blood, tissue and gas bubbles and hence doesn't participate in gas transfer gradients. Carbon dioxide is highly soluble, chemically active and able to bind to haemoglobin and proteins as well as to convert to bicarbonate ions. Hence, carbon dioxide doesn't play a role in gas bubble formation either in the EOW. The elasticity of cells seems to keep nitrogen in solution to a minor degree too. The concept was designed to allow a new decompression profile. His calculations were validated in studies. The outcome was that an initial faster decompression rate is allowed, which minimises nitrogen uptake at greater depth and reduces decompression time.

However, from my understanding, pCO_2 needs to be excluded from the OW as venous pCO_2 is the dissolved content of the total CO_2. The dissolved pCO_2 is not involved in metabolic or chemical processes till reaching the lungs. Hence, in the venous system, pCO_2 can be expected to remain steady. According to Dalton's law, the sum of all partial pressures of gases are combined, and therefore pCO_2 has to be a part of gas bubbles. Water vapour theoretically can be excluded, as it is only a part of gas and not liquid. But when gas bubbles develop, water vapour suddenly appears in the gaseous phase. This makes it complicated in calculations, and therefore modern diving algorithms include water vapour as it adds extra security. By critically reviewing all theories of the OW, it needs to be noted that in none of those theories, blood pressure changes are included. Having a mean arterial blood pressure of 100 mmHg or a venous blood pressure of 20 mmHg however is not insignificant to 60 mmHg of the OW. I would rather propose an OW, which includes water vapour and blood pressure changes. The total OW, which I think would be appropriate, would be 127 mmHg (OW_v 60 mmHg + BP_v 20 mmHg pH_2O 47 mmHg). For current dive computer algorithms, still water vapour might be excluded as it adds an extra safety gap.

The maximal allowable decompression rate ($rate^{max}$) is depending on the maximum persistently allowable elimination gradient from the limiting compartment (Δp^{max}) with the constant of proportionality k of the slowest compartment (k^{min}).

with

$$k^{min} = \frac{\ln(2)}{T_{1/2}^{max}}$$

$$rate^{max} = k^{min} \times \Delta p^{max}$$

At normal sea level, approximately 1.37 L nitrogen is dissolved in the body. After fully saturation at 2.8 bar, there is an excess of 2.5 L nitrogen in tissues, which needs to be eliminated. The decompression rate with normal air needs to be below the EWO to avoid gas bubble formation. It seems that values of Δp lower than PiO_2 are too restrictive and values greater than PiO_2 induce gas bubbles. The EOW allowed in Phase I of the decompression a faster rate. This also reduces the total decompression time, as due to slow decompression with normal air in Phase I nitrogen reuptake occurs. In Phase 1, mainly compartments with shorter half-times are targeted, which are off-gassing faster, and hence a relatively increased decompression rate is possible. The slower compartments require more time for off-gassing, and hence the decompression rate has to be lowered to allow sufficient time for off-gassing. The Phase II of the EWO decompression profile and its decompression rate are similar to the Thalmann or US Navy profiles. Previously that concept has been proposed by several authors but never has been applied. The application of the EWO might be a new method of calculating saturation decompressions and risk assessments of DCI. It would also mean that treatment durations and pressure could be adjusted accordingly. This would reduce oxygen exposure to patients but also to tenders.

References

1. Behnke AR. The isobaric (oxygen window) principle of decompression. In the new thrust seaward. Trans. Third Marine Tech. Soc. Conf. 5–7 June 1967, San Diego. Washington DC: Marine Tech. Soc.
2. Carreau A, Bouchra El HR, Matajuk A, Grillon C, Kieda C. Why is the partial oxygen pressure of human tissues a crucial parameter? Small molecules and hypoxia. J Cell Mol Med. 2011;15(6):1239–53.

25

3. Kot J, Sicko Z, Doboszynski T. The extended oxygen window concept for programming saturation decompression using air and nitrox. Plos One. 2015. https://doi.org/10.1371/journal.ponr.0130835.

4. Reinertsen RE, Flook V, Koteng S, Brubakk AO. Effect on oxygen tension and rate of pressure reduction during decompression on central gas bubbles. 1996. http://jap.physiology.org/content/jap/84/1/351.full.pdf. Accessed 4 July 2017.

5. Severinghaus JW. Simple, accurate equations for human blood O2 dissociation computations. J Appl Physiol Respirat Environ Exercise Physiol. 1979;46(3):599–602. Revisions, 1999, 2002, 2007.

6. Vann RD, Thalmann ED. Decompression physiology and practice. In: Bennett PB, Elliott DH, editors. The physiology and medicine of diving. London: Saunders; 1993. p. 376–432.

7. West JB. Respiratory physiology. 5th ed. Baltimore: Williams & Wilkins; 1995.

Suggested Reading

Burton DA, Stokes K, Hall GM. Continuing education in Anaesthesia. Crit Care Pain. 2004;4(6):185–8.

Geers C, Gros G. Carbon dioxide transport and carbonic anhydrases in blood and muscle. Physiol Rev. 2000;80(2):681–715.

Guyton AC. A Concept of negative interstitial pressure based on pressure in implanted capsules. Circ Res. 1963;XII:399–414.

Kenney WL, Wilmore JH, Costil DL. Physiology of sport and exercise. 5th ed. Auflage: Human Kinetics; 2012.

Kerem D, Melamed Y, Moran A. Alveolar PCO2 during rest and exercise in divers and non-divers breathing O2 at 1 ATA. Undersea Biomed Res. 1980;7:17–26.

Lambertson CJ. Effects of excessive pressures of oxygen, nitrogen, helium, carbon dioxide, and carbon monoxide. In: Mountcastle VB, editor. Medical Physiology. Missouri: CV Mosby Co; 1980. p. 1901–46.

Mummery HJ, Stolp BW, De Dear L, Doar PO, Natoli MJ, Bosa AE, Archibald JD, Hobbs GW, El-Moalem HE, Moon RE. Effects of age and exercise on physical dead space during stimulated dives at 2.8 ATA. J Appl Physiol. 2003;94:507–17.

National Oceanic and Atmospheric Administration. Diving for science and technology. In: Noaa diving manual. Washington, DC; 1990.

Petterson J, Glenny RW. Gas exchange and ventilation-perfusion relationship in the lung. Eur Respir J. 2014;44:1023–41.

Respiratory Physiology. https://www.ucl.ac.uk/anaesthesia/people/RespPhysiolLong.pdf. Accessed 4 July 2017.

Segadal K, Gulsvik A, Nicolaysen G. Respiratory changes with deep diving. Eur Respir J. 1990;3:101–8.

Sharpe AG. Solubility explained. Educ Chem. 1964; 1(2):75–82.

Simons M. The physiology of compressed gas diving. http://www.navy.gov.au/sites/default/files/documents/THE_PHYSIOLOGY_OF_COMPRESSED_GAS_DIVING.pdf. Accessed 02 May 2015.

Stickland MK, Lovering AT. Exercise-induced intra pulmonary arteriovenous shunting and pulmonary gas exchange. Exrec Sport Sci Rev. 2006;34(3):99–106. American College of Sports Medicine.

Intoxication of Breathing Gases During Diving

© Springer International Publishing AG, part of Springer Nature 2018
O. Rusoke-Dierich, *Diving Medicine*, https://doi.org/10.1007/978-3-319-73836-9_26

26

A part of diving accidents are caused by effects of breathing gases during diving. Normal air contains approx. 78% nitrogen (N_2), 21% oxygen (O_2), 0.9% argon (Ar), 0.03% carbon dioxide (CO_2) and 0.01% helium (He), neon (Ne), krypton (Kr), hydrogen (H), xenon (X) and ozone (O_3). All gases except oxygen and carbon dioxide are inert gases. Inert gases are only slightly chemical reactive. They don't participate in physiological processes and hence will be at the same level expired as they were inhaled. Normally carbon monoxide isn't included in the normal air. However, with insufficient burning of fossil fuels, carbon monoxide is produced and causes problems during diving.

All gases are affected by *partial pressure*, the *time of exposure*, the *solubility coefficient* and its *toxicity*. Gases dissolve physically more or less in correspondence with the ambient pressure. Oxygen and carbon monoxide additionally bind onto haemoglobin with a reversible chemical reaction. This makes these two gases different from the inert gases.

26.1 Nitrogen or Inert Gas Narcosis (IGN) (◘ Fig. 26.1)

A delirious state is a subjective sensation caused by substances, which are not present in the body under physiological conditions. This sensation can exhibit differently in each person in regard to its intensity and quality. An altered state of mind doesn't have to be recognised as such by the affected person. Self-control, self-overestimate, high tolerance or adaptation to the substance can convey a feeling of not being affected by the narcotic effects of the substance. Usually, the concentration of inert gases increases slowly and the body and mind can adapt to increased levels up to a certain degree. At a certain point however, it becomes noticeable and thus can occur gradually or suddenly.

Inert gas narcosis is an occult stress for divers. If external (exogenous) or internal (endogenous) factors like stress or anxiety arise, still

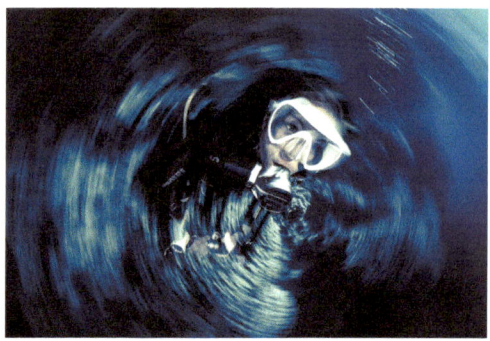

◘ **Fig. 26.1**   Inert gas narcosis. (Mares)

tolerated or occult inert gas narcosis can come to a level, which may affect consciousness and behaviour of the diver. This may result in potentially dangerous behaviour during diving. Moreover, inert gas narcosis itself could provoke a stress reaction of the diver and might lead to a panic attack. *Inert gas narcosis* is also referred as *nitrogen narcosis*. It accounts for approximately 6% of death in diving.

26.1.1 Aetiology and Pathogenesis

Pathomechanisms of inert gas narcosis or general anaesthetic are not fully understood. Some theories try to elucidate this process. There are however few scientific facts. Anaesthetic effects causing unconsciousness, immobilisation and amnesia are a quite complex matter. Inert gas narcosis is caused by inhaled gases under high pressure with elevated partial pressures. Hence, it has similarity to other inhalation anaesthetics. It is obvious that inert gas narcosis is caused by the increase in the partial pressure of various breathing gases. Inert gas narcosis is mainly triggered by nitrogen. However, other inert gases, even in small concentration, may contribute to IGN. Carbon dioxide appears to have an additive role in it. Normally, CO_2 is not expected to have strong narcotic effects by itself under these conditions. However, it can significantly increase in greater depth, as in exposures to pressure more than 5 bar airflow in airways becomes increasingly turbulent. The resulting hypercapnia triggers the sensation of suffocation and leads to panic attacks and increasing respiration as well as cardiac output. As a result of hyperventilation and increased cardiac output, more nitrogen may enter the bloodstream at a faster rate. The combination of hypercapnia and IGN together may cause loss of consciousness. Inert gase. The MAC value of nitrogen is approximately 110% [19] is compared to Xenon, which is a relative strong anaesthetic, with only 71% [28].

The best way to understand IGN is to compare it to effects of other inhaled anaesthetics. Still, the mechanism of anaesthetics is not fully understood. But there is a consensus that their action is produced by enhancing inhibitory channels and attenuating excitatory channels. A way of describing their efficiency is the minimum alveolar concentration (MAC). The MAC is the alveolar concentration at which 50% of patients will not show a motor response to a standardised surgical incision. MAC is an ED_{50} concentration. That means that 50% of all patients achieve the proposed goal, e.g. being awake or not responding to pain stimuli. In

praxis this means that MAC has to be exceeded by factor 1.3 to allow anaesthetic effect for most of patients to prevent a response to a surgical incision (MAC-BAR). The 0.3 resembles 3SD where 97% of patients do not respond to pain stimuli on incision. A MAC with the factor 0.4–0.6 will prevent a response to verbal/tracheal stimulation and a 0.1–0.5 MAC is associated with wakening (MAC awake). All anaesthetics cause amnesia. This is usually achieved by 0.06–0.3 MAC (MAC amnesia). All MAC values vary in species or substance. The MAC is usually expressed as % of 1 atm. However, the MAC value is measured in atm. The MAC value in correlation to the oil solubility is reflected in the Meyer-Overton correlation (☐ Fig. 26.2) (☐ Table 26.1). Therefore, MAC can be estimated by taking the oil-gas partition (λ) in consideration [1, 8]:

$$MAC \cdot \lambda \approx 1.82 \, atm$$

However, not all anaesthetics, like nitrogen, follow the Meyer-Overton correlation. Additionally, the MAC is age dependent and

☐ **Fig. 26.2** Meyer-Overton correlation. (Tonner and Lutz [31], Abb 2.3.)

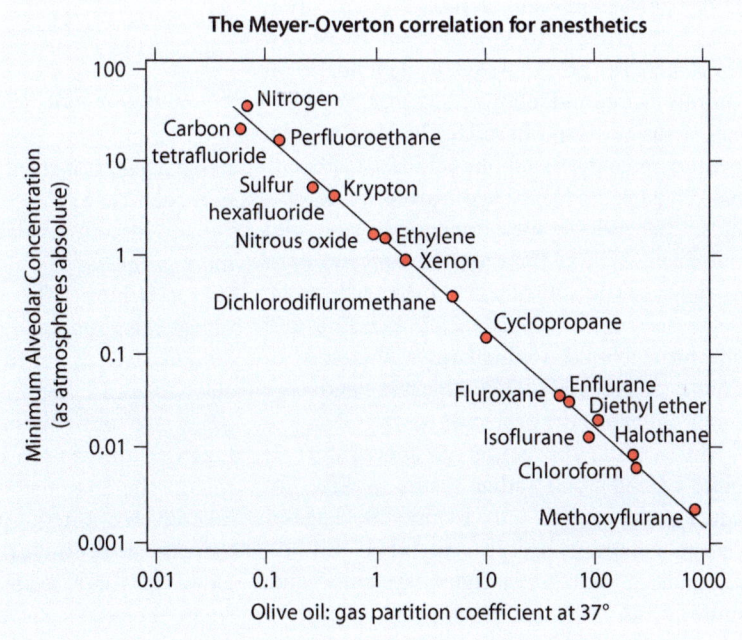

26

26

■ **Table 26.1** Correlation between the relative narcotic potency of inert gases, solubility in lipid, their molecular weight and their oil-water solubility of different phases

Gas	Molecular weight	Solubility in lipid	Oil-water solubility ratio	Relative narcotic potency
Xe	131.3	1.7	20	25.6
Kr	83.7	0.43	9.6	2.5
CO_2	44	0.876	1.6	20
Ar	40	0.14	5.3	2.3
N_2	28	0.067	5.2	1
Ne	20	0.019	2.07	0.3
He	4	0.015	1.7	0.2
H_2	2	0.036	2.1	0.5

decreases with age. It also has an additive effect, which means that one anaesthetic gas lowers the MAC of another anaesthetic gas. In general, all inhaled anaesthetics decrease the respiratory tidal volume and increase the ventilation rate, both leading to greater dead space and thus increase pCO_2. MAC is dependent on various factors and follows a sigmoid, not a linear, curve. Hypothermia, hyponatraemia, hypo-osmolality, metabolic acidosis, hypercarbia, anaemia, increased age, nitrous oxide, opioids, benzodiazepine, increased age and intoxication lower the required concentration of the narcotic substance, and hyperthermia, decreased age, amphetamine, cocaine and chronic alcohol abuse increase it. Therefore, in diving hypercarbia, hypothermia and age might influence the development of IGN.

In general, the action of anaesthetics is quite complex and rather seems to affect an entire pathway than only a single blockage of certain receptors or cell structures only. As anaesthesia affects various systems, like motoric as well as nociceptive function,

consciousness and memory, it seems to act on multiple levels. Main focus has been on synapses. It may mainly act on neurotransmitter release at presynaptic level but also might affect impulse alterations at postsynaptic levels. It seems rather that excitation is impaired much more than inhibitory transmission.

The uptake of inhalative anaesthetics is subject to the transfer from air to alveoli, the transfer from alveoli to blood and to the transfer from blood to tissue. Factors influencing this are concentration of the gas, alveolar ventilation, blood-gas partition, blood-tissue partition, cardiac output, alveoli to venous pressure difference and tissue perfusion.

26.1.2 Hypothesis of Narcotic Substances, Which Can Be Applied to IGN

■ **Meyer-Overton Theory**

For more than 100 years, the anaesthetic potency was commonly correlated with the lipid solubility (Meyer-Overton correlation). In humans the product of the anaesthetising partial pressure and oil-gas partition coefficient varies little over a ~100,000-fold range of anaesthetising partial pressures:

$$p_g \cdot \tau_{O:G} \sim 1.28 \pm 0.09 \, bar$$

p_g = partial pressure of gas, $\tau_{O:G}$ = oil-gas partition coefficient.

The highest relative anaesthetic potency of inert gases has the noble gas xenon and the lowest helium. The anaesthetic potency of nitrogen is about in the middle range. However, quantitatively it has the biggest part in normal air. Nitrogen composes 78% of the air. Noble gases are only accounted for about 0.1%. Likewise, the molecular weight seems to play a role in the anaesthetic potency too [24]. The relative anaesthetic potency is thought to increase with increasing molecular weight. However, there seems to be a cut-off effect, where molecules above a certain size lose their anaesthetic effect despite increasing lipid solubility. Moreover, newer studies showed that the Meyer-Overton correlation has exemptions and the narcotic potency, which are not solely explained by lipid solubility. Anaesthetic substances may bind to the membrane and proteins. Helium itself has a narcotic effect only for dives of more than 400 m, if one would apply the increased lipid solubility. But somehow high ambient pressure seems to counteract the narcotic effect. The symptoms of helium narcosis are probably not only caused by anaesthetic properties themselves and are therefore referred to as high-pressure nervous syndrome (HPNS), which will be mentioned later.

■ **Lipid Hypothesis (Critical Volume Hypothesis)**

A physical explanation proposes that the site of the IGN is on a lipophilic (fat-soluble) portion of the cell membrane. The cell membrane consists of a lipid bilayer. Due to their lipophilicity, nitrogen and inert gases bind to membranes. This is thought to cause swelling of the membrane. If a certain critical volume of the membrane is exceeded, narcotic effects may be triggered. Therefore, this is also referred as the "critical volume hypothesis". In this theory, the way how pressure affects narcotic potency is linear. This means that the narcotic potency of inert gases or nitrogen increases with increasing pressure. However, in case of helium,

increased ambient pressure seems to counteract the volume increase and thus the narcotic effect. This hypothesis was regarded valid for a long time but now has been replaced by the neurophysiological explanation. The majority of studies showed that there was no significant increase of the thickness of the membrane. Other studies, which have been conducted, used partial pressures far beyond anaesthetic concentrations that are clinically relevant. Moreover, nitrogen seems to gather rather on the surface of the bilayer, not inside. Therefore, this mechanism couldn't explain IGN (■ Fig. 26.3).

Ion channels may be affected in their function by alterations of membrane thickness. If the thickness changes in proximity to channels, it might distort them and interfere with ion transport. It may lead to a change of the bilipid layer configuration, increased fluidity of the cell membrane or increased lateral pressure. It is thought to be most relevant when narcotic substances bind closely to ion channels. Ion channels are very sensitive to changes in the double lipid membrane. This reaction is unspecific to the triggering substance, as it does not lead to a change of ion channels' configuration themselves. It is the structural change in the vicinity of ion channel, which might trigger their effects. The configuration change seems to inhibit the opening of the ion channel and therefore a reaction of the nerve cell (■ Fig. 26.4).

■ **Fig. 26.3** Hypothesis of volume changes of the double lipid layer

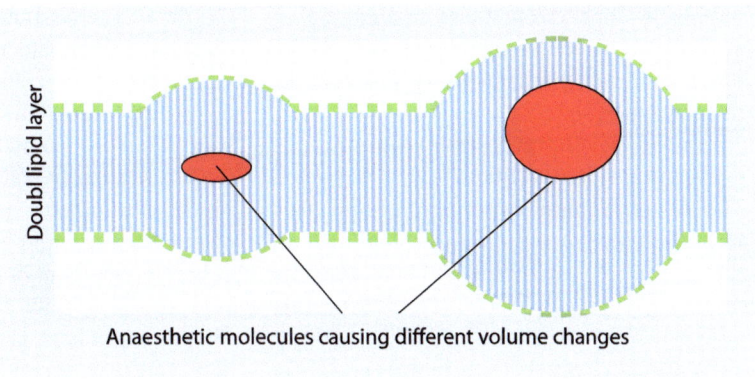

Anaesthetic molecules causing different volume changes

Fig. 26.4 Configuration change of the lipid layer in proximity of ion channels

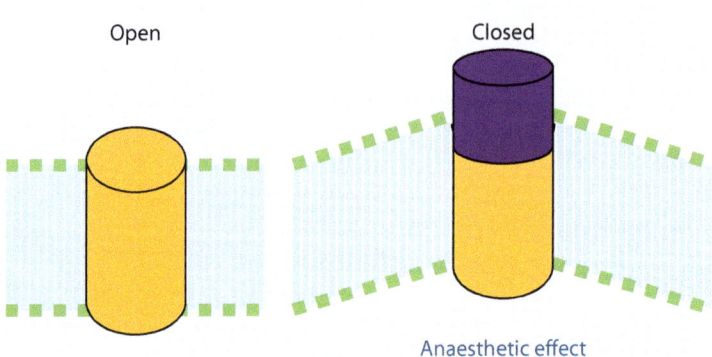

Open   Closed

Anaesthetic effect

■ **Biochemical Hypothesis**

Over a long period, different theories have emerged, which attempt to explain the anaesthesia at the biochemical level. Many of them failed to thrive. The theory of Quastel postulates that the anaesthetics intervene in the intracellular oxidation by preventing the energy transfer in the respiratory chain. Another theory describes that anaesthetics interfere with the neurotransmitter system. A combination of the lipid and biochemical approach suggests that a decrease of the oxygen availability in the cells reduces the energy production. This was supposed to lead to a lack of supply from the capillary bed to the neuron. The result would be a suppression of the central nervous system activity. Another theory assumed that water molecules form around the inert gas molecule. These gaseous microcrystals (hydrate) should prevent the transmission of excitation in the synaptic region. Some anaesthetics such as halothane don't create these hydrates. Their anaesthetic properties seem to be effective on different sites or mechanisms. Helium too can't form hydrates.

■ **Neuro- or Physiochemical Hypothesis**

The neurochemical hypothesis is the most recent and most commonly accepted theory of the action of narcotic substances. On the inhibitory side, substances can bind on proteins affecting Cl channels (GABA$_A$ and glycine) and K channels (K$_{2P}$, K$_V$ and K$_{ATP}$). On the excitatory side, inhibition of glutaminergic ion channels activated by acetylcholine, excitatory amino acids (AMPA, kainate and NMDA receptors) and serotonin is thought to be responsible off anaesthetic effects [15, 35, 38]. For example, anaesthetic substances binding to the α-subunit of the GABA$_A$ transmembrane receptor lead to opening of Cl channels. This leads to increased Cl conductance as well as hyperpolarisation of the cell membrane and thereby increasing the depolarisation threshold as well as inhibiting postsynaptic neural excitability. The neurochemical explanation proposes a disruption of the ion transport or a direct impact on receptors. This reaction influences anaesthetic potencies rather in a sigmoidal fashion, compared to the lipid hypothesis. This mechanism seems to be more selective in its action in regard the response of different anaesthetic agents. Trials with increased pressure showed that nitrogen decreased dopamine and glutamate but increased serotonin levels. On the other hand, helium seems to increase serotonin, glutamate and dopamine. Nitrogen seems to concentrate around ion channel under hyperbaric conditions [37]. It seems to bind directly on proteins of receptors, like on GABA$_A$ receptors acting as a co-agonist or a so-called allosteric modulator. This mechanism therefore could be a possible explanation of the development of IGN. At increased pressure, the sensibility of GABA$_A$ and GABA$_B$ receptors seems to increase in the substantia nigra reticulata (SNr) [25, 27]. In the substantia nigra compacta (SNc), this increase of sensitivity leads to a greater response by the $GABA_A$ postsynaptic receptors on the GABAnergic nigrothalamic pathway in the SNr and in the GABAnergic interneurons of the SNc. With recurrent exposure, the response seems to get milder, which reminds of responses of tolerance or addiction [20, 21].

26.1.3 Symptoms

There are individual differences in regard to symptoms, receptivity and depth, in which symptoms of inert gas narcosis occur. These differences don't necessarily depend on the diving experience but rather on the physiological disposition. The impact of the IGN is only to a certain extent influenced by diving experience, as experienced diver only handles better the subjective symptoms of IGN. Their subjective adaptation results in a greater depth tolerance and symptom mitigation. However, adaption to IGN, likewise as to alcohol, leads to the false belief that critical thinking and reasoning as well as self-control are still preserved. This misjudgement can have disastrous, even fatal, consequences for the diver. Stress symptoms can be aggravated by IGN and symptoms of IGN can be aggravated by stress. Generally speaking, symptoms of IGN can be always expected at 50 m and below. The first symptoms may occur in some divers as early as in 20 m depth or less. At 60–70 m depth, significant symptoms of IGN can be expected (▶ Box 26.1). Effects of IGN may resemble those of hallucinogenic drugs. The first signs are a feeling of well-being, arousal, drowsiness and increased satisfaction [3–5, 16–18]. As well, increased susceptibility for panic attacks may result. Higher brain functions such as memory, appropriate decision-making, reasoning, concentration, learning and attention are affected first. Further signs of increasing IGN are restricted ability of targeted actions, increasing disorientation, inability to determine the body position (temporo-spatial disorientation), increasing deterioration of abstract thinking, automatisms, idea fixation, partial amnesia, hallucinations and eventually

> **Box 26.1   Stages of the Inert Gas Narcosis**
> — *Stage I (3–6 bar/20–50 m)*
>   — Dizziness, increased sense of well-being, increased tendency for panic attacks, euphoria, mood changes
>   — Disturbance of higher cerebral functions (memory, reason, decision-making capabilities, concentration, learning, attention)
>   — Temporo-spatial disorientation
>   — Decline of ability for abstract thinking (calculating, creating)
>   — Increasing disorientation
>   — Partial amnesia
> — *Stage II (5–8 bar/40–70 m)*
>   — Hallucinations
>   — Fixation of ideas
>   — Sensorimotor disturbance (saccadic pursuit, paraesthesia, dysaesthesia, disturbance in the fine motor skills, ataxia)
>   — Automatism, impaired neuromuscular coordination
>   — Hysteria
> — *Stage III (from 5 bar to 40 m)*
>   — Loss of consciousness

unconsciousness. Phenomena of narrowing of the peripheral visual fields (tunnel vision), saccadic pursuit, altered body awareness, paraesthesia increasing rapidly from the body periphery to the centre of the body (tingling sensation, numbness) and motor disturbance (fine motor skills, ataxia) may occur. The transition from stage II to stage III can develop rapidly. That's why the diver should ascend immediately when symptoms of stage II appear. In addition to the possibility of becoming unconscious, IGN can be life-threatening because of inappropriate actions, which puts the diver or the dive partner at risk. IGN can be reinforced by fear, unusual environmental conditions, cold, fatigue, medication affecting the central nervous function and drugs.

Experiments with an electroencephalogram (EEG) were made to determine changes in brain activity with IGN. In contrast to the expectation, signs of a neural hyperexcitability of the cortex were seen. This includes an increase in the voltage of the basal rhythm and a regular occurrence of spikes in the low voltage range not showing up at normal atmospheric pressure. There were two other neurophysiological changes. Alpha waves, which prevail in the relaxed waking state, are normally interrupted by optical, acoustic and sensitive stimuli or through mental activity (alpha block). The development of an alpha block decreases a certain time (T) of elevated pressure exposure (P) inversely proportional to the square of the pressure. This means that the relaxed waking state is less likely to be interrupted by stimuli or through mental activity. As well, the frequency increase of the EEG in flickering light is subject to pressure changes. The frequency decreased after a certain period of elevated pressure exposure. This means that external stimuli are less perceived. Therefore, the ability to create an adequate response to the situation of the environment decreases.

- **Correlation of Exposure Time and Pressure Causing EEG Changes**

$$T \sim \frac{1}{P^2}$$

Studies of cortical evoked potentials, in particular the visually evoked potential, showed changes during pressure exposure with normal air. Initial EEG changes decreased within a certain period of time, so that one can assume an adaptation. That effect is reflected in practice for divers who are frequently exposed to greater depth. Other human studies with limited numbers could prove adaptation to nitrogen narcosis. These studies included the choice-reaction time (RT) [9].

26.1.4 Treatment and Prophylaxis

Occurrence and intensity of inert gas narcosis are dependent on the ambient pressure and the rate of the ambient pressure increase.

The deeper the dive and the faster the diver reaches this depth, the stronger are the effects of IGN. Extreme environmental conditions, such as poor visibility, darkness, currents, etc., as well as discomfort and fear are strong factors that favour the IGN. IGN does not depend on the exposure time, which means that the existing symptoms at a certain depth don't increase with the exposure time. Deep dives require long preparation because divers have to be accustomed gradually to depth and have to get to know themself and their reactions during deeper dives. If inert gas narcosis occurs, symptoms diminish when ascending from that depth. Often only a few meters are needed for this to happen. It is very important to avoid panic actions. Also uncontrolled ascent should be avoided. Physiological effects of elevated arterial carbon dioxide partial pressure might increase the heart rate and the respiratory rate. These symptoms as well can be minimised by reducing the depth. The increase of carbon dioxide partial pressure and the inert gas narcosis act synergistically together and reinforce symptoms. The increase of heart rate and respiratory rate should be considered as a serious sign of hypercapnia or an inert gas narcosis. The deeper the dive, the more attention should be paid to these symptoms, because personal limits can be exceeded unintentionally. At greater depth, it needs to be considered that inflating the BCD takes a significant longer time than in shallow water, and the resulting downforce can't be compensated as quick. Hence, divers can descend deeper as planned. Therefore, care should be taken during the descent with frequent inflating of the BCD, to prevent uncontrolled rapid descends. Scuba divers' international diving organisations have set a dive limit of 40 m depth. Dive tables go up to 42 m, to allow a certain safety gap. Every dive below 30 m depth is regarded as a deep dive. To these diving limits should be adhered for safety reasons.

26.2 High-Pressure Neurological Syndrome (HPNS)

Helium is used as a substitute for nitrogen for commercial divers when working at greater depths to avoid inert gas narcosis. During helium dives greater than 200 m depth, changes of the mental state were noticed. Many attempts had been made to explore this phenomenon. The deepest dive with 686 m was achieved in 1981 with an ascent time of more than 28 days. HPNS is the limiting factor of diving depth to this day. The development of HPNS is dependent on the compression rate, the absolute pressure and gas composition. HPNS is not specifically regarded as a narcotic effect of helium. The symptoms might be caused by changes in the cell and the cell permeability, which in turn affect the nervous system. There are individual differences in sensitivity to pressures, such as to inert gas narcosis. The slower the descent, the less is the probability of occurrence of HPNS. Trimix (oxygen, helium, nitrogen) turned out as the best combination, as it reduces the tremor, which is typical for HPNS (▶ Box 26.2). The record of 686 m was reached with a trimix of 5–10% nitrogen in the gas mixture. Nitrogen was added, to relieve dyspnoea and to reduce the tremor. Helium itself is regarded to have only little narcotic effects. It seems to have narcotic effects only below 400 m. HPNS symptoms in less than 400 m are regarded to be caused by pressure itself, as pressure counteracts the weak narcotic potency of helium [3, 14]. Hydrogen seems to be less suitable because it has a higher narcotic potency than helium. Narcotic sensations with hydrogen seem to appear in dives greater than 240 m. Moreover, hydrogen is highly explosive with gas mixtures of more than 4% oxygen. It is therefore technically impractical to use.

Bühlmann described three stages of HPNS [5]:
1. Dizziness, mild vestibular disturbance, unsteadiness of standing on one foot

> **Box 26.2   HPNS Symptoms**
> ▬ Dizziness and vestibular disturbance
> ▬ Nausea, vomiting
> ▬ Cognitive impairment and visual disturbance
> ▬ Tremor
> ▬ Muscle fasciculations
> ▬ Dyspnoea
> ▬ Hallucinations
> ▬ Dizziness
> ▬ Limitation of abstract thinking
> ▬ Somnolence
> ▬ EEG changes:
>   ▬ Increase in slow waves (theta and delta waves) [33]
>   ▬ Decrease in high-frequency activities (alpha wave) [33]
>   ▬ Changes in evoked potentials in cortical excitability cycle [34]
>   ▬ Sleep: increase in stages 1 and 2, decrease in stage 3 and 4, REM [26]
>   ▬ Hyperreflexia

2. Nausea, visual disturbance, significant vestibular disturbance, unable to stand on one foot
3. Vomiting, diaphoresis, tremor

Stages 1 and 2 seem to appear within minutes but are reversible with pressure reduction. Stage 3 seems to have a latency of 30–60 min or longer and eases with pressure reduction. However, this is often followed with fatigue and apathy.

26.3 Oxygen Intoxication

Cells need oxygen to function. Oxygen is the fuel for the cell's processes such as oxidative phosphorylation and respiratory chain. These processes are localised in the mitochondrial wall. At normal levels, oxygen is a vital part of metabolism. In high concentrations, it can be harmful. Oxygen in high concentrations for humans is toxic. Important factors for the toxicity are *partial pressure and exposure time.*

26

Rebreather using 100% oxygen, exclusively used in the military, can be used for several hours at a maximum depth of 7 m. But also for sport and professional divers, oxygen poisoning may occur. Dives with pure oxygen at more than 10 m or dives with different gas mixtures, such as heliox, trimix or nitrox with varying proportion of oxygen, can cause oxygen toxicity. The main organs, which are sensible for oxygen intoxication, are the central nervous system, lungs, blood, eyes, enzymes, and cells themself. CNS effects of oxygen toxicity were first described by Paul Bert in 1878. Few years later, Smith noticed severe effects on the lungs in 1899.

26.3.1 Aetiology and Pathogenesis

Oxygen is a part in our normal breathing air and has a fraction of about 21%, which corresponds to a partial pressure of 0.21 bar at atmospheric pressure. The partial pressure of oxygen increases with ambient pressure or changes in gas composition with different oxygen fractions. The increase of oxygen partial pressure can cause damage in various parts the body. Short exposures cause in general only reversible effects. Long exposures rather result in irreversible damages. There is no absolute limit for the O_2 partial pressure, since toxicity depends on several factors.

■ **Factors for the Oxygen Intoxication**
— Duration of exposure
— Partial pressure of oxygen
— Individual differences in susceptibility
— Protective and enhancing factors

These factors have a synergistic effect and therefore can accumulate. However, the possibility of occurrence of oxygen intoxication in breathing normal compressed air increases drastically below 70 m or 8 bar. At this depth, the oxygen partial pressure is 1.68 bar. Even a relatively short exposure at this depth can cause CNS symptoms.

The formula for the determination of oxygen partial pressure under water is

$$PO_2 = \left(\frac{d}{x}+1\right) \bullet FO_2.$$

PO_2 = oxygen partial pressure; FO_2 = oxygen fraction in the gas mixture; d = depth; x = either 10 (m)/33 (feet) in seawater or 10.3 (m)/34 (feet) in freshwater

Oxygen toxicity results in:
— Inhabitation of enzymes with SH groups
— DNA damage
— Destruction of lipid membranes via lipoperoxide production

■ **Free Oxygen Radicals**
A major factor in oxygen toxicity may be the increased formation of *oxygen radicals or radical oxygen species (ROS)* at elevated oxygen partial pressure. Oxygen radicals include O_2^-, HO, HO_2^-, H_2O_2, OH^-, O_3, OCL^- and $^1O_2$. The formation of oxygen radicals is a physiological process. Oxygen radicals play a role in many diseases but also in the defence response against microorganisms. Oxygen radicals are affecting membrane lipids, proteins, nucleic acids and cytosol-molecules. Normally, oxygen radicals are intercepted by various protection mechanisms. These include superoxide dismutase, catalase, glutathione peroxidase, cytochrome-oxidase system and antioxidants (e.g. vitamins E, C and A, mannitol, thiols, cysteine, magnesium, zinc, selenium, etc.). Oxygen radicals produce lipoperoxides, which affect enzymes with SH groups, cause disruption of membranes and lead to impaired energy production via oxidative processes of glutathione and pyridine nucleotides. This causes cell injury or cell death and DNA destruction [13].

During ischaemia-reperfusion (IR) injury, ROS are generated by xanthine oxidase of skeletal muscle endothelial cells and neutrophils, which are recruited to the blood-endothelial cells.

■ CNS Effects ("Bert Effects")

Oxygen influences the regulation of perfusion, oxygenation of the tissue and the metabolism of the CNS. The exact mechanism of toxicity is still not fully understood, because oxygen interferes in many places of the metabolism and cellular functions. In vitro studies showed that just enzymes with hydrogen sulfide (-SH) groups seem to be sensitive to oxygen. The reason for this is thought to be the oxidation of – SH – S – S -, which leads to *inactivation of various enzymes*. Enzymes including phosphate dehydrogenase (key enzyme of glycolysis), flavoproteins of respiratory chain and enzymes of oxidative phosphorylation seem to be mainly affected. Increased oxygen levels were described to cause *decreased secretion of the inhibitory transmitter GABA* (gamma-amino butyric acid) and *increased production of the excitatory transmitter glutamine* in the brain [6, 13]. The reduction of GABA and the increase of glutamine in the brain are thought to influence the development of epileptic seizures. Increased generation of radical oxygen species (ROS) may lead to increased oxygen consumption and hence to oxygen-induced convulsions. ROS and increased oxygen levels on the other hand cause vasoconstriction in cerebral arterioles. Increased NMDA activity and NO production counteract this and allow excessive oxygen delivery to the brain, which in return may cause convulsions. A combination of enzyme inhibition, NO production and ROS generation may cause irreversible damage to cells as well as DNA and may result in delayed neurological damage. Another cause for CNS effects might be CO_2 retention and accumulation of acid metabolites secondary to maldistribution of cerebral blood flow. In HBOT venous blood is completely saturated with oxygen. Due to the Haldane effect, this results in a reduced transport of CO_2 as carbonic acid in the erythrocytes and increased transport in carbamino compounds and dissolved CO_2. This causes a slight respiratory acidosis, which is compensated by increased ventilation. The increased ventilation increases slightly the alveolar oxygen partial pressure and hence the oxygen uptake. CO_2 response is not the same in all vascular beds. It causes an increased blood flow in the brain, which seem to be a significant contributing factor in CNS toxicity of oxygen.

■ Pulmonary Effects ("Smith Effects")

The *pulmonary toxicity* of oxygen results from the increased formation of oxygen radicals and the inactivation of enzymes [13]. This causes an inflammatory response of the lung tissue. In the acute phase, alveolar oedema develops as a result of proteinaceous exudation, destruction of capillary endothelial cells as well as alveolar cells causing bleeding from the lung tissue. These manifestations are still reversible. In the chronic phase, which usually only occurs with increased oxygen exposure over time, a progressive fibrosis of the lung tissue, caused by proliferation of type II epithelia cells as well as fibroblast, might develop. Bleomycin seems to support this process for an unlimited duration. Increased oxygen exposure can also cause damage to other organs. Increased oxygen partial pressure can cause haemolysis, a destruction of red blood cells. Likewise, it results in narrowing of retinal blood vessels, which results in a reversible decrease in vision. Increased oxygen partial pressure is also suspected of being a factor in development of dysbaric osteonecrosis.

Similar to pulmonary damages, other tissues and organs such as the heart, liver, spleen and kidneys can be affected by oxygen radicals. Depending on exposure time at increased oxygen partial pressure, symptoms occur in chronological order, with first affecting the central nervous system, then pulmonary tissue and followed by other organs. Short-term reversible symptoms of oxygen intoxication in the form of epileptic seizures may occur at 1.5 bar oxygen partial pressure or at 60 m and more with normal air. Already a relatively short-term exposure is sufficient to cause seizure. Hyperbaric oxygenation

26

(HBOT), which is performed typically at 2.8 bar absolute by breathing 100% oxygen, has air breaks with normal air to reduce the likelihood of seizures. The likelihood of oxygen toxicity of the central nervous system is increased at oxygen partial pressures above 1.7 bar and of the lung or other organs pulmonary above 0.5 bar. To cause cellular damage, increased oxygen exposure times at oxygen partial pressure are needed. The exposure time for cell damages is usually in the range of hours. With increasing duration, the risk of permanent injury to organs increases. Because of long exposure times in saturation dives, in HBOT (medical staff as well as patients) and long-term mechanical ventilation, cell damages may contribute to pulmonary damages.

26.3.2 Symptoms

CNS symptoms vary in their presentation and intensity. It depends on the diver's predispositions and activity level. The most common symptoms are dizziness, drowsiness, pallor, bradycardia, palpitations, vertigo, nausea, changes in behaviour, euphoria, apprehension, fidgeting, loss of acuity, constriction of visual field, acoustic sensations (e.g. music, bell ringing, knocking), olfactory and gustatory sensations and perioral muscle fasciculations followed by seizures. Donald 1947 has summarised the incidence of symptoms (◻ Table 26.2 and ▶ Box 26.3) [7]. He described the "end point" as the onset of the first symptoms. Manifestations of oxygen toxicity increase with activity, immersion in water and an increase in carbon dioxide partial pressure. There also seems to be intra-individual oxygen sensitivity. The symptoms can either occur suddenly without warning or be initiated by warning signs (◻ Figs. 26.5 and 26.6).

Pulmonary oxygen toxicity is dependent on partial pressure, length of exposure and individual sensitivity. First signs are tracheal irritation (tracheobronchitis) with cough. This

◻ **Table 26.2** Incidence of CNS symptoms with increased oxygen partial pressure to the "end point"

Symptoms	Incidence in %	
	At rest	With activity
Perioral fasciculations	60.6	50
Tonic-clonic seizure	9.2	6.8
Dizziness/vertigo	8.8	20.8
Nausea	8.3	17.5
Dyspnoea	3.8	5
Other muscle fasciculations	3.2	1.7
Neuropsychological effects	3.2	
Visual disturbance	1	
Acoustic hallucinations	0.6	
Paraesthesia	0.4	

Donald (1947)

Box 26.3   Main Symptoms of CNS Oxygen Toxicity
– *Early signs*
  – Perioral muscle fasciculations
  – Finger tremor
  – Generalised muscle fasciculations
  – Restlessness
– *Warning signs*
  – Dizziness, nausea
  – Visual disturbance (tunnel vision)
  – Acoustic hallucinations
  – Distal dysesthesia/paraesthesia
– *Seizures*

symptom intensified during forced inspiration. Pleuritic pain behind the sternum, which increases by forced inspiration is another sign associated with shortness of breath. The symptoms appear faster and more intense, if the

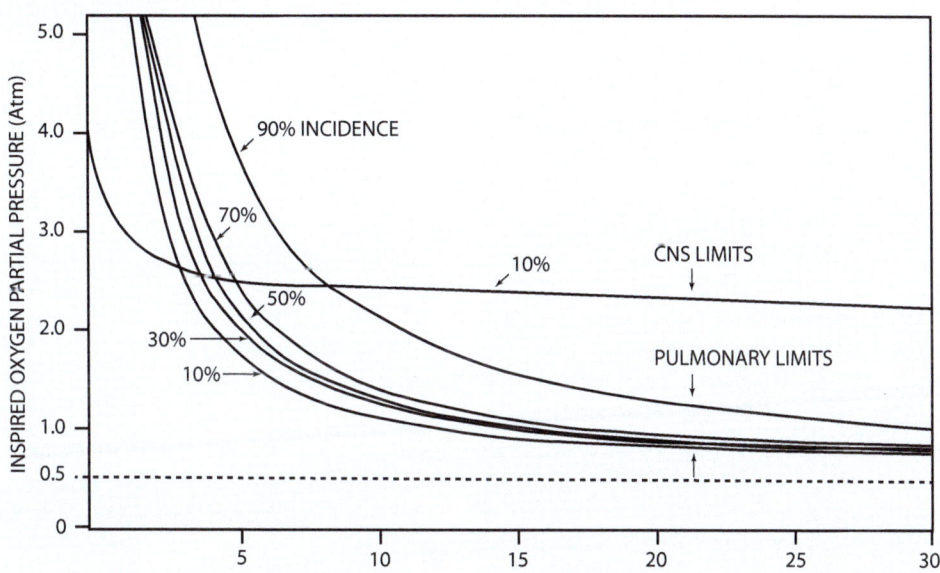

■ **Fig. 26.5**   Oxygen tolerance curves. Adapted from Davis JC, Hunt TK Hyperbaric oxygen therapy, Bethesda, MD, Undersea and Hyperbaric Medical Society 1977

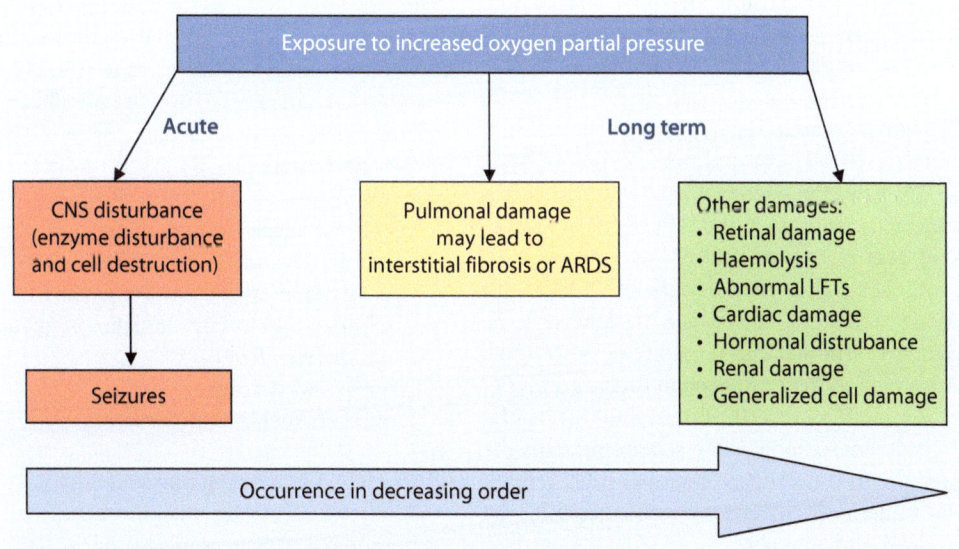

■ **Fig. 26.6**   Propability of symptoms of the oxygen intoxication of the CNS, the lung and other tissues in correlation to exposure time and oxygen partial pressure

oxygen partial pressure is higher. In its extreme form, pulmonary oxygen toxicity can lead to ARDS (adult respiratory distress syndrome). The ARDS is also known as acute lung failure, which well describes the seriousness of this syndrome. In the ARDS the lung function is severely impaired. Chronic changes include lung fibrosis and widespread alveolar damage.

26

■ **Main Symptoms of the Pulmonary Oxygen Intoxication**

‒ Tracheal irritation
‒ Cough
‒ Pleuritic retrosternal pain
‒ Shortness of breath

26.3.3 Treatment

Oxygen poisoning can occur when a critical increase of oxygen partial pressure is exceeded. Scuba diving in extreme deep with normal breathing gas and the use of nitrox contribute to this. Extreme deep diving over 70 m increases the likelihood to suffer an acute reversible oxygen intoxication of the central nervous system. Because the 40-m limit with scuba divers should not be exceeded, this factor doesn't matter to recreational divers. By using nitrox, where the oxygen-nitrogen ratio shifts in favour of oxygen, the calculated depth that is dependent on the nitrox composition shouldn't be exceeded. First and foremost, the oxygen partial pressure must be reduced in individuals with symptoms of oxygen intoxication. This means the diver has to ascend to a lower depth. Convulsive seizures under water bear a risk to suffer a hyperbaric pulmonary barotrauma. In this case, the seizure must be ceased before starting ascending. In the HBOT, the first measurement in case of a convulsive seizure is to avoid the traumas caused by the convulsion and pressure changes. The oxygen mask needs to be removed. The patient shouldn't be restrained. Administration of midazolam (0.15–0.3 mg/kg iv, 0.2 mg/kg at; 5–10 mg intrabuccal) can be considered. As long as the seizure persists, the pressure in the pressure chamber must remain the same, and any pressure changes must be stopped immediately.

26.3.4 Prophylaxis

The best prevention is to avoid critical oxygen partial pressures. For diving with pure oxygen, the Royal Navy and the Royal Australian Navy

■ **Table 26.3** Maximal oxygen time according to the diving depth [32]

Depth		Maximum oxygen time (min)
25 fsw	7 msw	240
30 fsw	9 msw	80
35 fsw	10 msw	25
40 fsw	12 msw	15
50 fsw	15 msw	10

impose a limit of 9 m for dives at rest and 7 m for dives in activity. The US Navy recommends following single-depth oxygen exposure limits (■ Table 26.3).

The critical limit for oxygen toxicity to occur is diving with normal breathing air beyond 70 m. Since the oxygen sensitivity from person to person is different, it could be considered to test oxygen sensitivity for professional divers. In nitrox the maximum O_2 partial pressure is 1.6 bar under normal conditions and 1.4 bar at extreme conditions. However, even in less than 1.4 bar, pO_2 seizures are possible.

It is recommended for divers who use pure oxygen, and someone who works under hyperbaric conditions, to avoid the following:

‒ Increased oxygen exposure during fever
‒ Medications and drugs, which increase the CO_2 of tissue, such as carbonic anhydrase inhibitors, barbiturates, opiates, benzodiazepines and alcohol
‒ Aspirin and steroids
‒ Stimulants such as caffeine or energy drinks

Other factors enhancing oxygen toxicity are:

‒ Medication (insulin, disulfiram, aspirin, paraquat, steroids, amphetamines)
‒ Gases (carbon dioxide, nitrous oxide)
‒ Exercise
‒ Hyperthermia

Protective factors are:

‒ Antioxidants
‒ Chemicals (e.g. coenzyme A)

☐ Table 26.4 OTU scale

Day	1	2	3	4	5	6	7	8	9	10	>11
OTU	850	650	600	520	450	420	400	350	330	320	300

In order to reduce the toxicity of oxygen during the HBOT, 100% oxygen is supplied intermittently. In contrast to short-term administration of 100% normobaric oxygen for an hour, HBOT at 2.5 bar increases the release of free radicals. For HBOT oxygen treatment times, treatment depth and treatment intervals need to be taken into consideration. HBOT with 100% oxygen is usually performed at a maximum pO_2 of 2.8 bar (equivalent to 18 m depth). Duration and frequency of HBOT are also limited to avoid oxygen-related damages. Oxygen can't be given unlimited as it is toxic. Long-term exposure mainly causes pulmonary damages. Safe unlimited pO_2 levels are regarded below 0.5 bar (375 mmHg), which equal approx. 60% normobaric oxygen. Lambertsen developed the oxygen tolerance unit (OTU) to prevent damages by oxygen toxicity [11]:

$$OTU = t \cdot \left(\frac{p_{O_2} - 0.5}{0.5} \right)^{0.83}$$

A similar oxygen toxicity unit, the unit pulmonary toxic dose (UPTD), was also introduced by Lambertsen, which is quite similar:

$$UPTD = t \cdot \left(\frac{0.5}{p_{O_2} - 0.5} \right)^{-\frac{1}{1.2}}$$

The Repex approach (Hamilton, Kenyon and Petersen 1988; Hamilton, Kenyon, Petersen, Butler and Beers 1988) empirically determined the maximal OTU [10]. It sets the tolerable dose with 850 OTU on the first day, reducing it

☐ Table 26.5 Overview of OTUs of common treatment tables

Treatment table	OTU
5	327
9	300
6	634
6a	785
Comex 30	1108
Each extension on 2.8 bar for 20 min	71
Each extension on 1.9 bar for 60 min	141

gradually and levelling out to 300 OTU after 11 days (☐ Table 26.4).

For example, the USN Table 6 has a total OTU of 634. That leaves another 216 OTU for normobaric oxygen treatment on the first 24 h. This could be used for, e.g. 60% normobaric oxygen for 720 min (12 h) (☐ Table 26.5).

There was also a reduction in vital capacity (VC) with increased pO_2 at certain exposure times (t) proposed. The original calculations from Lambertsen were reviewed by Harabin and colleagues at the Navy Medical Research Institute (1987) [10].

■ **Harabin Equation**

$$\%VC\,drop = -0.011 \times (PO_2 - 0.5) \times t$$

The "NOAA oxygen partial pressure and exposure time limits" chart (NOAA Diving Manual 1991) specifies oxygen exposure limits (☐ Table 26.6) [23].

26

■ Table 26.6   NOAA oxygen partial pressure and exposure time limits [23]

pO_2 in bar	Maximum single exposure time in minutes	Daily limit: maximum total duration for any 24-h day in minutes
1.6	45	150
1.5	120	180
1.4	150	180
1.3	180	210
1.2	210	240
1.1	240	270
1	300	300
0.9	360	360
0.8	450	450
0.7	570	570
0.6	720	720

26.4   Carbon Dioxide (CO_2) Intoxication

Carbon dioxide (CO_2) is a normal content of the air we breathe. CO_2 is the main trigger for respiratory drive in a healthy person. It is a gaseous end product of the aerobic cell metabolism. It is transported via the blood to the lungs. There, it passes via diffusion in the alveoli and is exhaled. Its content in the air is only 0.03–0.04% (0.0003–0.0004 bar). In the alveoli the CO_2 content is usually around 40 mmHg (0.053 bar) but can increase briefly during vigorous exercise briefly to approx. 90 mmHg. As the ventilation rate increases during exercises, alveolar CO_2 regresses to normal levels or even below.

Under water we face significant changes in the respiration mainly due to the change in gas density as well as viscosity and its effect on the ventilation of the lungs. Linear with ambient pressure, the density of gases increases. With increasing density, laminar airflow might turn into turbulent flow in the airways. Under physical exertion, lung ventilation has an approxi-

mate efficiency of only 75%. At increased ambient pressure that might be even less. This means that previous optimal flow patterns change to less favourable ones. Depending on the density, residual air is less exchanged and carbon dioxide might accumulate.

26.4.1   Aetiology and Pathogenesis

Carbon dioxide intoxication is described as an increase of carbon dioxide partial pressure (pCO_2) in blood (hypercapnia). There are different reasons for an increase of pCO_2:

- *Air contamination* with CO_2 that might occur during the filling process of scuba tanks.
- *Disturbed ventilation in closed circuit breathing systems*, e.g. helmet diving and HBOT. All these systems require an appropriate elimination of CO_2.
- *Voluntary reduced air consumption* results in an accumulation of CO_2 as its elimination is reduced due to reduced ventilation. However, increased pCO_2 triggers the respiratory reflex, which increases the respiratory rate.
- *Increased resistance in airways or air supply*. The rise of ambient pressure causes increasing density of the breathing gases. The density increases linear to the ambient pressure and varies in different gases or gas mixtures. The airway resistance seems to increase in proportion to the square root of the gas density. This might result in turbulent airflow. This is effective in small and bigger airways. The small diameter of the small airways and the turbulent flow of the bigger airways cause increased resistance. The airflow is predominantly affected during expiration in the bigger airways. In the bigger airways, the laminar flow turns into a turbulent one. This leads to a relative hypoventilation as the alveolar gas exchange is reduced. The maximal expiratory flow in 20 msw is reduced by approx. 1/3 and in 90 msw by approx. 2/3 (Wood and Bryan 1978 [36]). Reduced expiration in return leads to accumulation

of CO_2. This again increases the respiration rate due to central respiratory stimulation. As a result, the increased respiratory rate leads to an increased airflow and deteriorates the already unfavourable turbulent airflow. Exercise in greater depth can therefore increase dramatically the alveolar CO_2 and hence the arterial CO_2, which may lead in its extreme to unconsciousness due to CO_2 intoxication (■ Figs. 26.7 and 26.8).

━ *Faulty CO_2 absorption in rebreather systems.*
━ *Increased activity and metabolism* increases the CO_2 production of the body.

Increase of resistance in the airways with turbulent flow patterns and attempting to save breath arbitrarily are the most common causes of CO_2 build-up in the body of recreational divers. Carbon dioxide in the body is the most powerful respiratory stimulus. However, in extreme levels of 100–200 mmHg (0.13–0.26 bar) and above, it depresses respiration. The carbon dioxide concentration is sensed by central chemoreceptors of the medulla oblongata and is an important factor in the respiratory regulation. In addition to the influence on the regulation of respiration, CO_2 affects the acid-base balance. A pH level of 7.4 is an important prerequisite for a variety of the body's functions. A change in pH causes deterioration in effectiveness of enzymes, disruption of the metabolism, changes in permeability for electrolytes and proteins of cell membranes and disturbance of the electrolyte metabolism.

The maximum voluntary ventilation (MVV) is one way of quantifying the effects of

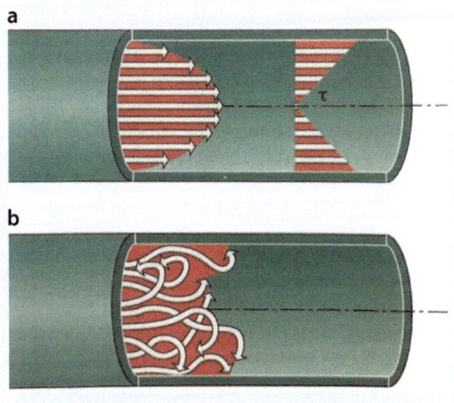

■ **Fig. 26.7** Laminar and turbulent flow patterns. (From Schmidt 2010 [29])

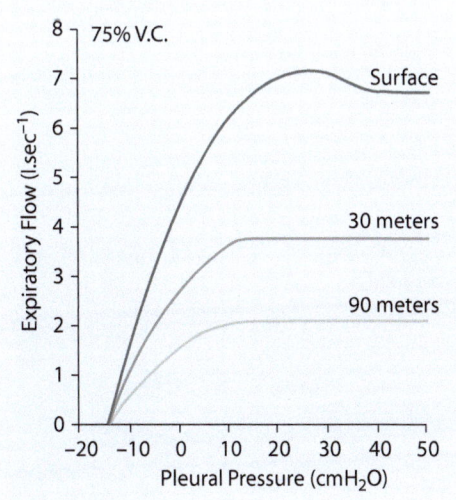

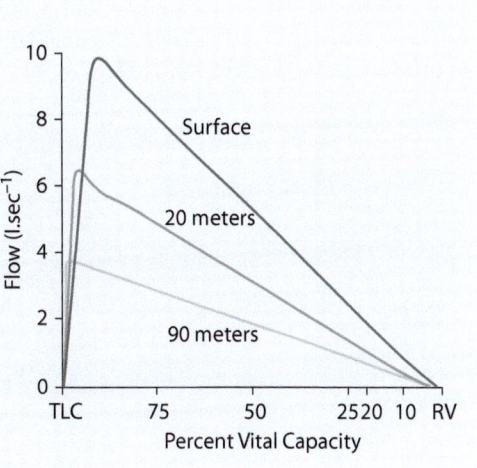

■ **Fig. 26.8** Expiratory flow-volume curves at various depths in a dry chamber breathing air. (SPUMS Journal Volume 27, No. 4, December 1997/Data from Wood and Bryan)

26

increased gas density on the respiration. MVV can be described as [22].

$$MVV_p = MVV_0 \rho^{-k}$$

MVV_p = maximum voluntary ventilation at pressure, MVV_0 = MVV at the surface, ρ = gas density [g/l], k = constant (0.3–0.5)

At approximately 40 m, the MVV is reduced by 50%. At this depth the ventilation required to eliminate metabolically produced CO_2 may exceed the maximum possible ventilation.

The normal arterial carbon dioxide partial pressure ($PaCO_2$) is 35–45 mmHg (0.046–0.06 bar). The venous carbon dioxide partial pressure is approximately 5 mmHg (0.0066 bar) higher. It is partially physically dissolved in the blood and is eliminated via the lungs. It is 25 times more lipid soluble than nitrogen. However, its narcotic effects don't seem to be related to that factor.

26.4.2 **Symptoms**

Symptoms of increased CO_2 levels (hypercapnia) or carbon dioxide intoxication are dependent on the arterial pCO_2. Mild elevation to 70–75 mmHg (0.093–0.099 bar) pCO_2 might cause dizziness. Levels of 100–200 mmHg (0.133–0.26 bar) cause unresponsiveness, and 220–300 mmHg (0.29–0.39 bar) is considered to produce general anaesthesia (◘ Table 26.7).

Symptoms might range from mild respiratory acidosis to severe derailment in the acid-base balance. The initial symptoms are usually very discreet. The first symptoms are increased respiration, drowsiness, restlessness, disorientation, diaphoresis, shortness of breath and flushing. Further symptoms of increased pCO_2 are muscle fasciculation, altered level of consciousness, tremor, seizures and respiratory arrest caused by central nervous system depression. The possibility of CO_2 intoxication increases significantly in depth greater than 40 m with increased exercise and may lead to unconsciousness. Duration and intensity of the exercise are influencing factors in CO_2 production and retention (◘ Fig. 26.9).

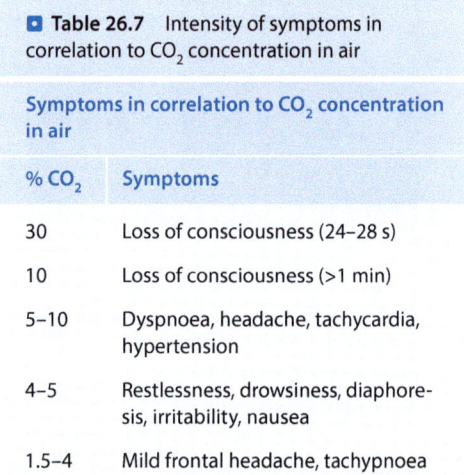

◘ **Table 26.7**   Intensity of symptoms in correlation to CO_2 concentration in air

Symptoms in correlation to CO_2 concentration in air	
% CO_2	**Symptoms**
30	Loss of consciousness (24–28 s)
10	Loss of consciousness (>1 min)
5–10	Dyspnoea, headache, tachycardia, hypertension
4–5	Restlessness, drowsiness, diaphoresis, irritability, nausea
1.5–4	Mild frontal headache, tachypnoea

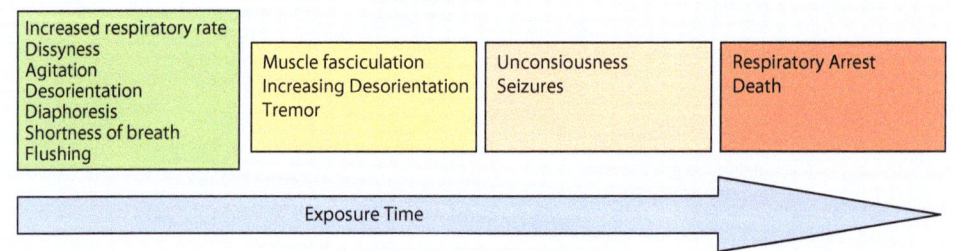

◘ **Fig. 26.9**   Carbon dioxide intoxication in relation to exposure time

However, the most important sign of CO_2 intoxication a diver may experience is shortness of breath!

26.4.3 Treatment and Prophylaxis

In case of carbon dioxide intoxication, the causes for elevated CO_2 should be minimised. The diver should reduce muscular activity to a minimum and breathe at a normal rate but emptying the lungs completely, so that the CO_2 can be exhaled to the maximum extent. In more severe intoxications associated with coma and respiratory failure, vital functions should be stabilised (e.g. resuscitation, maintain respiratory function, etc.). Severe acidosis causes short-term hyperkalaemia due to cellular potassium outflux. Usually it is enough to stabilise the general condition of the patient and restore normocapnia to reduce acidosis. Usually the potassium normalises then without further medical intervention.

The best prophylaxis is to avoid an increase of CO_2. This includes a detailed maintenance of good-quality diving equipment. Long snorkels with small diameters should be avoided, as the functional dead space or the respiratory resistance increases. The snorkel should be about 35 cm long and have a diameter of 1.5–2.5 cm. Recreational diving limits shouldn't exceed 40 m as the maximum voluntary ventilation (MVV) is reduced by 50% and turbulent expiratory airflow leads to a relative hypoventilation due to reduced ventilation with the effect of inadequate elimination of metabolically produced CO_2. Diving deeper than 40 m, in particular during exertion, with normal air poses a risk of reduced CO_2 elimination. Gas mixtures with helium or hydrogen improve the ventilation due to their lower densities. With normoxic gas mixtures with helium or hydrogen, several hundreds of meters can be reached.

26.5 Carbon Monoxide (CO)

The odourless carbon monoxide is an end product from incomplete combustion of carbons, such as fuel engines. Some of the compressors for filling scuba tanks are powered by fuel. By its own exhaust fumes or using contaminated air in garages or near roads for filling, CO may get into scuba tanks. CO is also present in cigarette smoke, especially in smoke from filtered cigarettes. Heavy smokers have haemoglobin loaded with carbon monoxide (HbCO) up to 20% of the total haemoglobin. Carbon monoxide of a single cigarette is present in blood for about 12 h.

26.5.1 Aetiology and Pathogenesis

Carbon monoxide has a 200–300 times higher affinity to haemoglobin in red blood cells compared to oxygen. Usually 1% of haemoglobin is HbCO under normal conditions. Carbon monoxide binds to haemoglobin not only much easier but also stronger compared to oxygen. Carbon monoxide haemoglobin (HbCO) has therefore a longer half-life of about 4–6 h. This means that once absorbed, carbon monoxide stays in the body for a prolonged time. Oxygen is displaced by CO in haemoglobin. As haemoglobin facilitates oxygen transport, this process is interrupted, and the body lacks significantly of oxygen and "suffocates endogenously". Another factor of the toxicity of carbon monoxide is that there is a left shift of the O_2 dissociation curve of oxygen haemoglobin (HbO_2). This increases the oxygen affinity to haemoglobin, resulting in a lower rate of releasing oxygen molecules. Various degrees of oxygen deficiencies may develop, which can also be fatal. CO binds to cytochrome a3 oxidase reversibly. Due to the inactivation of this enzyme oxygen, utilisation of mitochondria is interrupted. This results in more oxygen radical (O_2^-) release.

After Thom (1990), there is an increase of lipid peroxidase in the brain due to free O_2 radicals [30]. This leads to a disruption of the cerebral metabolism and brain tissue and thus to the brain function itself. Carbon monoxide, which may be present at sea level in non-toxic concentrations, may, for example, exceed toxic limits at a depth of 30 m, as the CO concentration is fourfold compared to the surface. Hence, great care needs to be taken when the scuba tanks are filled to avoid air contamination.

26.5.2 **Symptoms**

First symptoms of carbon monoxide poisoning are headache, visual disturbance, drowsiness and a decreased respiratory rate. With increasing concentration, symptoms progress into blurred vison, collapse, loss of consciousness, coma and death (◙ Table 26.8). A pink skin and "bright red" lips of the patient are visible signs aside from signs of suffocation. Developing Parkinsonism may be a late complication after severe carbon monoxide poisoning.

◙ **Table 26.8**   Symptoms of CO intoxication in correlation with % HbCO to total Hb

Content of HbCO in %	Symptoms
5–10	Visual disturbance
10–20	Headache, dizziness (concentration of a normal smoker)
20–30	Intense headache, drowsiness
30–40	Significant visual disturbance, collapse
40–50	Loss of consciousness
50–60	Coma, fatal within 10 min to 1 h
>60	Profound coma, fatal within minutes

26.5.3 **Treatment and Prophylaxis**

To avoid a carbon monoxide contamination in scuba tanks, air used for filling should be clean. The air intake hose of the compressor should be placed at a suitable distance from the compressor's engine. The compressor should not be in the vicinity of any combustion engines, garages or roads. Some compressors have filters to isolate contaminants. But even having them, it is better to avoid any pollutant sources. Also smoking adversely affects divers. Apart from many other adverse health effects, such as irritation of the respiratory tract, arteriosclerosis, coronary vascular diseases and lung cancer, the elevation of HbCO can be detrimental on the diver. The exchange of oxygen with carbon monoxide reduces the ability of blood to carry oxygen. Oxygen deficit of tissue in combination with gas embolisms can be enhanced with carbon monoxide.

Patients require cardiac monitoring as arrhythmias, tachycardia, hypotension and cardiopulmonary arrest might evolve. Pulse oximetry might be misleading as HbCO absorbs light almost identically as oxyhaemoglobin. Venous HbCO is an important measure. Levels of >40% HbCO and above or in combination with neurological or cardiovascular impairment are regarded serious and require HBOT. Levels below might be managed with normobaric 100% oxygen only. However, patients with cardiovascular or respiratory or psychological signs are at higher risk and are recommended to receive HBOT regardless of the carboxyhaemoglobin levels. Pregnant women with symptomatic CO intoxication and/or >20% HbCO are recommended to receive HBOT [2, 12]. Common signs are confusion, coma and cerebral oedema. If there are any neurological signs, fundoscopy and CT or MRI should be performed to investigate for cerebral oedema. Acidosis should not be corrected as it causes a right shift of the oxyhaemoglobin dissociation curve. The acidosis corrects usually itself after treatment. In case of increased cranial pressure head elevation, mannitol and a moderate hyperventilation with PCO_2 of 28–30 mmHg could be considered.

In carbon monoxide poisoning, 100% oxygen is recommended to be given immediately as a first-line treatment. This reduces oxygen deficit and at the same time half-life of HbCO. These effects are reinforced by HBOT. The half-life of HbCO with breathing of 100% oxygen is approximately 30 min, and with HBOT at 2.8 bar absolute pressure only 10–20 min. Recurrent HBOT might be necessary, depending on symptoms or progression.

HBOT treatment for CO intoxications is either TS 300-90 or TS 280-60 (USN-table 6), TS 280-40 (USN-table 5) or TS 240-90 (USN-table 9). The HBOT varies depending of the severity but also is handled differently in different countries. The last resort is a blood transfusion to restore functional haemoglobin.

CO intoxication can have short- and long-term consequences. Late complications are neurological symptoms, like impaired fine motor skills, cortical blindness, psychiatric diseases, pulmonary oedema, myocardial infarction, hepatic lobar necrosis, renal failure, rhabdomyolysis, compartment syndrome and ophthalmological problems like retinal haemorrhage, papilloedema and floaters.

26.6 Air Contamination

Oil may enter the scuba tanks by using old filters, faulty compressors or insufficient draining of the oil condensate mixture. The air tastes rubbery and has an unpleasant smell. Oil particles in the air can cause pneumonia or pneumonitis. Even lower concentrations can trigger an asthma attack. Solid particles can get through defective equipment in the respiratory tract. Oil as well as solid particles can provoke coughing. Such hazards can be avoided by regular inspections and maintenance of the diving equipment.

References

1. Aranake A, Mahour GA, Avidan MS. Minimum alveolar concentration: ongoing relevance and clinical utility. Anaesthesia. 2013;68:512–22.
2. Aubard Y, Magen I. Carbon monoxide poisoning in pregnancy. Bri J Obstet Gynocol. 2000;107:833–8.
3. Bennett P. Inert gas narcosis and HPNS. In: Bove A, editor. Bove and Davis' diving medicine. 4th ed. Philadelphia: WB Saunders; 2004. p. 225–40.
4. Bennett PB, Rostain JC. Inert gas narcosis. In: Brubakk AO, Neuman TS, editors. Bennett and Elliott's physiology and medicine of diving. 5th ed. Toronto: Saunders; 2003. p. 300–22.
5. Bühlmann AA, Voelmm EB, Nussberger P. Tauchmedizin, Barotrauma, Gasembolie, Dekompensation, Dekompensationskrankheit. 5th ed. Berlin: Springer; 2002.
6. De Martino G, Luchetti M, De Rosa RC. Toxic effects of oxygen. In: Michael M, Marroni A, Longoni C, editors. Handbook of hyperbaric medicine. New York: Springer; 1996. p. 59–68.
7. Donald KW. Oxygen poisoning in man. Brit MEC J. 1947;1:667–712. 712–717.
8. Eger EI 2nd, Ionesco P, Laster MJ, et al. Minimum alveolar anaesthetic concentration of fluoridated alkanols in rats: relevance to theories of narcosis. Anaesth Analg. 1999;88:867–76.
9. Hamilton K, Laliberte MF, Heslegrave R, Khan S. Visual/vestibular effects of inert gas narcosis. Ergonomics. 1993;36:891–8. https://doi.org/10.1080/00140139308967954.
10. Hamilton RW. Tolerating exposure to high oxygen levels: Repex and other methods. MTS J. 1989;23(4):19–25.
11. Hamilton RW. Tolerating oxygen exposure. SPUMS J. 1997;27(1):43–7.
12. Hampson NB, Dunford RG, Kramer CC, Norkool DM. Selection criteria utilized for hyperbaric oxygen treatment of carbon monoxide poisoning. J Emerg Med. 1995;13(2):227–31.
13. Jain KK. Chapter 6 Oxygen toxicity. In: Textbook of hyperbaric medicine. 5th ed: Springer; 2017. p. 49–60.
14. Jain KK. High-pressure neurological syndrome (HPNS). Acta Neurol Scand. 1994;90:45–50.
15. Karsowski MD, Harrison NL. General anaesthetic actions on ligand-gated ion channels. Cell Mol Life Sci. 1999;55(10):1278–303.
16. Kneller W, Hobbs M. Inert gas narcosis and the encoding and retrieval of long-term memory. Aviat Space Environ Med. 2013;84:1235–9.
17. Kneller W, Hobbs M. The levels of processing effect under nitrogen narcosis. Undersea Hyperb Med. 2013;40:239–45.

26

18. Koblin DD. Inhaled anesthetics: mechanisms of action. In: Miller R, editor. Anesthesia. 4th ed. New York: Churchill-Livingstone; 1994. p. 67–99.

19. Koblin DD, Fang Z, Eger E, Laster MJ, Gong D, Ionescu P, Halsey MJD, Trudell JR. Minimum alveolar concentrations of noble gases, nitrogen, and sulfur hexafluoride in rats: helium and neon as nonimmobilizers (nonanesthetics). Anesth Analg. August;87(2):419–24.

20. Lavoute C, Weiss M, Rostain JC. Alterations in nigral NMDA and GABAA receptor control of the striatal dopamine level after repetitive exposures to nitrogen narcosis. Exp Neurol. 2008;212:63–70. https://doi.org/10.1016/j.expneurol.2008.03.001.

21. Lavoute C, Weiss M, Sainty JM, Risso JJ, Rostain JC. Post effect of repetitive exposures to pressure nitrogen-induced narcosis on the dopaminergic activity at atmospheric pressure. Undersea Hyperb Med. 2008;35:21–5.

22. Moon R, Bryant S. Diving and the lung. SPUMS J. 1997;27(4):218–27.

23. National Oceanic and Atmospheric Administration. Diving for science and technology. In: NOAA diving manual. Washington, DC; 1990.

24. Overton CE. Studien über die Narkose zugleich ein Beitrag zur allgemeinen Pharmakologie. Jena: Gustav Fischer; 1901.

25. Rostain JC, Balon N. Recent neurochemical basis of inert gas narcosis and pressure effects. UHM 2006;33, No. 3-Neurochemical bases of narcosis and HPNS.

26. Rostain JC, Gardette-Chauffour MC, Naquet R. EEG and sleep disturbances during dives at 450 msw in helium-nitrogen-oxygen mixture. J Appl Physiol. 1997;83:575–82.

27. Rostain JC, Lavoute C, Risso JJ, Vallee N, Weiss M. A review of recent neurochemical data on inert gas narcosis. Undersea Hyperb Med. 2011;38:49–59.

28. Sanders RD, Franks NP, Maze M. Xenon: no stranger to anaesthesia. BJA: Br J Anaesth. 2003;91(5):709–17. https://doi.org/10.1093/bja/aeg232

29. Schmidt RF, Lang F, Heckmann M, Physiologie des Menschens, 31. Auflage, Springer; 2010

30. Thom SR, Elbuken ME. Oxygen-dependent antagonism of lipid peroxidation. Free Radic Biol Med. 1991;10:413–26.

31. Tonner PH, Lutz H. Pharmakotherapie in der Anaesthesie und Intensivmedizin. Berlin: Springer; 2011.

32. US Navy Diving Manual. www.uhms/images/DCS-and-AGE-Journal-Watch/recompression_therapy_usn_di.pdf. Accessed 04.10.2015.

33. Vaernes R, Bennett PB, Hammerborg D, Ellertsen B, Peterson RE, Toonjum S. Central nervous system reactions during heliox and trimix dives to 31 ATA. Undersea Biomed Res. 1982;9:1–14.

34. Wada S, Yokota A, Matsuoka S, Kadoya C, Mohri M. Effects of hyperbaric environment on human auditory middle latency response (MLR) and short latency somatosensory evoked potential (SSEP). J UOEH. 1989;11:441–7.

35. Weir JC. The molecular mechanisms of general anaesthesia: dissecting the GABAA receptor. Contin Educ Anaesth Crit Care Pain. 2006;6(2):49–53.

36. Wood LD, Bryant AC. Exercise ventilators mechanics at increased ambient pressure. J Appl Physiol. 1978;44:231–7.

37. Zhang M, Gao Y, Fang H. A new understanding of inert gas narcosis. Chin Phys B. 2016;25(1):013602.

38. Zhou C, Liu J, Chen XD. General anaesthesia mediated by effects on ion channels. World J Crit Care Med. 2012;1(3):80–93.

Suggested Reading

Behnke AR, Thompson RM, Motley EP. The psychologic effects from breathing air at 4 atmospheres pressure. Am J Physiol. 1935;112:554–8.

Canlas CG, Cui T, Li L, Xu Y, Tang P. Anesthetic modulation of protein dynamics: insights from a NMR study. J Phys Chem B. 2008;112(45):14312–8.

Cantor RS. The lateral pressure profile in membranes: a physical mechanism of general anesthesia. Biochemistry. 1997;36(9):2339–44.

Cantor RS. Breaking the Meyer-Overton rule: predicted effects of varying stiffness and interfacial activity on the intrinsic potency of anesthetics. Biophys J. 2001;80(5):2284–97.

Elayan IM, Axley MJ, Prasad PV, Ahlers ST, Auker CR. Effect of hyperbaric oxygen treatment on nitric oxide and oxygen free radicals in rat brain. J Neurophysiol. 2000;83(4):2022–9.

Fang XL, Mai J, Choi ET, Wang H, Yang X. Targeting mitochondrial reactive oxygen species as novel therapy for inflammatory disease and cancers. J Hematol Oncol. 2013;6:19.

Farmery S, Sykes O. Neurological oxygen toxicity. Emerg Med J. 2012;29:851–2. https://doi.org/10.1136/emermed-2011-200538.

Fothergill DM, Hedges D, Morrison JB. Effects of CO2 and N2 partial pressures on cognitive and psychomotor performance. Undersea Biomed Res. 1991;18:1–19.

Fowler B, Ackles KN, Porlier G. Effects of inert gas narcosis on behavior—a critical review. Undersea Biomed Res. 1985;12:369–402.

Franks NP, Lieb WR. Do general anaesthetics act by competitive binding to specific receptors? Nature. 1984;310(16):599–601.

Franks NP, Lieb WR. Molecular and cellular mechanisms of general anesthesia. Nature. 1994;367(17):607–14. Franks NP, Lieb WR .Where do general anaesthetics act? Nature. 1978;274(5669):339–42.

Franks NP, Lieb WR. Mapping of general anesthetic target sites provides a molecular basis for cutoff effects. Nature. 1985;316(6026):349–51.

Franks NP, Lieb WR. Molecular and cellular mechanisms of general anesthesia. Nature. 1994;367(17):607–14.

Franks NP, Lieb WR. Stereospecific effects of inhalational general anesthetic optical isomers on nerve ion channels. Science. 1991;254(5030):427–30.

Geers C, Gros G. Carbon dioxide transport and carbonic anhydrases in blood and muscle. Physiol Rev. 2000;80(2):681–715.

Gelfand R, Lambertsen CJ, Peterson RE. Human respiratory control at high ambient pressures and inspired gas densities. J Appl Physiol. 1980;48:528–39.

Grover CA, Grover DH. Albert Behnke: nitrogen narcosis. J Emerg Med. 2014;46:225–7.

Hamilton K, Laliberte MF, Fowler B. Dissociation of the behavioral and subjective components of nitrogen narcosis and diver adaptation. Undersea Hyperb Med. 1995;22:41–9.

Harless E, von Bibra E. Die Ergebnisse der Versuche über die Wirkung des Schwefeläthers. Erlangen: Verlag von Carl Heyder; 1847.

Hobbs M, Higham PA, Kneller W. Memory and metacognition in dangerous situations: investigating cognitive impairment from gas narcosis in undersea divers. Hum Factors. 2014;56:696–709.

Hobbs M, Kneller W. Effect of nitrogen narcosis on free recall and recognition memory in open water. Undersea Hyperb Med. 2009;36:73–81.

Hobbs M. Subjective and behavioural responses to nitrogen narcosis and alcohol. Undersea Hyperb Med. 2008;35:175–84.

Hugh C, Jr H. Molecular targets of general anaesthetics in the nervous system, Chapter 2. In: Supressing the mind, contemporary clinical neuroscience: Humana Press; 2010.

Janoff AS, Miller KW. A critical assessment of the lipid theories of general anaesthetic action. Biol Membr. 1982;4(1):417–76.

Janoff AS, Pringle MJ, Miller KW. Correlation of general anesthetic potency with solubility in membranes. Biochim Biophys Acta. 1981;649(1):125–8.

Kandel L, Chortkoff BS, Sonner J, Laster MJ, Eger EI. Nonanesthetics can suppress learning. Anesth Analg. 1996;82(2):321–6.

Kiessling RJ, Maag CH. Performance impairment as a function of nitrogen narcosis. Rep US Navy Exp Diving Unit. 1960:1–19.

Koblin DD, Chortkoff BS, Laster MJ, Eger EI II, Halsey MJ, Ionescu P. Polyhalogenated and perfluorinated compounds that disobey the Meyer-Overton hypothesis. Anesth Analg. 1994;79(6):1043–8.

LaBella FS, Stein D, Queen G. Occupation of the cytochrome P450 substrate pocket by diverse compounds at general anesthesia concentrations. Eur J Pharmacol. 1998;358(2):177–85.

Lawrence JH, Loomis WF, Tobias CA, Turpin FH. Preliminary observation on the narcotic effect of xenon with a review of values for solubilities of gases in water and oils. J Physiol. 1945;105:197–204.

Lerner RA. A hypothesis about the endogenous analogue of general anesthesia. Proc Natl Acad Sci U S A. 1997;94(25):13375–7.

Liu J, Laster MJ, Taheri S, Eger EI, Koblin DD, Halsey MJ. Is there a cutoff in anesthetic potency for the normal alkanes? Anesth Analg. 1993;77(1):12–8.

Liu R, Loll PJ, Eckenhoff RG. Structural basis for high-affinity volatile anesthetic binding in a natural 4-helix bundle protein. FASEB J. 2005;19(6):567–76.

Lofdahl P, Andersson D, Bennett M. Nitrogen narcosis and emotional processing during compressed air breathing. Aviat Space Environ Med. 2013;84:17–21.

Lugli AK, Yost CS, Kindler CH. Anaesthetic mechanisms: update on the challenge of unravelling the mystery of anaesthesia. https://www.ncbi.nlm.nih.gov/pmc/articles/PMC2778226/#!po=43.7500. Accessed 23.7.2017.

Lüllmann H, Mohr K, Ziegler A. Taschenatlas der Pharmakologie, 6. Auflage, Thieme Stuttgart; 2008.

Ma D, Brandon NR, Cui T, Bondarenko V, Canlas C, Johansson JS, Tang P, Xu Y. Four-α-helix bundle with designed anesthetic binding pockets. Part I: structural and dynamical analyses. Biophys J. 2008;94(11):4454–63.

Mathieu D, Nolf M, Durocher A, et al. Acute carbon monoxide poisoning. Risk of late sequelae and treatment by hyperbaric oxygen. J Toxicol Clin Toxicol. 1985.

Mekjavic IB, Savic SA, Eiken O. Nitrogen narcosis attenuates shivering thermogenesis. J Appl Physiol. 1995;78:2241–4.

Meyer HH. Welche eigenschaft der anasthetica bedingt ihre narkotische Wirkung? Arch Exp Pathol Pharmakol. 1899;42(2–4):109–18.

Meyer HH. Zur Theorie der Alkoholnarkose. Arch Exp Pathol Pharmacol. 1899;42(2–4):109 18.

Meyer KH. Contributions to the theory of narcosis. Trans Faraday Soc. 1937;33:1062–8.

Mihic SJ, Ye Q, Wick MJ, Koltchine VV, Krasowski MD, Finn SE, Mascia MP, Valenzuela CF, Hanson KK, Greenblatt EP, Harris RA, Harrison NL. Sites of alcohol and volatile anaesthetic action on GABA(A) and glycine receptors. Nature. 1997;389(6649):385–9.

Miller JW, Bachrach AJ, Walsh JM. Assessment of vertical excursions and open-sea psychological performance at depths to 250 fsw. Undersea Biomed Res. 1976;3(4):339–49.

Miller KW. The nature of the site of general anesthesia. Int Rev Neurobiol. 1985;27(1):1–61.

Miller KW, Paton WD, Smith RA, Smith EB. The pressure reversal of general anesthesia and the critical volume hypothesis. Mol Pharmacol. 1973;9(2):131–43.

Mitchell SJ, Cronjé FJ, Meintjes WA, Britz HC. Fatal respiratory failure during a "technical" rebreather dive at extreme pressure. Aviat Space Environ Med. 2007;78(2):81–6.

26

Mohr JT, Gribble GW, Lin SS, Eckenhoff RG, Cantor RS. Anesthetic potency of two novel synthetic polyhydric alkanols longer than the n-alkanol cutoff: evidence for a bilayer-mediated mechanism of anesthesia? J Med Chem. 2005;48(12):4172–6.

Morrison JB, Florio JT, Butt WS. Effects of CO_2 insensitivity and respiratory pattern on respiration in divers. Undersea Biomed Res. 1981;8:209–17.

Mullins LI. Some physical mechanisms in narcosis. Chem Rev. 1954;54(2):289–323.

Pringle MJ, Brown KB, Miller KW. Can the lipid theories of anesthesia account for the cutoff in anesthetic potency in homologous series of alcohols? Mol Pharmacol. 1981;19(1):49–55.

Raub JA, Benignus VA. Carbon monoxide and the nervous system. Neurosci Biobehav Rev. 2002;26(8):925–40.

Rogers WH, Moeller G. Effect of brief, repeated hyperbaric exposures on susceptibility to nitrogen narcosis. Undersea Biomed Res. 1989;16:227–32.

Slater SJ, Cox KJ, Lombardi JV, Ho C, Kelly MB, Rubin E, Stubbs CD. Inhibition of protein kinase C by alcohols and anaesthetics. Nature. 1993;364(6432):82–4.

Taheri S, Laster MJ, Liu J, Eger EI II, Halsey MJ, Koblin DD. Anesthesia by n-alkanes not consistent with the Meyer-Overton hypothesis: Determinations of solubilities of alkanes in saline and various lipids. Anesth Analg. 1993;77(1):7–11. Tang P, Xu Y. Large-scale molecular dynamics simulations of general anesthetic effects on the ion channel in the fully hydrated membrane: the implication of molecular mechanisms of general anesthesia. Proc. Natl. Acad. Sci. U.S.A. 2002;99(25):16035–40.

Talpalar AE. High pressure neurological syndrome. Rev Neurol. 2007;45(10):631–6.

Trudell JR. A unitary theory of anesthesia based on lateral phase separations in nerve membranes. Anesthesiology. 1977;46(1):5–10.

Trudell JR, Koblin DD, Eger EI 2nd. A molecular description of how noble gases and nitrogen bind to a model site of anesthetic action. Anesth Analg. 1998;87:411–8.

Unsworth IP. Inert gas narcosis—an introduction. Postgrad Med J. 1966;42:378–85.

Vaes WHJ, Ramos EU, Hamwijk C, van Holsteijn I, Blaauboer BJ, Seinen W, Verhaar HJM, Hermens JLM. Solid phase microextraction as a tool to determine membrane/water partition coefficients and bioavailable concentrations in in vitro systems. Chem Res Toxicol. 1997;10(10):1067–72.

van Wijk CH, Meintjes WA. Complex tactile performance in low visibility: the effect of nitrogen narcosis. Diving Hyperb Med. 2014;44:65–9.

Varene P, Vieillefond H, Lemaire C, Saumon G. Expiratory flow volume curves and ventilation limitation of muscular exercise at depth. Aerosp Med. 1974;45:161–6.

Waters RM. Toxic effects of carbon dioxide. New Orleans Med Surg J. 1937;90:219–24.

Yogev D, Mekjavi IB. Behavioral temperature regulation in humans during mild narcosis induced by inhalation of 30% nitrous oxide. Undersea Hyperb Med. 2009;36:361–73.

Apnoea Diving

© Springer International Publishing AG, part of Springer Nature 2018
O. Rusoke-Dierich, *Diving Medicine*, https://doi.org/10.1007/978-3-319-73836-9_27

27

Apnoea diving or freediving is diving with no air supply. It requires only basic equipment like mask, fins and snorkel. Freediving equipment is specifically designed to assist in apnoea diving. The lips of freediving masks usually have a single instead of a double sealing lip and a smaller air volume. This reduces the additional functional dead space caused by the mask. The fins have larger blades and made out of carbon. With long unbroken stokes and good efficiency due to the shape of the fins, energy consumption is reduced. Also, monofins are commonly used for freediving. With them divers have different movements compared to conventional fins and hence exert different muscles. In general, both fin types are equally suitable for freediving. The choice is more or less a personal preference. Snorkels should have a sufficient diameter (1.5–2.5 cm) and should not be too long (35 cm). With regular snorkels alone, normal respiration approximately is reduced by 70%. Therefore, snorkels are not used in freediving competitions. If the diameter is too small, CO_2 elimination may be decreased as airflow resistance might be increased. This results in poor ventilation. In contrast, a too wide and long snorkel increases functional dead space and leads to CO_2 retention. Diving with snorkels of 1 m or longer causes an increased pulmonary negative pressure in immersed divers. This can result in inability of respiratory muscles to expand the lungs against the ambient pressure. This might result in increased respiratory rate, as breathing reflexes are reinforced by chest compressions. Additionally, inhalation is significantly reduced by the increased ambient pressure. Moreover, on exhalation, the lower limit of the residual volume is exceeded. Hence, pulmonary hypobaric barotrauma may develop. The maximum length of the snorkel should not exceed 50 cm (■ Fig. 27.1).

Freediving is limited by duration and diving depth. With a bit of practice, 1–2 min in breath-holding can be easily achieved. At rest, of course, less oxygen is needed. Due to the fact that the body consumes less oxygen on slow movements, slow movements are recom-

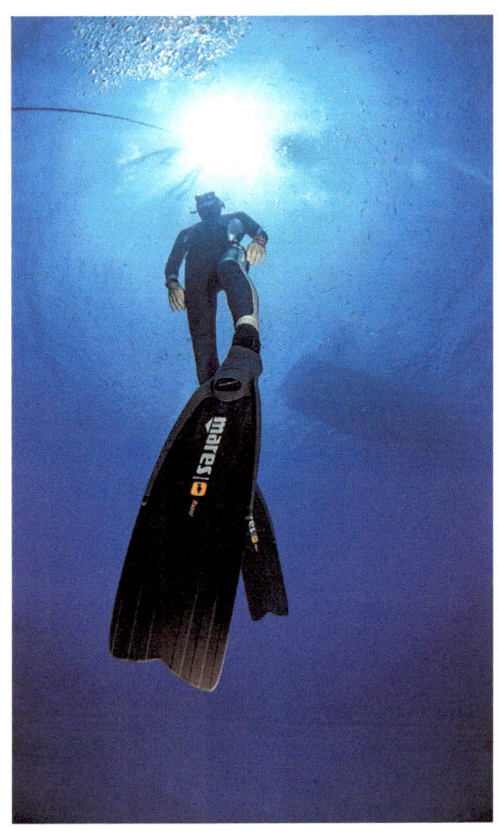

■ **Fig. 27.1**   Apnoea diver. (Mares)

mended during freediving, as they are more energy efficient than fast ones. Thus, breath-holding time can be extended. The diving depth is usually limited by the capacity of the lung to reduce their volume. Compression of the chest wall due to negative pressure in the lungs triggers an inspirational reflex, which is stimulated by activation of inspirational neurons. This trigger is caused by narrowing of rib spacing and curvature of the diaphragm.

27.1 Unconsciousness Underwater

Any condition with ceased psychological functions but obtained somatic functions is specified as unconsciousness. Unconsciousness underwater is quite dangerous, because of the risk of drowning. Unconsciousness in freediving is mainly caused by arterial cerebral oxygen deficit. The threshold before losing consciousness is usually a cerebral arterial pO_2 of approximately 33 mbar (25 mmHg) [4]. Oxygen deficiency is often a result of false estimation of the diver's capability of holding breath. As hyperventilation before diving reduces the carbon dioxide content in blood (hypocapnia), the central respiratory trigger may come too late and critical hypoxia may develop before reaching the surface. Other factors for unconsciousness during freediving are hypobaric pulmonary barotrauma, DCS, congestive heart failure, arrhythmia and congenital and acquired vascular changes that reduce blood flow to the brain, redistribution of blood volume during diving (e.g. orthostasis, Valsalva manoeuvre), hypothermia and trauma or injury caused by marine creatures.

■ **Causes for Unconsciousness During Freediving**
 – Oxygen deficit (hypoxia)
 – Hyperventilation
 – Hypothermia
 – Valsalva manoeuvre
 – Hypobaric pulmonary barotrauma
 – Heart failure
 – Arrhythmia
 – Congenital or acquired vascular disease
 – DCS
 – Orthostatis
 – Trauma or injury cause by marine creatures

After scuba diving, freediving should be avoided for at least 2–6 h. After each dive, gas bubbles are present in blood and tissue. Keeping in mind, that repetitive freediving to only 10 meters by itself causes dissolved and undissolved nitrogen to increase. DCI has been even observed on pearl divers just with freediving ("Taravana"). At the usually relatively fast ascent during freediving, gas bubbles increase in size. At repeated descending and ascending, the body may be unable to outgas completely and gas bubbles accumu-

late. Hence, freediving should be done before scuba diving and not after.

Hyperventilation is particularly dangerous in freediving. It increases oxygen uptake only a little as the blood has already oxygen saturation of approx. 97–98%. This is the main mechanism of oxygen transport in blood. One Hb molecule can carry up to four oxygen molecules. With hyperventilation, only a small increase of alveolar and arterial pO_2 is achieved. It increases O_2 only by 25% to approx. 130 mmHg but reduces CO_2 by 50% to 20 mmHg. Both alveolar and dissolved arterial pO_2 prolong only to a certain degree an oxygen supply. The main supply of O_2 during diving is the lung itself, as it acts as storage for O_2. In the alveoli, usually the pO_2 is 101 mmHg, which gradually diffuses during breath-holding and can last for approx. 1–2 min at rest till the venous pO_2 equals the alveolar pO_2. In the alveoli the pO_2 is usually 101 mmHg. During breath-holding, oxygen gradually diffuses into the blood. At rets, it can take up to approx. 1–2 min till the venous pO_2 equals the alveolar pO_2. End-tidal alveolar pO_2 levels in competitive divers are approx. 27 mmHg [5]. Hyperventilation favours mainly CO_2 elimination. The result is hypocapnia. This can be in freediving quite dangerous. Low CO_2 can also occur with normal oxygen level. During freediving, oxygen levels decrease due to apnoea. CO_2 represents the most important central respiratory trigger. Hyperventilation reduces CO_2 levels and delays the sensation of running out of breath (◻ Table 27.1). The signal to return to the surface may be perceived too late. Oxygen deficiency is additionally reinforced by oxygen partial pressure changes. During descend alveolar and arterial pO_2 relatively increases. Due to the continuous oxygen consumption and additional reduction of ambient pressure during ascending, alveolar and arterial pO_2 have a steeper than expected decline. The usual oxygen consumption continues and partial pressures are decreasing with changing ambient pressure. That means oxygen suddenly is missing in the blood and loss of consciousness due to hypoxia may develop. As

External factors	Breath-holding time in seconds
Moderate exertion, normal breathing air	30
At rest, 3 min hyperventilation, normal breathing air	Up to 120
At rest, 100% O_2 for 5 min, normal breathing	Up to 180
At rest, 100% O_2 for 6 min, normal breathing	Up to 330
At rest, 100% O_2 for 10 min, hyperventilation	Up to 700
At rest, 100% for 7 min, hyperventilation with normal breathing air and some deep breath 100% O_2	1205 (unofficial record)

Table 27.1 Correlation between breath-holding time and external factors (Mithoefer 1964) [7]

pressure differences increase exponentially towards the surface, the last meters below the surface are the most critical zone for unconsciousness to occur (sallow water blackout). Divers should not hyperventilate or perform rapid movements to avoid hypoxia (■ Fig. 27.2).

As we know, patients suffering from chronic obstructive airway disease can adapt to higher carbon dioxide levels. CO_2 tolerance can increase from normal levels of 0.03% by 10–100-fold to 0.5–4%. This might explain why in frequent freediving the respiratory response is impaired. CO_2 tolerance is associated with a reduced stress response and a reduced adrenergic response. This evolves within the first 24 h with increased respiratory volume and decreased respiratory rate. It is also associated with an increase in serum calcium levels and other electrolytes. Initially, H^+ − ions and bicarbonate ions are rising and chloride ions are decreasing. These changes are reversing again over time. In the first 3–5 days of building up CO_2 tolerance, a mild compensated

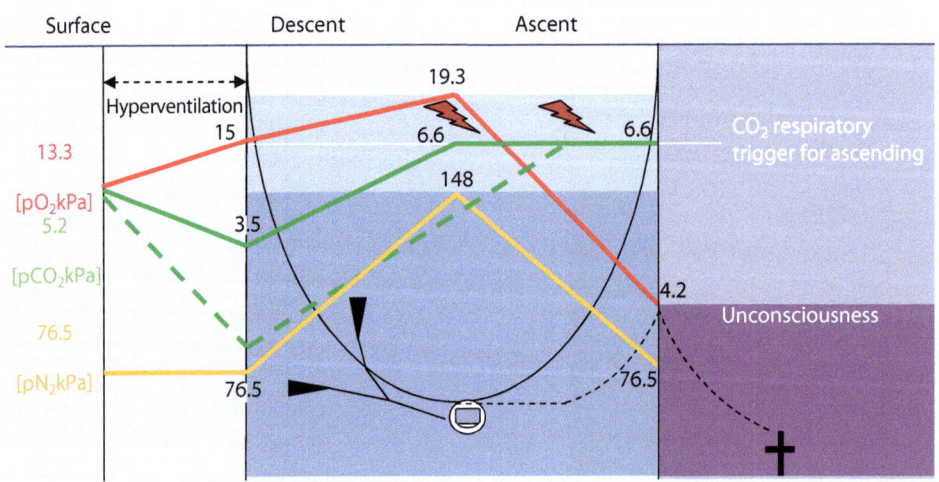

Fig. 27.2 Partial pressure of the breathing gases during freediving at 10 meters depth; pO_2, red; pCO_2, green; pN_2, orange; diving profile, black; with hyperventilation (pCO_2 and diving profile), dashed; without hyperventilation, solid line [9]

acidosis can be expected. After 5 months of freediving break, the CO_2 tolerance is expected to be completely lost again. With frequent freediving, lower levels of hypoxia are tolerated (normal blackout level of cerebral arterial pO_2 = 0.042 bar = 4.2 kPa = 31 mmHg) as well.

The duration of apnoea increases with physical training and diving technique. Muscle activity becomes more efficient with training. Oxygen demand of the body reduces. The result of physical training is an increase of the total lung capacity, a decrease in residual volume (→ increased vital capacity). Increased oxygen supply via respiration and lower oxygen demand due to increased muscle efficiency are beneficial in freediving. Additionally, the tolerance to pCO_2 increases with increasing pO_2.

In certain circumstances, divers can experience loss of consciousness due to cardiovascular dysregulation. Valsalva manoeuvres or strenuous activities such as heavy lifting with breath-holding can temporarily increase the intrathoracic pressure. This leads to reduction of the venous blood flow to the heart, caused by obstruction of pulmonary vessels resulting in a temporary drop in blood pressure. If the blood pressure isn't compensated, cerebral blood flow may be reduced and lead to unconsciousness. Normally, after normal thoracic pressure is restored, a short-term blood pressure increase is followed before normalizing again. Reduced perfusion may be enhanced by immersion-induced bradycardia causing a decreased cardiac output (approximately 12% less cardiac output) during freediving. Bradycardia is a result of parasympathetic activation (vagal stimulation) cold stimulus, centralization and redistribution of blood volume. Centralization and redistribution of blood volume (→ relative hypervolaemia) are caused by the shift of the peripheral blood volume into the pulmonary vessels. Because lower levels of oxygen cause vasodilatation of peripheral vessels, decreasing pO_2 during apnoea diving

causes increasingly a blood shift from central to peripheral. During ascending, pO_2 decreases rapidly. This may result in a further temporary drop in blood pressure with increased cardiac output. Hypotension together with hypoxia could be a cause to lose consciousness during fast ascents.

❯ Therefore, always plan a steady ascend!

Furthermore, reversible ECG changes, such as various forms of arrhythmias, P-wave changes, bundle branch blocks and ventricular ectopics might occur during freediving. These changes normalise spontaneously after diving.

The physical response of the body in water is called *immersion*. The classic diving reflex (*submersion*) as seen in sea mammals is to a small proportion still rudimentary present in humans. Body reactions of submersion are triggered directly through contact with water or by pressure changes.

- Immersion
  - Vasoconstriction of peripheral vessels
  - Elimination of hydrostatic forces
  - Hydrostatic pressure on peripheral vessels
  - Blood shift into pulmonary vessels
  - Cold stimulus

❯ Centralisation and relative increase of the blood volume

❯ Bradycardia (may be as little as only 8–10 beats per minute!)

- Submersion
  - Decrease of the heart rate
  - Peripheral vasoconstriction
  - Centralization
  - Reduction of cardiac output
  - Decrease of in body core temperature
  - Switching from aerobic to anaerobic metabolism

Another phenomenon is the *immersion pulmonary oedema (IPO)*, which can affect swimmers, snorklers and divers the same way. IPO affects everyone, but it depends on immersion time [7], external factors and intra-individual disposition. IPO occurs shortly after the start of a dive, and divers develop symptoms like shortness of breath and dizziness up to more pronounced symptoms associated with productive pink, frothy cough. It is often perceived by the diver of having faulty equipment. Initially, it was believed to be related to cold-water immersion only and centralisation of the blood. However, it also occurs in warm water immersion. The mechanism is not completely understood, but it seems that a combination of several factors leads to it. During water immersion, orthostatic forces are drastically reduced, and it comes to a redistribution of the blood. The approximately 500–800 mL blood from the legs are added to the central blood volume and reduce the lung volume. Additionally, exercise increases cardiac output and blood flow. Even cold-water stimulus is not the main facture, but it may contribute to the blood pooling. The pulmonary vascular system functions as a blood reservoir and can accommodate the "extra" blood. It increases the pulmonary capillary pressure with unchanged vascular protein content and leads to transudation of fluid from the alveolar capillaries into the extravascular lung tissue and alveoli. People with high left ventricular filling pressures, e.g. with hypertension, heart diseases or excessive pre-hydration, are at greater risk. Exertion increases the filling pressure even more. Diving equipment (SCUBA and snorkel) may contribute to the IPO. In particular upright position, where the pressure at mouth level is lower than the pressure at lung level, produces an increased negative pressure in the lungs, which promotes IPO.

27.2 Freediving Limits

There are currently two organisations that regulate the freediving disciplines: *AIDA International* (International Association for development of apnoea) and *CMAS* (World Underwater Federation).

There are different disciplines [1–3]:

- **Deep dive**
  - Constant weight apnoea (CWT): descending and ascending with the same weight with fins (world record, ♀101 m, ♂128 m); AIDA
  - Constant weight apnoea without fins (CNF): descending and ascending with the same weight, no fins (world record, ♀71 m, ♂101 m); AIDA
  - Free immersion apnoea: descending and ascending with the same weight using a vertical guide robe (world record, ♀91 m, ♂121 m); AIDA
  - Variable weight (VWT): descending with weighted sled, independent ascent (world record, ♀130 m, ♂146 m); AIDA
  - No-limits apnoea (NLT): descending with weighted sled; diving using a balloon for the ascent (world record, ♀214 m, ♂160 m); AIDA

- **The jump blue**
  - Also called "the cube", descending in a cubic form of 15 x 15 meters to a depth of 10 meters and swimming as far as possible along this cube (world record, ♀201 m; ♂190 m); CMAS

- **Pool discipline**
  - Static apnoea (STA): breath-holding underwater (world record, ♀11 min 54 s; ♂9 min, 02 s); AIDA
  - Dynamic apnoea with fins (DYN): distance diving underwater with fins (world record, ♀237 m; ♂281 m); AIDA and CMAS
  - Dynamic apnoea without fins (DNF): distance diving underwater without fins (world record, ♀182 m; ♂226 m); AIDA (◘ Fig. 27.3)

In the past, physicians tried to determine a theoretical depth limit for freediving. However, it was quite difficult to determine this. In 1960,

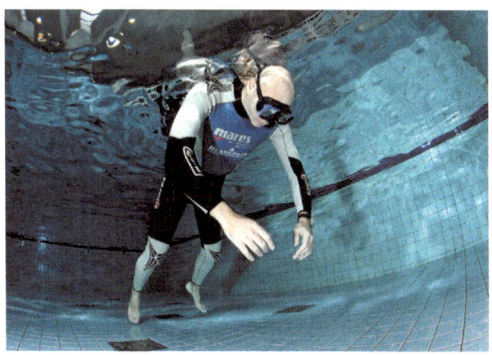

Fig. 27.3 Static apnoea. (Mares)

the 29-year-old Enzo Majorca exceeded the former deep diving limit of 50 meters. Jacques Mayol an him persued one record after another. In 1981, the then 54-year-old Jacques Mayol reached 101 meters, in 1983 105 meters, exceeding the magical 100-meter mark. In 1996, Francesco Ferrera Rodriguez ("Pipin") reached 130 meters. Herbert Nitsch reached 214 meters (no-limits apnoea) in 2007. His later attempt to reach 253 m in 2012 ended in a severe DCI. Tanya Streeter currently holds the record among women with 160 meters (no-limits apnoea).

A simplified theoretical depth limit in freediving depends on the residual volume and is about 30 meters. This value results from the volume reduction of the total lung capacity. An average total lung capacity of 6 litres with negligible functional dead space shrinks at diving to 30 meters depth (without a mask) by 3/4 of the initial volume to 1.5 litres. This corresponds approximately to the residual volume. It was suspected that if the pulmonary air volume is less than the residual volume, pulmonary hypobaric barotrauma develops. Wearing a mask increases the functional dead space. To replace the mask volume, the diver must fill that space with the pulmonary air volume, to prevent hypobaric barotrauma in the mask area. The loss of this air volume further reduces diving time and depth.

The formula for the theoretical depth limit in freediving in correlation to the lung capacity with residual volume as a limit is

$$V_n = \left(TLC - FDS\right)\frac{1\,bar}{n \bullet bar_{abs}}$$

TLC = total lung capacity; FDS = functional death space; V_n = lung volume in correlation of the ambient pressure; bar_{abs} = absolute pressure; 1 bar = surface pressure

This formula however wasn't supported in praxis, as freediving records exceeded that limit. With training diving depth can be increased. With gradual adaption to increasing depth, elasticity of the diaphragm increases. Additionally, the filling capacity of the lung vessels increases. Thus, the pulmonary airspace is reduced by tissue expansion, and blood volume shifts into the pulmonary vessels (up to approx. 700 ml). Hence, the total lung capacity and residual volume are reduced. The vacuum can partly be compensated by this volume exchange of gas with liquid or solid and prevent a hypobaric pulmonary barotrauma.

The formula for the practical depth limit in freediving in correlation to the lung capacity is

$$V_n = \left(TLC - FDS\right)\frac{1\,bar}{n \bullet bar_{abs}} + BV$$

TLC = total lung capacity; FDS = functional death space; V_n = lung volume in correlation of the ambient pressure; bar_{abs} = absolute pressure; 1 bar = surface pressure; BV = blood volume of the pulmonary vessels

Another accepted calculation of the maximal diving depth is

$$\text{Predicted maximal diving depth}\,[bar] = \frac{TLC}{RV}$$

RV = residual volume

An estimated BV value of 1.0 L pushes the practical freediving limits well beyond the initially expected theoretical limit. In more extreme freediving beyond 30 m, commonly exudation into the alveolar space due to blood shift into the pulmonary vessels occurs. That is why it is not safe to perform repetitive deep freediving. Almost everyone who has learned the right technique can easily reach more than 10 meters depth within a short time. Freediving over 15 meters must be approached with care. The best way is to extend the diving depth meter by meter and try to prolong the duration underwater gradually. Apnoea with physical activity above water can safely be practiced building up resistance to oxygen deficiency. In general, after each freediving, at least 2-min break should be taken. Keeping in mind, it takes at least a minute for blood to complete a full cycle in the body's circulation.

There are a variety of exercises to improve the effectiveness of breathing. Most breathing exercises are similar to certain yoga exercises. It not only trains breathing techniques but also the mind. Continuous practice causes reduced oxygen consumption by minimizing metabolism and increasing self-control. In addition, good physical fitness reduces skeletal muscle oxygen consumption. Therefore, physical fitness is essential for freediving. Trained freedivers seem to have a reflex of the autonomic nervous system shifting blood volume by peripheral vasoconstriction to vital organs. The total lung capacity can be increased by special breathing techniques, called "lung packing" or "buccal pumping" (glossopharyngeal insufflation). These are advanced breathing techniques used by freedivers. By using the mouth and throat, additional air is pumped into the lungs. The total lung capacity increases by 0.6–4.16 L (7–47%). Disadvantages are that it might increase the heart rate and causes damage by overinflating the lungs. Deep freediving increases the risk of DCS or inert gas narcosis. Herbert Nitsch suffered from an inert gas narcosis during his freediving record of 253 meters. During the standard protocol of wet recompression with 100% oxygen, he developed additionally severe DCS symptoms. Extreme freediving can lead to pneumomediastinum, pneumothorax, AGE and alveoli damage. Symptoms like loss of consciousness, chest pain, tracheal pain, cough and haemoptysis might have no preceding warning signs. To avoid damage through lung packing, regular exercises like lung stretches or yoga should be performed and the number of packs should be only slowly increased over time. To reduce the residual volume, techniques of "reversed packing" (glossopharyngeal exsufflation) can be used. The mouth and throat acts hereby as a vacuum pump to empty the lungs after exhalation. The residual volume can be reduced by 0.1–0.44 L (8–26%). Normally, the lung capacity is 4–6 L. Through these techniques, it can be increased up to 9–11 L. Herbert Nitsch has achieved approx. 15 L.

CO_2 is the main trigger for the respiratory reflex, which provokes inspiration. Respiratory reflex can be delayed by a reduction of CO_2 via hyperventilation. However, this increases the risk of unconsciousness. As described in the previous chapter, freediving can cause unconsciousness. Therefore, hyperventilation and rapid, high intensity movements should be avoided. Even intense shortness of breath should not mislead to fast movements to reach the surface, as oxygen deficit grows even faster by doing that. The feeling of shortness of breath is often complemented subjectively by the inability of breathing underwater. Freediving requires adaption to depth and apnoea duration. To dive to 20 meters or more initially, dives should be less deep and gradually built up by dives to increasing depth. This allows the body to adjust to immersion, hypercapnia and the oxygen deficiency. Special care should be taken in disciplines with no fins and the blue jump, as frequent blackouts occur.

Freediving should be never carried out alone. Alternate descent increases security of freediving because the other person can intervene in the event of loss of consciousness underwater (�‍ Fig. 27.4).

❯ Never, ever dive alone! Never, ever!!!

As loss of consciousness occurs usually in the last meters before surfacing, it is very important to take great care during this part of ascent. By falling unconscious, movements like few fin strokes might be initially still possible, until muscles begin to relax. During the initial reflex to inhale, water is aspirated, which

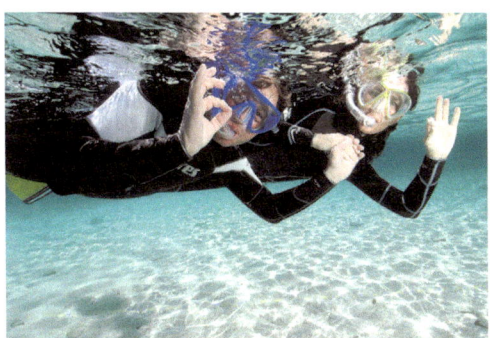

Fig. 27.4 Diving with a buddy also applies for free diving. (Mares)

leads to laryngospasm. The laryngospasm resolves after approx. 20–30 s. If the diver is not rescued and the head is above water within this time, further aspiration occurs and the diver will drown.

27.3 Drowning [8]

Common causes of drowning are unconsciousness (due to hypothermia, panic, suicide, inert gas narcosis, gasping for breath, hyperventilation, poisoning by CO, CO_2 and O_2), disruption of air supply from the scuba tank or misjudgement of own abilities to hold breath. Some of the drowning accidents are also attributed to alcohol or use of drugs. The use of alcohol and drugs increases the risk of suffocation by vomiting, peripheral vasodilation, weakening of the protective laryngeal reflexes and risky behaviour.

It needs to be distinguished between salt water aspiration syndrome, near-drowning and drowning. *Drowning* is defined as death by water aspiration. Aspiration of water occurs approximately 20–30 s after the onset of unconsciousness. In the first 20–30 s underwater, laryngospasm prevents further inspiration (inspiratory apnoea). Laryngospasm is usually released completely after 1–2 min. In rare cases, laryngospasm remains. The increased arterial CO_2 levels are a strong inspirational trigger, which leads eventually to asphyxiation. This is followed by seizures. 3–5 min later, the last reversible respiratory failure (preterminal apnoea) develops. Just before the final cardiac arrest, there might be some gasping (agonal respiration).

Fresh water drowning causes fluid shift from the extravascular into the intravascular space. Fresh water has lower electrolytes concentrations. Due to oncotic forces, fluid is drawn into the blood. The fluid influx from the alveoli into the blood vessels leads to an electrolyte shift, as blood is "diluted" (haemodilatation). Sodium, chloride and protein concentrations are decreasing, and simultaneously volume in blood vessels is increasing (hypervolaemia). Potassium may be released from red blood cells due to haemolysis and cause their levels in serum to increase. Normal potassium levels are 3.5–5 mmol/L. Levels above are classified as hyperkalaemia and levels above 7 mmol/L represent severe hyperkalaemia. High levels of potassium (hyperkalaemia) can cause ECG changes (peaked T waves, shortened QT, ST segment depression, followed by bundle-branch blocks, increased PR interval, decreased amplitude of P wave), ventricular fibrillation and cardiac arrest. Oedematous swelling of bronchial cells causes bronchial obstruction. The fluid in the alveoli is trapped and gets absorbed into the blood stream. Therefore, lungs may remain "dry" even for a long time after the death. Hence, a synonym for drowning in fresh water is "dry drowning" (emphysema aequosum). But dry drowning can also occur in sea water, if laryngospasm persists.

Drowning in *salt water* causes a fluid shift from the blood vessels into the lungs due to the hypertonic salt water (approximately fourfold higher osmotic pressure than blood). Pulmonary fluid loss leads to decreased blood volume, increased blood concentration (haemoconcentration) and pulmonary oedema. Even some time after death, fluid can be found in the lungs. That's why drowning in salt water is called "wet drowning" (oedema aequosum). Serum electrolyte changes are minimal and have therefore no effect on the heart conduction (**Fig. 27.5**).

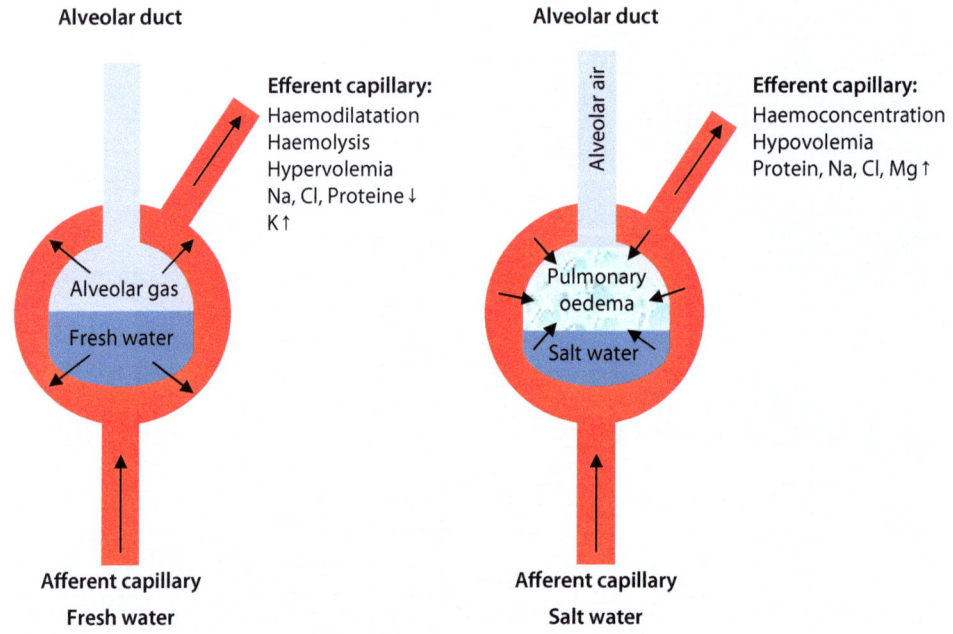

Alveolar duct

Efferent capillary:
Haemodilatation
Haemolysis
Hypervolemia
Na, Cl, Proteine ↓
K ↑

Alveolar gas

Fresh water

Afferent capillary
Fresh water

Alveolar duct

Alveolar air

Efferent capillary:
Haemoconcentration
Hypovolemia
Protein, Na, Cl, Mg ↑

Pulmonary
oedema

Salt water

Afferent capillary
Salt water

■ **Fig. 27.5** Effects of drowning in fresh and sea water

Near-drowning is drowning, which is prevented by early resuscitation and not causing death. Prognostic factors for recovery are age, time period until commencing resuscitation and ambient temperature. The time period until commencing resuscitation is an important factor for organ or cerebral damages. The earlier vital functions are stabilized, the better is the prognosis. Regaining consciousness and spontaneous breathing are positive signs. The probability of the occurrence of irreversible brain damage increases with the duration of hypoxia. Irreversible brain damage occurs after about 5–10 min of absolute hypoxia. Therefore, it is important that resuscitation is commenced as soon as possible. With the correct use of CPR, blood flow and oxygen supply are partially provided, which delays the time of irreversible damages. Also, the age of the affected person and ambient temperatures affect the time of irreversible organ damage. It is reported that children were revived without further damages, after cardiac arrest caused by drowning lasting for an hour. Near-drowning in fresh and salt water can cause a washout of the surfactant, which leads to a collapse of the alveoli. Pulmonary oedema of sea water drowning delays alveoli to unfold to a greater extent than in fresh water drowning. Hence, the lungs take longer to recover. Results are massive respiratory complications. Within hours up to 2 days after the alveoli damage, exudative inflammatory responses can develop. Due to exudation, secondary drowning is possible. Hence, patients with water aspiration should be monitored for 48 h. Through forceful respiration at the initial phase of drowning in combination with pharyngeal and bronchial fluids, specific foam can form in the nasopharynx. This kind of foam can be found in salt and fresh water drowning, as well as in near-drowning.

Salt water aspiration syndrome can even occur with aspiration of only small amounts of salt water. Aspiration can happen through accidental inhalation of salt water during snorkelling, swimming or scuba diving. In mild cases, the only symptoms are coughing. In severe cases, haemoptysis might occur. Other symptoms might be rigor, tremors, chills, vomiting, dyspnoea, cough and headache. The symptoms disappear in general after 2–15 h. By administering 100% oxygen and bed rest, symptoms subside usually spontaneously.

References

1. AIDA International. AIDA International World Records. International Association for Development of Apnea. Available at https://www.aidainterna-tional.org/WorldRecords. Accessed 5 Oct 2007.
2. AIDA International. www.aidainternational.org. Accessed 11.9.2015.
3. CMAS. www.CMAS.org. Assessed 14.7.2015.
4. Lindholm P, Lundgren CE. The physiology and pathophysiology of human breath-hold diving. J Appl Physiol. 2009;106(1):284–92.
5. Lindholm P, Lundgren CEG. Alveolar gas composition before and after maximal breath-holds in competitive divers. UHM. 2006;33(6):463 – Hypocapnia and Static Apnea.
6. Otteni CE, Kernagis DN, White WD, Freiberger JJ. Swimming-Induced pulmonary edema pathophysiology and risk reduction with sildenafil. Circulation. 2016;133:988–996; originally published online February 16, 2016; https://doi.org/10.1161/CIRCULATIONAHA.115.019464
7. Mithoefer JC. Breath holding. In: Handbook of physiology. Section 3: respiration, vol. II. Washington DC: AmericanPhysiologicalSociety; 1964. p. 1011 25.
8. Riede UN, Werner M, Freudenberg N. Basiswissen Allgemeine und Spezielle Pathologie. 2nd ed. Stuttgart: Georg Thieme Verlag; 2009.
9. Silbernagel S, Despopuluos A. Taschenatlas der Physiologie. 7th ed. Stuttgart: Thieme; 2007.

Suggested Reading

Lundgren CEG. Freediving science. In: Lindholm P, Pollock NW, Lundgren CEG, editors. Breath-hold diving. Proceedings of the Undersea and Hyperbaric Medical Society/Divers Alert Network 2006 June 20–21 Workshop. Durham, NC: Divers Alert Network; 2006.
Gempp E, Blatteau JE. Neurological disorders after repetitive breath-hold diving. Aviat Space Environ Med. 2006;77(9):971–3.
Gold D, Aiyarak S, Wongcharoenyong S, Geater A, Juengprasert W, Gerth WA. The indigenous fisherman divers of Thailand: diving practices. Int J Occup Saf Ergon. 2000;6(1):89–112.
Gold D, Geater A, Aiyarak S, Wongcharoenyong S, Juengprasert W, Johnson M, et al. The indigenous fisherman divers of Thailand: diving-related mortality and morbidity. Int J Occup Saf Ergon. 2000;6(2):147–67.
Lewis PR. Skin diving fatalities in New Zealand. N Z Med J. 1979;89(638):472–5.
Mangge H, Plecko B, Grubbauer HM, Popper H, Smolle-Jüttner F, Zach M. Late-onset miliary pneumonitis after near drowning. Pediatr Pulmonol. 1993;15(2):122–4.
Moon RE, Martina SD, Peacher DF, Potter JF, Wester TE, Cherry AD, Natoli MJ, Eng M, Orlowski JP. Drowning, near-drowning, and ice-water submersions. Pediatr Clin N Am. 1987;34(1):75–92.
Papa L, Hoelle R, Idris A. Systematic review of definitions for drowning incidents. Resuscitation. 2005;65(3):255–64.
Suominen P, Baillie C, Korpela R, Rautanen S, Ranta S, Olkkola KT. Impact of age, submersion time and water temperature on outcome in near-drowning. Resuscitation. 2002;52(3):247–54.

Damage Caused by External Factors

© Springer International Publishing AG, part of Springer Nature 2018
O. Rusoke-Dierich, *Diving Medicine*, https://doi.org/10.1007/978-3-319-73836-9_28

28.1 Thermal Damages

28.1.1 Hypothermia

Water has a 25 times higher thermal conductivity than air. Water removes more heat from the body compared to air. Wet or dry suits are used to protect against hypothermia. The thickness of wetsuits ranges from 2 mm up to 8 mm. The insulating effect is based on tiny air pockets in the rubber. A thin layer of water sits between skin and neoprene, which is heated up by the body. The water film is merely exchanged and remains stationary. As a result, convection is reduced and body heat is preserved. Convection is the process of enhanced heat transfer to another medium that has a different temperature. It can add or remove heat from one medium to the other. The water layer under the neoprene has usually only little exchange with water of the environment. If however the wetsuit is too big, the gap widens between the skin and neoprene, which facilitates the exchange of the already heated water under the neoprene and the cold water of the environment. This causes further heat loss. The insulating effect is decreasing with increasing depth as air bubbles in the neoprene become smaller, which decreases its insulating effect. Dry diving suits prevent the diver's skin from any direct contact with water at all. The insulating effect is caused by warm clothing under the dry suit and the reduction of conduction. To maintain neutral pressure within the dry suit, air needs to be supplied and released to inside of the dry suit. Unlike the neoprene suit, the dry suit is a closed system and does not have direct exchange with the environment. This results in less heat loss due to convection. The insulating effect is better in dry suits than in wetsuits. To avoid hypothermia during diving, the head should be covered as well. As skin vessels of the scalp have limited ability to contract, body heat can be lost significantly. At lower water temperatures, gloves and boots should be used as well, to minimise the area of convection.

Hypothermia causes vasoconstriction of peripheral blood vessels. Blood is shifted to the body's centre to maintain normal body core temperature and to ensure adequate perfusion of organs (centralisation). The right body temperature is necessary for the metabolism. At rest heat is produced by metabolic processes. Approximately 25% is produced by the liver, 20% by the brain, 8% by the heart, 7% by the kidneys and 25% by muscular activity. To maintain core body temperature in a cold environment, the body starts to shake. Energy in form of heat is released by chemical processes in muscles during its activity. Oxygen in return is required to produce this energy. The oxygen demand may increase it by up to 300% in hypothermia. If the body core temperatures sink below 33 °C, the metabolism slows down and regulatory heat production by muscle rigours ceases.

Initial symptoms of hypothermia are rigours and tachycardia. Heart rate decreases exponentially with decreasing core body temperature. At 32 °C the heart rate decreases to 83% at 30 °C to 67% and at 28 °C on 58% of the normal heart rate. Blood pressure increases to counteract the bradycardia, which returns to normal levels at 28 °C. Temperatures below 32–30 °C can cause arrhythmia. The lower the core body temperature is, the more likely ventricular fibrillation is to develop. However, even at 25–23 °C, ventricular fibrillation may not appear. The cause of ventricular fibrillation in hypothermia is yet unclear. It is believed to be caused by electrolyte shifts (hypokalaemia) due to pH level changes. A possible ECG change might be prolongation of the vulnerable phase (R-T interval). A delay in electric conduction of the bundles causes a shift of electrical impulses into the vulnerable phase and thus may trigger ventricular fibrillation. Hypothermia itself seems to trigger atrial and ventricular arrhythmias caused by coronary vasoconstriction and disturbance of electric conduction such re-entry mechanisms. Exposure in cold environment or exposure to cold water initially causes hyperventilation with a refractory respiratory alkalosis. CO_2 production of the body is halved every 8 °C body core temperature. This leads to reduction of respiratory stimulus, which explains respiratory failure in extreme hypothermia. During hypothermia CNS metabolism is reduced. Cerebral blood flow decreases steadily with decreasing temperature. Oedematous swelling of the brain may develop. Lactate and bicarbonate accumulates and pH decreases. Due to the decreased metabolism of the brain, the point of irreversible damage is delayed. EEG changes are rarely in temperatures above 28 °C. Form 25 °C on, EEG slowdown and disorganisation delta waves may develop. EEG zero lines appear at 17–18 °C. There is also a volume shift into cells and interstitial space. In the intestines, this volume shift leads to diarrhoea. The shift of blood volume to the body core results in stimulation of central volume receptors and thus increases diuresis. These effects on the intestines and kidney lead to a decrease of blood volume (hypovolemia) and a significant haemoconcentration.

Mild hypothermia causes hyperkalaemia, increases cortisol as well as serum chloride and magnesium levels. In advanced hypothermia hypokalaemia and hyponatraemia develop. It may cause leukopenia and thrombocytopenia.

- ■ **Hypothermia Can Be Divided into Three Stages**

I mild (core body temperature 32–35 °C)
- Rigours
- General feeling of pain, especially in the knees and the genitals
- After initial tachycardia reduction of the heart rate
- Initially still oriented, later increasing disorientation, confusion
- Later central nervous system involvement (slurred speech, memory disturbance, idea fixation, etc.)
- Increased reflexes

II moderate (core body temperature 28–32 °C)
- General muscle rigidity
- Reduction in the tidal volume
- Bradycardia (approx. 30–40 beats per minute)
- Arrhythmia
- Decreased reflexes
- Hypoglycaemia
- Decrease of standard bicarbonate
- Stupor
- No rigours with core body temperatures below 31 °C
- Termination of reflexes and the pupillary light response with core body temperatures starting from below 28–30 °C

III severe (core body temperature < 28 °C)
- Symptoms of apparent death, respiratory failure and paralysis
- Increasing hypotension
- Pulmonary oedema
- Coma

Stage I is specified as mild hypothermia. Patients are shaking and disoriented and muscular activity is restricted. Stages II and III are specified as moderate to severe hypothermia causing death without adequate clinical treatment. In stages II and III, ECG changes (Q-T extension or full distortion of the ECG) can be found. Therefore, if any ECG activities are present in an unresponsive patient with hypothermia, this should be interpreted as a sign of life. ECG changes can't be interpreted reliably till the normal core body temperature is restored. Even after a prolonged cardiac arrest, recovery may be possible. Vital signs are hardly recognisable with core body temperatures below 27 °C.

The main aim in the *treatment* of hypothermia is to restore normal core body temperatures. Complications of increasing body temperature are a breakdown of centralisation, which keeps the patient alive. External warming causes dilatation of skin vessels. This leads to shift the relatively warm blood of the body centre into the cold periphery. Mixing warm central blood with cold blood of the periphery results into further drop of core body temperature. The lower the core body temperature is, the more likely are cardiac arrhythmias. Moreover, dilatation of cutaneous vessels (peripheral vasodilatation) due to external warming leads to a decrease in blood pressure.

28

Therapy of stage I is replacement of wet clothes through dry ones followed by wrapping in warm blankets and internal warming including hot drinks to increase core body temperature. Warm baths carry the risk of a short-term decrease of the core body temperature (see above) and of burning the skin. Burning of cold skin requires lower temperatures than skin of normal temperature. Warming increases the risk of DCS, too. Since gas at increased temperatures is less dissolved in fluids, bubble formations are more likely.

In stages II and III, wet clothes should not be replaced by dry ones, since any movement of the victim can redistribute blood volume. This redistribution is causing further decrease of the core body temperature. Rewarming of the body has to be carried out carefully and slowly. Sudden warming or heating can be fatal. Sudden changes of the patient's position and manipulation such as passive movement of muscles or rubbing of the skin as well as inserting intravenous lines have to be avoided too as this can break down centralisation and warm centralised blood and cool peripheral blood mix, which lowers further the overall core body temperature. The best warming methods are using the body's own heat production. The *Hibler method* is a method which can be even used in remote areas. Hereby, the body is tightly wrapped with three layers, a vapour-tight, insulating layer on the outside, an insulating blanket in the middle and an additional wet layer inside. The inner layer is wrapped tightly around the chest of the patient, moistened with warm water. Heat packs may be applied additionally around the neck, axilla or groin. The warm, wet layer should be never applied directly on the skin. The wet layer can be replaced several times with new warm water. Just as tightly an insulating blanket, with the silver side facing towards the body, is wrapped around the inner wet layer. This reflects up to 80% of the heat. Then, patients are wrapped with multiple layers of tightly wrapped blankets and/or a sleeping bag. Initially, before applying the Hilbert method, patients should be protected by plastic foil

from further heat loss through evaporative cooling. Another option in hospital is cautious warming by specific heating blankets filled with warm air. During warming, there is a risk of causing further hypotension. Extracorporeal rewarming represents another more invasive method. Blood from central vessels is extracted to the outside of the body to being warmed up and redirected into the body (e.g. femoral vein) again. Peritoneal dialysis (exchange of fluid in the peritoneal space) with warmed electrolyte solution or respiration with preheated air (CBRM central body, rewarming method) is an alternative method for severe hyperthermia. Last resort in case in hypothermia with cardiac arrest is opening of the chest and direct heating of the heart via a preheated electrolyte solution. Invasive methods should be applied, only if other methods failed. Slower rewarming is preferred over fast one. If the patient requires resuscitation, it is absolutely vital to continue CPR until normal body temperature is achieved. *Don't stop until warm!* Only at normal temperature vital signs can be assessed accurately.

- ▪ **Overview over Treatment Options of Hypothermia**

Acute

- ▬ Careful removal of wet clothes (only body core temperatures >30 °C)
- ▬ Apply dry and warm clothes
- ▬ Avoid unnecessary manipulations and position changes
- ▬ Warm drinks
- ▬ Hibler Pack (body core temperature < 30 °C; do not undress!)
- ▬ Protection against further heat loss
- ▬ At cardiac arrest only intubation, respiration and chest compressions; no defibrillation, no infusions, no $NaHCO_3$, no aggressive rewarming

Follow-up

- ▬ Protection against heat loss, Hilbert Pack first-line therapy
- ▬ Rewarming by baths with increasing temperature (only the torso without limbs)

— Thoracic warming by ventilation with preheated air
— Extracorporeal warming, peritoneal dialysis
— Thoracotomy and applying warm saline solution onto the heart
— Monitoring

28.1.2 Hyperthermia

Hyperthermia has three different presentations, heat exhaustion, heat stroke and sunstroke. Heat exhaustion and heat stroke vary in their severity. While heat exhaustion despite strong subjective symptoms is rather harmless, heat stroke is potentially life-threatening. Heat stroke represents a combination of shock and overheating. There are two forms of heat-related injuries: at physical activity (EHS = exertional heatstroke) and at physical inactivity (NEHS = non-exertional heat stroke). The former occurs under extreme physical exertion at high ambient temperatures. The latter is more common in elderly or chronically ill.

Short-term increases of in body core temperatures are usually well tolerated. Even with body core temperatures of 46 °C [4], full recovery was achieved in some cases. However, temperatures above 41.1 °C are regarded as life-threatening and should be treated aggressively. Hyperthermia is caused by a lack of complete or partial removal of the excess body's heat. Excess heat is transferred to the body's periphery and leaves the body via radiation or via evaporation from sweat. Heat radiation makes up to 65% of the heat release and depends on clothes, humidity and ambient temperature. At high ambient temperatures, release of heat via skin is the main mechanism. Core body temperature is mainly regulated by blood circulation or sweating. A lower percentage of heat is released via the lung. Air humidity over 75% reduces heat release via sweating. Acclimatisation to high temperatures is also an important factor. At insufficient acclimatisation, the body can only produce 1 L/h of sweat. After sufficient acclimatisation

that can increase up to 2–3 L/h. A complete acclimatisation is usually achieved after 7–10 days. The use of air conditioning actually reduces acclimatisation.

28.1.2.1 Heat Stress and Heat Exhaustion

■ **Symptoms**

Arousal, confusion, delirium, psychosis, dyspnoea, increased rigidity, nausea, vomiting, diarrhoea, hyperventilation, shock, decreased urinary output, exhaustion, thirst, headache, muscle pain (myalgia)and cramps, oedema (lower legs, forearms), profused sweating, dilated pupils, normal or increased temperature (37–40 °C), rhabdomyolysis and cold, pale and clammy skin.

28.1.2.2 Heat Stroke

■ **Symptoms**

Altered level of consciousness; hypoglycaemia; behavioural disturbance; loss of consciousness; coma; shock; convulsions; photophobia; severe headache; neck stiffness; hypotension; hypoglycaemia; cyanosis; fixed pupils; arrhythmias; rigidity; acute renal failure; nausea; vomiting; myalgia; dyspnoea; diarrhoea; hyperventilation; *body temperature > 40.5 °C (hyperpyrexia) with neurological symptoms*; tachycardia; urinary incontinence; hot, red, dry or damp skin; constricted pupils; faecal incontinence; and rhabdomyolysis. Temperature might not be a reliable sign of heat stroke, as symptoms can be still present after lowering core body temperature.

■ **Complications**

Delirium, coma, death, heart failure, heart attack, cor pulmonale, pulmonary oedema, atelectasis, pulmonary infarction, liver damage (mostly short-lived and reversible), rhabdomyolysis with renal failure.

■ **Therapy**

Treatment for heat exhaustion or heat stroke is the same and is depending on the severity of symptoms (◘ Table 28.1). Both represent a medical emergency and have to be treated immediately. Target is to reduce the core body

▣ Table 28.1 Therapy of hyperthermia

	Decrease of body core temperature/min (°C)	Procedure
Non-invasive cooling methods		
Misting [6]	0.3 (less in patients with heat stroke, approx 0.05–0.09)	Removal of all clothes, misting with cold water of 15 °C, constant airflow via fan at room temperature
Ice water immersion [6]	0.15–0.35	Removal of all clothes, immersion of the entire body in ice water
Whole body ice packs [2]	0.03	Removal of all clothes, cover the person with a plastic foil and then cover with ice
Targeted ice packs [2]	0.02–0.03	Removal of all clothes, ice pack in groin and axilla
Invasive cooling methods		
Gastric lavage [5]	0.15	Gastric lavage with ice water 10 m//kg bw), removal of the ice water after 30–60 s
Peritoneal lavage [2]	0.5	Cooling of isotonic sodium solution in ice water, peritoneal lavage with 500–1000 mL

temperature below 39 °C as quickly as possible. When 39 °C is reached, external and internal cooling methods should be ceased, to avoid iatrogenic hypothermia. Temperatures should be measured rectally, because other methods are too inaccurate. All patients should be treated also for dehydration. Complications associated with hyperthermia must be treated additionally. Hypoglycaemia, which often is associated with hyperthermia, needs to be treated with glucose or dextrose infusions. As upper GI bleeding is a common complication, prophylactic PPIs may be given.

28.1.3 Sunstroke

Increased sun exposure on the uncovered head can cause sunstroke. Through meningeal irritation, headaches, dizziness, intracranial hypertension as well as increase in protein and cell numbers in the cerebrospinal fluid, sunstroke can develop. Headaches may last for several days. Treatment remains the same as hyperthermia. If shock develops, corticosteroids can be used additionally to the normal shock treatment.

■ **Symptoms**
Loss of consciousness, red hot head, drowsiness, vertigo, tinnitus, nausea, vomiting, diarrhoea, shock, hyperthermia and meningism.

■ **Therapy**
The patient should be positioned with head slightly elevated in a cool environment; cooling of the head; cooling of body's core temperature as hyperthermia; corticosteroids can be considered.

During diving hyperthermia can occur due to wearing a diving suit outside the water. Therefore, diving suits should be put on just before diving and be removed directly after diving. Since usually it is windy at the seaside, strong sunlight might not be noticed. By not wearing a hat, sunstroke can develop.

◻ Table 28.2 Water balance of the body			
Uptake approx. 2.5 L/day		**Loss approx. 2.5 L/day**	
Oxidation	0.3 L	Faeces	0.1 L
Meals	0.9 L	Breathing	0.4 L
Drinks	1.3 L	Skin	0.5 L
		Urine	1.5 L

28.1.4 Dehydration

The human body contains approx. 45–80% water depending on age and gender (◻ Table 28.2). Infants have a water content of 70–80%. At a young age, women have a water content of approximately 53%, which decreases to 46% later on in life. Men have a water content of about 64% at a young age and 53% when they are older. The body receives its water from oxidation, fluids or meals. It eliminates water by breathing, sweating, via urine and faeces.

Fluid loss through breathing and skin depends on the water content of the ambient air. *Dry air*, such as compressed air, extracts more moisture via breathing compared to moist air. Release of fluid through the skin via sweating provides cooling of the body at increased core body temperatures. At high humidity sweat can't evaporate sufficiently. In dry, hot weather, the water evaporates immediately without being noticed as sweating. Loss of fluid through the skin may increase up to 20 times (10 L/day) under certain conditions. Electrolytes are also excreted via sweat. With excessive sweating, water and minerals have to be subsidised to the body. Hormonal control of water balance is achieved over three different pathways, by ADH (adiuretin = vasopressin), aldosterone, ANP (atriopeptin = atrial natriuretic peptide) and BNP (brain natriuretic peptide). *ADH* is secreted by the hypothalamus. ADH causes water reabsorption in kidneys (medullary section of the collecting tubes) and thus concentrates urine. With the help of renin, which is produced in the liver, angiotensin I is converted from angiotensinogen. Angiotensin I is then transformed with the help of ACE (angiotensin-converting enzyme) to angiotensin II. *Aldosterone* is released from the adrenal cortex triggered by angiotensin II. Aldosterone prevents excretion of sodium in the ascending part of the loop of Henle and promotes sodium reabsorption. *ANP and BNP* are excreted by the heart itself (◻ Fig. 28.1).

During diving, blood volume is redistributed within the body by elimination of hydrostatic forces. Additionally, cold ambient temperatures can cause peripheral vasoconstriction, which redirects blood to central regions. Both factors together cause a blood shift from peripherally towards centrally. Blood vessels of the lungs can herby take up to 300–500 mL of blood. The redistribution of the body's blood volume leads to relative hypervolaemia, which is sensed by volume receptors of the heart. Particularly, ANP and BNP increase and ADH decreases. The result is increased diuresis mainly caused by ANP and BNP. All these factors cause an increased production of urine, which is noticeable after diving. Because of its delayed effect, aldosterone plays probably only a minor role in diving.

Diving-induced diuresis and hot ambient temperatures, in combination with wind, lead to dehydration. Additionally, diarrhoea, which is not an uncommon during travelling, can deplete fluid of the body. The body responds to dehydration with thirst. Age and adaptation to chronic dehydration reduce the sensation of thirst, so that a fluid depletion is no longer noticed. Dehydration increases the risk of developing DCS. When the body is dehydrated, fluid needs to be replaced. A good indicator for sufficient hydration is the urine colour and production. It should be clear and have a light colour. The normal amount of fluid intake is approx. 2 L/day. Heat or diarrhoea may increase it to more than 3–4 L per day. Extreme exercise and heat can increase the fluid demand up to 10 L/day. Preferably, drinks shouldn't be cold. Cold drinks can cause internal cooling

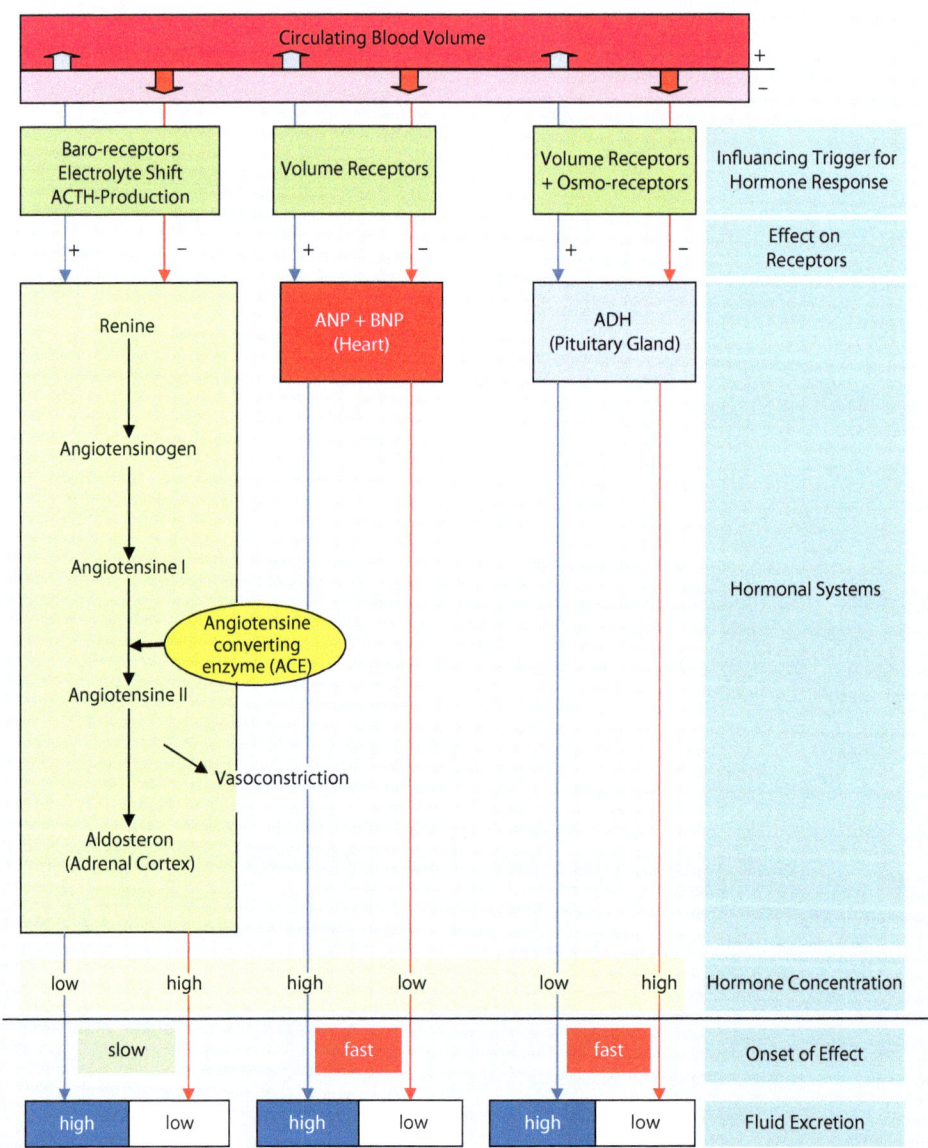

Fig. 28.1 Regulation of the fluid balance; blue, increasing circulating blood volume; red, decreasing circulating blood volume

and mislead the central regulation of core body temperature. As the body falsely senses a cooler core body temperature the body's cooling mechanism with sweating fails and the body overheats.

Dehydration is defined as a negative fluid balance in the body (□ Table 28.3). This negative balance can occur because of decreased fluid intake, increase fluid output or extravascular fluid shift (ascites, effusion, burns or sepsis).

Table 28.3 Symptoms of dehydration	Mild dehydration	Moderate dehydration	Severe dehydration
Fluid deficit	0–5%	5–10%	>10%
State of consciousness	Normal	Lethargy	ALOC
Capillary refill	<2 s	2–4 s	>4 s
Tongue appearance	Normal	Dry	Dry, swollen
Tears	Normal	Reduced	Absent
Heart rate	Normal or slightly elevated	Elevated	Tachycardia
Respiratory rate	Normal	Elevated	Tachypnoeic
Blood pressure	Normal	Slightly low	Hypotension
Eyes	Normal	Slightly sunken	Severly sunken
Urine output	Low	Oliguria	Oliguria/anuria
Skin turgor	Normal	Reduced	Severely reduced

28.1.4.1 Forms of Dehydration

■ **Isotonic Dehydration (Serum Sodium 130–150 mmol/L)**

Isotonic dehydration causes sodium and water loss of the intercellular space and body fluids (blood, lymph and cerebrospinal fluid). However, fluids inside cells remain unaffected. Osmolarity of blood remains the same. Isotonic dehydration can have renal and extrarenal causes. Renal causes include polyuric phase of acute and chronic renal failure, M. Addison and diuretic treatment. Extrarenal causes are vomiting, diarrhoea and fistulas. Losses into the intercellular space are promoted by pancreatic inflammation (pancreatitis), peritoneal inflammation (peritonitis) and bowel obstruction, as well as by burns with losses via skin. Symptoms of fluid deficiency (hypovolaemia) are thirst, tachycardia, orthostatic dysregulation, postural drop of blood pressure, headache and oliguria.

■ **Hypotonic Dehydration (Serum Sodium <130 mmol/L)**

Hypotonic dehydration has a greater loss of minerals than of water, resulting in hyponatremia. Sodium and fluid disappear into the intercellular space and the body fluids (blood, lymph and cerebrospinal fluid). There is a fluid shift to the inside cells (intracellular oedema). The cause is usually excessive administration of sodium solutions. Symptoms are similar as in the isotonic dehydration with pronounced tendency to an orthostatic dysregulation. Additionally, there are cerebral symptoms such as dizziness, headaches, delirious states and convulsions.

■ **Hypertonic Dehydration (Serum Sodium >150 mmol/L)**

Hypertonic dehydration has general extra and intracellular volume depletion, resulting in hypernatremia. Causes can be lack of water supply, cutaneous (excessive sweating), pulmonary (dry air, hyperventilation), renal (diabetic coma, diabetes insipidus) and gastrointestinal (vomiting, diarrhoea) water loss.

Fluid input and output, weighing, monitoring of electrolytes and renal function, probable regulation of derailed electrolytes and fluid substitution are necessary in the therapy of dehydration. Mild to moderate dehydration can be treated by oral fluid intake (□ Table 28.4).

■ **Table 28.4**   Oral rehydration therapy (ORT) recommendation by WHO and UNICEF

Glucose, anhydrous in mmol/L	Na⁺ in mmol/L	K⁺ in mmol/L	Cl⁻ in mmol/L	Citrate in mmol/L	Osmolarity in mmol/L
75	75	20	65	10	245

Box 28.1   Stages of Volume Substitution
- *Stage I: Volume substitution (stat)*
  - 20 mL/kg bw stat
- *Stage II: Substitution of the regular fluid demand (over 2–4 days)*
  - < 10 kg = 100 mL/kg bw per day
  - 10–20 kg bw = 1000 + 50 mL/kg bw for each kg > 10 kg per day
  - 20 kg bw = 1500 + 20 mL/kg bw for each kg > 20 kg per day
  - Volume substitution = % of dehydration x kg bw x 10 – initial stat dose (stage I) divided by the amount of days of rehydration
- *Stage III: Substitution of the ongoing fluid losses (additional with stage II)*
  - Volume substitution = volume loss

Moderate to severe dehydration requires intravenous treatment and monitoring (■ Box 28.1). Isotonic dehydration requires isotonic fluids (e.g. Ringer's solution). Acute dehydration generally can be quickly treated with IV fluid administration. Fluid substitution of chronic dehydration has to be given slowly.

- **Fluid substitution has three stages**
  - Volume substitution
  - Substitution of the regular fluid demand
  - Substitution of the ongoing fluid losses

For hypotonic dehydration, a 0.9% NaCl solution is used for rehydration. In stage I volume replacement is given as 20 mL/kg bw stat. In stage II the daily fluid demand will be calculated. To the daily fluid demand, the amount of the missing fluids due to dehydration will be added. However, sodium loss has

to be corrected in addition over 24 h. The sodium correction should be <0.5 mmol/l/h. The sodium loss can be calculated:

$$Na_{loss} = \left(Na_{reference\ value} - Na_{actual\ value} \right) \times volume\ of\ distribution\ kg\ bodyweight$$

Too rapid intravenous sodium replacement can cause central pontine myelinolysis, a fatal complication. Longer persisting hyponatremia causes a shift of the cerebrospinal fluid into the blood when fluid replacement is administered too rapidly. This can lead to insufficient energy supply of nerve cells in the CNS, resulting in degradation of myelin.

For hypertonic dehydration, the initial volume replacement is 20 mL/kg bw stat. The infusion can be given in the form of 5% glucose solution. Infusions in stages II and III should be administered over 48 h, and the sodium correction rate of 10 mmol/L / in 24 h shouldn't be exceeded, as rapid volume resuscitation may lead to a strong influx of fluid and cell swelling or rupture, resulting in cerebral oedema. Osmotically active fluids (plasma expanders, such as Dextran) for dehydration should be avoided, as they increase extracellular fluid deficit.

28.2 Sea or Motion Sickness

There are individual dispositions to sea or motion sickness. Irritation of the inner ear causes nausea and vomiting during a boat trip. Sensitive people should be located on the boat in a place with the least movements. This is usually the centre of the boat close to sea level. The affected person should look rather into the distance than to close structures of the boat or the horizon. There are several drugs available, which are recommended to prevent sea sickness. It is important that these drugs are taken before the boat ride and not just when symptoms occur. Drugs, which can be used, are promethazine, dimenhydrinate or hyoscine hydrobromide (scopolamine). All these medications have a sedative effect and may therefore result in temporary unfitness for diving.

28.3 **Infections**

During a diving holiday, overseas various infections may be contracted. They might be caused by direct contact with water, through injuries, food, drinking water or tropical and subtropical pathogens. The skin and mucous membranes surfaces are covered with a combination of bacterial flora, oily secretions and dead skin cells that prevents pathogens from entering the skin. There is also a lymphatic network in the skin, respiratory tract and gastrointestinal tract, which is involved in the immune response. Infections occur, if the skin barrier is damaged, the immune system is weakened or after a highly exposure to pathogens. There are a wide variety of pathogens in seawater (◘ Table 28.5). The water of non-polluted areas can already cause infection of skin, mucous membranes, upper respiratory tract or intestinal flora. In

◘ **Table 28.5** Potentially bacterial pathogens in normal and contaminated seawater

Normal seawater	Contaminated seawater
Acinetobacter lwoffii	Bacteria
Actinomyces species	Aeromonas species
Aeromonas sobria	Bacteroides species
Alcaligenes faecalis	Campylobacter
Bacillus cereus	Citrobacter
Bacillus subtilis	Chromobacterium
Clostridium botulinum	Eubacterium
Edwadsiella tarda	Fusobacterium
Enterobacter aerogenes	Yersinia
Enterobacter species	Virus
Enterococcus faecalis	Enterovirus
Erysipelothrix species	Reovirus
Escherichia coli	Adenovirus
Flavobacterium species	Hepatitis A virus
Klebsiella pneumoniae	Protozoa
Micrococcus sedentarius	Entamoeba
Micrococcus tetragenus	Giardia
Mycobacterium marinum	Acanthamoeba
Neisseria catarrhalis	Naegleria
Plesiomonas shigelloides	Hartmannella
Proteus mirabilis	
Pseudomonas aeruginosa	
Pseudomonas species	
Salmonella enteritidis	
Serratia species	
Staphylococcus epidermidis	
Staphylococcus aureus	
Staphylococcus citreus	
Streptococcus species	
Vibrio alginolyticus	
Vibrio cholerae	
Vibrio parahaemolyticus	
Vibrio vulnificus	

contaminated waters, highly infectious pathogens or increased numbers of pathogens can be found. This makes it more likely to contain infections.

Large parts of self-cleaning mechanisms of the sea (shore region, deep sea and microorganisms) are sensitively disturbed. Not only disposing waste water but also the worldwide pollution of industrial waste, eutrophication and overfishing are destroying sensitive maritime ecosystems. With increasing pollution, the number of pathogens in seawater increases.

28.3.1 Skin

The fatty substances produced by sebaceous glands and secretions of sweat glands form a protective layer on top of the skin with a pH usually ranging between 4.0 and 5.1. This protective layer can be destroyed by chemical or mechanical irritation. Damaged skin allows pathogens to enter and cause an inflammatory or infective reaction. Continuous irritation or progression of infections can result in ulcerations. Ulcerations are surrounded by an inflammatory area. If bacteria are involved in the infection, pus and a solid, whitish and fibrin-containing slough could be a visible sign of infection. Without treatment, ulcers expand. Pathogens entering the blood stream may develop into sepsis. Infections close to bones may progress to infections of the bone (osteomyelitis).

Ointments or creams can be used for dry and flaky skin to maintain its protective features. Damaged skin should be cleaned only with water. Especially after diving or swimming in seawater, damaged areas should be rinsed with clear water without rubbing or using soap. Even purulent wounds should be cleaned with water only. In severe cases, a broad-spectrum antibiotic may be applied. In general, antibiotics are not required in normal wounds. Furthermore, overuse of topical antibiotics might create antibacterial resistances. Wounds can be treated with silver dressings and other disinfectant agents. Often crusts form on top of wounds. These crusts prevent disinfectants reaching pathogens, which remain underneath the crust. Therefore, formation of crusts should be avoided. A waterproof dressing is usually sufficient to keep the wound moist. Sometimes it is advisable to cover the wound with wound gel, before dressings are applied. If a wound is present, further water contact should be avoided, especially seawater, which is rich in bacteria and hence promotes infections. Abrasions and wounds can be caused by tight-fitting diving suits, heel straps of the fins, or by hard and sharp objects. In particular coral cuts can cause infections as they have specific pathogens. The symptoms appear after approx. 1–2 days and usually disappear after 3–7 days. Fungal infections can be transmitted through poorly cleaned wetsuits or booties. The usually sharply demarcated, itchy and irritated skin rash is often located in moist areas of the body (between the toes, knee, groin, neck, etc.). Application of antifungal creams provides relief from symptoms. Diving gloves, diving suits and boots especially in diving schools should be cleaned regularly. Hanging up the suits inside out and exposing it to sun light helps to prevent the transmission of diseases, because ultraviolet radiation itself has disinfecting properties. Treatment of skin infections (Erysipelas/cellulitis) depends on the pathogens. *Staph. aureus* and *Streptococcus pyogenes*, the usual pathogen of the skin, are well responsive to dicloxacillin 500 mg QID or flucloxacillin 500 mg QID [1]. Coral cuts are often infected by *Streptococcus pyogenes*, which usually respond well to dicloxacillin or flucloxacillin. Infection caused by seawater or marine animal bites contain often bacteria such as vibrio species, pseudomonas or mycobacterium. Aeromonas species is often found in freshwater or brackish water as well as in mud in almost all waters. *Mycobacterium marinum* is found in fish tanks and salt water. An infection caused by the vibrio species may be followed by exposure to warm brackish or salt water. Therefore, it may be necessary to add other antibiotics such as ciprofloxacin 500 mg BD for Aeromonas species and doxycycline 100 mg BD for Vibrio species [1]. For

Mycobacterium marinum infections, clarithromycin 500 mg BD, doxycycline 100 mg BD (vibrio and mycobacterium species) or trimethoprim/sulphamethoxazole 160/800 mg BD (mycobacterium species) should be used [1]. For unresponsive mycobacterium infections, a combination of clarithromycin and rifampicin or ethambutol might be considered. The usual course of antibiotics for Vibrio or Aeromonas infections is 14 days and for other simple skin infections 7 days. The duration of the treatment of mycobacterium infections is recommended for 1–2 months after resolution of the lesions (typically 3–4 month). Mycobacterium infections usually present with modular skin lesions and the diagnosis is made by biopsy.

28.3.2 Ear Infections

A common cause for an inflammation or infection of the *external ear* (otitis externa) is contact with contaminated water entering the ear canal. If the protective layer of the ear canal is compromised, pathogens can grow and inflammation or infection may develop. Usual pathogens are *Pseudomonas, Staphylococcus aureus* and *Proteus*. Main reasons of destruction of the protective layer are usually caused by continuous rinsing of the ear canal with bacteria-rich water during diving and swimming or by cleaning with ear buds. Symptoms include localised ear pain and tragus tenderness. The patient often describes a fullness and hearing loss of the affected ear. On inspection, there might be swelling and discharge of the ear canal and tympanic membrane. Sometimes the swelling extends to the external ear and to the neck. The application of oil (e.g. olive oil) in the ear as a prophylaxis before diving is not recommended, because the oil clogs the skin pores in the ear canal and thus promotes the growth of bacteria and fungi. It might be useful to rinse the ear gently with freshwater after each dive to remove contaminated water. Flushing should be simply done with running water. Irrigation with a syringe can cause damage to the eardrum or ear canal and removes

the protective layer on the skin. External antibiotic ear drops (Sofradex® or Otodex®) with anti-inflammatory and analgesic agents are used to treat otitis externa. If a fungal infection is associated with otitis externa, Kenacomb® might be considered. If pseudomonas as a causative pathogen is suspected, ciprofloxacin is the drug of choice. Sometimes inserting a wick might be supportive for treatment. More severe infections affecting the outer ear or causing an occlusion of the ear canal are treated with intravenous ciprofloxacin. Contact with water (swimming, diving and showering) of the ear canal is to avoid until symptoms subside. Diving is contraindicated during this time. To avoid water entering the ear canal, ear plugs or buts of cotton wool sealed with Vaseline can be used to block the opening of the ear canal.

Middle ear inflammation or infections (otitis media) are caused by bacteria entering the middle ear from pathogen-rich water or the nasopharynx through the nasopharyngeal cavity. Antibiotics (amoxicillin) can be given in severe cases or if symptoms persist more than 3 days. During this time, diving is temporarily prohibited. Decongestant nose drops (e.g. Otirven®) may accelerate the healing process.

28.3.3 Others

In general, all damaged body surfaces can become infected, if they come into contact with contaminated water. If the eye is affected, conjunctivitis may develop. Inflammation of the conjunctiva (conjunctivitis) may be bacterial, viral or allergic nature. Mostly, conjunctivitis is caused by viruses and bacteria. Rarely, conjunctivitis is caused by fungal infections. In the tropics, lack of hygiene often causes conjunctivitis, which is also known as trachoma, a chlamydial infection. Trachoma can lead to blindness due to scarring. Trachoma is commonly found in Egypt. Other severe infections have to be treated with antibiotics (e.g. chloramphenicol 0.5% for normal infections or ciprofloxacin for corneal ulcers) or antivirals (e.g. acyclovir systemic or topical), depending on the pathogens.

28.4 UV-Related Damages

In holiday destinations, the sun is usually more intense than in the home country. Sunlight is intensified by reflection of the water surface at sea, which produces additional horizontal UV exposure. Swimming or snorkelling intensifies sunlight as the thin water layer acts like a magnifying glass. Vulnerable areas are shoulders, neck, ankles, nose and ears. A protection mechanism of the skin against sunlight is hyperpigmentation with melanin, callus formation and repair mechanisms.

The ultraviolet radiation is subdivided: $UV\text{-}A_{I} = 340–400$ nm; $UV\text{-}A_{II} = 320–340$ nm; $UV\text{-}B = 320–290$ nm; $UV\text{-}C = 200–290$ nm.

Radiation below 200 nm is almost completely filtered by the atmosphere. The most common and obvious injury caused by UV radiation is sunburn. It is mainly caused by UV-B. DNA of skin cells are hereby damaged, which leads to inflammation and apoptosis. Redness of sunburns is caused by the release of inflammatory mediators like histamine, serotonin, TNF, prostaglandins, leukotrienes and cytokines. The erythema develops over the first 4 h and reaches its maximum after approximately 24 h. The damage is similar to a burn. UV-A rays can penetrate into deeper skin layers. The effects of UV-A rays are still not fully understood. Their role in sun allergies is however confirmed. It is believed that UV-A rays contribute in the development of skin tumours. Simple sunburns usually are first degree burns with redness and swelling only. More severe sunburns with blistering are second-degree burns. In particular severe sunburns and family or personal history of melanomas increase the later risk of melanoma. Basal carcinomas (BCC) and squamous cell carcinomas (SCC) are rather a result of accumulation of UV radiation in the course of life. With increasing exposure to UV radiation, the risk to develop BCCs and SCCs increases. Fair-skinned people with blond or red hair are especially at risk for any kind of skin cancer.

Skin protection with sunscreens, which have a specific sun protection factor (SPF), is dependent on skin type and sun exposure (◘ Table 28.6). The SPF is a multiplicator of

◘ Table 28.6   Fitzpatrick classification [3]

Skin type	UV sensitivity	Skin colour	SPF in general	SPF for outdoor activities
I	Always burns, extremely sensitive, never tans	Extremely fair – pale, white, freckled	15	25–30
II	Easily burns, sensitive, rarely tans	Fair – White, sometimes freckled	12–15	25–30
III	Moderately burns, sensitive, usually tans	White, light brown	8–10	15
IV	Occasionally burns, less sensitive, tans well	Olive coloured, medium brown	6–8	15
V	Rarely burns, minimal sensitive, tans profusely	Dark brown	6–8	15
IV	Almost never burns, minimal sensitive, deeply pigmented	Very dark brown to black	6–8	15

SPF sun protection factor

▣ Table 28.7 Glogau photoageing classification

Glogau photoageing classification	Skin features
Type I	"No wrinkles", early photoageing, minimal wrinkles, mild pigmentary changes, no keratosis, younger patients, 20–30s, minimal or no makeup
Type II	"Wrinkles with motion", early to moderate photoageing, early senile lentigines visible, keratosis palpable but not visible, parallel smile lines begin to appear, patient age late 30s or 40s
Type III	"Wrinkles at rest", advanced photoageing, obvious dyschromia, telangiectasis, visible keratosis, always wears heavy foundation
Type IV	"Only wrinkles", severe photoageing, yellow-grey colour of skin, prior skin malignancies, wrinkles throughout, no normal skin, patient age 60s or 70s, can't wear makeup: "cakes and cracks"

the maximal tolerated sun exposure before skin erythema appears. In other words, the time to develop erythema with a sunscreen with SPF 30 extends from 10 min to up to 5 h. A sunscreen with SPF 15 filters approximately 93% and with SPF 30 approximately 95% of the UV-B radiation. Now, SPF 50 is readily available. However, the photoprotective properties of a sunscreen also depend on external factors like sweating, UV Index or water contact. Moreover, the time guide for prolonging sun exposure can be misleading, as erythema is only caused by UV-B. The vast majority of the UV radiation is UV-A, which takes up to 95–98% around midday! In general, sunscreens should contain ingredients blocking UV-A (oxybenzone, avobenzone) and UV-B (para-aminobenzoic acid, octyl methoxycinnamate and octyl salicylate) or physical blockers like titanium oxide or zinc oxide. Topical vitamins C and E seem to have an additional effect on to the photoprotective properties. Studies suggest that daily use of sunscreen might reduce melanoma risk by 5%. Sunscreens should be water resistant and need to be reapplied every 2 h.

Repeated exposure in particular to high amount of UV light causes photoageing.

Photoageing often adds onto intrinsic ageing. Photoageing causes wrinkling, roughness, dryness, telangiectasia, cancerous lesions, precancerous lesions and pigmentary alterations (▣ Table 28.7). Pigmented alterations include hyper- or hypomelanosis. Mottled hyperpigmentation, ephelides, lentigines and seborrheic keratosis are the primary lesions of hypermelanosis. Photoageing is also dependent on the individual skin type. Glogau described different levels of photoageing (▣ Fig. 28.2).

28.5 Accidents

Injuries caused by boats during ascent are another risk for divers, especially in free diving. Divers should obtain a 360° overview during ascent before reaching the surface, to detect approaching boats. Due to the higher sound conductivity of water compared to air, distance and direction can be not recognised. Areas with high boat traffic should be avoided for diving and snorkelling. To be visible for boat divers can use a buoy for safety reasons. The buoys are tied to the diver to indicate the position of divers on the surface.

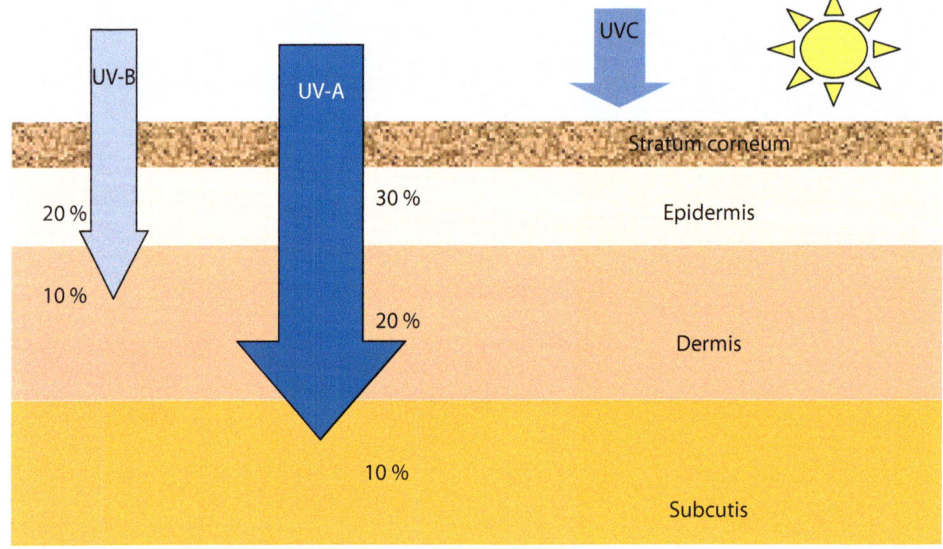

Fig. 28.2 UV-mediated skin damages

References

1. Antibiotic Expert Group. Therapeutic guidelines: antibiotic. Version 14. Melbourne: Therapeutic Guidelines Ltd; 2010.
2. Erickson TB, Prendergast HM. Procedures pertaining to hyperthermia. In: Roberts JR, Hedges JR, Chanmugan AS, et al., editors. Clinical procedures in emergency medicine. 4th ed. Philadelphia: WB Saunders; 2004. p. 1358–70.
3. Fitzpatrick TB. The validity and practicality of sun-reactive skin types I through VI. Arch Dermatol. 1988;124(6):869–71.
4. Helman RS. Heatstroke. http://emedicine.medscape.com/article/166320-overview. Accessed 14 Oct 2015.
5. Syverud SA, Barker WJ, Amsterdam JT, et al. Iced gastric lavage for treatment of heatstroke: efficacy in a canine model. Ann Emerg Med. 1985;14(5): 424–32.
6. Webb P. The physiology of heat regulation. Am J Phys. 1995;268(4 Pt 2):R838–50.

Suggested Reading

Akhtar MJ, Al-Nozha M, Al-Harthi S, Nouh MS. Electro-cardiographic abnormalities in patients with heat stroke. Chest. 1993;104(2):411–4.
American College of Sports Medicine Joint Statement. National Athletic Trainers' Association. Inter-association task force on exertional heat illnesses consensus statement. 2003.. Available at https://www.nata.org/ sites/default/files/inter-association-task-force-exertional-heat-illness.pdf. Accessed 13 Aug 2010.
Armstrong LE, De Luca JP, Hubbard RW. Time course of recovery and heat acclimation ability of prior exertional heatstroke patients. Med Sci Sports Exerc. 1990;22(1):36–48.
Ash CJ, Cook JR, McMurry TA, Auner CR. The use of rectal temperature to monitor heat stroke. Mo Med. 1992;89(5):283–8.
Bettari L, Fiuzat M, Shaw LK, Wojdyla DM, Metra M, Felker GM, et al. Hyponatremia and long-term outcomes in chronic heart failure--an observational study from the Duke Databank for Cardiovascular Diseases. J Card Fail. 2012;18(1):74–81.
Bouchama A, Dehbi M, Chaves-Carballo E. Cooling and hemodynamic management in heatstroke: practical recommendations. Crit Care. 2007;11(3):1–17. [serial online]. 05/12/07. Accessed 02 Mar 07. Available at http://ccforum.com/content/11/3/R54.
Bouchama A, Knochel JP. Heat stroke. N Engl J Med. 2002;346(25):1978–88.
Brothers RM, Bhella PS, Shibata S, Wingo JE, Levine BD, Crandall CG, et al. Am J Physiol Heart Circ Physiol. 2009;296(4):H1150–6.
Burgess CM. Cosmetic dermatology. Berlin/Heidelberg: Springer; 2005.
Centers for Disease Control and Prevention. Extreme heat: a prevention guide to promote your personal health and safety. Updated July 31, 2009. Available at http://emergency.cdc.gov/disasters/extreme-heat/heat_guide.asp.

Chou YT, Lai ST, Lee CC, Lin MT. Hypothermia attenuates circulatory shock and cerebral ischemia in experimental heatstroke. Shock. 2003;19(4):388–93.

Davis JC, Kizer KW. Diving medicine. In: Auerbach PS, Geehr EC, editors. Management of wilderness and environmental emergencies. 2nd ed. St. Louis: CV Mosby; 1989. p. 879–905.

Dean R, Mulligan J. Management of water incidents: drowning and hypothermia. Nurs Stand. 2009;24(7):35–9.

Decraemer WF, Funnell WRJ. Anatomical and mechanical properties of the tympanic membrane. In: Ars B, editor. Chronic otitis media. Pathogenesis-orientated therapeutic management. The Hague: © Kugler Publications; 2008. p. 51–84.

DeFranco MJ, Baker CL 3rd, DaSilva JJ, Piasecki DP, Bach BR Jr. Environmental issues for team physicians. Am J Sports Med. 2008;36(11):2226–37.

Denoble PJ, Caruso JL, Dear Gde L, Pieper CF, Vann RD. Common causes of open-circuit recreational diving fatalities. Undersea Hyperb Med. 2008;35(6):393–406.

Easterling DR, Meehl GA, Parmesan C, Changnon SA, Karl TR, Mearns LO. Climate extremes: observations, modeling, and impacts. Science. 2000;289(5487):2068–74.

El-Kassimi FA, Al-Mashhadani S, Abdullah AK, Akhtar J. Adult respiratory distress syndrome and disseminated intravascular coagulation complicating heat stroke. Chest. 1986;90(4):571–4.

Epstein Y, Moran DS, Shapiro Y, Sohar E, Shemer J. Exertional heat stroke: a case series. Med Sci Sports Exerc. 1999;31(2):224–8.

Gasparro FP, Brown D, Diffey BL, Knowland JS, Reeve V. Sun protective agents: formulations, effects and side effects. In: Freedberg IM, editor. Fitzpatrick's dermatology in general medicine. 6th ed. New York: McGraw-Hill; 2003. p. 2344–52.

Ginsberg MD, Busto R. Combating hyperthermia in acute stroke: a significant clinical concern. Stroke. 1998;29:529–34.

Hadad E, Rav-Acha M, Heled Y, Epstein Y, Moran DS. Heat stroke a review of cooling methods. Sports Med. 2004;34(8):501–5611.

Han A, Maibach HI. Management of acute sunburn. Am J Clin Dermatol. 2004;5(1):39–4.

Heled Y, Rav-Acha M, Shani Y, Epstein Y, Moran DS. The "golden hour" for heatstroke treatment. Mil Med. 2004;169(3):184–6.

Huang KL, Wu CP, Chen YL, Kang BH, Lin YC. Heat stress attenuates air bubble-induced acute lung injury: a novel mechanism of diving acclimatization. J Appl Physiol. 2003;94(4):1485–90.

Hubbard RW, Gaffin SL, Squire DL. Heat-related illnesses. In: Auerbach P, editor. Wilderness medicine: management of wilderness and environmental emergencies. 3rd ed. St. Louis: Mosby Year Book; 1995. p. 167–212.

Hubbard RW, Matthew CB, Durkot MJ, Francesconi RP. Novel approaches to the pathophysiology of heatstroke: the energy depletion model. Ann Emerg Med. 1987;16(9):1066–75.

Hubbard RW. The role of exercise in the etiology of exertional heatstroke. Med Sci Sports Exerc. 1990;22(1):2–5.

Lomax P, Schonbaum E. The effects of drugs on thermoregulation during exposure to hot environments. Prog Brain Res. 1998;115:193–204.

Lowe NJ. An overview of ultraviolet radiation, sunscreens, and photo-induced dermatoses. Dermatol Clin. 2006;24(1):9–17.

Maier T, Korting HC. Sunscreens - which and what for? Skin Pharmacol Physiol. 2005;18(6):253–62.

Mazerolle SM, Ganio MS, Casa DJ, Vingren J, Klau J. Is oral temperature an accurate measurement of deep body temperature? A systematic review. J Athl Train. 2011;46(5):566–73.

Mazerolle SM, Pinkus DE, Casa DJ, et al. Evidence-based medicine and the recognition and treatment of exertional heat stroke, part II: a perspective from the clinical athletic trainer. J Athl Train. 2011;46(5):533–42.

McDermott BP, Casa DJ, Ganio MS, Lopez RM, Yeargin SW, Armstrong LE, et al. Acute whole-body cooling for exercise-induced hyperthermia: a systematic review. J Athl Train. 2009;44(1):84–93.

McGugan EA. Hyperpyrexia in the emergency department. Emerg Med (Fremantle). 2001;13(1):116–20.

MMWR. Heat-related illnesses, deaths, and risk factors–Cincinnati and Dayton, Ohio, 1999, and United States, 1979–1997. MMWR Morb Mortal Wkly Rep. 2000;49(21):470–3.

Moran DS, Gaffin SL. Clinical management of heat-related illness. In: Auerbach PS, editor. Wilderness medicine. 4th ed. St. Louis: Mosby; 2001.

Murphy C, Hahn S, Volmink J. Reduced osmolarity oral rehydration solution for treating cholera. Cochrane Database Syst Rev. 2004:CD003754.

Nalin DR, Hirschhorn N, Greenough W, et al. Clinical concerns about reduced-osmolarity oral rehydration solution. JAMA. 2004;291(21):2632–5.

Noonburg GE. Management of extremity trauma and related infections occurring in the aquatic environment. J Am Acad Orthop Surg. 2005;13(4):243–53.

Plattner O, Kurz A, Sessler DI, Ikeda T, Christensen R, Marder D, et al. Efficacy of intraoperative cooling methods. Anesthesiology. 1997;87(5):1089–95.

Polderman KH. Mechanisms of action, physiological effects, and complications of hypothermia. Crit Care Med. 2009;37(7 Suppl):S186–202.

Raju SF, Robinson GH, Bower JD. The pathogenesis of acute renal failure in heat stroke. South Med J. 1973;66(3):330–3.

Reid SR, Bonadio WA. Outpatient rapid intravenous rehydration to correct dehydration and resolve vomiting in children with acute gastroenteritis. Ann Emerg Med. 1996;28(3):318–23.

Roland PS, Belcher BP, Bettis R, Makabale RL, et al. A single topical agent is clinically equivalent to the combination of topical and oral antibiotic treatment for otitis externa. Am J Otolaryngol. 2008;29(4):255–61.

Roland PS, Stroman DW. Microbiology of acute otitis externa. Laryngoscope. 2002;112(7 Pt 1): 1166–77.

Schraga ED. Cooling techniques for hyperthermia. http://emedicine.medscape.com/article/149546-overview. Accessed 12 Oct 2015.

Shapiro Y, Seidman DS. Field and clinical observations of exertional heat stroke patients. Med Sci Sports Exerc. 1990;22(1):6–14.

Shibolet S, Lancaster MC, Danon Y. Heat stroke: a review. Aviat Space Environ Med. 1976;47(3): 280–301.

Squire DL. Heat illness. Fluid and electrolyte issues for pediatric and adolescent athletes. Pediatr Clin N Am. 1990;37(5):1085–109.

Stevens DL, Bisno AL, Chambers HF, Dellinger EP, Goldstein EJ, Gorbach SL, et al. Practice guidelines for the diagnosis and management of skin and soft tissue infections: 2014 update by the infectious diseases society of America. Clin Infect Dis. 2014;59(2):e10–52.

Tek D, Olshaker JS. Heat illness. Emerg Med Clin North Am. 1992;10(2):299–310.

Vicario SJ, Okabajue R, Haltom T. Rapid cooling in classic heatstroke: effect on mortality rates. Am J Emerg Med. 1986;4(5):394–8.

Van Laethem A, Claerhout S, Garmyn M, Agostinis P. The sunburn cell: regulation of death and survival of the keratinocyte. Int J Biochem Cell Biol. 2005;37(8):1547–53.

Walker SL, Hawk JL, Young AR. Acute effects of ultraviolet radiation on the skin. In: Freedberg IM, editor. Fitzpatrick's dermatology in general medicine. 6th ed. New York: McGraw-Hill; 2003. p. 1275–82.

Wyndham CH, Strydom NB, Cooke HM, Maritz JS, Morrison JF, Fleming PW, et al. Methods of cooling subjects with hyperpyrexia. J Appl Physiol. 1959;14: 771–6.

Yang YL, Lin MT. Heat shock protein expression protects against cerebral ischemia and monoamine overload in rat heatstroke. Am J Phys. 1999;276: H1961–7.

Yaqub B, Al DS. Heat strokes: aetiopathogenesis, neurological characteristics, treatment and outcome. J Neurol Sci. 1998;156(2):144–51.

Yarbrough B, Bradham A. Heat illness. In: Emergency medicine: concepts and clinical practice. 4th ed. St Louis: Mosby Year Book; 1998. p. 986–1002.

Yoder E. Disorders due to heat and cold. In: Goldman L, editor. Cecil textbook of medicine. 21st ed. Philadelphia: WB Saunders; 2001.

28

Venomous and Dangerous Marine Animals

© Springer International Publishing AG, part of Springer Nature 2018
O. Rusoke-Dierich, *Diving Medicine*, https://doi.org/10.1007/978-3-319-73836-9_29

29

A variety of different life forms arose throughout evolution. An important aspect for survival was defence and food supply. Protection was provided by camouflage or by defensive mechanism. Some animals developed venom or poison, so they became unattractive as prey. Some fish have spines, which contain venom; some other animals have poison within the body to make them unattractive for consumption. Especially sick, weak animals or carrion are preferred prey. By this, nature on the one hand is cleaned up, and on the other hand, it guarantees "strong, healthy" animals to survive and reproduce. At the end of the food chain are predators like sharks, barracudas and humans who are benefiting from marine food sources. A variety of marine animals could harm divers by their venom, electrocution or biting. But mainly carelessness is putting divers at risk. Either unintentional touching of venomous fish or provocation of marine life is a major cause of injuries by marine animals. But even if divers behave prudently, injuries and envenomation may occur.

29.1 Marine Invertebrates

29.1.1 Jellyfish

Jellyfish consist of 99% of water and are found in virtually all seas. In general their presence is seasonal. Due to ocean currents and nutrient supply, jellyfish are mainly restricted to coastal areas. Occasionally they travel large distances into the open sea during their different life cycles.

Tentacles are found at the bottom of jellyfish. While it is safe to touch them from above, a contact with tentacles can have serious consequences. Tentacles have capsules (nematocysts) containing venom, which serves to protect or to catch prey. They can be quite long, depending on the species. Single cell formations that produce and store venom in small vesicles are located on the tentacles. Inside these cell formations are thorns, which are spirally pulled together. They remain permanently under tension. After contact they are discharged, and the venom literally gets catapulted out. The thorn penetrates the

skin, and venom is injected in varying quantities. Contacts with harmless jellyfish are only uncomfortable. Usually localized, painful skin reactions are the result of it. Commonly a string-like, reddish purple rash is visible. However, in some jellyfish the reaction is more serious. Further physical symptoms, such as fever, fatigue, restlessness, headache and respiratory problems, and gastrointestinal and cardiovascular symptoms may occur. Allergies to jellyfish venom can develop after previous disposition. It even can cause anaphylactic reactions with shock or airways obstruction. All reactions to jellyfish can also occur, if there is a contact with dead animals lying on the beach (◘ Fig. 29.1).

The most venomous jellyfish is the *box jellyfish*. With quite small bodies of 20 cm, they may have up to 3 m long tentacles. They are found in the warm waters of north-east Australia, close to shore. They are usually not found within the Great Barrier Reef or open waters. However, in an opportunistic deep-sea video study, large numbers had been found at depths of 39–56 m. As the juvenile form hatches in tidal rivers, they are frequently present around areas where rivers

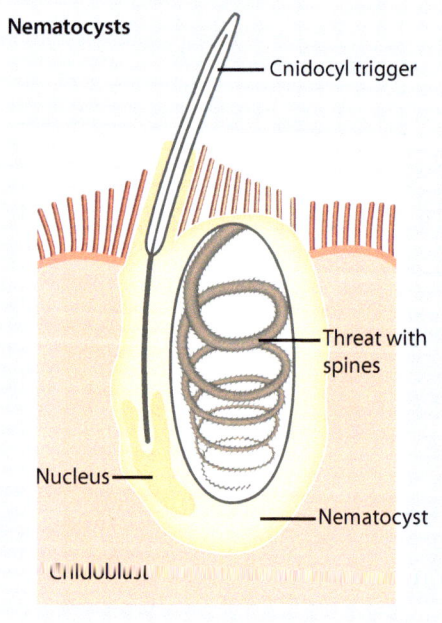

◘ **Fig. 29.1** Nematocysts (Wikipedia)

enter the sea. They appear commonly in warm seasons from November to April, particularly after rain and strong winds. The times vary, depending on local conditions. Unprotected swimming or diving should be avoided around this time. It is little known about its venom. But we know it is cardio- and neurotoxic and potentially fatal. Symptoms appear within seconds. Deaths occur commonly within the first 10 min as a result of cardiac arrest (initially tachycardia, then transition to bradycardia and cardiac arrest) and respiratory problems, particularly if welts caused by tentacles are longer than 70 cm. People with a pre-existing heart and lung conditions are particularly at risk. After contact, small, reddish-brownish spots as well as welts, blisters and rapid swelling of the affected area occur. Strong pain persists for 4–12 h. After about 7–10 days, deep wounds and tissue destruction may appear. Necrosis may occur after 1–2 weeks. Healing of these wounds takes sometimes up to several months. Hypo- or hyperpigmentation can develop later (■ Fig. 29.2).

A similarly dangerous jellyfish species is the *Irukandji*. The Irukandji is found at the north and north-eastern coast of Australia, Indonesia, Pacific and Gulf of Mexico. Its venom is a sodium channel agonist and causes an enormous release of noradrenalin, which is responsible for the adrenergic symptoms. It is only about 12–20 mm in size but can be fatal. The tentacles are only a few centimeter long when contracted but can be extended 10 times of their length. The contact is initially painless (first 5–40 min). After that severe pain devel-

ops, first in the abdominal, lumbar and sacral area and then spreads over the rest of the body. Sweating, headache, anxiety, tachycardia and extreme hypertension, which can lead to heart failure or cerebral haemorrhage, may occur. The pain peaks are typically intermittent. Localized goose bumps may develop at the injection site. Approx. 10–18 h later, pulmonary oedema can develop as a complication (■ Fig. 29.3).

Other jellyfish species are the *bluebottle* and the *lion's mane jellyfish*. The bluebottle is distributed in the Atlantic and Pacific Ocean. Individual tentacles can even reach up to 50 m. The lion's mane jellyfish is found in the North Sea and Baltic Sea and Mediterranean Sea. Lion's mane jellyfish of 2 m in diameter had been sighted. Contact with tentacles of both jellyfish causes a stringlike rash. Pain and tissue swelling, spreading over the rest of the body, may develop, starting from the affected area (■ Fig. 29.4).

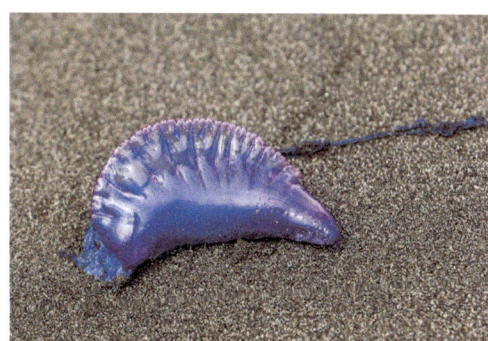

■ **Fig. 29.3** Bluebottle (Copyright Martin Schlecht/ Fotofolia)

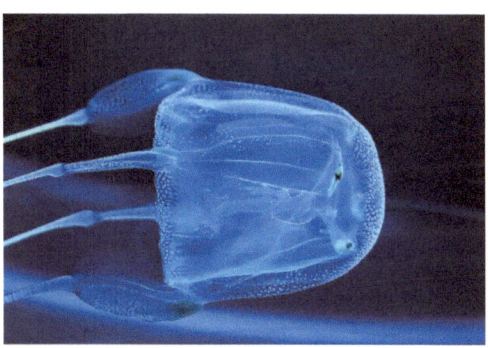

■ **Fig. 29.2** Box jellyfish (Copyright linkie/ Fotofolia)

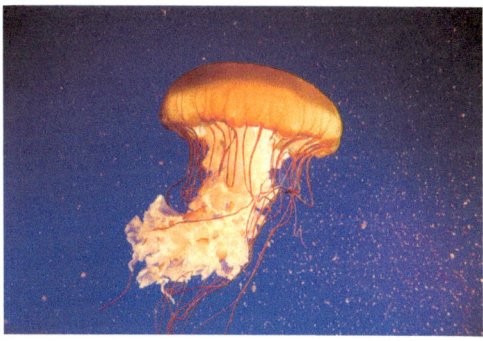

■ **Fig. 29.4** Lion's mane jellyfish (Copyright flippi/ Fotofolia)

An allergic reaction may develop with all jellyfish contacts, even with harmless jellyfish. This means that the otherwise rather harmless jellyfish can trigger a severe shock reaction in humans. Some venom is more likely to cause cross allergies. Especially the venom of more dangerous jellyfish has the tendency to do so. Direct effects of the venom in combination with allergic reactions potentiate highly venomous jellyfish. Each of those can cause a significant drop in blood pressure and tachycardia. Allergic reactions require corresponding predisposition to allergens. To become allergic to a substance, at least single contact to activate the typical immune response for an allergic reaction has to take place. Sometimes, also cross-reactions are possible, where an allergic reaction occurs when an allergy to a similar substance exists. Hence, even without having ever had a contact to this particular substance, allergic reactions can occur.

■ **Treatment**

A person, who got in contact with *box jellyfish*, should be removed from the water as quickly as possible to prevent drowning but also to start resuscitation, if required. If the person suffers from cardiac arrest, resuscitation should be commenced at once. The initial treatment for injuries caused by the box jellyfish is application of vinegar to the affected area for at least 30 s (but can be applied until ambulance arrives) after removal of the tentacles. Studies have shown that application of 4–6% vinegar reduces the excitability of the remaining undischarged nematocysts (▶ Box 29.1). Thus it prevents that potential excessive amount of nematocysts fire off and inject more venom. There may be only as little as 20% of the nematocysts discharged. Hence, the toxic load is significantly reduced by disabling the remaining 80%. New findings challenge the conventional therapy recommendations. As shown in recent in vitro studies by Seymour (2014) [5], nematocysts apparently do not completely empty. Treatment with vinegar seems to cause further depletion of the previously discharged nematocyst and therefore increases up to 69% (± 32%) of their venom

> **Box 29.1   Initial Treatment for Box Jellyfish and Irukandji** [1]
> — *Box jellyfish management*
> — Retrieve victim
> — Start CPR if necessary
> — Remove tentacles, if possible
> — Pour for at least 30 s vinegar on tentacles
> — Send for help/ambulance

load. However, vinegar treatment prevents the release of venom of the remaining undischarged nematocyst. Compared to that, hot water application may reduce only the venom load of the already undischarged nematocyst. Additionally hot water treatment poses the risk of releasing more venom from the remaining undischarged nematocyst. Therefore, vinegar treatment is still the first-line treatment. However, hot water application after the vinegar treatment and removal of tentacles can be considered. Hot water application or heat packs require 39–45 °C to be effective. They have to be applied after application of vinegar and removal of tentacles for 20 min. Complications might be burns and scalding. This makes the hot water application as a treatment rather unpractical. Cardiac arrest can occur, especially in the initial phase of envenomation and requires immediate resuscitation. Tentacles of jellyfish should not be brushed off, as they may discharge further and increase the toxin load. Washing of the tentacles with fresh water or alcohol also worsens the symptoms. It might cause more nematocysts to discharge and additional venom to be injected into the skin. It is recommended either to pull off the tentacles or wash them off with salt water. After manual removal of the tentacles, the helper should wash carefully the hands, to avoid discharge of nematocysts, which might be still attached to the hands. The thick skin of fingers seems to prevent the box jellyfish nematocysts from penetrating the skin of the helper, which means that remaining tentacles can be plucked off using the fingertips. It is still safer to avoid any contact with the tentacles. Antidote is available for box jellyfish envenomation. In unresponsive cardiac arrest, a vial of box jellyfish antivenom should be administered over 5–10 min. Maximum of six vials can be given. For cardioprotection magnesium sulphate 50% may be given iv over 5–15 min. After about 5–10 min after a box jellyfish sting, the chance of survival is approx. 100%. Because box jellyfish injuries are very painful, a sufficient quantity of analgesia should be given. Local anaesthetics (lidocaine) and narcotics (morphine or fentanyl) are recommended.

The initial treatment of an *irukandji* contact is similar to the one of the box jellyfish. The follow-up treatment includes mainly pain relief and treatment of hypertension as these are the main symptoms. If hypertension persists after administration of appropriate analgesia, aggressive arrhythmic and antihypertensive treatment (GTN) may be considered. Extreme hypertension could cause end organ damage (especially the brain, heart, liver and kidney). Therefore ECG monitoring and regular blood test (troponin and ELFTs) are necessary. Regular CK and troponin should be checked within the first 48 h. CXRs are required after 24 h to check for signs of pulmonary oedema [2]. Administration of intravenous magnesium may be considered for the irukandji syndrome, but there are no strong evidence of its effectiveness. For nausea slow iv promethazine 10–25 mg is the preferred choice, as a side effect of promethazine is lowering the blood pressure. In pulmonary oedema GTN infusions, CPAP or intubation could be considered.

A general measure in all other *jellyfish injuries* (box jellyfish and irukandji excluded) is hot water applications for 20 min instead the previous recommendation of ice application [4]. Ice reduces pain though but doesn't inactivate venom. Because jellyfish venom is unstable to heat, hot water applications help to destroy their protein structure. Because some toxins reduce skin sensitivity, water should be tested on other body parts before using it in the sting area, to avoid burns and scalding. The water should exceed 39 °C and should be as hot as tolerated.

Adrenalin, intravenous steroids and rapid volume replacement is recommended for

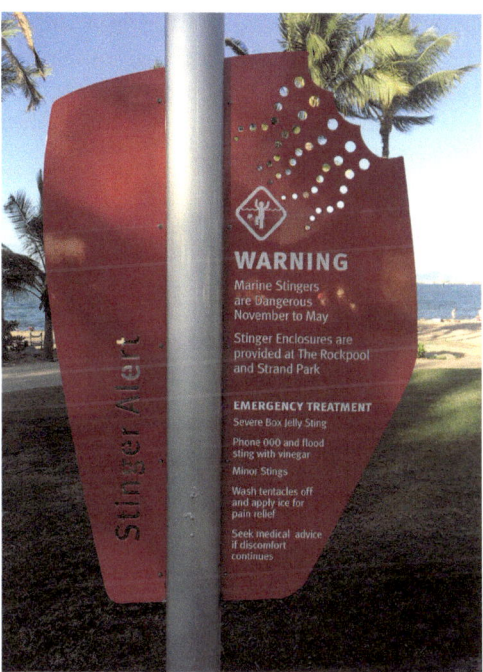

Fig. 29.5 Warning signs for stingers in Australia

anaphylactic reactions. In milder cases, antihistamines and oral steroids can be used. Wounds should be disinfected and dressed. Sulfadiazine silver cream and gauze dressing can be applied. If the wound becomes necrotic, surgical intervention may be necessary (**Fig. 29.5**).

29.1.2 Fireworm, Annelids, Sea Anemones, Sponges and Sea Cucumbers

Some fireworms, annelids, sea cucumbers, starfish, sea anemones, molluscs and sponges can cause itching, pain and swelling after skin contact. Symptoms usually don't remain for long. However, the more often contact with these animal occurs, the more severe reactions become. These animals contain similar to jellyfish venom for protection against other animals. Sea cucumbers, for example, can turn their insides out, so that the attacker is exposed to the venomous mucus from the gastrointestinal tract. This mucus adheres well to the skin and

29

is difficult to be washed off. Also sea anemones have venom. Some fish, like the clown fish, have a layer of mucus that neutralises the venom, so that they are able to live symbiotically with them (◘ Figs. 29.6, 29.7, and 29.8).

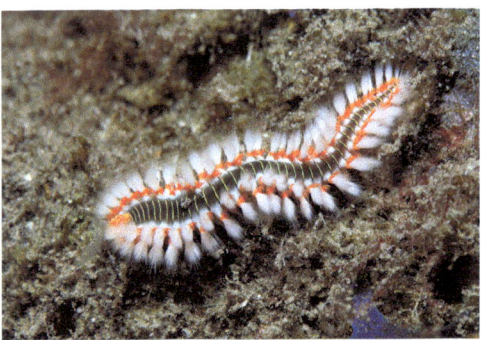

◘ **Fig. 29.6**   Fireworm (Copyright aquapix/Fotofolia)

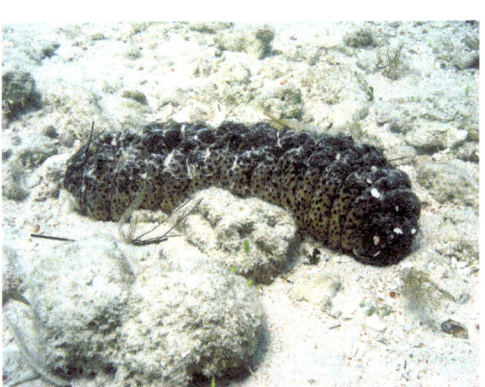

◘ **Fig. 29.7**   Sea cucumber (Copyright Christian Schoettler/Fotofolia)

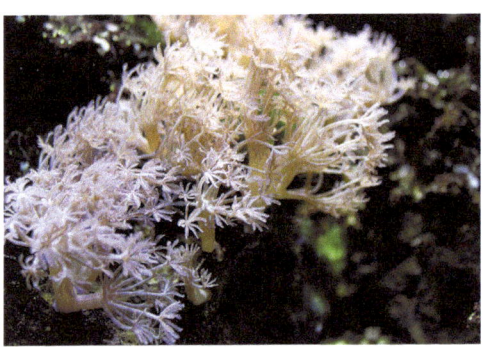

◘ **Fig. 29.8**   Sea anemone (Copyright rbkelle/Fotofolia)

■ **Treatment**

The skin reactions can be treated with antihistamines. More severe reactions might require steroids or treatment for anaphylaxis.

29.1.3 Corals

Simple cuts from corals are the main cause of coral injury. Directly after the injury, only a cut might be visible (◘ Fig. 29.9). After a few hours, discrete redness around the wound may develop. Within the next few days, the whole area might become swollen and reddened. Coral cuts commonly cause infections.

Many corals have nematocysts like the jellyfish. Likewise in jellyfish, they have different level in toxicity. Especially *fire corals* can cause severe reactions. It ranges from localised swelling to severe systemic reactions. Symptoms are worse, if the skin is penetrated additionally. Due to cuts, venom may enter directly the bloodstream and cause strong anaphylactic reactions.

The wound should be thoroughly cleaned and foreign material removed. For infection prophylaxis, topical antibiotic ointments (e.g. Bactroban®) can be applied. Itching can be eased by additional calcium (3 x 1 effervescent tablets daily) or ordinary mosquito bites ointments and antihistamines. Cuts of corals

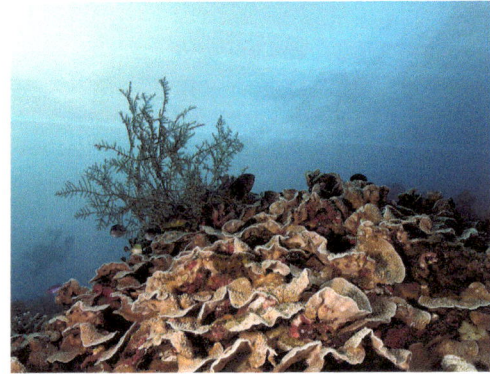

◘ **Fig. 29.9**   Fire coral (Copyright scubaluna/Fotofolia)

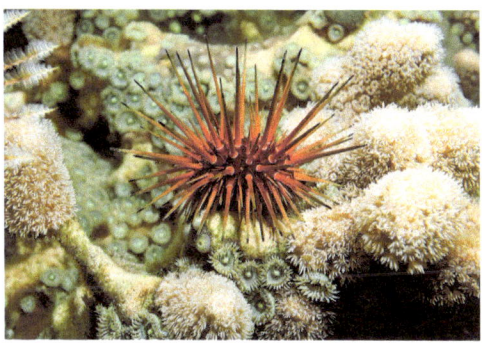

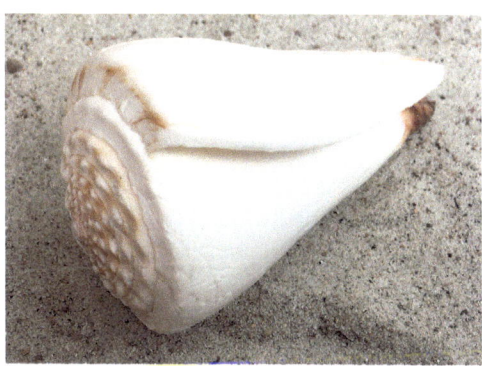

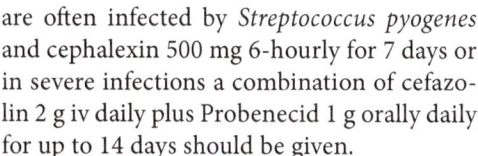
■ **Fig. 29.10**   Sea urchin (Copyright seaphotoart/Fotofolia)

■ **Fig. 29.11**   Cone Shell

are often infected by *Streptococcus pyogenes* and cephalexin 500 mg 6-hourly for 7 days or in severe infections a combination of cefazolin 2 g iv daily plus Probenecid 1 g orally daily for up to 14 days should be given.

29.1.4 Sea Urchins

Most *sea urchins* can be found close to shore (■ Fig. 29.10). About 14% of sea urchins are venomous. Strong symptoms of envenomation are however rare. Characteristics are their more or less thick spines that can inflict painful injuries on divers or swimmers. The thin spines penetrate easily the skin and break off. Parts of the spine may remain in the wound. Commonly spikes find their way out by themself. But if spikes remain in the skin, they have to be removed. Prior to removing the spikes, it is advisable to soak the affected area with warm soapy water. This is recommended only in acute injuries. The spines can be better removed of the skin as skin softens by using warm water. The soap also makes the water more alkaline, which prevents premature softening of the calcareous spikes. The spikes can be then removed using a forceps and needle. Sometimes surgical removal is necessary, if the spikes are in deeper layers of the skin and not visible. An ultrasound can be used to localise the spikes in the skin prior to surgical removal.

29.2 Cone Shell

Cone shells can eject a spike on their narrow end (■ Fig. 29.11). Great care should be taken by picking up seemingly "empty" snails, because the shell can withdraw into its housing and might not be visible. Thus, just by looking at it, it cannot be figured out, whether the shell is alive or not. Twenty-five percent of cone snail stings are fatal. Cone snails often are found in shallow waters. Their size varies from 2–10 cm. As the name implies, its structure is cone-shaped. Their venom (conotoxin) affects sodium channels of skeletal muscles. Others block calcium – channels and nicotinic transmitters on the postsynaptic membrane in cardiac and nerve tissues. This leads to paralysis with or without muscular pain (myalgia). The first symptoms may occur as early as 10 min. Paralysis and paraesthesia commences usually in the perioral area and lips. Then, the symptoms continue to spread over the entire body. In mild envenomations, paralysis can mimic general muscle weakness. Neurological symptoms, like double vision, dysarthria, and ataxia, may develop. Severe envenomation may lead to generalised paralysis with respiratory and cardiac failure. Respiratory paralysis and the resulting lack of oxygen cause cyanosis (bluish discoloration especially lips and fingernails). The victim still has a strong respiratory thrive, but cannot breathe due to the paralysis of respiratory muscles. Within 24 h, the paralysis disappears completely. However, other neurological symptoms and the local reaction at the injection site can remain for many more weeks.

The wound should be covered immediately with hot compresses (up to 45 °C) for 20 min. A consistently high temperature is achieved by continuously changing compresses. Animal venom, which consists of protein, can be denatured by high temperatures. Distribution of the venom throughout the body can be reduced by pressure compression bandages and splinting, to minimise lymphatic flow. Pressure immobilisation is recommended [3]. Compression bandages are applied initially distally of the wound and then extending proximally. If no paralysis is present, patients should be only immobilised. If paralysis is present, patients may need to be ventilated. The paralysis usually resolves after 12–36 h. A mouth to mouth resuscitation, which might have to be carried over hours, can save the patient's life. Cardiac compressions only have to be performed in cardiac arrest. There is no antivenom available for conotoxin. There are some suggestions that edrophonium can be used for the treatment of paralysis. An initial test dose of 2 mg iv followed by 8 mg iv might be effective. In case of an adverse reaction to edrophonium, atropine 0.6 mg can be used. 2 to 4 mg naloxone might be effective for treatment of hypotension.

29.3 "Giant Clams"

The giant clam (Tridacna gigas) is referred by many as killer clams (■ Fig. 29.12). It is the largest bivalve organisms that ever lived. The giant clams can be found in the warm waters of Australia, Micronesia and the southern Japanese islands. Other giant clams can be found all over of the world. However, they are much smaller. Giant clams can grow up to 1 m in length and 430 kg in weight. Sought after as souvenirs and for its tasty meat, they were almost extinct. Australia began to breed them and gradually reintegrate them again into their

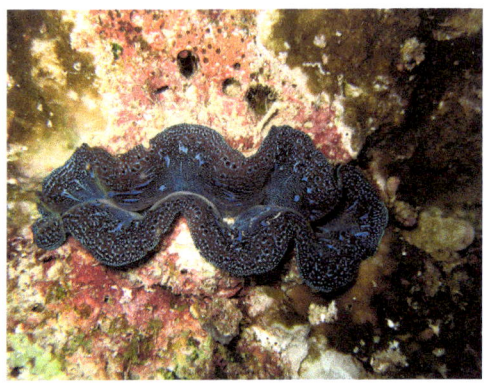

■ **Fig. 29.12** Giant clam (Copyright Wernerrieger/Fotofolia)

natural habitat. They cause no harm to humans. In particular, large specimens close very slowly, as they have to displace large amount of water during closing. Even when the large clam is closed, it is possible to pull out an object with the size of an arm. The smaller the clams are actually "more dangerous" for divers, as the gab becomes increasingly smaller on smaller clams. If divers get caught in a clam, which is attached to the reef, they might get trapped. This of course could have disastrous consequences. However, the likelihood is negligible.

29.4 Blue-Ringed Octopus

The blue-ringed octopus (Hapalochlaena lunulata) lives off the Australian coasts and the Indo-Pacific region (■ Fig. 29.13). It lives close to shore at a depth of 0–10 m. It is often found in rock pools, in cracks, mussels or other items. It is yellow-brown, has a ring-shaped drawing on its tentacles and is only about 2–20 cm in size. The rings become intense blue under stress and feeding. Its main toxin is tetrodotoxin (TTX) and more toxic than all known toxins. It was previously described as maculotoxin. The TTX is found in the saliva glands of the octopus. The octopus doesn't produce this toxin by itself. Actually, large amounts of bacteria harboured within the salivary glands are producing the TTX. One blue-ringed octopus has enough

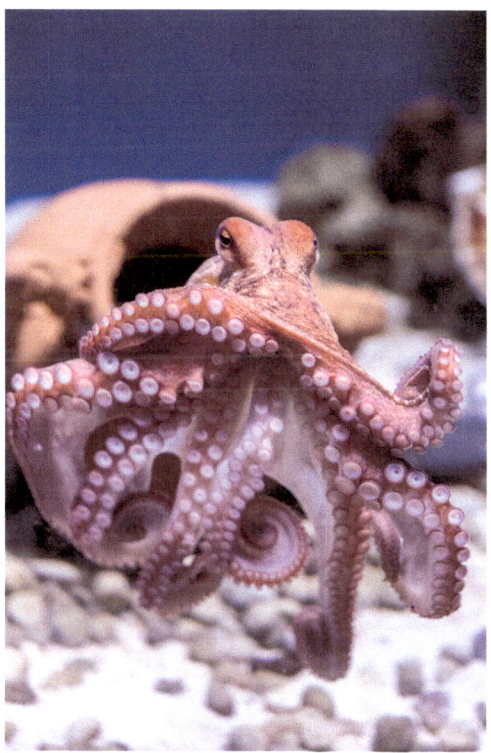

■ Fig. 29.13 Blue-ringed octopus (Copyright Andrea Lzotti/Fotofolia)

venom to kill ten adult humans. The venom has similar effects as the tetrodotoxin from the pufferfish's bile. TTX blocks sodium channels and causes paralytic symptoms. It doesn't affect the heart or brain. The octopus bite occurs usually accidental. It is rarely felt, as it causes no or minimal pain. The bite marks are hardly recognisable. The area swells within 5–10 min and blood blisters may appear. Then paralysis develops after a few minutes. Initially, it may cause abnormal sensations in the area of the mouth, neck and head. Double vision, slurred speech, nausea and vomiting may develop next, followed by rapid onset respiratory distress, dilatation of the pupils (mydriasis) and progressive paralysis of the entire body. The paralysis lasts usually for 4–12 h. Some other octopuses produce also similar venom. But their venom is much weaker and causes only local reactions.

■ **Treatment**

Due to the high toxicity, immediate transport to the nearest hospital is recommended after a bite of a blue-ringed octopus. To prevent a wider distribution of the venom, pressure bandage and splinting should be supplied on the affected limb. *Maintaining sufficient respiration by assisting ventilation until arrival of medical personal is lifesaving.* The use of antihistamines and cortisone is only indicated for allergic reactions. Bradycardia may be treated with atropine, if required. In severe cases ventilation is required for up 2 to 5 days. However, recovery is usually less than 24 h.

29.5 Fish

29.5.1 Venomous Fish

A number of fish, especially in tropical waters, are venomous. The venom is predominantly in their spines. Usually, contacts with their spines are accidental, as venomous fish usually are not aggressive. They often reside in shallow water. Some species, such as, for example, the extremely venomous scorpion- and stonefish, are very well camouflaged and easily be confused with a stone or a piece of coral. *Stonefish* have a round shape and may be up to 30 cm in length. Its venom is located in the dorsal fins. The venom of one spike is sufficient to kill an adult horse. The colour and texture of its skin can adjust to the surrounding. In addition, the skin has a mucus layer that makes algae, pieces of coral, stones and others stick to it. Thus, the camouflage is perfect. Often, stonefish only can be detected by their U-shaped mouth. Stonefish are the most venomous fish. Obviously they are aware of it. Even coming close to them, they won't move. They are bad swimmers and rather hop over the ground and swim only short distances. Its venom is neurotoxic, myotoxic, cardiotoxic and cytotoxic (■ Fig. 29.14).

The *scorpionfish* is a close relative of the stonefish. He also is a camouflage artist. Its shape is elongated, and it can swim quite well and quickly. If it swims, his bright orange-red

29

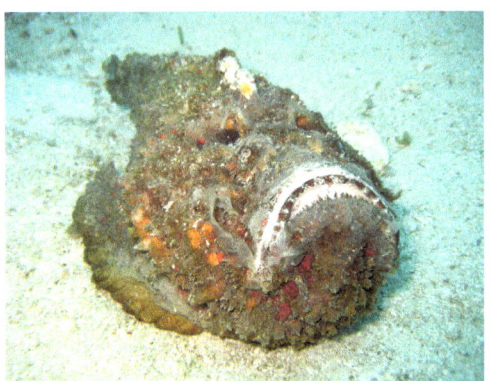

■ **Fig. 29.14** Stonefish (Copyright wenerrieger/Fotofolia)

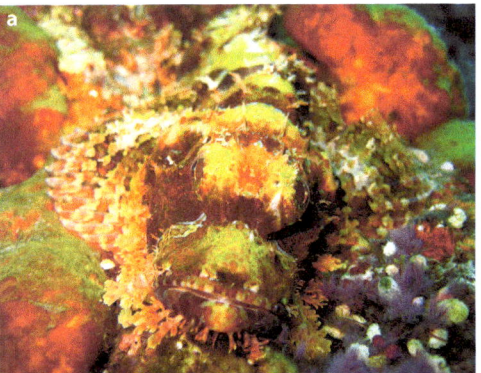

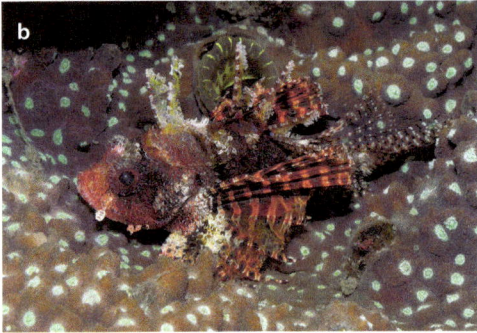

■ **Fig. 29.15** Scorpionfish. **a** (Copyright wenerrieger/Fotofolia) + **b** (CopyrightFotofolia)

pectoral fins can be seen. Usually it is stationary and not aggressive. Stone- and scorpionfish lie flat on coral and stones or burrow in sand (■ Fig. 29.15a, b).

Another relative is the *lionfish*. It is easy to recognise by its red and white stripes and

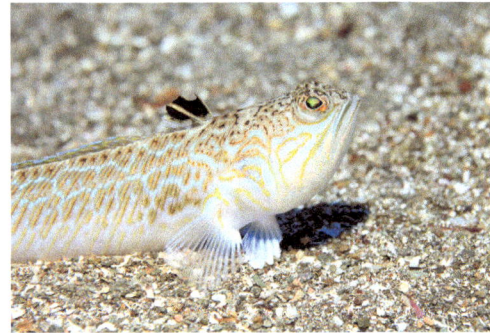

■ **Fig. 29.16** Weever fish (Copyright aquapix/Fotofolia)

its magnificently large pectoral fins. He often floats behind coral blocks. Stonefish, scorpionfish and lionfish can be found in tropical waters.

Some scorpionfish and the *weever fish* are to be found in temperate waters. The weever fish stays on the ground of sandy shore areas. If it is irritated or feels threatened, it can attack. Weever fish swim with the dorsal fins pointed along the alleged attacker and stabs them several times with their dorsal fins (■ Fig. 29.16).

Scorpionfish of temperate seas lay mostly motionless on the ground. It is to be found mainly on rocky shores close to shore. They are quite common, and sometimes you will be surprised when you snorkel and see how many scorpionfish you just passed by walking in.

The most venomous fish are stonefish. Less venomous are scorpionfish (tropical), lionfish, followed by weever fish and scorpionfish of temperate seas. According to their toxicity, symptoms vary. Stings of venomous fish are extremely painful. Pain appears immediately and increases over the next 10 min and radiates along the lymphatic pathways. Poor blood supply with white discoloration of the skin and swelling in the wound area develop. Diaphoresis, hypotension, loss of consciousness, fever, chills and fatigue are following symptoms. Stonefish can cause paralysis, arrhythmias, bradycardia and cardiovascular failure with pulmonary oedema. The reduction in respiratory function results from pulmonary oedema and cerebral respiratory depression. Wound healing in venomous fish-related injuries can take up to months. Injured area can become necrotic and persist for months. In severe cases tissue necrosis can lead to amputation of the affected limb.

■ **Treatment**

Hot water or hot compresses at temperatures up to 45 °C should be applied at the injury site for 30 to 90 min or till the pain subsides. It is an important treatment soon after the injury as the venom denaturates and becomes ineffective. Compression bandages and splinting may be applied. Administering pain medication provides symptom relief within few minutes. Local anaesthetic can be given for pain relief. If available, stonefish antidote can be administered with severe stonefish injuries.

■ **Venomous Fish Injury Treatment**

Acute

- Rescue
- Immediate application of hot water (up to 45 °C) on the bite area for approx. 30–90 min, till pain subsides
- Pressure bandage, splinting
- Resuscitation

Medical

- Local anaesthetic (lidocaine 1–2%, without adrenaline, can be combined with bupivacaine to prolong half-life)
- Pain control (opiates)
- Maintaining vital functions
- Administration of antidote (2000 U per 2 spine punctures, max. 6000 U; undiluted as im, diluted with 100 mL normal saline over 20 min iv, repeat 2000 U till local and systemic symptoms subside)

To prevent venomous fish injury, barefoot wading and touching coral or rocks should be avoided. As stonefish sometimes are burried in the sand or sitting on sandy ground, divers should inspect the place before settling down on the ground.

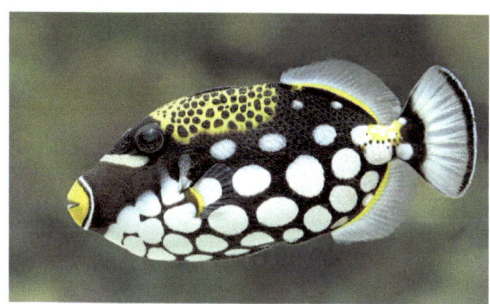

☐ **Fig. 29.17** Triggerfish (Copyright Herber Damke/Fotofolia)

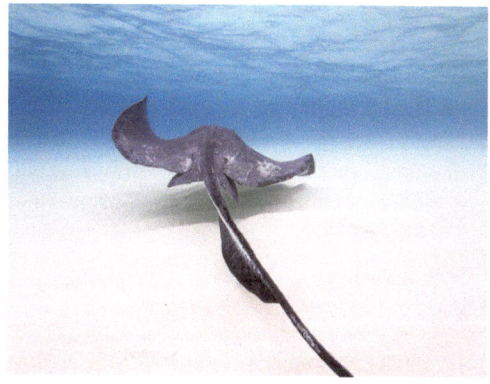

☐ **Fig. 29.18** Stingrays (Copyright penacino/Fotofolia)

29.5.2 **Triggerfish**

Triggerfish are found in all tropical waters (☐ Fig. 29.17). They are usually not aggressive. But when it comes to breeding season, they become territorial. Everyone who comes close to their nest gets attacked. They have strong jaws with sharp front teeth. Depending on the size of the triggerfish, bite injuries can be few centimeters big. The sparkling, round eggs are often found in funnel-shaped hollows of the sandy ground. The eggs can be also laid on corals.

29.6 **Rays**

Stingrays are cartilaginous fishes closely related to sharks (☐ Fig. 29.18). Their distribution is worldwide. However, they are

29

rather found in warmer waters. Some species swim constantly, and some burrow in sandy soil close to shore. Most stingrays have one or more toxins stored in their tail end. Stingrays are not aggressive, but they defend themselves, if they feel threatened. They can swing their tail like a whip and put a blow to the alleged attacker. Even without venom the thorn of the tail can cause fatal injuries, if the trunk area or large blood vessels are hit. The barbs of the thorn cause significant tissue damage, and the thorn may remain in the wound. These thorns contain additionally venom. The venom is based on proteins and can denaturate in hot water. Pain due to the venom commences immediately after the injury and increases within the next 1–2 h. It starts to decline after 6–10 h but will remain for several days. Generalised symptoms such as nausea, vomiting and unconsciousness can occur. The venom can cause arrhythmias (I-III degree AV block) and severe hypotension. Other symptoms that occur occasionally are respiratory depression, cough, agitation, confusion and delirium. Stingray envenomations can be also fatal in someone with pre-existing cardiovascular diseases. Wounds are often accompanied by tissue destruction and an infection, leading to delayed wound healing.

■ **Treatment**

As the thorn has barbs and can't be removed without causing major damage and hence should be removed only surgically in hospital. Initially, the tail of stingray may have to be cut off. With inadequate treatment, the wound can remain for months. Treatment against the venom is corresponding to treatment of venomous fish injuries, with hot water. The wound itself should be thoroughly cleaned and flushed. Foreign bodies should be removed. Wound infection is a common problem. Mild wound infections can be treated with Amoxicillin+Clavulanate 875 + 125 mg BD orally. Severe infection can be treated with iv

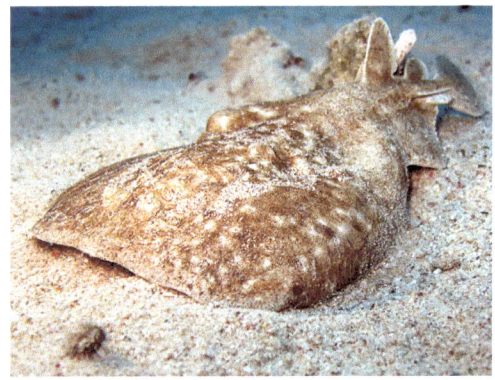

■ **Fig. 29.19**   Electric ray (Copyright lilithlita/Fotofolia)

cefazolin 2 g 8-hourly +500 mg metronidazole 12-hourly or Ticarcillin+Clavulanate 3 + 0.1 g 6-hourly. If vibrio species is suspected, a treatment of doxycycline as monotherapy or in combination with ceftriaxone is recommended. Wounds have to be dressed and disinfected on a daily base. If severe bleeding of wound occurs, blood loss control has priority (■ Fig. 29.19).

A different kind of rays uses electric shocks to hunt for prey or defence. *Electric rays* vary from 20 cm up to over 1–2 m in size depending on the species. They have the ability to unload voltage of up to 750 V, but usually it is around 20–50 V. Their electrocytes are usually arranged in columns in within their electric organs close to the head. The electricity usually gets discharged on the dorsal part, where the resistance is lower. These electrocytes act like batteries placed in a row, and the tension is created by summation. The electric ray hunts at night and recharges during the day. If threatened the shocks are mostly used to deter the potential attacker. However, electrical shocks can be dangerous for divers. An electric shock in the vulnerable period (ascending part of the T wave) of the cardiac excitation may be fatal under certain circumstances. But serious injuries are rather rare.

29.7 **Predators**

Sharks, moray eels and barracudas are among the maritime predators. The risk for divers is however far exaggerated. A diver is only attacked if it fits the pattern of prey, when predator is provoked or if the diver violates the territory. All marine animal bites need to be considered for antimicrobial treatment.

29.7.1 **Sharks**

Sharks are certainly not as voracious as assumed (■ Fig. 29.20). Sharks of 2.5 m in length eat about 70 kilograms prey per year, which is not a lot. The typical food of bigger sharks is sick animals and cadaver. The most sharks might be curious but not aggressive. There are, however, some sharks which display more aggressive behaviour than others. These include especially great white sharks, mako sharks, tiger sharks, blue sharks, bull sharks and hammerhead sharks. Shark attacks seem to be more frequent in specific areas. Especially on the coast of San Francisco, South Africa and South and Western Australia are among the most affected areas. Often surfers are attacked in areas where seals can be found. Others are in places with increased risk of shark attacks are where shark feeding is performed, as their natural fear of humans diminishes. Paradoxically, most shark attacks occur in knee-deep water. Divers are less at risk because they do not necessarily conform to the schema of prey. Sharks can perceive electromagnetic waves through special receptors on their muzzle over several kilometers. Hectic movements and blood attract them. Bright orange-red colour and silver glittering items are also subordinate key stimuli. The summation of all stimuli causes a shark to attack. The threshold is lower for the more aggressive sharks. Reef sharks have a pronounced territorial behaviour and may mistake divers as putative rivals. Invading their territory is provoking its aggressive behaviour. If divers remains in the area, they risk to get a warning bite to be deterred. The wounds caused by sharks are ragged wounds. Their prey is being held with the teeth. By fast back and forth shaking, a piece is pulled out. Their teeth are razor sharp and have small blades on their edges.

29.7.2 **Moray Eels**

Moray eels are normally not aggressive (■ Fig. 29.21). They are extremely short sighted and limited to perceive their environment visually. They only bite if provoked or if divers carelessly put their hands into a cave, where a moray eel resides. If they bite, they wedge

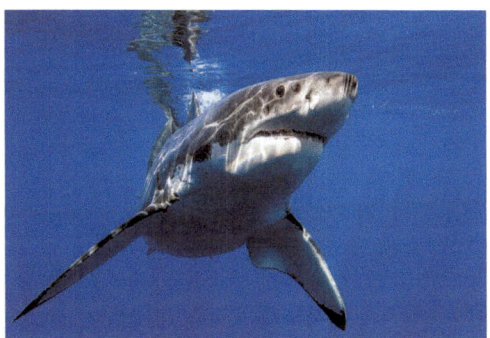

■ **Fig. 29.20** Shark (Copyright Andrea Lzotti/Fotofolia)

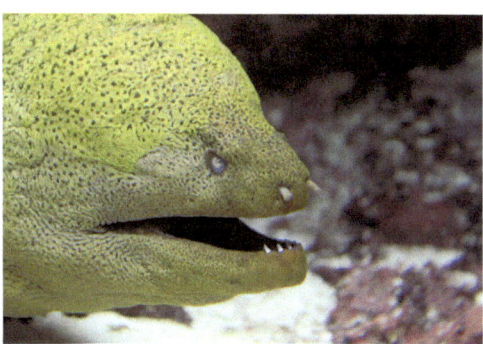

■ **Fig. 29.21** Moray eel (Copyright tino fotografie/Fotofolia)

29

themselves in their cave and don't let go. In case of a larger animal, this might be quite dangerous, as it will be difficult to get free to reach the surface. Moray eels are not toxic, as often falsely believed. However, leftovers of their meal can be located between their teeth, which can become toxic by decomposition.

29.7.3 Barracudas

Barracudas form schools at young age. Later in their life, they become individual hunters and grow up to more than 2 m long. They remain often motionless in the water, and caused by their camouflage they often might not be seen. Therefore, their attacks can be quite unexpected. They attack only after they have inspected their prey and have recognised it as such or if they feel threatened. In schools, they revolve around their victims to observe it. If it matches their prey pattern, they attack. Divers however don't really match their prey pattern. So no panic, but respect for the predator! The wounds caused by them have smooth edges as barracudas in contrast to the sharks with their razor-sharp teeth bite pieces out easily (■ Fig. 29.22).

■ Treatment

Bite injuries can cause in addition to organ injuries large blood losses. The result of the blood loss is hypovolemic shock or death. Blood loss over 3 l in an adult is fatal. But despite the blood loss, an attack with bite injuries is enough to cause shock symptoms. Injured divers need to be removed from the water first. Pressure bandages and pressure on large blood vessels proximal to the wound of the corresponding extremity can reduce the blood loss. The injured person should be recovered in a shock position. Blood loss initially can be replaced with intravenous fluids like normal saline solution and later with transfusions, if possible. Bites of morays are usually not extensive. But these bite injuries easily get infected. Such contamination can easily lead to a septicaemia.

■ Measures in Case of Bite Injuries
Acute
- DRCABD (see ▶ Chap. 31)
- Keep calm and reassure the injured person
- Bleeding control via pressure of the corresponding major blood vessels
- Shock treatment

Medical
- Volume substitution
- Primary wound care
- Stabilisation of the cardiovascular and respiration function
- Shock treatment
- Long-term wound care

29.8 Sea Snakes

Sea snakes belong to the family of Elapidae (■ Fig. 29.23). They are found in all tropical waters around the world. Their sensitivity to changes in temperatures limits their natural habitat. They do not tolerate water temperatures below 20 °C. On the other hand, body temperatures above 33–36 °C are fatal for sea serpents. Therefore, sea snakes may reside in the tropics sometimes far below the surface to avoid overheating. Snakes are well adapted to salty sea water and can stay long time under water. Excess salt is secreted by glands below their tongue. Their great lungs, which extend throughout the entire body, and their ability to

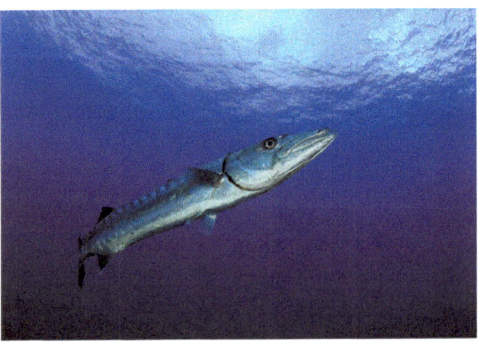

■ **Fig. 29.22**   Barracuda (Copyright Richard Carey/ Fotofolia)

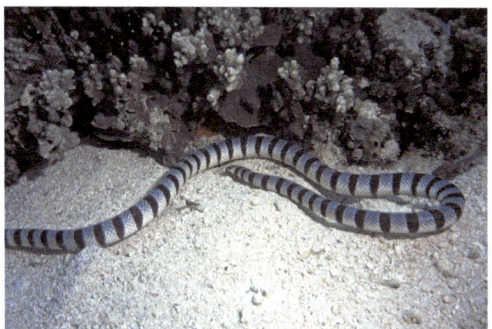

Fig. 29.23 Sea snake (Copyright RICO/Fotofolia)

tolerate low oxygen levels enable them to dive for a long period of time. Its highly effective venom is injected through fangs of the maxilla into the prey. Their venom is 2–20 times stronger than that of Cobras. However, often only a small amount of the venom is injected. Sea snakes seem to have a regulatory mechanism to dose the amount of venom. Eventually only a quarter of people who have been bitten show symptoms of envenomation. The injection of venom itself is often without significant symptoms and painless. The bite site has 1 to 20 entry points caused by their fan and other teeth. First symptoms appear in average after 30–90 min. Mild symptoms like vomiting, nausea and euphoria occur first. Stronger envenomation causes paralysis first with ptosis and double vision followed by muscle weakness, which spreads first to the respiratory muscles than over the rest of the body. Because the venom is myotoxic, it can cause myalgia due to disintegration of muscles (rhabdomyolysis), myoglobinuria (brown colouration of the urine) and hyperkalemia. Hence, monitoring of CK and renal function is essential. To avoid acute renal failure, early aggressive fluid therapy should be initiated. Sea snake venom in general doesn't affect the coagulation to a significant degree. The heat-stable toxin inhibits postsynaptic transmission in nerve cells. Initial treatment consists of applying of pressure bandages, splinting and immobilising of the limb. The bandage is applied with an elastic bandage directly over the wound. After that, the bandage is tightly fitted (as in sprains) distally (to the body periphery) and then proximally (towards the body centre). The limb then should be splinted to produce immobilisation. As venom spreads via lymphatic pathways, movement should be avoided as they trigger lymphatic flow. The location of the bite site should be marked as venom testing is directly performed of the penetration site. Bandages should not be taken off for venom testing in the hospital. The bandage should be only opened locally at the bite site. Snake bite envenomation can be also detected by urine testing. The patient should be transported immediately into the next hospital. Main initial treatment aim is to maintain vital functions and correct effects on the blood until toxicity subsides or an antidote is given. Antidotes should be only administered, only if significant symptoms of envenomation are present. Administration of antidote has a high risk of causing allergic reactions or subsequent allergies. Frequent administration of antivenom bears a higher risk of severe allergic reactions and administration hence should be considered carefully. After 4–14 days after receiving the antivenom, the person might suffer from a delayed serum sickness, with fever, rash, myalgia, arthralgia and nonspecific systemic features. For a moderate to severe serum sickness, 25–50 mg prednisolone for 7 days can be given.

29.9 Crocodiles

Crocodiles are creatures, which exist since the age of dinosaurs (Fig. 29.24). They have hardly changed in their appearance and behaviour since that time. However, it is not a "stupid" dinosaur but rather a highly differentiated animal with relatively large brain, measured against its body size. It has sophisticated hunting techniques but also pronounced social behaviour in bringing up their children. In many species the young animals find protection in the mother's mouth. Crocodiles are cold blooded, which means they need warmth from the outside, to maintain their body

29

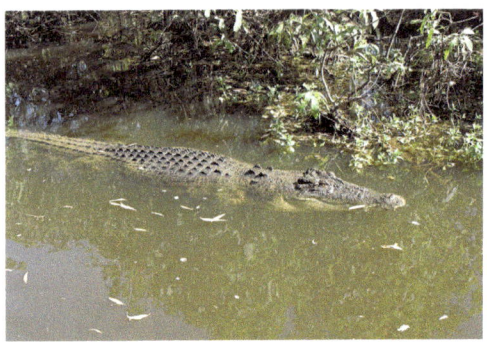

■ **Fig. 29.24** Crocodiles (Copyright alfotokunst/Fotofolia)

temperature. Crocodiles or alligators can be found in Northern Australia, in the tropical area of the Asia, Papua New Guinea, Africa, South and Central America and Florida. They vary in size depending on the species. Smaller species measure just 1 m, with the largest species reaching over 5 m. Most crocodiles are found in freshwater, where they usually are motionless or sunbathing on sand banks. Some species in Australia, Papua New Guinea and America reside in coastal salt water. Crocodiles can get up instantaneously from complete rest to catch prey. Over short distances, a full-grown animal can reach a speed of about 50 km/h. A crocodile attack results in severe and often fatal injuries. The best way to avoid crocodile injuries is widely to avoid contact with them. Crocodiles are active at night. Local warnings or warning signs should be taken seriously. An injury of a crocodiles should be treated as soon as possible as there is often substantial flesh and bone destruction and significant blood loss.

29.10 **Consumption of Marine Animals**

29.10.1 **Shellfish**

Planktonic toxins like *saxitoxin*, *brevetoxin and okadaic acid* can accumulate in *clams and mussels* (■ Fig. 29.25). Saxitoxin is produced by certain species of algae that occurs worldwide. This algae species gets absorbed by shellfish and

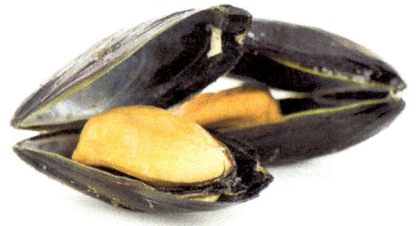

■ **Fig. 29.25** Intoxication may develop by consumption of shellfish (Copyright ppi09/Fotofolia)

other marine life and accumulates. Saxitoxin is a very strong poison that blocks sodium-potassium channels. Saxitoxin is the most potent toxin responsible for causing paralytic symptoms. Brevetoxin causes usually gastroenteritis and minor neurological symptoms. Okadaic acid mostly produces gastroenteritis. There are various ways such poisoning manifests. Mild forms show cutaneous signs (redness, swelling, itching and sensation of heat) and generalised symptoms (diarrhoea, vomiting and nausea). However, it can cause more severe symptoms like with paralysis too. Decisive for this poisoning is that they occur quite soon after the meal. The sooner symptoms begin, the stronger the poisoning is to be expected. As long as the poison remains in the body, symptoms will occur. As long as patients are symptomatic they should be observed. Saxitoxin can be detected in urine tests. Because algae bloom in warm seasons, consumption of shells and mussels should be limited during these months.

■ **Symptoms of Shellfish Poisoning**
Gastroenteritis
- Incubation 10–12 h
- Diarrhoea
- Vomiting
- Nausea

Skin
- Incubation of 2–3 h
- Erythema
- Itching of skin and swelling of face and neck
- Sensation of heat

- Headache
- Conjunctivitis
- Glottis oedema with stridor and obstructed breathing!

Neurological symptoms (mainly saxitoxin and brevetoxin)

- Incubation period 1–30 min
- Affects the entire body in up to 6 h
- Paralysis starting at the mouth, spreading all over the body
- Paraesthesia (face, limbs)
- Ataxia
- Epileptic seizures
- Dizziness
- Headache
- Palpitations
- Thirst
- Duration of 24 h and more

Therapy

- Immediately seek medical attention
- Increased fluid intake
- Stabilisation of vital functions
- Hydration

29.10.2 Pufferfish

Symptoms of intoxication can occur after consumption of improperly prepared *pufferfish* (☐ Fig. 29.26). Poorly gutted pufferfish can contaminate the entire fish with its bile. *Tetrodotoxin* can be mainly found in the bile but also found in the intestine, skin and gonads of the pufferfish. Tetrodotoxin

- **Symptoms of Poisoning by Consumption of Improperly Prepared Pufferfish**
- Occurs within 20 min to 8 h but mostly between 4–6 h
- Paralysis starting at the mouth, spreading all over the body
- Paraesthesia face and extremities
- Double vision
- Nausea, vomiting and diarrhoea
- Headache
- Dyspnoea and cyanosis

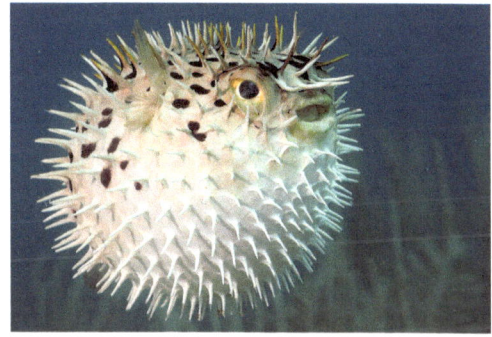

☐ **Fig. 29.26** Pufferfish (Copyright ftlaudgirl/ Fotofolia)

- Hypotension
- Arrhythmia
- Respiratory arrest
- Death

Therapy

- Seek immediate medical help.
- Stabilisation of vital functions.
- Treatment of hypotension (naloxone can be considered).
- Ventilation until paralysis subsides (up to 5 days).

29.10.3 Ciguatera

Ciguatera is another toxin that occurs with about 300 other fish families (doctor fish, parrotfish, triggerfish, perch, barracudas, butterfly fish, moray eels, snapper, street sweeper, wrasse, mackerel etc.). The toxin is caused by the marine microalgae (dinoflagellate) called *Gambierdiscus toxicus*, which accumulates in fish. The highest concentrations are found in the liver, gonads and intestines. Ciguatera is much less toxic than tetrodotoxin. It colonises on algae and is food of smaller fish. Ciguatera accumulates in larger fish at the end of the food chain (shark, mackerel, tuna, rays, eels, barracuda, red snapper, etc.). Ciguatera toxin acts as an inhibitor of sodium-dependent channels at neuromuscular end plates. It is not affected by heating or freezing. It is odourless and tasteless. No test is available for ciguatera; it is a clinical diagnosis.

Symptoms

- Incubation time 0–12 h (usually within minutes)
- Duration between 6 to 10 days (sometimes persists for months to years)
- Numbness of extremities
- Arthralgia
- Paraesthesia in the mouth (pain in teeth or feeling the teeth are loose)
- Metallic mouth taste
- Blurred vision or temporary blindness
- Paradoxical perception of temperature (hot is as perceived cold and vice versa)
- Nausea, vomiting and diarrhoea
- Cramps
- Pruritus
- Headaches
- Bradycardia
- Hypotension
- Pulmonary oedema
- Rigors
- Diaphoresis
- Coma, death

Therapy

- Atropine in bradycardia
- Mannitol (iv) only effective if commenced promptly
- Vitamin B complex and vitamin C
- Calcium
- Antihistamines
- Stabilisation of vital functions

29.10.4 Scombroid

Scombroid is created by bacteria in certain fish. Such species include mackerel and tuna. It is more likely when fish is left out in a warm environment for several hours. This toxin produces a histamine-like reaction likewise allergies. Histidine is converted to histamine by bacterial overgrowth. This occurs mainly in fish, which is not refrigerated properly. Burning around the mouth, facial flushing, palpitations,

nausea vomiting, diarrhoea, skin rash, confusion, shortness of breath (asthma), itching and anaphylactic shock may occur. The symptoms usually resolve by themselves. The skin reactions can be reduced by antihistamines. Severe intoxication requires in-hospital treatment.

Occurrence

- Tuna, mackerel, dolphin, anchovies, herring, bluefish, amberjack, sardine and marlin
- After extended in proper storage at warm temperatures

Toxin

- Scombroid
- Allergic reactions with mild to severe symptoms (rash, headache, palpitation, itching, blurred vision, abdominal cramps and diarrhoea)

Treatment

- Antihistamines (H1 and H2 receptor blockers)
- Steroids (prednisolone or hydrocortisone)
- Adrenalin (only in anaphylaxis)

29.10.5 Fish and Meat Poisoning

Meat and fish poisoning occur mostly due to contamination of food with bacteria and other pathogens. The symptoms such as nausea, vomiting, diarrhoea and fever usually occur after 2–48 h. The therapy depends on the severity of symptoms and the duration of the disease. Usually the treatment is symptomatically, and only in rare cases antibiotics are required.

References

1. Australian Resuscitation Council – ARC Guideline 9.4.5. Envenomation—Jellyfish stings 2010.
2. Fenner PJ, Williamson JA, Burnett JW, et al. The "Irukandji syndrome" and acute pulmonary oedema. Med J Aust. 1988;149(3):150–6.
3. Halford ZA, Yu PYC, Likeman RK, Hawley-Molly JS, Bingham CT, Bingham JP. Cone Shell envenomation: epidemiology, pharmacology and medical care. Diving Hyperb Med. 2015;45(3):200–7.

4. Loten C, Scokes B, Worsley D, et al. A randomised controlled trial of hot water (45 °C) immersion versus ice packs for pain relief in blue bottle stings. Med J Aust. 2006;184:329–33.

5. Ramasamy S, Isbister GK, Seymour JE, Hodgson WC. The IN VITRO effects of two (CHIRONEX FLECK-ERI and CHIROPSALMUS sp.) venoms: efficacy of box jellyfish antivenom. Toxicon. 2003;41:703–11.

Suggested Reading

Antibiotic Expert Group Therapeutic Guidelines: Antibiotic. Version 14 Melbourne: Therapeutic Guidelines Ltd; 2010.

Auerbach PS. Marine envenomations. N Engl J Med. 1991;325(7):486–93.

Australian Resuscitation Council – ACR9.4.7. Envenomation – fish stings July 2014.

Resuscitation Council – ARC Guideline 9.4.1. Australien Snake Bite 2011.

Australian Resuscitation Council – ARC Guideline 9.4.1. Australien Snake Bite 2011.

Australian Resuscitation Council – ARC Guideline 9.4.8. Pressure Bandage Technique 2011.

C. Dangerous Marine Creatures: Field Guide For Medical Treatment. 2nd ed. 1995. 63–68, 75–79, 239–249.

Edmonds C. Dangerous Marine Creatures: Field Guide For Medical Treatment. 2nd ed. Flagstaff: Best Pub. Co.; 1995. p. 63–68, 75–79, 239–249.

Fenner PJ, Lewin M. Sublingual glyceryl trinitrate as prehospital treatment for hypertension in Irukandji syndrome. Med J Aust. 2003;179(11–12):655.

Friedman MA, Fleming LE, Fernandez M, Bienfang P, Schrank K, Dickey R, et al. Ciguatera fish poisoning: treatment, prevention and management. Mar Drugs. 2008;6(3):456–79.

Gwee MC, Gopalakrishnakone P, Yuen R, et al. A review of stonefish venoms and toxins. Pharmacol Ther. 1994;64(3):509–28.

Habermehl G. Gift-Tiere und ihre Waffen. 5th ed. Berlin: Springer; 1994.

Isbister GK, Kiernan MC. Neurotoxic marine poisoning. Lancet Neurol. 2005;4(4):219–28.

Lalwani K. Animal toxins: Scorpaenidae and stingrays. BJA: Br J Anaesth. 1995;75:247.

Mers D. Gifte im Riff, vol. 1989. Stuttgart: Wissentschaftliche Verlagsgesellschaft; 1989.

Moczydlowski EG. The molecular mystique of tetrodotoxin. Toxicon. 2013;63:165–83.

Morrow JD, Margolies GR, Rowland J. Evidence that histamine is the causative toxin of scombroid-fish poisoning. N Engl J Med. 1991;324(11):716–20.

Stommel EW, Watters MR. Marine Neurotoxins: Ingestible Toxins. Curr Treat Options Neurol. 2004;6(2):105–14.

Sun KO. Management of puffer fish poisoning. Br J Anaesth. 1995;75(4):500.

Tiong K. Irukandji syndrome, catecholamines, and midventricular stress cardiomyopathy. Eur J Echocardiogr. 2009;10:334–6.

Watters MR, Stommel EW. Marine neurotoxins: Envenomations and contact toxins. Curr Treat Options Neurol. 2004;6:115–23.

Welfare P, Little M, Pereira P, Seymour J. An in-vitro examination of the effect of vinegar on discharged nematocysts of Chironex Fleckeri. Diving and hyperbaric medicine : the journal of the South Pacific Underwater Medicine Society. 2014;44(1):30–4.

Williamson JA, Fenner PJ, Burnett JW. Venomous and poisonous marine animals: medical and biological handbook. Sydney: U NEW SOUTH WALES P; 1996. p. 106–17, 374–87, 418–22

Winkel KD, Tibballs J, Molenaar P, Lambert G, Coles P, Ross-Smith M, Wiltshire C, Fenner PJ, Gershwin LA, Hawdon GM, et al. Cardiovascular actions of the venom from the Irukandji (CARUKIA BARNESI) jellyfish: effects in human, rat and guinea-pig tissues in vitro and in pigs IN VIVO. Clin Exp Pharmacol Physiol. 2005;32:777–88.

Assessment for Diving Fitness for Recreational Divers

© Springer International Publishing AG, part of Springer Nature 2018
O. Rusoke-Dierich, *Diving Medicine*, https://doi.org/10.1007/978-3-319-73836-9_30

Diving is different to most other sports as divers are exposed to different ambient pressures. This affects mainly air-filled organs in regard to barotrauma. Considering DCI, a holistic assessment including cardiovascular, respiratory, constitutional, endocrinological, comorbidities and pharmacological treatment needs to be conducted. Diving can also be a physical strenuous exercise on occasions. Therefore, physical fitness is very important in diving. As certain medical conditions increase the risk of DCI, diving fitness assessments are supposed to determine whether safety is ensured during diving. Diving fitness assessments are aiming for minimising medical risk factors in diving. There are different guidelines for recreational and commercial divers. Recommendation and guidelines vary from country to country.

Diving fitness assessments should be performed as followed:

30

- Every 3–5* years for divers between 18 and 40 years of age
- 1–3 years* in divers younger than 18 and older than 40 years of age
- Annually for any commercial divers
- Annually for divers who suffer from any chronic disease

*Depending on national requirements and recommendations

Contents of a diving fitness assessment

All Diving Fitness Assessments
- Level of diving experience (beginner, advanced) and reason for the dive medical (recreational or commercial)
- General fitness
- Medical and surgical past history
- Psychiatric history
- Medication
- Allergies
- Smoking, drugs and alcohol
- Full body examination, BP, pulse, weight, height, BMI, waistline and pregnancy

- Neurological examination (e.g. sharpened Romberg, reflex, nystagmus, cranial and peripheral nerves)
- Skeletal examination
- Cardiovascular and respiratory examination
- ENT examination (particularly Valsalva)
- Dental examination
- Tympanometry
- Spirometry
- Urinalysis

Initial Diving Fitness Assessments for Commercial Divers or Additional Assessments
- ECG
- Exercise stress test if there is a clinical concern, in divers above age 45, optional in professional divers
- Bloods like FBC, fasting lipids and sickle cell screen (optional at initial examination or if required)
- CXR (initial for all commercial divers or if required)
- Long-bone XR, (initial assessment for commercial divers)
- Audiometry
- Visual acuity testing

The initial examination for diving fitness should be detailed and thorough. Additionally, the initial dive fitness examination should include visual acuity testing, spirometry, audiometry and ECG. Tympanometry should be performed, if there is a suspicion of Eustachian tube dysfunction. Commercial divers should be tested for colour blindness on the initial examination (◘ Table 30.1). Exercise testing may be recommended to determine training status and to detect exercise-related cardiovascular disorders. In particular in divers above 40, exercise testing should be considered, if there is any concern. On initial examination or in the presence of respiratory diseases, a CXR may be considered to exclude structural changes of the lungs. Periodic CXRs are not necessary and therefore are not recommended for recreational or

■ **Table 30.1** Investigations during a fitness for diving assessment

Investigation	Recreational		Commercial	
	Initial	Regular[a]	Initial	Regular[b]
Audiometry	✓	Optional[c]	✓	Optional
Weight, BMI, waistline	✓	✓	✓	✓
BP, pulse	✓	✓	✓	✓
Colour blindness	✗	✗	✓	✗
CXR	Optional	✗	✓	Optional
Drug screen	✗	✗	✓	✓
ECG	✓	✓[c]	✓	✓
Exercise stress test (EST)	✗	✓[c]	Optional	✓[c]
Exercise testing	Optional	Optional[c]	✓	✓[c]
Fasting lipids	Optional[c]	Optional[c]	✓	✓[c]
FBC, ELFTs	Optional	✗	✓	✓
Long-bone XR	✗	✗	✓	✗
Pregnancy test	✓	✓	✓	✓
Sharpened Romberg	✓	✓	✓	✓
Sickle cell screen, thalassaemia	Optional	✗	✓	✗
Spirometry	✓	✓	✓	✓
Tympanometry	Optional	Optional	Optional	Optional
Urinalysis	✓	✓	✓	✓
Valsalva	✓	✓	✓	✓
Visual acuity	✓	Optional	✓	✓

[a]1–5 years dependent on age and medical status
[b]Annually
[c]Recommended above age 45 or any diving accident (barotrauma or DCI)

commercial divers. However, annual CXRs may be required for some professional divers. In particular divers working in areas where TB is likely and annual CXR might be considered. An alternative might be QFG (QuantiFERON®-TB gold) blood test to rule out latent TB. Only if positive, CXR would be required. Long-bone XRs are recommended in the initial assessment for commercial saturation divers as a baseline, as DON is a common workplace-related injury in these divers. Blood tests at the initial examination can be performed to determine diabetes, sickle cell anaemia, thalassaemia or other abnormalities of the blood. Extra investigations may be necessary for follow-up assessments, if the diver has underlying medical conditions. In general, audiometry and visual acuity testing are not necessary for consecutive dive medicals. However, it might be advisable to perform them regularly in divers over 45 and after ear barotraumas or inner ear DCI. It needs to be taken in consideration that criteria for recreational and professional diving fitness are not the same. The following recommendations are mainly aimed for recreational divers. For the assessment of professional divers, country-specific guidelines should be followed. Moreover, the requirements for commercial diving vary greatly. There are different demands for underwater research, military or saturation divers. Hence, not only national requirements but also job-specific requirements differ. Under certain circumstances, dive medicals could be issued but limited for a specific time period only, as some conditions need to be followed up more closely.

> In general, if in doubt, always refer to a specialist for clearance!

30.1 Respiratory Disease

All diseases that interfere with respiration or cause structural pulmonary changes can affect diving fitness, mainly due to the risk of pulmonary barotrauma.

- **Relative Contraindications (but Might Be Considered Fit for Diving)**
  - Asymptomatic well-controlled asthma and stable asthma with or without regular steroids containing medication (ICS) with FEV_1, PEF and FVC > 80% and FEV_1/FVC > 75% and negative exercise test (FEV_1-decline <15%) as well as asthma symptoms <10 years and equivocal or negative bronchial provocation test are advise of diving with care and annual review required*
  - Mild COPD with FEV_1, PEF and FVC > 80% and FEV_1/FVC > 75%
  - Pleuritis
  - Pneumothorax secondary to trauma >3 months requires a clearance of a respiratory physician
  - Spontaneous pneumothorax treated by bilateral surgical pleurectomy with normal

spirometry and CT requires a clearance of a respiratory physician
  - Sarcoidosis in remission (radiological) with normal spirometry
  - Strong smoker with no morphological changes

*Stable but active asthma, requiring relief medication in 48 h preceding the dive, has a reduced PEF (peak expiratory flow) > 10% of the best value or a PEF with >20% diurnal variation should not dive

- **Absolute Contraindications**
  - Acute asthma, asthma precipitated by exercise, colds or emotions, asthma with high airway variability, poorly controlled asthma
  - Asthma symptoms <10 years and positive bronchial provocation test
  - Acute obstructive pulmonary disease
  - All acute pulmonary disease
  - Asthma with regular medication containing leukotriene receptor antagonists
  - Chronic pulmonary disease with limitation in exercise
  - COPD (chronic obstructive pulmonary disease), FEV_1, PEF and FVC < 80% and FEV_1/FVC < 75%
  - Cystic fibrosis
  - Emphysema with bullae (increased risk of pulmonary barotrauma), cysts, bronchiectasis or caverns
  - Lung surgery
  - Pneumothorax with known cause
  - Spontaneous pneumothorax
  - Pneumothorax secondary to trauma <3 months
  - Pulmonary vascular disease
  - Respiratory deficiency
  - Restrictive pulmonary disease-like pulmonary fibrosis
  - Thorax surgery with pneumomediastinum
  - Untreated tuberculosis or tuberculosis with radiological changes
  - Active sarcoidosis
  - Neoplasm affecting the lung

In addition to the general lung examination (auscultation and percussion), a spirometry should be performed to exclude asthma, COPD or any air-trapping. Spirometry is indicative of possible lung diseases. In the interpretation of the individual values, in particular the functional vital capacity (FVC), forced expiratory volume in 1 s (FEV_1), peak expiratory flow (PEF) and forced expiratory flow at 25%, 50% and 75% (FEF_{25-75}) are important components. However, spirometry values shouldn't be interpreted on its own. The flow volume curve has to be taken in consideration too. An early expiratory kink indicates unstable airway passages. FEV_1 and PEF are user-dependent, and the lung function test should be repeated, if a low performance is expected. FEV_1, FEF_{25-75}, PEF and FEV_1/FVC ratio are usually reduced in obstructive lung diseases. If obstructive lung disease is suspected, spirometry should be repeated 5 min after administration of 5 mg salbutamol via nebulizer, to see whether an improvement occurs. Restrictive lung diseases often have obstructive elements but have additionally a reduced FVC. Besides the values, the shape of the spirometry curve can give directions for interpretations (◘ Fig. 30.1).

Standard CXR is not recommended as it has little diagnostic value and causes unnecessary radiation exposure. In commercial divers a CXR in the initial examination is required. Further CXRs are optional and depend on the country's requirements. In countries with risk of exposure to tuberculosis, annual CXR might be required. However, CXRs have a low sensitivity for detecting cavities. HRCT of the lung would be the preferred investigation method for lung diseases.

Asthma is a chronic disease requiring ongoing treatment. It involves airway inflammation, intermittent airflow obstruction and bronchial hyperresponsiveness. The inflammatory process causes airway oedema and mucus secretion. The bronchial hyperreactivity is an exaggerated response to endogenous or exogenous stimuli, leading to bronchial constriction via direct or indirect stimulation of the smooth muscles. Inflammatory processes and bronchial constriction result in airway obstruction and limited airflow. Asthma is defined by excessive variation in lung function and respiratory symptoms like wheezing, shortness of breath, cough and chest tightness. Asthma is often associated with a strong personal or family history of asthma and allergies. It often begins in childhood. It presents with an audible wheeze, which can occur spontaneously, is most often worse at night and early morning hours and can be triggered by exertion, cold air, irritants, medications like aspirin, beta

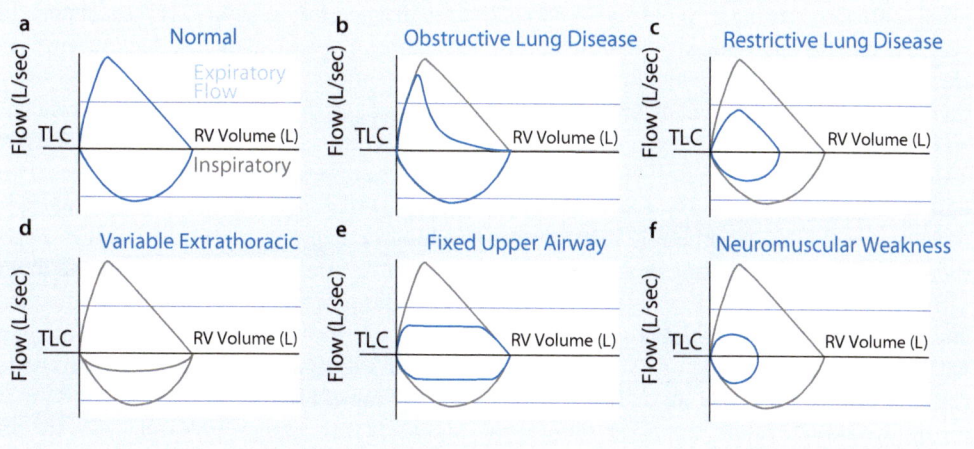

◘ **Fig. 30.1** Spirometry variations. (Wikipedia)

blockers or NSAIDs, respiratory infections or laughter. Asthma can be also triggered underwater by inhaling the dry air from the tank, which is mixed with saltwater particles. These symptoms may vary over time. Additionally, the diagnosis of asthma is more likely, with unexplained raise of IgE, a lowered FEV_1 and PEF without other explanation or if symptoms rapidly improve with SABA bronchodilators. The variable expiratory airflow limitation in adults can present in:

- FEV_1 of >200 mL or >12% from baseline after administration of bronchodilator
- Clinical variation in lung function change >20% in FEV_1 on various spirometries
- Decrease of FEV_1 > 200 mL or 12% in FEV1 after exercise (different criteria apply to formal laboratory-based exercise testing)
- Increase of FEV_1 > 200 mL or 12% from baseline after a trial of 4 weeks of treatment with an inhaled corticosteroid (ICS)
- Diurnal variation of peak expiratory flow >10%
- Positive exercise challenge test or bronchial provocation test

Asthma is mainly a clinical diagnosis, which is based on history, physical examination and consideration of differential diagnosis and testing. Any symptomatic or poor controlled asthma represents a contraindication in diving. Well-controlled asthma with normal or acceptable spirometry and negative indirect bronchial provocation testing may grant fitness for diving with the restriction of annual review and strict advice against diving, if symptoms of asthma are present or the PEF is <10% of the best value. Any symptoms of asthma need review prior diving. If asthma is suspected or there is a history of wheezing or asthma medication is taken in the last 10 years, a spirometry after exercising or a bronchial provocation test with a direct (metacholine, histamine, acetylcholine) or indirect active ingredient (mannitol or hypertonic saline solution) should be performed. The indirect testing is the preferred method in the assessment for diving fitness.

The metacholine test can be regarded as a measure for a bronchial hyperresponsiveness (BHR) or airway hyperresponsiveness (AHR) and as exclusion test for asthma. However, there are some doubts about its use in the assessment for fitness in diving, as this test is nonspecific. In this test increasing doses of metacholine are administered. To determine the severity of BHR depends on the required dose to produce a decline of FEV_1 of 20%:

- Positive test: FEV_1 decrement >20%
- >16 mg/ml normal
- 4–16 mg/ml borderline BHR
- 1–4 mg/ml mild BHR
- <1 mg/ml moderate to severe BHR
- High sensitivity with low specificity (exclusion test for asthma)

The mannitol test with recurrent administration of increasing doses of inhaled mannitol is rather an asthma confirmation test:

- Positive test: FEV_1 decrement >15% or <15% increment after bronchodilator
- Mild BHR >155 mg of mannitol
- Moderate BHR 35–155 mg of mannitol
- Severe BHR < 35 mg of mannitol
- Low to moderate sensitivity with high specificity (confirmation test of asthma)

Mannitol is an osmotic agent which depletes the cells of fluid and causes bronchoconstriction. This causes calcium to be released, which is a trigger for inflammatory mediators like histamines, prostaglandins, leukotrienes and neuropeptides. Hence, the mannitol test is regarded as the standard indirect bronchial provocation test for asthma or BHR. Other indirect bronchial provocation tests are dry air hyperventilation during exercise eucapnic voluntary hyperpnea, distilled water, hypertonic or hypotonic saline or adenosine monophosphate (AMP). In exercise-induced asthma, indirect bronchial provocation tests with exercise or eucapnic voluntary hyperventilation cause a fall of FEV1 of >10% or a positive mannitol test with a fall of FEV1 of >15% are considered diagnostic. Exercise challenge tests are similar to cardiac exercise stress tests. However,

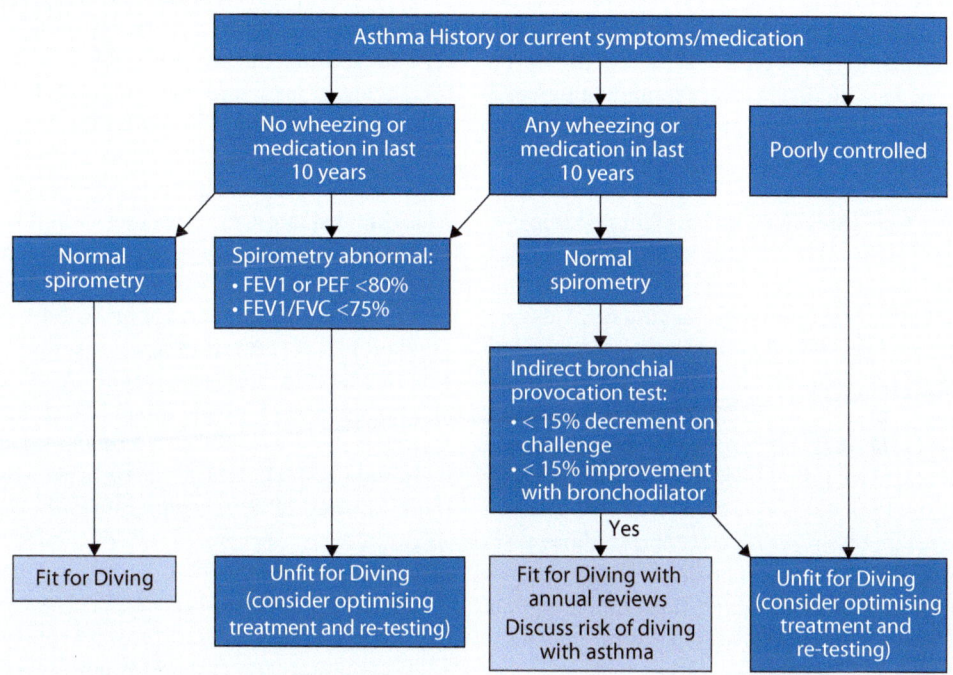

◻ Fig. 30.2   Asthma and flowchart (SPUMS) [3]

dry air at a temperature of 20–25 °C is used for inhalation during increasing exercise levels. The test has a total duration of 6–8 min. The exercise speed and grade are advanced in the first 2–3 min till 80–90% of the predicted maximum heart rate (calculated as 220 age in years) is achieved. A spirometry is performed 5, 10, 15, 20 and 30 min after cessation of exercise. A decline in FEV_1 > 10% is considered to be diagnostic. An AMP test is positive with a fall of FEV1 of >20% or a dose of >400 mg/mL.

These and other investigations, such as whole-body plethysmography, blood gas analysis, CT, etc. should be organised by respiratory physicians. After careful consideration, a conditional fitness for diving can be considered in divers with nonsymptomatic and well-controlled asthma. This is different to the approach to an unfit for diving approach in general in the past. Asthma precipitated by exercise, colds or emotions, asthma with high airway variability and poorly controlled asthma are still a contraindication for diving.

A useful guideline is the SPUMS flowchart in the management of asthma in diving (◻ Fig. 30.2) [3].

30.2 Cardiovascular Disease

Heart disease such as valvular diseases or PFO can increase the risk of DCI, as gas bubbles can bypass the lungs and enter the arterial system. Other heart disorders cause a reduced exercise tolerance and do not meet the high physical demands of diving. Cardiovascular examination includes the auscultation of the heart to check for murmurs. On the initial assessment, an ECG can be performed but is not mandatory. For commercial divers, an ECG is required on all annual examinations. In recreational divers above age 40, an ECG is recommended on regular dive medicals. An exercise stress test (EST) is only recommended, if there is a concern of lack of fitness or a suspicion of cardiovascular heart disease.

In recreational divers above age 40, with cardiovascular problems or obesity, an EST is a reasonable investigation to assess diving fitness. As a guidance divers should either reach stage 4 of the Bruce protocol or 13 METS. In commercial divers, the initial assessment should include an EST or a basic exercise fitness test. This can be either a Chester Step Test (CST), an army physical fitness test, a master two-step test, a cycle ergometer test/treadmill test (direct or indirect assessment of oxygen uptake) or a timed swimming test. An ECHO could be arranged, if there is a concern of valvular diseases or morphological abnormalities. The CST is an easily arranged and inexpensive test, which gives a good estimate of the individual VO_2 max. The VO_2 max is a measure of aerobic capacity and cardiorespiratory fitness. Commercial divers should achieve a VO_2 max of >45 mL/kg/min. A VO_2 max of at least 25–35 mL/kg/min in recreational diver might be reasonable. AVO_2 max of >40–45 mL/kg/min is guidance for optimal lifetime fitness. However, the VO_2 max needs to be taken in context with the general condition. A stress ECHO is a useful tool to assess the cardiac function under exercise. If there is any concern of cardiac abnormality in particular IHD, the diver should be referred to a cardiologist. In case of a suspicion of an IHD, a myocardial perfusion scan or an angiogram may be arranged by the cardiologist. Above the age of 30, a cardiovascular risk assessment should be done. A useful guide in assessing cardiac risk disease factors is the coronary heart risk factor prediction chart of the American Heart Association (AHA) (◘ Fig. 30.3). If the coronary risk factor scores (CRFS) are above 15, the diver should see a cardiologist to get clearance for diving.

Hypertension, with levels above 140 mmHg systolic and 90 mmHg diastolic, is a contraindication for diving. However, in mild hypertension (150 mmHg systolic and 95 mmHg), limited fitness for diving for 1 year might be granted after clearance from a cardiologist. It needs to be mentioned that hypertension is a risk factor for intrapulmonary oedema (IPE). IPE can occur in any in water immersion to anyone. Hypertension and cardiac diseases increase the risk of IPE. Condition for diving fitness and hypertension is that either no medication is required or the prescribed medication has no impact on diving. Beta blocker and Ca channel blocker may lead to an inadequate cardiovascular response to exertion. Therefore, these medications may not be suitable as antihypertensive treatment options in regard to diving, if orthostatic dysregulation and reduced exercise tolerance are experienced. In the absence of these side effects, fitness for diving might be granted. Diuretics require careful attention in regard to hydration and electrolyte disturbance. ACE inhibitors and AT II receptor antagonist don't seem to have any major adverse effect in diving.

Routine investigations for PFO are not required. However, any diver with previous DCI symptoms, migraine with aura, cryptogenic stroke or with a family history of PFO or ASD should be investigated with bubble contrast transthoracic echocardiogram (TTE) but also to establish the quantity of the shunt, if a PFO, ASD or VSD is present [5]. The bubble contrast is produced by pushing approximately 8 mL of normal saline, 1 mL or air and 1 mL of the patients' blood back and forth into another syringe till no bubbles are visible anymore. The blood is necessary to stabilise the microbubbles. Their mixture can be then used as contrast for the TTE. The screening has to include provocation manoeuvres to promote right-to-left shunt like Valsalva release and sniffing. The injections of contrast can be repeated several times at rest and with provocation manoeuvres. A normal two-dimensional and colour flow echocardiogram doesn't seem to be sufficient to assess the diving fitness in divers with PFO. Also transoesophageal echocardiography (TOE) is less sensitive to detect shunts as the patient is sedated and unable to perform provocation manoeuvres. Fitness for diving with PFO might be granted, if the diver has no previous history of DCI and no unprovoked or large shunt. After a closure of a PFO, testing

Fig. 30.3 Risk factor prediction chart (American Heart Association, April 2002). (From Ref. [1])

Age (female)		Age (male)		HDL		Total cholesterol		Systolic blood pressure		Others	
30	−12	30	−2	0.65–0.68	7	3.60–3.99	−3	98–104	−2	Cigarettes	4
31	−11	31	−1	0.69–0.76	6	4.00–4.30	−2	105–112	−1	Diabetic (M)	3
32	−9	32–33	0	0.77–0.84	5	4.31–4.69	−1	113–120	0	Diabetic (F)	6
33	−8	34	1	0.85–0.90	4	4.70–5.19	0	121–129	1	ECG-LVH	9
34	−6	35–36	2	0.91–0.99	3	5.20–5.69	1	130–139	2	No other	0
35	−5	37–38	3	1.00–1.09	2	5.70–6.19	2	140–149	3		
36	−4	39	4	1.10–1.19	1	6.20–6.79	3	150–160	4		
37	−3	40–41	5	1.20–1.30	0	6.8–7.49	4	161–172	5		
38	−2	42–43	6	1.31–1.43	−1	7.50–8.19	5	173–185	6		
39	−1	44–45	7	1.44–1.56	−2	8.20–8.55	6				
40	0	46–47	8	1.57–1.70	−3						
41	1	48–49	9	1.71–1.89	−4						
42–43	2	50–51	10	1.90–2.07	−5						
44	3	52–54	11	2.08–2.25	−6						
45–46	4	55–56	12	2.26–2.49	−7						
47–48	5	57–59	13								
49–50	6	60–61	14								
51–52	7	62–64	15								
53–55	8	65–67	16								
56–60	9	68–70	17								
61–67	10	71–73	18								
68–74	11	74	19								

needs to be repeated 3 months after surgery. If the surgery was successful and no shunt is present, fitness for diving can be granted. If fitness for diving is considered, advice should be given and documented to limit dives in diving times less than the recommended no-decompression limit as well to 15 m maximum and one dive per day. Preferably nitrox should be used, safety stops should be extended and advice to avoid heavy lifting, straining or heavy exercise during and after diving needs to be given.

■ **Relative Contraindications (but Might Be Considered Fit for Diving)**
- AMI or cardiac surgery >12 months and not symptomatic, normal ECG and ECHO; requires cardiologist clearance
- Atrial and ventricular septal defects without shunt require cardiologist clearance
- Hypertension (140–159 mmHg systolic 90–99 mmHg diastolic), if there is no evidence of end organ damage and no

medication is taken or the medication has no impact on diving; requires cardiologist clearance [2]

- Medication (antiarrhythmics, antihypertonics)
- Minor arrhythmias (<1st degree, RBBB with no morphological changes, LBBB with negative thallium scan and angiogram
- Myokarditis >6 months requires cardiologist clearance
- Pericarditis requires cardiologist clearance
- PFO with no or unprovoked shunt and no history of DCI
- Supraventricular tachycardia and not symptomatic for >6 months, after elimination of the cause and cardiologist clearance
- WPW syndrome and not symptomatic for >6 months, after ablation and cardiologist clearance

30

■ **Absolute Contraindications**
- All cardiac diseases unless cleared by cardiologist
- Angina
- Aortic aneurysm, dissection of the aorta
- Atrial and ventricular septal defects with shunt
- Asymmetric septal hypertrophy (can cause LOC)
- AV block ≥2 degree
- Cardiomyopathy
- Coarctation
- Complex ventricular disorder
- Congenital heart diseases
- Cor pulmonale, pulmonale hypertension
- Coronary heart disease with angina
- Large AMI with persisting symptoms and increased risk of further cardiac events
- LBBB with morphological cardiac disease
- Myocarditis for 6 months
- Pacemaker
- Paroxysmal tachycardia
- Recurrent syncopes
- Rendu-Osler syndrome
- Severe aortic and mitral valve stenosis

- Sick sinus syndrome
- Submaximal EST depending on the age and gender
- Supraventricular tachycardia
- Symptomatic cardiac failure
- Untreated hypertension (>140 mmHg systolic >90 mmHg diastolic)
- Valvular disease with haemodynamic effects
- Valvular replacement
- WPW syndrome

30.3 Vascular Diseases

Some vascular diseases increase the risk for DCI, as they have an impact in perfusion. Peripheral pulses should be checked on all dive medicals.

■ **Relative Contraindications (but Might Be Considered Fit for Diving)**
- DVT for 6 months requires haematologist or vascular surgeon clearance
- Pulmonary embolism >3 months with normal spirometry; requires respiratory physician as well as haematologist or vascular surgeon clearance

■ **Absolute Contraindications**
- Acute DVT
- All vascular disease influencing perfusion of any organs
- Pulmonary embolism for the first 3 months
- Symptomatic peripheral vascular disease
- Varices, which reduced perfusion

30.4 Neuropsychiatric Disorders

Psychiatric disorders may cause a reduction in the ability for adequate reactions and judgments. They can lead to an increased risk-taking, particularly during manic or depressive disorders. All acute mental health disorders, in particular Axis I disorders, are a contraindication for diving. Mental health disorders have often relapses. Hence, clearance for diving should be only issued for divers, which are cleared from any acute disorders, and sufficient time has to be elapsed between symptom remission and the time of assessment to establish a stability of the diver's mental health. Fitness for diving with pre-existing mental health conditions should only be attested temporally for up to 1 year. Diving might be possible, if depression is successfully treated on medication under the condition that the medication doesn't cause significant side effects, that the person has insight to potential effects of condition and medication as well as is compliant, and that the condition is stable over a substantial period. If there is any history of mental health disorder or a suspicion of mental health disorder, a mental state examination (MSE) should be performed. This includes:

- Appearance (clothing, grooming, hygiene)
- Behaviour (facial expression, behaviour, gestures, eye contact, response, social engagement and rapport, level of arousal, anxious or aggressive behaviour, psychomotor activity and movement)
- Mood and affect (range, appropriateness, stability, happiness, irritability)
- Speech (rate, volume, tonality, quantity, ease)
- Cognition (level, orientation, memory, literacy and arithmetic skills, visuospatial processing, attention and concentration, general knowledge, language, ability to deal with abstract concepts)
- Thoughts (content, process)
- Perception (assessing for dissociative symptoms, illusions, hallucinations)
- Insight and judgement

- **Relative Contraindications (but Might Be Considered Fit for Diving)**
- Adjustment disorders in remission
- Anxiety
- Isolated psychotic episode
- Phobia

- Self-harm
- Single depressive episode in remission

- **Absolute Contraindications**
- All acute psychiatric disorders
- Anorexia, bulimia
- Any mental health disorder, asymptomatic due to pharmaceutical treatment
- Asymptomatic psychiatric disorders requiring medication
- Bipolar affective disorders
- Claustrophobia
- Drug and alcohol dependency
- Narcolepsy
- Panic attacks, generalised anxiety disorder
- Recurrent depressive episodes
- Recurrent hyperventilation syndrome
- Unipolar affective disorder (major depressive disorder)
- Schizophrenia
- Suicidal risk

30.5 Central Nervous System

The central nervous system should be functional and structurally normal. Neurological examination should include cranial nerves, motor and sensory functions, coordination, reflexes, gait, balance, sense of vibration and two-point discrimination. Some neurological diseases like epilepsy or brain damage increase the risk of having seizures and are contraindications for diving. Moreover, higher oxygen partial pressure during diving might trigger seizures. Migraine can lead directly to an increased risk of DCI due to its patho-mechanism (vasoconstriction). Migraine can be triggered directly by diving and thus may affect divers and put them at risk. PFO seems to have a higher incidence in patients with migraine, in particular migraine with aura. Disorders with increased risk of unconsciousness represent also a contraindication to scuba diving. DCI without permanent neurological deficit results only in a temporary unfitness for diving. DCI with remaining symptoms however results in permanent unfitness for diving.

■ **Absolute Contraindications**
– All acute neurological disorders
– All severe brain trauma, with post-traumatic amnesia or loss of consciousness for >30 min, re-evaluation of each following 4 weeks is required
– CVA and TIA
– DCI with permanent neurological deficit
– Epilepsy (exemption is epilepsy-free interval of >10 years or more without medication and clearance by a neurologist)
– Migraine, with visual, sensory or motor disturbance and excessive daytime fatigue
– Intracranial surgery or trauma
– Intracranial tumour or aneurysm
– Neurological disorder like multiple sclerosis, Parkinson's disease and stroke
– Peripheral neuropathies
– Recurrent unprovoked loss of consciousness without diagnosis
– Severe motion sickness
– Spinal cord injuries

30.6 ENT

Diving fitness assessments should include the assessment of the mobility of the tympanic membrane. This can be done using tympanometry or, if not available, by simple otoscopy. During the Valsalva manoeuvre, the tympanic membrane bulges out and the light reflex on the tympanic membrane usually disappears. At the initial examination, an audiometry with the range from 500 Hz to 8 kHz could be considered. Further audiometries for recreational divers are only necessary, if required. Commercial divers might be asked for an audiometry on every assessment. The ear canal should be free from earwax. ENT diseases are a common cause for ear or sinus barotraumas.

■ **Absolute Contraindications**
– Acute and chronic otitis media and externa
– Acute or chronic vestibular disorders
– Acute or recurrent perforation of the tympanic membrane
– Atresia or stenosis of the eartube
– Attic or posterior marginal perforation of the tympanic membrane
– Atticotomy
– Cholesteatoma
– Costochondral graft (risk of pneumothorax)
– Disorders of the labyrinth (e.g. Meniere's disease)
– Facial paralysis secondary to baro-trauma
– Functional limiting disorders of the glottis
– Grommets
– Inability to equalise (fixed tympanic membrane during Valsalva manoeuvre)
– Incompetent larynx
– Inner ear surgery
– Labyrinthitis
– Laryngocele
– Mastoidectomy (radical) involving the external canal
– Nasal septum disorders with eustachian tube dysfunction
– Ossicular surgery
– Ossiculoplasty
– Otospongiosis
– Perilymphatic fistula
– Petrous temporal bone fracture
– Rupture of the round window
– Significant bilateral and unilateral loss of hearing
– Stapedectomy
– Tympanoplasty other than myringoplasty (Type I)
– Tracheoplasty
– Vestibular DCS
– Vestibular deficiency >50%: 6 months

30.7 Endocrine Disorders

■ **Absolute Contraindications**
- Phaeochromocytoma
- Insulin-dependent diabetes mellitus
- Any decompensated or not treated endocrine disorder
- Deficiency of the anterior lobe of the pituitary gland
- Deficiency of the adrenal glands
- Cryoglobulinemia

Diabetes poses a risk in diving by increasing risk or outcome of DCI, hypoglycaemia and ischemic events. Following criteria may allow recreational diving [3]:
- \>18 years of age
- \> 6 months or initiation of oral treatment or >1 year of insulin; both with appropriate 3 months "observation period" after changes in medication
- \> 1 year of no hypoglycaemia
- HBA1c ≤ 9% (HBA1c > 9% might be an indication for suboptimal managed diabetes)
- no hypoglycaemic unawareness
- no severe complications leading to hospital admission for at least 1 year
- Absence of retinoneuropathy, significant nephropathy, neuropathy, coronary artery disease or peripheral vascular disease
- ability of accurate use of blood glucose monitoring and good understanding of external factors (diet, stress, temperature and exercise) influencing the blood glucose levels
- annual review required
- written consent to diabetic diving protocol (limitations of diving and blood glucose monitoring prior and after diving)
- In divers older than 40 years of age, cardiological clearance is required, in particular taking in consideration silent ischaemia

Sulfonylureas pose a risk of hypoglycaemia and should be omitted at the day of diving. The diabetic diver should be well hydrated and avoid alcohol during the time of diving. The blood sugar should be closely monitored during that time. Any devices like pumps or continuous glucose monitors should be removed prior diving.

30.8 Blood Disorders

Some blood disorders increase the risk of DCI, or an acute exacerbation of the underlying condition can be triggered by diving, e.g. thalassemia major or sickle cell anaemia.

■ **Absolute Contraindications**
- Acute Anaemia
- Haemophilia (dependent on severity)
- Peripheral thrombocytopenia
- Sickle cell anaemia
- Thalassemia major
- Thrombocytic defects

30.9 Gastrointestinal Tract

As air can get trapped in any kind of hernia, it is important to check for hernias in abdominal, umbilical and groin regions during examination.

■ **Absolute Contraindications**
- All acute bowel diseases
- Antireflux plastic surgery (e.g. lap-band)
- Bowel obstruction (acute or chronic recurrent)
- Chronic inflammatory bowel disease
- Hernia
- Pancreatitis
- Peptic ulcer or severe GERD with continuous medication
- High-grade gastric outlet obstruction
- Blocked enterocutaneous fistula
- Oesophageal diverticula
- Hiatus hernia
- Achalasia
- Dumping syndrome

30.10 Eye

- ■ **Relative Contraindications (but Might Be Considered Fit for Diving)**
- ▬ Acute ocular diseases
- ▬ Chronic severe reduction of the visual field >80% horizontal and >50% vertical
- ▬ Primary open-angle glaucoma

- ■ **Absolute Contraindications**
- ▬ Acute severe reduction of the visual field >80% horizontal and >50% vertical: 4 months
- ▬ Angle-closure glaucoma or traumatic narrow angle glaucoma after known acute glaucoma
- ▬ Binocular uncorrected vision <6/12 or one eye <6/60 and the other eye <6/10
- ▬ Cataract surgery <4 months
- ▬ Keratoconus stage 2
- ▬ Corneal graft: 8 months
- ▬ Corneal surgery 3–12 months
- ▬ Hollow ocular prosthesis or implant
- ▬ Intraocular surgery: 1–3 months
- ▬ Persistent symptoms after ocular trauma
- ▬ Phacoemulsification-trabeculectomy and vitreo-retinal surgery: 2 months
- ▬ Photoreactive keratectomy and LASIK <1 month
- ▬ Retinal, choroidal or papillary vascular disorders, unstabilised and likely to bleed

30.11 Orthopaedic Disorders

Because of the heavy weight of scuba tanks, diving requires good mobility to safely operate diving equipment above and under water. Hence, diving fitness examinations require the assessment of the musculoskeletal system.

- ■ **Absolute Contraindications**
- ▬ Aseptic osteonecrosis
- ▬ All injuries, which reduce severe motility (amputations, back pain, stiffening of joints)
- ▬ Scoliosis reducing respiratory function

30.12 Medications

Some medications like bleomycin can directly affect divers of patients in HBOT. Others pose a risk during diving due to their side effects. Mainly sedative side effects of medications may affect fitness for diving. In general, if the divers suffer from the sedative effects of a medication, diving should be avoided. A medication, which interferes with commercial driving or operating of heavy machinery, should also not be taken during diving. Some medications cause sedation, if taken occasionally, like antihistamines, antidepressants or narcotics. That might interfere with cognitive functions and response. However, taking them long term might not cause significant side effects anymore, and diving might be possible. A psychiatrist assessment and clearance might be required. Still, underlying conditions of why the medication is taken need to be assessed.

- ■ **Contraindications**
- ▬ Bleomycin promotes oxygen radicals at elevated oxygen partial pressure and hence increases risk of organ damage, in particular of the lungs (pneumonitis). This may result in unfitness for diving [4].
- ▬ Insulin (risk of hypoglycaemia); but might be considered fit for diving (see endocrinology)
- ▬ Anticoagulation, e.g. with warfarin, rivaroxaban, dabigatran, apixaban (risk of haemorrhage)
- ▬ Sedatives, including some medication for sea sickness
- ▬ Hypnotics
- ▬ Opiates
- ▬ Antipsychotic medication
- ▬ Anticonvulsants
- ▬ Doxorubicin is cardiotoxic
- ▬ Mefloquine (Lariam®) may cause psychiatric symptoms and reduction in alertness

Disulfiram blocks superoxide dismutase, which is a protective factor against oxygen intoxication. This might need to be considered when diving with gas mixtures containing larger amounts of oxygen, as it might pose a higher risk of oxygen intoxication. Disulfiram is a contraindication for HBOT.

30.13 Pregnancy

Diving during pregnancy is contraindicated at any stage. Venous bubbles may cause a disruption of the foetal blood supply.

30.14 Obesity

Obesity with BMI > 35 and BMI > 30 in combination with a waist circumference > 102 cm (males) or 88 cm (females) is a contraindication for diving [2]. If BMI is between 30 and 34.9 and the waist circumference is 94–102 cm in males or 80–88 cm in females, a temporary fitness for diving can be given for a short term of approx 3 months. In particular high fat contents of more than 30% could result in N_2 accumulation in the body and therefore increase the risk of DCI. Obesity and decreased exercise tolerance should be viewed critically in diving fitness assessments. Fitness for diving with BMI > 30 should only granted for 1 year. BMI > 30 might become complex obesity, if certain diseases (e.g. cardio vascular, DM, hypercholesterolaemia, musculoskeletal disorders or injuries) exist. This means that obesity multiplies the risk of pre-existing conditions and accelerating present as well as future health risks. The combination of various factors together might lead to being unfit for diving.

30.15 Children and Adolescents

Scuba diving is becoming increasingly attractive for the younger generation. Diving under the age of 14 is generally not recommended. However, diving courses for children are offered from the

□ Table 30.2 Youth scuba diving programs and recommendations

Age	Diving depth in meter	Maximum diving time in minutes
8–9	2 (first dive)	15
8–9	4 (following dives)	15
10–11	12	30
12–14	18 (open water)	30
12–14	21 (advanced +)	30
Over 15	Like adults	45

age of 8 and above (□ Table 30.2). The allowed diving depth and time depend on age and diving experience. In general, children are only allowed to go diving accompanied by an experienced adult. As bones are still growing, the dive profile should be limited to ensure that slow compartments like bones aren't getting saturated with nitrogen. This means that diving depth and time are limited. Repetitive dives should be avoided as they pose the risk of saturating slow compartments. Children are more likely to suffer from ear and sinus barotraumas, as the connecting ducts are smaller. Mental maturity could also be a limiting factor and has to be involved in the consideration of diving fitness in children. Maturity cannot be linked to a specific age as there are individual variations. But immaturity can result in unfitness for diving. At the diving fitness assessment, a legal guardian must be present and give consent for the child diving. It is also beneficial in the assessment as the guardian might give more information in regard to the maturity of the child or adolescent.

30.16 Diving Accidents

After diving accidents, temporary unfitness for diving exists for a specific time period (□ Table 30.3). Persisting symptoms of a DCI

30

■ **Table 30.3**   Overview of recommendations for minimal time intervals for unfitness for diving[a]

Mild DCI

Limb pain, or unspecific manifestations (e.g., headache, fatigue, nausea, loss of appetite)[b]	7 days [6, 7]
Recurrence or relapse requiring further HBOT	14 days [6]

Moderate to severe DCI and/or AGE

DCI Type II or AGE[b] with normal/unchanged MRI of brain and/or spine within 7 days	30 days [7], requires cardiologist clearance excluding PFO/ASD [7]
DCI Type II or AGE with residual symptoms, neurological deficits, or abnormal MRI of brain and/or spine	May be considered fit for diving, if subsequent treatments including MRIs are well documented, a neurology consultation, and an assessment and recommendation of a diving medicine specialist [7]
Residual neurological manifestations	Unfit for diving [6]
Sensory disturbance only (paraesthesia of loss of sensation)	28 days [6], review of a diving medicine specialist
All other neurological or pulmonary symptoms	3 months [6], review of a diving medicine specialist
Cutaneous or lymphatic manifestations without neurological involvement	28 days [6], review of a diving medicine specialist
Recurrent DCI and AGE	Unfit for diving [7]

[a]All patients with history of DCI or AGE require a review of an experienced diving medicine specialist
[b]Resolved completely and remained asymptomatic after the initial HBOT

lead to permanent unfitness for diving. In general, for DCI unfitness for diving applies until medical clearance allows diving again.

References

1. Coronary Heart Disease Risk Factor Prediction Chart, Modified from chart, modified from chart by the American Heart Association. 2002. https://www.casa.gov.au/sites/g/files/net351/f/_assets/main/manuals/regulate/dame/riskchrt.pdf.
2. Health and Safety Executive (HSE) Standarts for Medical Assessment of Divers (MA1).
3. SPUMS – Guidleines on medical risk assessment for recreational divers. 2010. http://www.spums.org.au/sites/default/files/member_downloads/SPUMS%20Medical%204th%20edition-July%202011_0.pdf. Accessed 2 Mar 2017.
4. Van Hulst RA, Rietbroek RC, Gaastra MTW, Schloesser NJJ. To dive or not to dive with bleomycin: a practical algorithm. Aviatr Space Environ Med. 2011;82:814–8.
5. Wilmhurst P. Practice guidline– Detection of a persistent foramen ovale using echocardiography. Diving Hyperb Med. 2016; 46(1).
6. The Diving Medical Advisory Committee. Fitness to return to diving after decompression illness, DMAC 13 Rev. 2 Nov 2017.
7. Bureau of Medicine and Surgery, US Navy, Manual of the Medical Department (MANMED), NAVMED P-117, Article 15–102, updated 1 June 2018.

Suggested Reading

ADC international (Association of Diving Contractors International). International consensus for commercial diving and underwater operations, 6th edition 2016; www.adc-int.or/files/C12181_International%20Consensus%20Standards.pdf.
Bove AA. Medical aspects of sport diving. Med Sci Sports Exerc. 1996;28(5):591.
Bove AA. Medical evaluation for sport diving. In: Bove AA, Davis JC, editors. Diving medicine. 4th ed. Philadelphia: Saunders; 2004. p. 519–32.
Brannan JD, Koskela H, Anderson SD. Monitoring asthma therapy using indirect bronchial provocation tests. Clin Respir J. 2007;1:3–15.

Ehm OF. Tauchtauglichkeitsuntersuchung bei Sporttauchern, vol. 1989. Berlin: Springer; 1989.

FFESSM. www.cmp.fr/resources/Taucher-Kontraindikationliste-Est.pdf. Accessed 6 Mar 2015.

French Underwater Federation Guidelines. Recreational scuba diving contraindications, 2008: http://medical.ffessm.fr/wp-content/uploads/scubadiving_contraindication2009.pdf; (Accessed 13 May 2016).

Godden D, Currie G, Denison D, Farrell P, Ross J, Stephenson R, Watt S, Wilmhurst P. British Thoracic Society guidelines on respiratory aspects of diving. Thorax. 2003;58:3–13.

Harrah JD, O'Boyle PS, Piantadosi CA. Underutilization of echocardiography for patent foramen ovale in divers with serious decompression sickness. Undersea Hyperb Med. 2008;35(3):207–11.

Jette M, Sidney K, Blümchen G. Metabolic equivalents (METS) in exercise testing, exercise prescription and evaluation of functional capacity. Clin Cardiology. 1990;13:555–65.

Kontraindikationen Sorttauchen nach Empfehlung der GTUM, OGTH, SGUHM. http://www.tauchtauglichkeitsuntersuchungen.de/kontraindikationen/.

Kyi M, Paldus B, Nanayakkara N, Bennett M, Johnson R, Meehan C, Colman P. Insulin-requiring diabetes and recreational diving: Australian Diabetes Society position statement, Diving and diabetes – ADS position statement 2016.

Lafay V. The heart and underwater diving. Arch Mal Coeur Vaiss. 2006;99(11):1115–9.

Miller MR, Hankinson J, Brusasco V, Burgos F, Casaburi R, Coates A, Crapo R, Enright P, van der Grinten CPM, Gustafson P, Jensen R, Jphnson DC, MacIntyre N, MacKay R, Navajas D, Pedersen OF, Pellegrino R, Viegi G, Wagner J. Standardisation of spirometry. Eur Respir J. 2005;26:319–38.

Morgan WP, Raglin JS, O'Connor PJ. Trait anxiety predicts panic behavior in beginning scuba students. Int J Sports Med. 2004;25(4):314–22.

Pollock NW. Aerobic fitness and underwater diving. Diving Hyperb Med. 2007;37(3):118–24.

Sade K, Wiesel O, Kivity S, Levo Y. Asthma and scuba diving: can asthmatic patients dive? Harefuah. 2007;146(4):286–90, 317.

Scott DH, Marks AD. Diabetes and diving. In: Bove AA, Davis JC, editors. Diving medicine. 4th ed. Philadelphia: Saunders; 2004. p. 507–18.

Sporting Goods Manufacturers Association. 2007 sports and fitness participation report. Washington, DC: Sporting Goods Manufacturers Association; 2007.

Tauchtauglichkeitsuntersunchungen. www.tauchtauglichkeitsuntersuchungen.de. Accessed 5 June 2015.

Taylor DM, O'Toole KS, Ryan CM. Experienced, recreational scuba divers in Australia continue to dive despite medical contraindications. Wilderness Environ Med. 2002;13(3):187–93.

Tetzlaff K, Klingmann C, Muth CM, Piepho T, Welslau W. Checkliste Tauchtauglichkeit, vol. 2008. Stuttgart: Gentner Verlag; 2014.

Wendling J, Elliott D, Nome T. Fitness to dive standards, guidelines for medical assessment of working divers. 2003; www.edtc.org/EDTC-Fitnesstodivestandard-200.pdf. (Accessed 24/06/2003).

First Aid

© Springer International Publishing AG, part of Springer Nature 2018
O. Rusoke-Dierich, *Diving Medicine*, https://doi.org/10.1007/978-3-319-73836-9_31

First aid includes life-sustaining measures up to the point of hospital admission. The most important thing is to recognise an acute emergency and to distinct between non-life-threatening and life-threatening conditions. It is vital to distinguish, if there is immediate danger and if the injury poses a risk of rapid deterioration or dangers to life. Emergencies during diving are all types of DCI, arterial gas embolism, pulmonary barotrauma, drowning, hypo- or hyperthermia and injuries of marine creatures.

Important signs to look out in the assessment of a critically ill person are changes in:
- State of consciousness
- Cardiovascular activity
- Breathing

A person, who does not respond to tactile or acoustic stimuli, is classified unconscious. Arteries of the neck (carotid artery) or groin (femoral artery) can be used to assess pulses. While peripheral pulses at the wrist might not be palpable, central pulse of the neck (carotid pulse) or groin (femoral pulse) may be still present. Decreasing blood pressure first is noticeable with fading pulses in the periphery. In contrast, central blood pressure may be still maintained. Because pulses are a weak sign of cardiovascular activity, no *more than 10 s* should be wasted for their assessment during first aid. This may otherwise lead to unnecessary delay of CPR. Heartbeat and activity can also be assessed with stethoscope or ECG. However, pulseless ECG activity is also possible. Movements of the chest and breath sounds may be a sign of respiratory activity. But validation of respiration might be difficult. Most environmental noises prevent perceiving already quiet breath sounds. Breathing can be auscultated with the stethoscope. Synchronously chest movements should be observed, to see whether the movements correspond to the breathing sounds. Since the review of respiratory function is difficult and time-consuming, the respiratory assessment was taken out of the current

guidelines for CPR. Moreover, people suffering a cardiac arrest may have abnormal breathing pattern (such as grunting), which might be falsely interpreted as breathing activity and hence delay CPR. Therefore, abnormal breathing should not be interpreted as a vital sign. In the initial phase of cardiopulmonary arrest, convulsions are common. This can be mistakenly interpreted as epileptic seizure and not as a sign of cardiopulmonary arrest.

> **An unconscious person with abnormal or no breathing requires immediate resuscitation!**

The important question for the primary assessment is *whether to start CPR or not*. If no CPR is required, patients need to be provided with the necessary care prior arriving to hospital. This includes the protection of airways and cardiovascular function. For transport or positioning, airways need to be cleared from vomit, objects and the tongue, which may cause obstruction. However, this should not be performed by using the fingers of the helper, since bite injuries can occur and further vomiting may be provoked. In supine position the tongue easily can obstruct the airways, which can lead to death by suffocation. During positioning, a gentle of hyperextension of the neck to the back prevents the tongue from falling back. This can be achieved by the jaw thrust or head tilt-chin lift (◻ Figs. 31.1 and 31.2).

The recovery position is to prevent any airway obstruction. It should be applied for any unconscious person or who is at risk of becoming unconscious. It enables the treating person to focus on other aspects of the patient's management and protects the patient from choking. Patients are turned to the left side of the body in recovery position, unless the patient has a right-sided pneumothorax. The left-sided position is preferred as the right side of the lung is relatively larger in comparison to the left side. The lung gets compressed on the side the patient is positioned on and is therefore restricted in its movement.

a   b   c

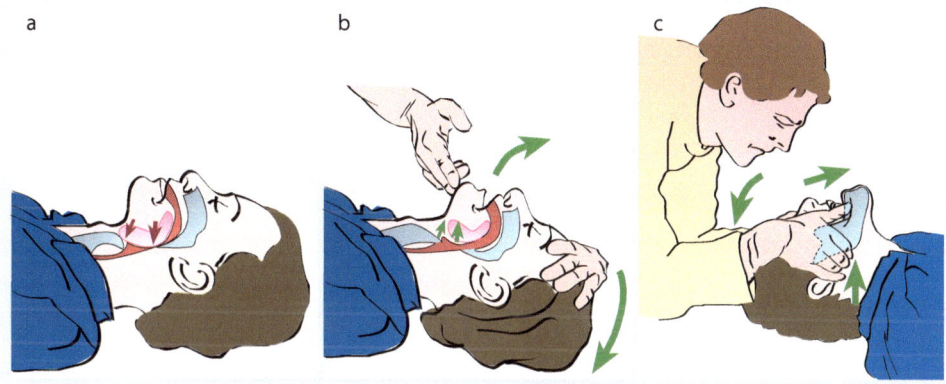

■ **Fig. 31.1** Opening of the airways **a** obstructed airways **b** head tilt-chin lift **c** jaw thrust. (From Ziegenfuss 2014)

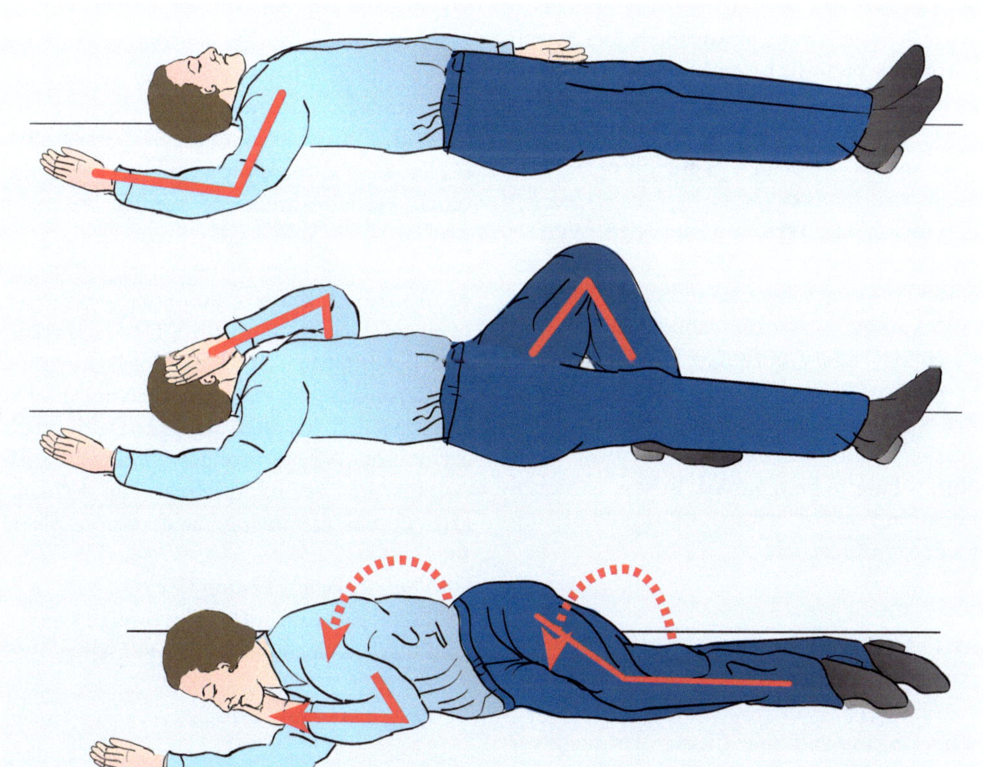

■ **Fig. 31.2** Recovery position. (From Ziegenfuss 2014)

Positioning on the smaller left lung would reduce its already smaller respiratory capacity. On the other hand, the larger right side can continue moving without restriction. In case of a unilateral pneumothorax, patients should be always positioned on the affected side to preserve the function of the unaffected side.

The recovery position is a stable position, enabling the unconscious person to breathe and avoid any airway obstruction with vomit or the tongue itself. Initially, the patient is placed on his back. Then the helper kneels down on the side of the patient, where he/she is supposed to be rolled over and places the arm, which is on the helper's side, slightly angled above the head. The hand of the opposite side has to be taken gently across to the other cheek, palm facing up. The opposite knee has to be lifted up, so that the food can be placed flat on the ground. The patient now can be easily rolled over towards the helper by supporting the opposite leg and the shoulder. As the patient roles onto the helper's knees, which are placed right next to the patient, this manoeuvre is controlled. Through a gentle tilt of the head to the back, the neck can be hyperextended, and thus airways are kept clear and open. With the palm facing down under the cheek, the hyperextension position is secured and stabilised.

Breathing and pulse should be checked in regular intervals during first aid to pick up changes in vital signs as early as possible. If the patient stops breathing, airways should be checked immediately and any obstructing objects have to be removed. In case of a respiratory and cardiac arrest, CPR should be commenced immediately.

31.1 Cardiac Arrest

Cardiac arrest can occur when entering the water, during and after diving. Although cardiac arrest is rare in diving, there is still a possibility. Training and mental preparedness assist in a quick response in critical situations and ensure an optimal outcome for the patient and a sufficient CPR.

31.1.1 Aetiology and Pathogenesis

There are various cardiovascular reasons for cardiac arrest. The most common ones are *ventricular tachycardia (VT), ventricular flutter or ventricular fibrillation (VF)*. Ventricular flutter can be regarded as an extreme form of VT. Both are caused by electrical re-entry or abnormal automaticity. Excitation is still coordinated, but the cardiac output is drastically reduced. Both forms quickly can turn into VF. In VF the heartbeat becomes so fast and uncoordinated that there is no sufficient cardiac output anymore. Approximately 50% of all VF is caused by acute myocardial infarction. Other causes of cardiovascular failure include atrial fibrillation (AF), WPW syndrome, long QT syndrome and cardiomyopathies. Cardiac arrest usually undergoes different stages ending up in VF and finally in asystole. ECG signs of VF initially have wide amplitude, which continuously narrows before turning into asystole. Primary asystole can be caused by occlusion of coronary arteries, advanced heart block, electric shock and cardiac trauma or may occur spontaneously. Secondary asystole may be found after hypoxia (e.g. suffocation or drowning), massive pulmonary embolism, myocardial infarction with VT/VF, hyperkalemia, hypothermia, stroke and "near drowning".

Cardiovascular failure is a failure of effective heart activity, often associated with cardiac arrhythmia, which produces reduced cardiac outputs in various degrees. The following arrhythmias are mainly held responsible for this:

- Ventricular fibrillation (VF)
- Pulseless ventricular tachycardia (VT)
- Pulseless electrical activity (PEA)
- Asystole
- Pulseless bradycardia

VT, ventricular flutter or VF can be reversed to normal rhythm by early defibrillation. Untreated VF converts to asystole just within few minutes. During VF cardiac cells are still excitable but in an uncoordinated fashion.

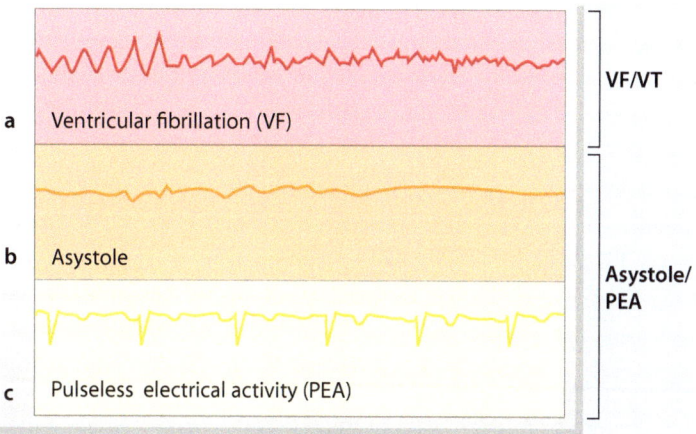

■ **Fig. 31.3** **a–c** ECG variations in cardiac arrest **a–c** VF/VT, **b** asystole and **c** pulseless electrical activity. (From Ziegenfuss 2014)

a Ventricular fibrillation (VF)

b Asystole

c Pulseless electrical activity (PEA)

VF/VT

Asystole/PEA

Therefore, immediate defibrillation is necessary to restore coordinated contractions of the heart. At asystole, heart cells are no longer excitable. Defibrillation "coordinates" only excitation and restores normal activity, but can't reactivate cardiac electric activity by itself. Hence, defibrillation in asystole is ineffective. In VF the time, at which defibrillation is still effective, can be prolonged by CPR. It even can be restored to a certain degree (■ Fig. 31.3).

VT, but in particular VF, leads to a drastic drop in cardiac output, reduced blood flow and reduced oxygenation of the body, especially of vital organs such as the brain or heart. Depending on age and body temperature, within a short period damages to vital organs are imminent. With advanced age cells have less tolerance to oxygen deficiency. Cell damages due to oxygen deficiency are quite dependent on body temperature. With increasing body temperature, biochemical processes are accelerated and vice versa. In general a time of 5–10 min of cardiac arrest leads to irreversible brain damage.

The 5 "Hs" and 5 "Ts" should be considered as reversible causes for cardiovascular failure and, where appropriate, need to be treated (■ Table 31.1).

— Asystole recorded on ECG for more than 20 min despite correct resuscitation (hypothermia excepted)

■ **Table 31.1** Reversible causes

H	T
Hypovolemia	Tension pneumothorax
Hypoxia	Tamponade, cardiac
Hydrogen Ion (Acidosis)	Toxins
Hypo-/Hyperkalemia	Thrombosis, pulmonary
Hypothermia	Thrombosis, cardiac

31.1.2 Treatment

Immediate action according to the guidelines of the AHA (American Heart Association) is required in cardiac arrest. Even for experienced medical professionals, resuscitation settings are challenging. Resuscitation is rarely 100% perfect. However, previous training and role plays improve skills, increase efficiency in real resuscitation, improve confidence and produce better outcomes.

Resuscitation protocols have been modified in recent years. Originally the ABC method for a single rescuer was the preferred sequence. With exception of newborns, this has is suggested to be modified to the CAB method.

Retrospective studies showed that the main problem of resuscitations was that CPR was not commenced at all or too late, resulting in increased mortality or poor outcome after a successful resuscitation. Each minute, in which resuscitation is delayed, the survival rate reduces by 7–10% without and approximately only 3–4% with CPR.

> CPR should be performed immediately on any unconscious person with no or abnormal breathing.

It is reasonable in resuscitation in primary cardiac arrest with a single person to commence with compression only without initial ventilation (compression only CPR = COCPR). Because blood is oxygenated to its maximum at the time of the cardiac arrest and the lungs still contain oxygen, additional ventilation contributes only little to maintain oxygenation in the initial phase. Hence, chest compressions without ventilation may be performed continuously for the first few minutes. Compressions combined with ventilation seem to be more effective and reduced neurologic complications after CPR. Also in cardiac arrest due to respiratory failure, it might be advisable to do compressions with ventilation as oxygen saturation in the blood is expected. To build up adequate blood pressure and perfusion, in particular of the coronary arteries (CPP coronary perfusion = pressure during the diastole), approximately 30 compressions are required. The blood pressure collapses immediately when compressions are ceased. Therefore, any interruption of chest compressions should be avoided, if possible. Even before defibrillation, interruptions in compression should be minimised to less than 5 s.

If more people assist during resuscitation, individual roles should be distributed. The most experienced person should be the team leader and maintain the airways. Only one person should give orders to avoid a poor coordination of the resuscitation process. Other helpers assist in chest compressions, administration of drugs and defibrillation. As the quality of chest compressions decreases along with fatigue, the person, who is giving compressions, needs to be exchanged every 2 min or five cycles.

Resuscitation scheme follows **DR SCABD:**
- **D = Danger** – check for hazards and risks; ensure safety
- **R = Response** – check for response
- **S = Send** for help
- **C = start CPR** – commence chest compressions
- **A = Airways** – clear and open
- **B = Breathing** – check for normal breathing, start ventilation
- **D = Defibrillation**

D = Danger check for hazards and risks; ensure safety   Initially, the accident scene needs to be scanned for safety hazards to ensure that no risks for the life-saver are identified.

In order to identify hazards, the following needs to be checked
- **Check up high**: overhead hazards
- **Check up eye**: insufficient visibility or light, traffic and people, smoke, fire gas and chemicals
- **Check down low**: ground stability, covered wires, sharp objects and animals
- **Check for specific hazards**: bystanders, bodily fluids and drugs

The person might to be relocated in a safe environment or hazards need to be eliminated. In case the person got in contact with stingers, it has to be searched for tentacles as they represent a hazard for the helper but also for the injured person.

R = Response check   A person, who does not respond to normal acoustic and tactile stimulation, is unconscious. The patient's response can be assessed by talking and touching. The patient can be asked to squeeze the hands, for example. If the person doesn't respond, a more firm pressure on the shoulders may be applied. Painful stimuli such as hard rubbing of the sternum or pinching are obsolete.

S = Send for help If the person does not respond, the rescue cascade should be activated. Others should be included in the resuscitation, and a request for help (ambulance, police and fire rescue) should be sent.

C = CPR – start chest compressions CPR should be started immediately, if a person is unconscious and has no or an abnormal breathing. A short attempt to check for the carotid pulse is acceptable, but that shouldn't take more than 10 s. There is no evidence whether the *praecordial thump* is effective. Hence, it is no longer recommended. It only might be recommended in a witnessed, monitored unstable VT or cardiac arrest. Patients should be placed on the back on a hard surface for chest compressions. A hard surface is important, since the substituted circulation is mainly due to compressions of the thorax. It is assumed that due to compressions of the thorax, pulmonary capacity vessels are compressed, which built up blood flow and blood pressure. To obtain a sufficient blood flow and blood pressure, at least 15–20 continuous compressions are necessary. The hands for the compression should be placed in the middle of the sternum. Compressions should be directed vertically to the patient. The compression rate should be 100–120 compressions per minute (*push hard, push fast*) in adults and children. The Bee Gees song "Stayin' Alive" can be used as rhythm guidance for the compression frequency. It is important for the effectiveness of chest compressions that after pushing down, the compression is fully lifted again. Incomplete lifting decreases the return blood flow to the heart and leads to reduced CPP (coronary perfusion pressure). The CPP is an important parameter for effectiveness of chest compressions. Proper CPR can establish 25–33% of the cardiac ejection performance (◘ Fig. 31.4, ◘ Table 31.2).

CPR
 ▬ Positioning on hard surface
 ▬ Hand position in the middle of sternum
 ▬ Vertical compression of the sternum

 ▬ Compression depth:
  ▬ Adults at least 5 cm or 1/3 of the chest
  ▬ Children at least 1/3 of the chest
 ▬ Compression rate

D = Defibrillation During resuscitation it needs to be distinguished between shockable or non-shockable rhythms. Shockable rhythms are VT, ventricular flutter and VF. The technical device for electrical therapy is the defibrillator. There are two types of defibrillators, biphasic and monophasic defibrillators. Biphasic defibrillators are preferred. Both are used with different voltage. Monophasic defibrillators use 360 V and biphasic 120–200 V (preferred initial shock with 150 V). Recently, automatic defibrillators (automated external defibrillator, AED) are made available in public places such as airports and department stores. The AED automatically detects shockable rhythms. The handling of the AED is simple and can be performed by anyone. The downside from an AED is that from analysis of the heart rhythm until defibrillation approx. 30 s may elapse. During this time no chest compressions are performed. Yet, survival rates are rising with AEDs, because of early defibrillation. There is a 49–75% survival chance, if chest compressions and defibrillation are applied within 3–5 min.

❯ Start chest compressions early and defibrillate as soon as possible!

Semiautomatic defibrillators can be converted from automatic to manual operation. The defibrillator's pads are placed right of the upper sternum (mid-clavicular line) and the other in the left mid-axillary line at level of the xiphoid process. Alternative positions are anterior-posterior (left of the lower sternum and below the left scapula) or do both chest walls in the mid-auxiliary line. Gel has to be applied between electrodes and the skin to avoid burns due to electrical surge. Adhesive pads have already integrated gel and don't require application of additional gel. Alcoholic substances can't be used, as they are highly inflammable and can catch fire during defibrillation. Oxygen masks have to be removed with each

31

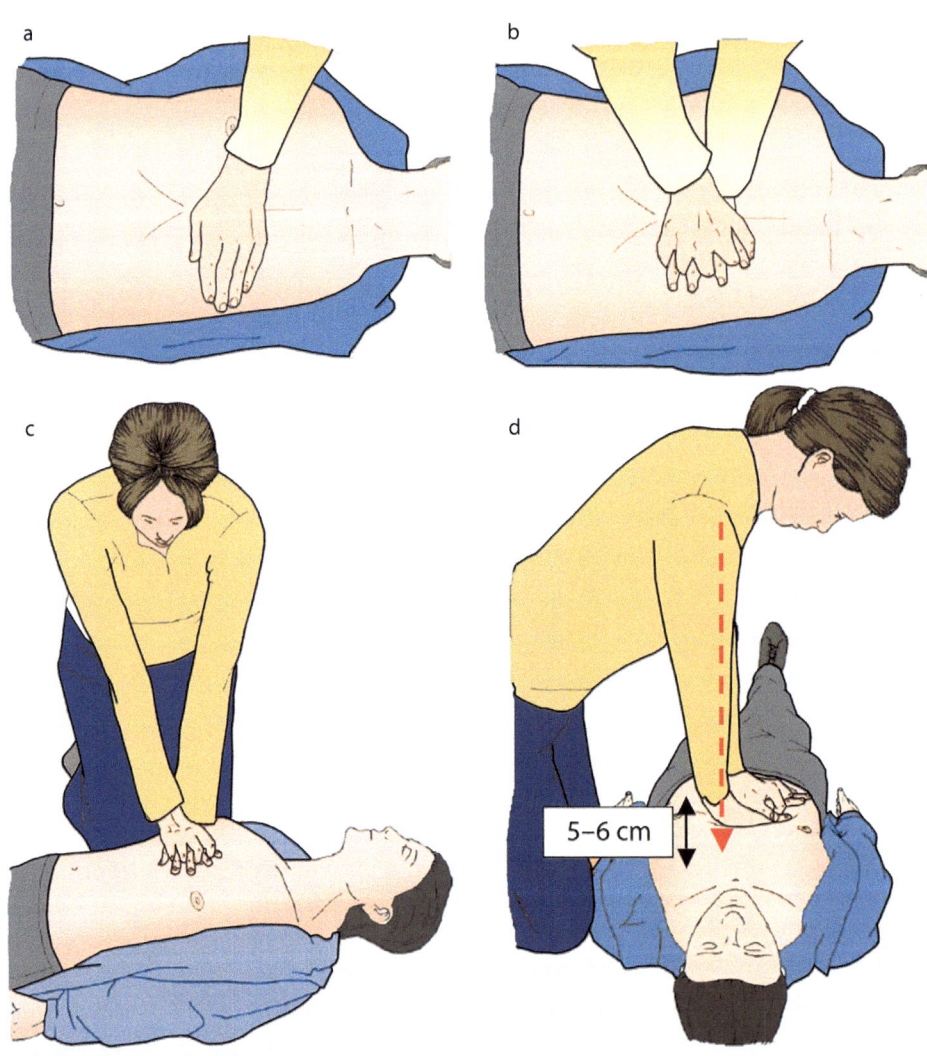

■ Fig. 31.4   CPR a + b Positioning and c + d body posture

	Frequency	Compression-ventilation ratio	Procedure
■ Table 31.2 Compression rates			
Adults and children >8 years	100/min	30:2	With both hands
Children (1–8 years)	100/min	30:2 (one person), 15:1 or 6–10 per minute (after placement of an ET)	With one hand
Infants (<12 months)	100/min	30:2 (one person), 15:2 (two trained person), after placement of an ET 10 ventilations per minute	With two fingers

defibrillation, as oxygen is highly flammable as well. Excessive hair must be removed prior to defibrillation, as it may lead to a gap between electrodes and the skin. Electric sparks can develop in this gap causing burns to the skin. At each defibrillation, the heart muscle suffers to a certain degree from damage, and therefore quantities of defibrillation are limited. During defibrillation direct or indirect contact with the patient or the electrodes (be careful on wet base) should be avoided. The interruption of chest compressions should be kept as short as possible (< 5 s) prior the defibrillation. Only *one set of defibrillation* for each cycle should be applied, as a sequence of three defibrillations leads to a long interruption of chest compressions and causes further unnecessary damage to the myocardium without having any benefits. The exception is a witnesses cardiac arrest with shockable rhythm. Here, 3 consecutive shocks can be given immediately (◘ Fig. 31.5).

A = Airways check, clear and open   Breathing is only possible, if airways are free. This means that air between the mouth or nose and lungs is not obstructed. Airways can be obstructed for a number of reasons. Obstruction through the tongue is the most common cause. But also vomit and foreign objects such as dentures or teeth could be responsible. The mouth should be inspected before ventilation. Items such as vomit should be completely removed. Clearance of the mouth shouldn't be performed with the helper's fingers since this may cause injury. Rather the patient's fingers should be used for that.

To open the airways, different methods are available. One is hyperflexion of the head. This is achieved by the *jaw thrust* or the *chin lift*. The jaw thrust is performed by simply lifting the posterior aspect of the mandible up while the thumbs are pushing down the chin to open the mouth. The chin lift is performed by tilting the head backwards by placing fingers under the chin. However, for airway management in spinal injuries, the jaw thrust is the preferred method.

■ **Ventilation**
During inhalation fresh, oxygen-rich air enters the lungs, and carbon dioxide-rich air is exhaled

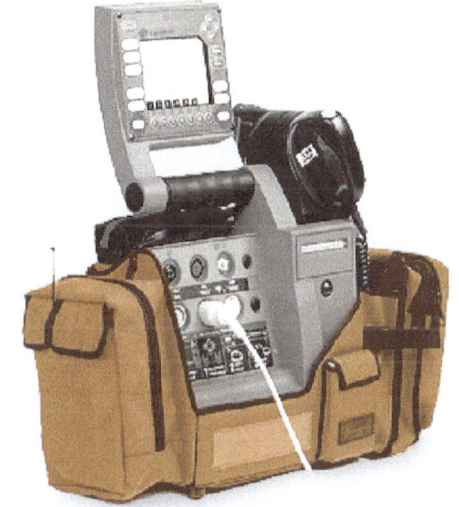

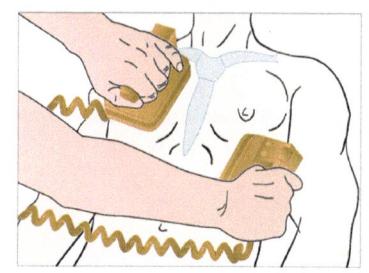

◘ **Fig. 31.5**   Positioning of the electrodes during defibrillation. (From Ziegenfuss 2014)

in return. Especially cardiopulmonary arrest in children or in drowning, where respiratory factors are the main causes, immediate restoration of ventilation is the most important treatment.

Ventilation can commence after clearing the airways. There are several ways for assisting ventilation. Methods of ventilation are mouth-to-mouth resuscitation, ventilation with mask, laryngeal mask airway (LMA) and intubation.

Mouth-to-mouth resuscitation can be performed in different ways. The "classic" mouth-to-mouth resuscitation is ventilation through the mouth with closing off the nose of the patient. The mouth-to-nose resuscitation is ventilation through the nose with closed mouth. The last variant is a combination of the two. Ventilation is applied through the mouth and the nose at the same time. To perform these ventilation methods, one hand is used to stabilise the hyperextension of the neck and the other hand to close the mouth or nose or for the additional stabilisation of the patient's position. To stabilise the neck in hyperextension, the hand is placed under the neck of the patient, so that the head can't slide back in the normal position. Depending on the method, the other hand is to be placed on the forehead and additionally occludes the nose or to be placed on the jaw to occlude the mouth. So far no cases of HIV transmissions through resuscitations have been recorded, but nevertheless care should be taken to reduce the risk. A protection device to prevent exposure to body secretions and blood is available in pharmacies. In general, application of cricoid pressure is not recommended.

During the *bag valve ventilation*, the helper should be positioned behind the patient's head. The head should be placed between the knees. After gentle hyperextension of the head, the mask is applied. The mask needs to be applied firmly onto the patient's face with the "E-C" technique. With the thumb and the index finger, a "C" is formed to apply downward pressure of the mask onto the face, including the mouth and nose. The jaw is lifted at the same time with the last three fingers, forming an "E". If air escapes next to the mask, the position of the mask needs to be corrected or the airways need to be cleared. Both lungs should lift and lower at the same time during ventilation. To make it easier for the person, who is ventilating, the bag can be placed on the thigh to be squeezed, resting on the thigh (■ Figs. 31.6, 31.7, and 31.8).

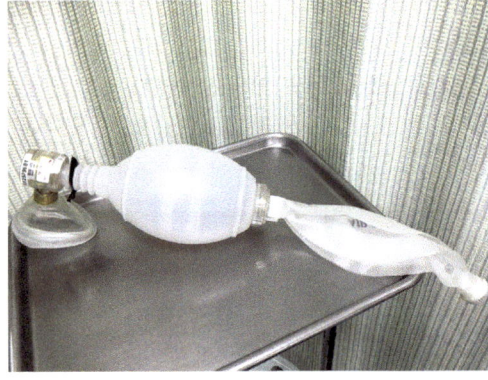

■ **Fig. 31.6**   Ventilation bag

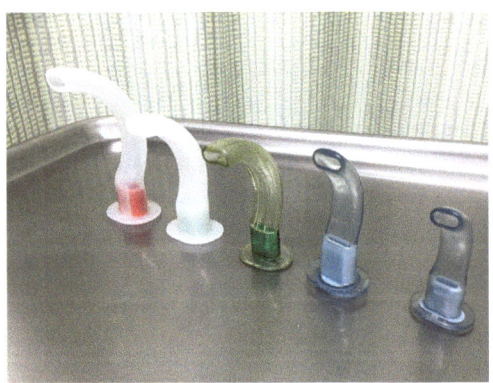

■ **Fig. 31.7**   Guedel

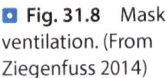

■ **Fig. 31.8**   Mask ventilation. (From Ziegenfuss 2014)

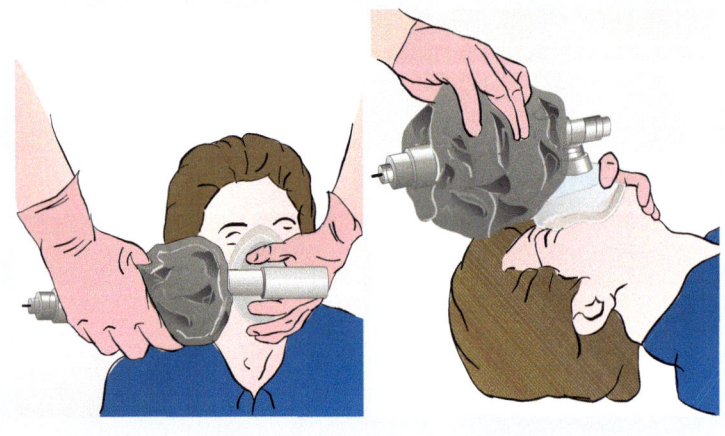

Oropharyngeal airway (Guedel) should be introduced to prevent the tongue of falling back. Guedels are inserted in inverted position and then turned around. The distance from the corners of the mouth to the ear of the patient can be used as guidance for the length of an appropriate Guedel. If the patient is not deeply unconscious or it is difficult to insert a Guedel, a *nasopharyngeal airway* may be used. Nasopharyngeal airways need to be lubricated with water-based lubrication before insertion. The direction of the insertion is vertically and not upwards, as this is the direction of the nasal cavity. The device needs to have the right size. Guidance for the right length of the nasopharyngeal airway is the distance between nostril and earlobe.

Another variant of ventilation is intubation with *endotracheal tubes (ETT)*. For this a slight hyperextension of the neck helps with visualising the vocal cords. The tube is placed as an artificial airway into the trachea. The end part of the tube should sit just before the bifurcation of the main bronchi and just behind the larynx. The tube has a cuff, which seals the airways once it is inflated. That ensures that no air passes next to the tube and no fluids enter the lungs. If HBOT is planned, the cuff should be filled with normal saline instead of air. On the other end, the bag or ventilator can be attached. Certain medications can be applied via the tube as well. This is the preferred ventilation in unconscious patients as it represents the best method for respiration, keeping airways open and preventing aspiration (◘ Figs. 31.9 and 31.10).

An alternative to intubation are supraglottic airway devices as the *i-gel®* and the *laryngeal mask airway (LMA)*. Laryngeal masks are easy and fast to use and don't require specific skills as for the ETT. The uninflated LMA is inserted via the mouth with its opening facing down. They are guided above the tongue, along the palate and advanced down to the larynx until resistance is felt. Before insertion the LMA needs to be lubricated, only on it's backside (to avoid aspiration/larynospasm). During insertion the LMA is held like a pen and guided with the index finger on the curved side under the lip. After the laryngeal mask is fully introduced, the cuff can be inflated. The mask seals the larynx sufficiently. The i-gel® doesn't require any inflation. It only needs to be removed from the cradle and be lubricated on it's backside (◘ Fig. 31.11).

During resuscitation, chest compressions are more important than ventilation. Intubation is time-consuming, and chest compressions are interrupted during inserting the ETT. The LMA can be introduced without interrupting chest compressions. The aim for all variants of ventilation is to establish as soon as possible a sufficient oxygen supply. Before attempting to intubate, the patient rather should be ventilated via bag valve mask or LMA. If possible, 100% oxygen should be supplied. The supply of 100% oxygen can be supplied with all ventilation methods. However, mouth-to-mouth resuscitation is sufficient enough, if there is no alternative. The oxygen content of the helper's exhaled air is still 17–18%. That is only 4% less oxygen than in the normal breathing air. This makes no real difference as the haemoglobin achieves still high levels of oxygen saturation.

After 30 compressions, two ventilations are followed in each resuscitation cycle. The inspiratory part of the ventilation should last 1 s, followed by 6–8 s break between the ventilations. Excessive ventilation should be avoided. Because of increased intra-pulmonary pressure, excessive ventilation reduces pulmonary blood flow to the heart. It also increases the risk of aspiration by overextending the stomach with air.

The breathing frequency is
- 30 compressions: two rescue breaths (mouth-to-mouth, mask or LMA), continuous compressions with ETT
- Ventilation volume approx. 600 mL (adults)
- One ventilation over 1 s; breath interval every 6–8 s, or 8–10 breaths/minute

■ **Drugs**

Medication during resuscitation can be given intravenously, intraosseous or intratracheal. The preferred ways to administer intravenous drugs are via proximal veins (cubical, femoral or central lines). If they can't be accessed, medication can be administered intraosseously.

□ Fig. 31.9 Instruments for intubation **a** laryngoscope handle, **b** laryngoscope blades, **c** Magill forceps **d** Magill-tubus **e** Oxford-tubus and **f** introducer. (From Ziegenfuss 2014)

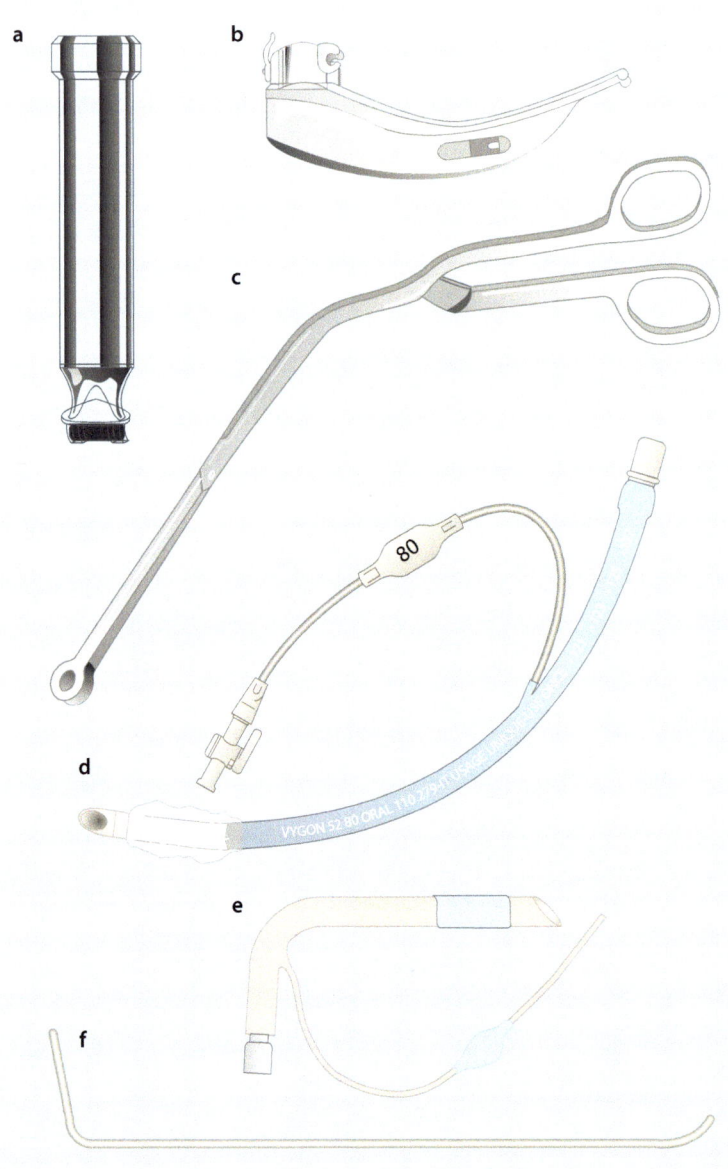

31

This method is equally efficient as intravenous administration. The preferred injection site of intraosseous cannulation is at the medial upper end of the tibia at the tibial tuberosity. Alternative sites are the distal tibia, proximal of the lateral malleolus or the proximal humerus.

Drugs for cardiac arrest
- Epinephrine/adrenaline 1 mg iv
- Amiodarone 300 mg iv bolus as a first dose, 150 mg iv bolus as second dose for refractory VF or VT

Adrenaline/epinephrine is the drug of choice. Adrenaline is a catecholamine, which acts on α- and β- receptors. The α-receptors cause vasoconstriction of peripheral blood vessels, which causes a volume shift into central vessels (visceral and cerebral vessels). β_1-receptors act chronotropic and inotropic. They increase the contractility of heart muscle cells, which eventually increases the success rate for defibrillation. However, they don't seem to increase CPP (cerebral perfusion pressure). Also O_2

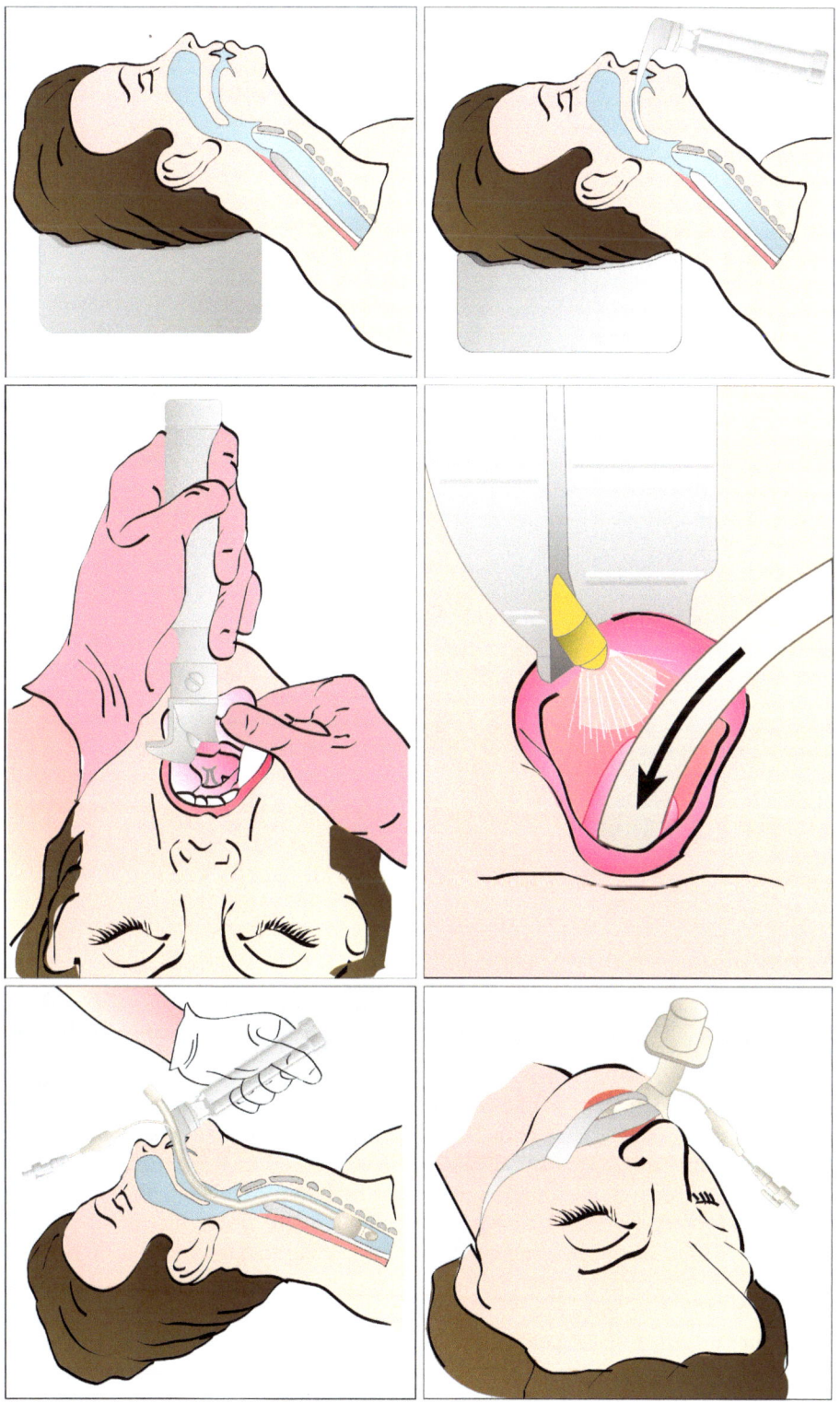

◨ **Fig. 31.10**   Intubation. (From Ziegenfuss 2014)

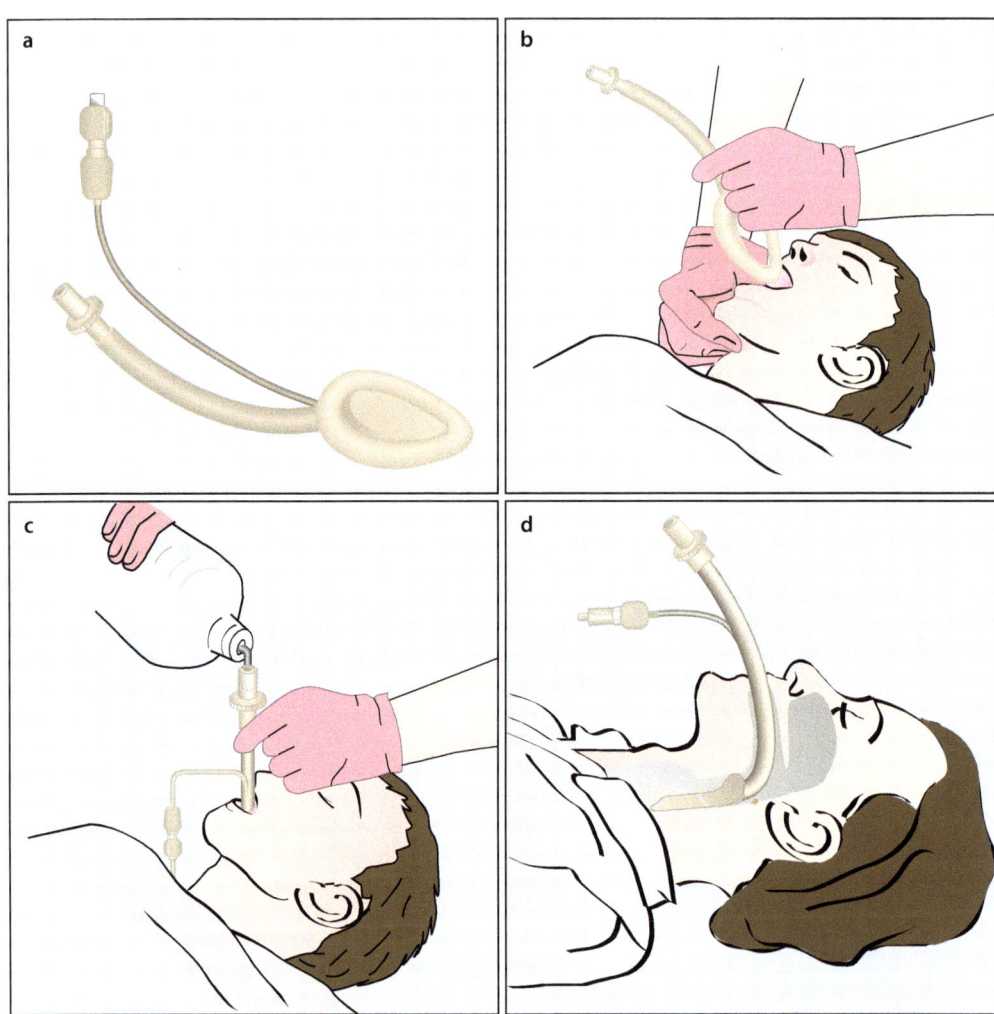

◻ Fig. 31.11   a Laryngeal mask airway (LMA) and **b–d** introduction of an LMA. (From Ziegenfuss 2014)

consumption of the cardiac muscle cells and the possibility of arrhythmias after resuscitation increase after adrenaline administration. Adrenaline 1 mg is administered with 10 mL of isotonic sodium chloride solution. Based on the ALS algorithm, it should be given every 3–5 min (after very second shock). It has a short half-life of 5–10 min. The single administration of vasopressin 40 IU is not reflected in the new AHA guidelines of 2015 anymore. Previously it was recommended as an alternative first or second dose instead of adrenaline. Vasopressin is an antidiuretic hormone that leads to vaso-

constriction in high doses. It causes peripheral vasoconstriction. At the same time, it leads to vasodilatation of cerebral vessels. It doesn't increases the O_2 consumption of the cardiac muscle cells. Amiodarone is a Class III anti-arrhythmic prolonging the action potential duration and hence the refractory period of myocardial tissue, which can be given for refractory ventricular fibrillation or refractory ventricular tachycardia (if no cardioversion is achieved with defibrillation). The first dose is 300 mg and second dose 150 mg, diluted in 10–20 mL 5% glucose over 1–2 min after at least three unsuccessful shocks. Amiodarone is contraindicated in polymorphic ventricular tachycardia, which is usually associated with a prolonged QT interval and is worsened by anti-arrhythmics. It has a half-life of 14–110 days.

All other drugs are obsolete. Atropine and bicarbonate are no longer used. However, in case of monochrome tachycardia with narrow QRS complex, adenosine 6–12 iv mg can be used. Intravenous fluid substitution reduces CPP and is therefore not recommended (except for cardiac arrest cause by hypovolaemia) (◘ Figs. 31.12 and 31.13).

Resuscitation runs in cycles. One cycle has 30 chest compressions and two breaths. The cycles are repeated five times. Five cycles make one loop. After every five cycles, or two loops, an evaluation of the resuscitation progress will be conducted. On each loop the ECG has to be analysed to determine whether a shockable rhythm is present or not. During the loops the team leader can gather useful information concerning the patient and organise the next steps of the resuscitation protocol (e.g. preparation for intubation, medication, transport, etc.). The chest compressions are to be continued immediately without delay after analysis or defibrillation. Proper implementation of five cycles takes about 3 min. The duration of 30 compressions is approx. 20 s. The duration of two breaths is about 12–16 s. Drugs, such as adrenaline and amiodarone, can be given according to the ALS-algorithm during the loops. The medication should be administered before ECG analysis and without interrupting chest compressions.

31.2 Shock

Shock is a result of physical or mental trauma. It results in decreased blood supply and oxygenation plus metabolic disturbance.

There are various forms of shock
— Hypovolemic shock
— Cardiogenic shock
— Obstructive Shock

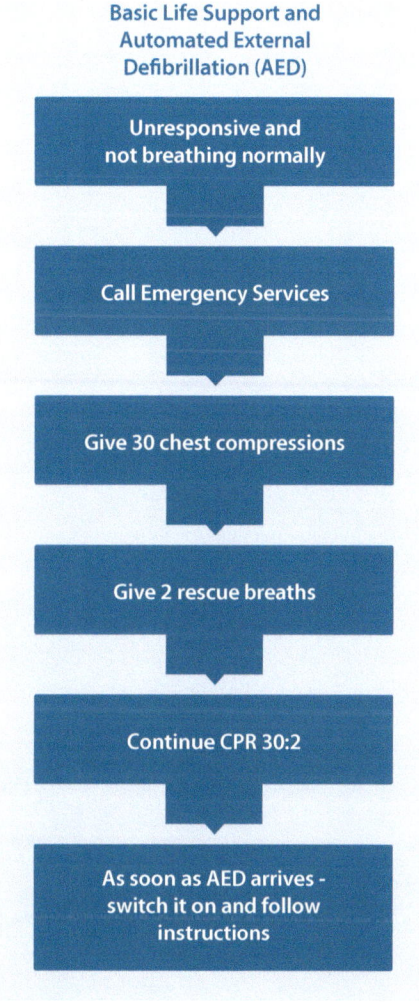

Basic Life Support and Automated External Defibrillation (AED)

Unresponsive and not breathing normally

Call Emergency Services

Give 30 chest compressions

Give 2 rescue breaths

Continue CPR 30:2

As soon as AED arrives - switch it on and follow instructions

◘ **Fig. 31.12**   BLS algorithm for adults. (© European Resuscitation Council, ERC 2015)

— Anaphylactic shock
— Septic shock
— Neurogenic shock

Causes of various forms of shock
— Hypovolemic Shock

Reduction of circulating blood volume causes hypovolemic shock. Reduction in blood volume can be caused by severe blood loss due to injury or dehydration (profuse sweating, severe vomiting and diarrhoea).

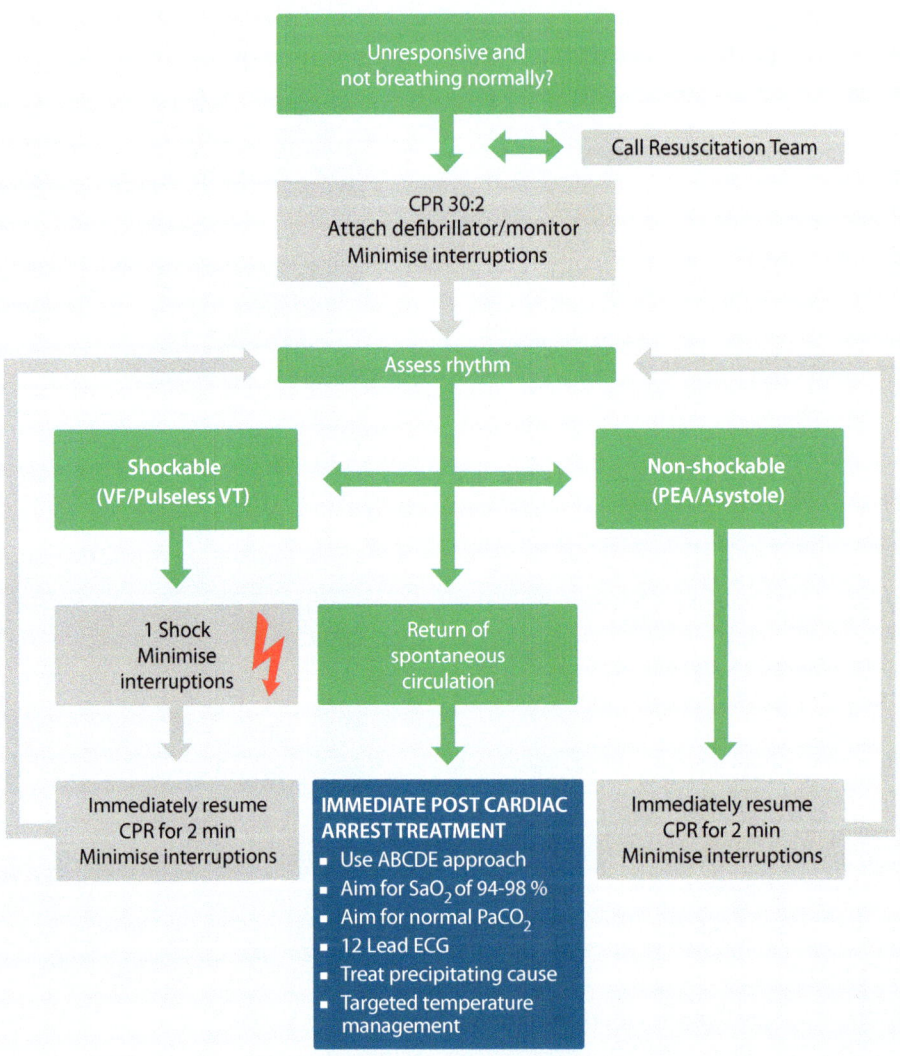

31

🔹 **Fig. 31.13**   ALS algorithm for adults. (© European Resuscitation Council, ERC 2015)

— Cardiogenic Shock

Cardiogenic shock is a result of a drastic decrease of the cardiac output. This can be caused by cardiac arrhythmia, acute myocardial infarction (AGE or DCI) or by heart failure.

— Obstructive Shock

Causes for an obstructive shock are pulmonary embolism and tension pneumothorax (massive pulmonary embolism due to VGE caused by severe DCI with, hyper- or hypobaric pulmonary barotraumas, tension pneumothorax and fat embolism triggered by serious injuries or by massive cutaneous DCS or barotrauma).

— Anaphylactic Shock

Sensitising substances like nettle or venom can cause allergies. This can in its extreme lead to anaphylactic shock. It results in failure of peripheral vascular regulation. Anaphylaxis is an allergy Type I (immediate type) reaction and is triggered by allergens. Previous contact with particular allergens is required to trigger this reaction. The first contact to allergens doesn't causes allergic reactions. After the body is sensitised and produces antibodies (IgE), an allergic reaction can be provoked. IgE has the ability to bind on antigens and at the same time on mast cells. This causes the mast cells to release histamine. Histamine dilates blood vessels, increases permeability of blood vessels, narrows bronchi and promotes formation of mucus in the lungs.

— Septic Shock

Septic shock can result from septicaemia. Sepsis is mainly caused by gram-negative bacteria. It also results in failure of peripheral vascular regulation and paralysis of vascular muscles by bacterial toxins.

— Neurogenic Shock

If centres for blood pressure regulation of the CNS (the brain and spinal cord, only in segments above T6) are damaged, neurogenic shock may develop. The result is cardiovascular dysregulation, which can end up in shock. Severe DCI may cause neurogenic shock during or after diving.

In all forms of shock, blood pressure drops and stress hormones are released (adrenaline, noradrenalin). Stress hormones cause increased heart rate and constriction of arterial and venous vessels (*reduction of microcirculation*). Therefore, blood pressure initially can be quite normal. Later vasodilatation develops, and blood pressure starts declining. Adrenaline and noradrenaline act on receptors of blood vessels in different ways (see physiologically basics/autonomic nervous system). Adrenalin acts equally on α- and β-receptors. Noradrenaline, which takes the majority, mainly affects α-receptors. Through α- and β-receptor distribution, blood volume shifts from peripheral to central areas (*centralisation*) to ensure a sufficient oxygen supply to vital organs like the heart and brain. The periphery of the body, which is now poorly perfused, acidifies. Through local tissue acidosis, the permeability of blood vessel increases, and fluid shifts from the inside of blood vessels into the surrounding extravascular tissue. Fluid shift and additional vasodilatation reduce significantly the blood pressure. The initial only localised tissue acidosis quickly turns into a generalised acidosis. Blood vessels lose their ability to contract and can't maintain a sufficient blood pressure. All these mechanisms lead to a vicious circle that accelerates the catastrophic effects of shock (Fig. 31.14).

31.2.1 Symptoms

Common features of all forms of shock are blood pressure reduction and increased heart rate. Often, peripheral pulses on the wrist or foot can't be felt, since blood pressure is insufficient or the pulse frequency is too high. The shock index is a value, which can indicate the presence of shock.

Shock index = pulse rate / systolic blood pressure

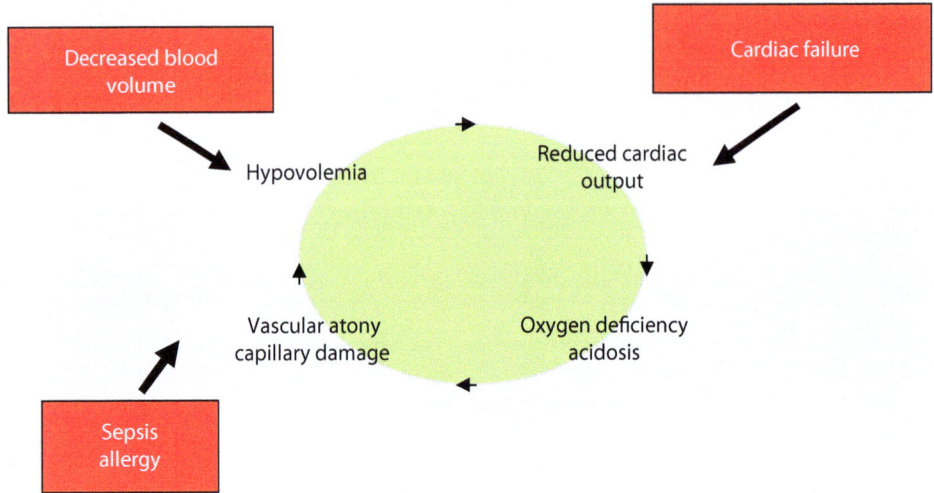

◘ **Fig. 31.14**   Shock cycle

❯ **Values over 1 is indicative for shock!**

■ **Hypovolemic Shock**

Blood loss of up to 1000 mL is still quite tolerated in adults. Blood loss of 2000–3000 mL is no longer compatible with life (◘ Table 31.3). As you can see, there is only a very narrow window between having no symptoms and actually dying from blood loss. Blood loss of small vessels is usually minimal, except if large areas are affected. Normally, blood loss is ceased with help of the coagulation cascade and local vascular constriction. However, if widespread superficial wounds persist for a prolonged time, blood loss may be sufficient enough to lead to shock. Blood losses of larger, deeper blood vessels, especially arteries, can be life-threatening even in a short time. Because arteries have more pressure than veins, blood gets lost on a faster rate. During venous bleeding, blood rather flows. During arterial bleeding blood is rather ejected in a pulsating way.

Signs for a successful CPR are palpable pulses, warming and regaining normal skin colour, constriction of the pupils, spontaneous breathing and regaining consciousness. If CPR is unsuccessful, cessation of CPR might be considered under following condition:

■ **Cardiogenic Shock**

Right or left heart failure can lead to cardiogenic shock. Both produce a reduced cardiac output. Left heart or global heart failure can be caused by cardiac arrhythmia or myocardial infarction. Pulmonary embolisms block pulmonary blood vessels to various degrees. This impedes the blood supply to the left heart and hence to the large circulation. At the same time in the right heart, pressure increases. This pressure increase puts a strain on the heart and ultimately leads to right heart failure.

Symptoms of left heart or global heart failure

- Systolic blood pressure < 80–90 mmHg
- Cardiac index < 1.8 L / min / m^2
- Left ventricular end-diastolic pressure > 20 mmHg
- Crackles mainly over the lower sections of the lungs
- Shortness of breath, increased by exercise
- Cyanosis
- Reduced palpable pulse

Damage to the lung parenchyma or pronounced pulmonary embolism causes venous back flow into the pulmonary circulation. As a result,

◻ Table 31.3 Signs and symptoms of haemorrhage by class

Parameter	Class I	Class II (mild)	Class III (moderate)	Class IV (severe)
Approximate blood loss	<15%	15–30%	31–40%	> 40%
Heart rate	↔	↔/↑	↑	↑/↑↑
Blood pressure	↔	↔	↔/↓	↓
Pulse pressure	↔	↓	↓	↓
Respiratory rate	↔	↔	↔/↑	↑
Urine output	↔	↔	↓	↓↓
Glasgow coma scale score	↔	↔	↓	↓
Base deficit[a]	0 to −2 mEq/L	−2 to −6 mEq/L	−6 to −10 mEq/L	−10 mEq/L or Less
Need for blood products	Monitor	Possible	Yes	Massive transfusion protocol

With kind permission from American College of Surgeons 2018
[a]Base excess is the quantity of base (HCO3−, in mEq/L) that is above or below the normal range in the body. A negative number is called a base deficit and indicates metabolic acidosis

massive right heart failure can develop. Shortness of breath, respiratory failure, retrosternal pain, tachycardia, arrhythmia (mainly AF), increased JVP, haemoptysis and general symptoms of shock may be features of this. Without treatment, sooner or later this results in a complete cardiovascular failure (◻ Table 31.4).

Symptoms of right ventricular failure
- Tachycardia
- Tachypnoea, haemoptysis and shortness of breath
- Increased JVP
- General shock symptoms
- Retrosternal pain
- Cyanosis

Typical signs of pulmonary embolisms
- Shortness of breath with increased respiratory rate
- Sudden pleuritic retrosternal pain
- Haemoptysis
- Right ventricular failure
- Tachycardia

◻ Table 31.4 Grading of the severity of pulmonary embolisms (Schulte 1987)

I	Small embolus (<25%), normal ABG and dyspnoea
II	Sub massive embolus (25–50%), pCO_2 < 35 mmHg and high respiratory rate
III	Massive embolus (50–80%), pCO_2 < 30 mmHg, pO_2 < 65 mmHg, cyanosis, tachycardia and cardiogenic shock
IV	Fulminant embolus (>80%), cardiac arrest and pO_2 < 50 mmHg

- Arrhythmia (mainly AF)
- LOC

■ **Anaphylactic Shock**
Symptoms arise almost immediately or within a short time after the contact with an allergen (◻ Table 31.5). An anaphylactic shock during diving may occur after contact of jellyfish or other venomous marine creatures.

31

■ Table 31.5   Severity grade of anaphylaxis

0	Local cutaneous reaction
I	Generalised symptoms (dizziness, anxiety, headache etc.) and skin reactions (itchiness, hives, flush etc.)
II	In addition to I hypotension, tachycardia, dyspnoea and gastrointestinal symptoms (nausea, vomiting, diarrhoea)
III	In addition to II bronchial spasms (asthma), shock, laryngeal oedema and life-threatening hypotension
IV	Respiratory or cardiac arrest

■ **Septic Shock**

Septic shock is always caused by infections. Sepsis originates from infections of the organs, skin, or abscesses. Septic shock may develop even within hours. Typical signs of sepsis are high fever, chills and confusion. Complications include abscess formations, damage to vital organs (mainly heart), multi-organ failure, ARDS and a high mortality rate of 30–50% even in treated sepsis. If left untreated, the mortality rate is 100%.

■ **Symptoms of Septic Shock**
General
– Fever, confusion and agitation
– Hyperventilation
– Cutaneous manifestation like pustules, purpura, tissue necrosis and blisters

Early phase (hyperdynamic phase)
– Warm, dry skin and rosy look
– Oxygen partial pressure in arterial blood gas analysis (ABG) and venous blood gas analysis (VBG) are matching increasingly
– Blood pressure normal or slightly decreased

Late phase (hypodynamic phase)
– Pale, moist cool skin
– Increasing oxygen difference between arteries and veins
– Hypotension, tachycardia and polyuria

■ **Neurogenic Shock**

The symptoms are similar as in the late phase of the septic shock.

31.2.2 **Complications**

Multi-organ failure may be a *complication* in all forms of shock:
– Kidney: oliguria and anuria
– Stomach: stress ulcers
– Lung: shock lung (ARDS)
– Heart: heart failure, caused by a decreased blood flow to the heart
– Immune system: highly disturbed function of the RHS with greatly increased susceptibility
– Coagulation: possibly there is a disseminated intravascular coagulation (DIC) with micro embolism and severe bleeding (haemorrhagic diathesis)

31.2.3 **Treatment and Prophylaxis**

In all forms of shock, the patient should be laid down in a flat position. Unconscious patients should be positioned in a left-side stable side position. Elevation of legs is no longer recommended because it might cause cardiac overload, which increases the risk of heart failure and myocardial infarctions. The patient should be remained calm, as agitation and anxiety additionally intensify shock symptoms. The body should be kept at normal temperature. In hot areas, the body should be protected from excessive heat such as direct sunlight. In cool environment, the body needs to be kept warm.

Injuries during diving, where blood loss might occur, can be caused by sharks, barracudas and also by motorboats during the ascent. Hence, diving buoys should be used where motorboats are present. The buoy is connected to the diver by a long robe. It follows the divers everywhere and is visible for others. In particular in free diving, the surface should be observed at any time during the ascent, by turning around 360° on its own axis. Because of the increased conductivity of sound underwater, divers cannot rely on their recognition of sounds underwater. Distance and direction of sound sources can't be predicted underwater.

In general wounds initially should be covered with dressings and bleeding should be controlled. A thorough cleaning of the wound can be conducted later in the hospital. Cleaning on site could delay suppression of blood loss and cause additional damage and contamination of the wound area. Bleeding should be contained by pressure bandages. Heavy bleeding of limbs can be reduced by compressing the supplying artery (femoral artery in the groin, brachial artery on the inside of the upper arm above the elbow joint). A ligature of the limbs is no longer recommended, as the damage to the tissue and nerves outweighs its benefits. A proper compression is completely sufficient. A blood pressure cuff might be applied proximal to the wound area.

Hypovolemic shock due to dehydration should be initially treated by drinking water. Due to the loss of water, blood volume decreases and the electrolyte concentration increases. Rapid drinking of large volumes should be avoided because water intake with its relatively low electrolyte content causes to a rapid influx into the "thickened" blood. It might also cause hyponatremia. The consequence can be destruction of red blood cells (haemolysis). The same applies to rapid infusions. Intravenous fluid replacement need to be carried out carefully. However, in hypovolemic shock rapid hydration might be required.

In cardiogenic shock excessive fluid replacement can cause great harm. In this condition, it is rather necessary to "reduce" the relative blood volume. This can be done through a so-called bloodless bleeding. It can be achieved by positioning the patient in an upright position. A part of the blood volume is shifted into the legs. Hence, the circulating blood volume decreases, which relieves the heart. Septic, anaphylactic and neurogenic shock are treated with general shock treatment for the time being.

The most important thing in treatment of a shock is to stabilise perfusion. Basic monitoring should be carried out:

Basic monitoring

- Pulse, blood pressure, central venous pressure (JVP), ECG monitor, respiratory rate, fluid input and output
- Full blood count, HB, HCT, lactate, coagulation factors, urea, creatinine, electrolytes
- Arterial blood gas analysis
- Pulse oximetry

■ **Volume Substitution**

For *hypovolemic shock,* volume substitution is essential. Substitution can be given intravenously. At least two large bore cannulas should be placed on opposite sites. This allows access on the one site for fluid substitution and medication administration. The other site is an alternative venous access in case the other one fails. It is often difficult to get intravenous accesses in severely sick patients. Hence, in every severely sick patient an alternative intravenous access is required to have an alternative venous access for fluid or medication administration, as this is essential for the treatment.

For *volume substitution,* there are different drugs available:

■ **Colloid: Plasma Expanders**

Plasma expanders are plasma substitutes with oncotic pressure more than plasma itself. This means that in addition to administered fluids, extravascular fluid is drawn into the blood vessels. Dextran, hydroxyethyl starch (HAES) and body plasma agents are available.

Dextrans have low molecular weight (MG 40000). Monovalent dextran (1000 MG) is injected to prevent anaphylactic reactions prior administration of dextran infusions. This ensures that pre-existing antibodies are bound to the extremely small molecules of the monovalent dextran, without causing a systemic reaction to the following dextran infusion. *Hydroxyethyl starch (HAES)* is preferred as a plasma expander, since the risk of severe anaphylactic reactions is less than in dextrans. There are 6% and 10% solutions, but 6% solutions are preferred. Red blood cells are more rigid in shock (sludge phenomenon). The normal diameter of red blood cells is already more than the diameter of normal capillaries. The physiological deformability of red blood cells is enhanced by plasma expanders like HAES and dextrans and counteracts the sludge formation. Red blood cells are therefore increasingly able to pass through capillaries. Human colloidal solutions (pasteurised human albumin, plasma protein solution, fresh frozen plasma) are less suitable for the use as emergency drugs because they expire quickly at room temperature, and their production is expensive. Fresh frozen plasma also poses a risk of infection.

■ Isotonic Crystalloid Salt Solutions

Normal saline solutions and Ringer-lactate or Ringer's solutions remain only a short time (approx. 30–40 min) in the vascular system compared to colloidal plasma expanders (HAES and dextran 40,000) with approx. 3–4 h. Isotonic crystalloid solutions can be used together with plasma expanders in severe volume losses. They are excellent first-line infusions in emergency situations.

■ Erythrocytes Infusion

Erythrocyte infusions are almost exclusively used in hospital settings during operations or for severe blood losses. The advantage of erythrocyte infusions is their ability to bind and transport oxygen. As a result, the body has an improved oxygen supply. Plasma expander and saline solutions only cover the volume deficit, but not transporting oxygen. The disadvantage of red cell preparations is their short expiry date, potential infection source, risk of hypersensitivity reactions and that they may lead to unnecessary delays due to blood group testing.

■ Hypertonic Saline (3%)

Hypertonic saline is only utilised in severely symptomatic hyponatremia (e.g. seizing, severe altered level of consciousness, focal neurological sign due to hyponatremia) and elevated cranial pressure. It is more commonly used for the later. It requires regular blood test every 4–6 h to monitor sodium levels as there is a risk of causing overcorrection. Hypernatremia or rapid correction in sodium of more than 8–10 mmol in a 24-h period might occur and has to be avoided. It preferably should be administered via a central venous catheter. Additionally, urine output needs to be measured. A urine output of >250 mL per hour raises the suspicion of diabetes insipidus.

■ Specific Treatment Options

In *anaphylactic shock*, the allergic reaction itself has to be treated, but also blood pressure needs to be restored. First of all, further exposure to allergens needs to be ceased. To stabilise blood pressure, colloid or crystalloid solutions can be given. To stabilise blood vessels, epinephrine/adrenaline is used. Cortisone and antihistamines are used to curb effects of inflammation and allergic reactions. However, they have only delayed effects. Antihistamines prevent further histamine release. H_1 –antihistamines are commonly used in mild to moderate allergic reactions. H_2 –antihistamines could be added, if needed. In anaphylaxis however antihistamines should be used with care as they can worsen hypotension. The role of cortisone in treating anaphylaxis is unknown. It mainly has its benefits in the treatment of respiratory symptoms. It increases the responsiveness of the β_2-receptors in the lungs and prevents a potential late-phase reaction in allergies. In an allergic-related asthma β_2-mimetics (salbutamol) as nebulisers or sprays or intravenous β_2-mimetics or theophylline as a short infusion can be utilised. Other catecholamines like dopamine may be used in persistent shock.

■ Medication for the Treatment of an Anaphylactic Reaction

- Adrenaline 0.01 mg/kg bw sc or im, 0.001 mg/kg bw iv, as a rule adults, 0.5 mg in the in the thigh, children depending on the body weight (e.g. at 30 kg bw = 0.3 mg im/sc); intramuscular or subcutaneous administration can be repeated every 20 min depending on the symptoms. The initial is intravenous administration in adults usually is 100–250 µg, with 25–50 µg every 5–15 min. Intravenous administration has to be given slowly.

31

- Fast volume substitution with isotonic saline solution.
- Cortisone (hydrocortisone 5 mg/kg bw but max. 200 mg iv or prednisolone 1 mg/kg bw max 50 mg).
- When shocks persist a continuous perfusion with dopamine can be given (initial dose 2–5 µg/kg bw/min with increasing dose up to 20–50 µg/kg bw/min).
- Antihistamines, such as promethazine 50 mg iv (handled with care in anaphylactic shock, may cause additional hypotension).
- H2-receptor antagonist, such as ranitidine 50 mg iv (handled with care in anaphylactic shock).
- For upper airways obstruction, 5 mg adrenaline as nebuliser.

Neurogenic shock mainly requires stabilisation of blood pressure. This can be achieved with catecholamines and fluid administration. If the CNS is affected, a systolic blood pressure of about 140 mmHg should be aimed for. Embolisms, which caused *obstructive shock*, need to be eliminated as quickly as possible to restore normal perfusion. If embolisms are caused by gas (decompression sickness) after diving, HBOT should be initiated as soon as possible. The most important general treatment is elevation of the upper body and oxygen administration. Elevation of the upper body reduces the preload and hence reduces the cardiac workload. Antiarrhythmics can be used in adjunction for cardiac arrhythmias.

Suggested Reading

Anthem, Medical Policies and Clinical UM Guidelines. 2008. https://www.anthem.com/medicalpolicies/policies/mp_pw_a049925.htm. Accessed 12 July 2015.

Berg RA, Hemphill R, Abella BS, Aufderheide TP, Cave DM, Hazinski MF, Lerner EB, Rea TD, Syre MR, Swore RA. Part 5: adult basic life support: 2010 American Heart Association guidelines for cardiopulmonary resuscitation and emergency cardiovas-

cular care science. Circulation. 2010;122(suppl 3): S685–705.

Berg RA, Sanders AB, Kern KB, et al. Adverse hemodynamic effects of interrupting chest compressions for rescue breathing during cardiopulmonary resuscitation for ventricular fibrillation cardiac arrest. Circulation. 2001;104(20):2465–70.

Cameron P, Jalinek G, Kelly AM, Murray L, Heyworth J. Textbook of adult emergency medicine. Edinburgh: Churchill Livingstone; 2000.

Field JM, Hazinski MF, Sayre MR, et al. Part 1: executive summary: 2010 American Heart Association guidelines for cardiopulmonary resuscitation and emergency cardiovascular care. Circulation. 2010;122(18 Suppl 3):S640–56.

Hayek DA, Veremakis C. Physiologic concerns during brain resuscitation. In: Civetta JM, Taylor RW, Kirby RR, editors. Critical care. 2nd ed. Philadelphia: Lippincott Williams & Wilkins; 1992.

Hazinski MF, Shuster M, Donnino MW, Travers AH, Samson RA, Schexanyder SM, Sinz EH, Woodin JA, Atkins DL, Bhanji F, Brooks SC, Callaway CW, de Caen AR, Kleinman ME, Kronick SL, Lavonas EJ, Link MS, Mancini ME, Morrison LJ, Neumar RW, O'Connor RE Singletary EM, Wyckoff MH. Highlights of the 2015 American Heart Association, Guidelines update for CPR and ECC, 2015.

Hupfl M, Selig HF, Nagele P. Chest-compression-only versus standard cardiopulmonary resuscitation: a meta-analysis. Lancet. 2010;376(9752):1552–7.

Link ML, Atkins DL, Passman RS, Halperin HR, Samson RA, White RD, Cudnik MD, Berg MD, Kudenchuk PJ, Kerber RE. Part 6: electrical therapies: automated external defibrillators, defibrillation, cardioversion, and pacing 2010 American Heart Association guidelines for cardiopulmonary resuscitation and emergency cardiovascular care. Circulation. 2010;122:S706–19.

Mentzelopoulos SD, Malachias S, Chamos C, Konstantopoulos D, Ntaidou T, Papastylianou A, et al. Vasopressin, steroids, and epinephrine and neurologically favorable survival after in-hospital cardiac arrest: a randomized clinical trial. JAMA. 2013 Jul 17;310(3):270–9.

MIMS online (Australia). Accessed 12/11/2017. www.mimsonline.com.au.

Morrison LJ, Verbeek PR, Vermeulen MJ, et al. Derivation and evaluation of a termination of resuscitation clinical prediction rule for advanced life support providers. Resuscitation. 2007;74(2):266–75.

Mutschler A, Nienaber U, Brockamp T, et al. A critical reappraisal of the ATLS classification of hypovolaemic shock: does it really reflect clinical reality? Resuscitation. 2013;84:309–13.

Neumar RW, Otto CW, Link MS, Kornick SL, Shuster M, Callaway CW, Kudenchuck PJ, Ornato JP, McNally B,

Silvers SM, Passman RS, White RD, Hess EP, Tang W, Davis D, Sinz E, Morrison LJ. American Heart Association guidelines for cardiopulmonary resuscitation and emergency cardiovascular care science; part 8: adult advanced life support. Circulation. 2010;122:S729–67.

Nolan JP, Hazinski MF, Aickin R, et al. Part 1: executive summary: 2015 international consensus on cardiopulmonary resuscitation and emergency cardiovascular care science with treatment recommendations. Resuscitation. 2015;12:e1.

Perki GD, Travers AH, Berg RA, Castren M, Considine J, Escalante R, Gazmuri RJ, Koster RW, Lim SH, Nation KJ, Olasveengen TM, Sakamoto T, Sayre MR, Sierra A, Smyth MA, Stanton D, Vaillancourt C, on behalf of the Basic Life Support Chapter 2: Resuscitation, Part 3: Adult basic life support and automated external defibrillation 2015 International Consensus on Cardiopulmonary Resuscitation and Emergency Cardiovascular Care Science with Treatment Recommendations, Elsevier, Resuscitation 95(2015)e43–e69.

Sayre MR, Berg RA, Cave DM, Page RL, Potts J, White RD. Hands-only (compression-only) cardiopulmonary resuscitation: a call to action for bystander response to adults who experience out-of-hospital sudden cardiac arrest: a science advisory for the public from the American Heart Association Emergency Cardiovascular Care Committee. Circulation. 2008;117(16):2162–7.

Travers AH, Rea TD, Bobrow BJ, Edelson DP, Berg RA, Sayre MR, et al. Part 4: CPR overview: 2010 American Heart Association guidelines for cardiopulmonary resuscitation and emergency cardiovascular care. Circulation. 2010;122:S676–84.

31

Travel Medicine

© Springer International Publishing AG, part of Springer Nature 2018
O. Rusoke-Dierich, *Diving Medicine*, https://doi.org/10.1007/978-3-319-73836-9_32

Before travelling to other countries, thorough travel advice should be provided. Not only information about diseases of specific countries but also general advice for travelling should be given on this consultation.

The following topics should be included in the travel advice consultation:

- Vaccinations (general and country specific)
- Country-specific diseases
- Malaria prophylaxis
- Mosquito prophylaxis (wearing bright long-sleeved clothes, avoiding perfume, staying in air-conditioned rooms, using a mosquito net, using insect repellents, staying inside at dawn and dusk)
- Food consumption and drinking overseas (no consumption of ice cubes, uncooked meals, salads and food, which is exposed to flies, limited alcohol consumption)
- UV protection (using sun cream, avoiding sun exposure between 11.00 and 15.00 o'clock, remaining in shaded areas, wearing a hat and covering skin)
- Fitness assessment for travelling, flying and diving
- Challenges of different climates and their effects on the personal health (dehydration, hyperthermia)
- Medications
- Thrombosis counselling
- Counselling on symptoms on return, which require review (fever, skin changes, abnormal bleeding, lymphadenopathy, diarrhoea)
- Sexual transmitted diseases
- Contraception
- Rabies

The following items should be asked to enable to give the appropriate advice:

- Risk assessment of the travel in a particular country (transport, area of stay/ rural or resort, reason for travelling, appropriate conduct overseas, pre-existing diseases and medications)
- Vaccination status
- Accomodation and stopovers
- Duration of the stay

The vast majority of up-to-date travel information and information about tropical disease are available on WHO (World Health Organization) or CDC (Centres for Disease Control and Prevention) websites. Information on these websites are frequently updated. Before giving appropriate advice based on these online resources, it should be checked, which medications are available in the particular countries. Hence, recommendations need to be adjusted individually. Usually, a medication record is required at the customs. However, it might be sufficient, if the original medication box has the patients and prescribing doctors details (■ Table 32.1).

32.1 Malaria

Malaria is a tropical disease transmitted by the female *Anopheles* mosquito. The distribution of malaria is primarily in the tropics and subtropics of Africa, Central and South America, Asia, Papua New Guinea and the Western Pacific Islands. As popular diving spots are located in these areas, malaria prophylaxis and advice should be given. The WHO (World Health Organization) estimates the worldwide number of people affected by malaria with about 198 million and 1,200,000 deaths (2013). The *Plasmodium* parasites need temperatures above 20 °C in order to complete the entire growth cycle. Therefore, malaria occurs in some places only seasonal. Additionally, there are differences in *Anopheles* species regarding the affinity to the host and their local distribution. Some genetic factors are protected against malaria. For example, sickle cell anaemia gives a certain protection against *P. falciparum* and Duffy negative blood group against *P. vivax*. It appears that after recurrent malaria infections, the body adapts to the disease. This means that an infection is possible, but the symptoms of malaria seem to be reduced. Children and pregnant women have an increased risk of being affected by malaria. Additionally, children have a high mortality rate. During pregnancy the resistance against malaria is reduced.

Table 32.1 DVT prophylaxis

Risk	Risk factors	Prophylaxis
Minimal risk	Age < 40, no health issues	a
Low risk	Age > 40, obesity, acute inflammation, minor surgery <3 days	aCompression stockings
Medium risk	Varicose veins, poorly controlled heart failure, acute myocardial infarction <6 days, oestrogen therapy and OCD, polycythemia, pregnancy and postpartum, injury or paralysis of the lower limbs <6 weeks	aAspirin (if there are no contra-indications; not in pregnancy; effectiveness not proven), compression stockings
High risk	Previous DVT or pulmonary embolism, thrombocytophilia (AT III, protein C and protein S deficiency, APC resistence, factor II-dimorphism, dysfibrinogenemia, hyperhomocysteinemia, factor V-Leiden, etc.), major surgery <6 weeks, previous stroke, neoplasia, family history of DVT and pulmonary embolism	a, bAnticoagulation with low molecular weight heparin (e.g. dalteparin 5000 IE, enoxaparin 40 mg) or an off label use of a single dose of rivaroxaban (Xarelto®) 10 mg before and 3 days after the flight

aExtension of legs and ankles, no luggage under seat in front of the passenger, frequent walking, avoiding sleeping crippled over, high fluid intake, avoiding alcohol, coffee or tea
bApproval of anticoagulants for VTE prophylaxis depends on national regulations; contraindications prior administration need to be excluded

It also poses an increased risk for the unborn child (low birth weight). *Anopheles* is active especially at sunrise and sunset. Different kinds of mosquitoes are rather active during the day and can transmit other diseases such as dengue. Especially *P. falciparum* and *P. vivax* have resistances against antimalaria drugs. There are different *Plasmodium* pathogens:

- *P. falciparum*: Worldwide tropical and subtropical distribution, mainly in Africa; pathogen of severe malaria causes 1 million deaths per year; rapid growth in the blood with haemolysis and emboli due to cytoadherence of affected erythrocytes; 7–30 days of incubation, irregular fever spikes.
- *P. vivax*: mainly in Asia, Latin America and some countries in Africa; the disease can be activated after months or years. Incubation period of 12–18 days; fever spikes every 2 days.
- *P. ovale*: mainly West Africa and the Western Pacific Islands. Similar to the *P. vivax*, it can also infect people with Duffy-negative blood group; incubation

period of 12–18 days; fever spikes every 2 days.
- *P. malariae*: worldwide distribution; typical 3-day cycle, untreated can lead to lifelong chronic malaria; incubation period 16–50 days; fever spikes every 3 days.
- *P. knowlesi*: Southeast Asia, mainly infected animals.

32.1.1 Aetiology and Pathogenesis

After the *Anopheles* mosquito aspirates with gametocytes infected blood, the gametocytes develop to gamete in the mosquito's intestines. In the blood of the mosquito, the microgametes (male) penetrate the macrogametes (female), forming zygotes. Then cells are changed to an elongated, motile ookinete. This evolves into an oocyst. After the oocyst bursts, sporozoites are released and get in the saliva of the mosquito. The entire cycle inside the mosquito takes 8–16 days. If sporozoites enter the human bloodstream through the saliva of the mosquito, liver cells via the bloodstream get infected. They penetrate liver cells and turn into schizonts (exo-erythrocytes cycle). With the exception of *P. oval*, merozoites are released in the bloodstream after the liver cycle (exo-erythrocytic cycle). *P. vivax* and *P. ovale* produce hypnozoites, which can stay dormant in liver cells. Merozoites enter red blood cells and multiply there asexually. By rupturing erythrocytes, merozoites are released, which some of them are infecting other erythrocytes. The cycle repeats every 2 or 3 days. The blood stage parasites are responsible of the typical malaria symptoms. Some merozoites differentiate into gametocytes, after being aspirated by the mosquitoes. Again, in a mosquito infected with the pathogen, transfer of the parasite to someone else is possible (◻ Table 32.2, ◻ Fig. 32.1).

32.1.2 Symptoms

Symptoms of malaria appear after the incubation period. The incubation period varies depending on the pathogen. It can be between a few weeks and also takes up to several months or even a year (*P. vivax* or occasionally *P. ovale*). Malaria can be divided in three different forms:
- *Malaria tertiana*: Pathogen: *P. vivax* and *P. ovale*; fever every second day with one day without fever, spontaneous remission after max. 5 years
- *Malaria quartana*: Pathogen: *P. malaria*; fever every third day with 2 days without fever, no spontaneous remission
- *Malaria tropica*: Pathogen: *P. falciparum*, irregular fevers due to the lack of synchronisation of the parasite reproduction, severe form of malaria (Malaria maligna) with high fatality, recurrence up to 2 years

The fever has a specific pattern. In the first hour, strong rigors and increasing fever typically develop. The fever can reach 40 °C and more for duration of about 4 h. It is often associated with flushing, vomiting and nausea. The fever stage is followed by an approximately 3-h stage of severe sweating with decreasing fever.

◻ **Table 32.2** Comparison of mild and severe malaria symptoms

Mild symptoms	Severe symptoms
Fever, rigors	Altered level of consciousness, confusion, coma,
Cough	GCS < 11 (adults), Blantyre coma scale <3 (children)
Malaise	Shock
Diaphoresis	Icterus (bilirubin >3 mg/dL or 50 μmol/L)
Myalgia, arthralgia	Acute renal failure (creatine >265 μmol/L, urea >20 mmol/L); oliguria (<400 mL/24 h)
Abdominal pain	Seizures >2/d
Headache	Hyperparasitaemia >2%
Vomiting, nausea	Extreme weakness (requires assistance for sitting up)
Diarrhoea	Shortness of breath (pulmonary oedema, shock)
Anorexia	SaO$_2$ < 92%, respiratory rate > 30/min
Hepatosplenomegaly	Acidosis (pH < 7,25, plasma bicarbonate <15 mmol/L)
Mild anaemia	Hypoglycaemia (<40 mg/dL), haematocrit >15% (children) and >20% (adults)
Mild thrombocytopenia (important parameter for the staging of severity)	Severe Anaemia (Hb < 5 g/dL)
	Severe thrombocytopenia with spontaneous bleeding

Severe forms of malaria can be fatal in within few days. Causes of death are cerebral malaria, respiratory failure with ADRS and kidney failure. The main reason of these complications is the cyto-adherence ("bonding") of the erythrocytes. It results in a failure of the microcirculation followed by ischaemia of vital organs.

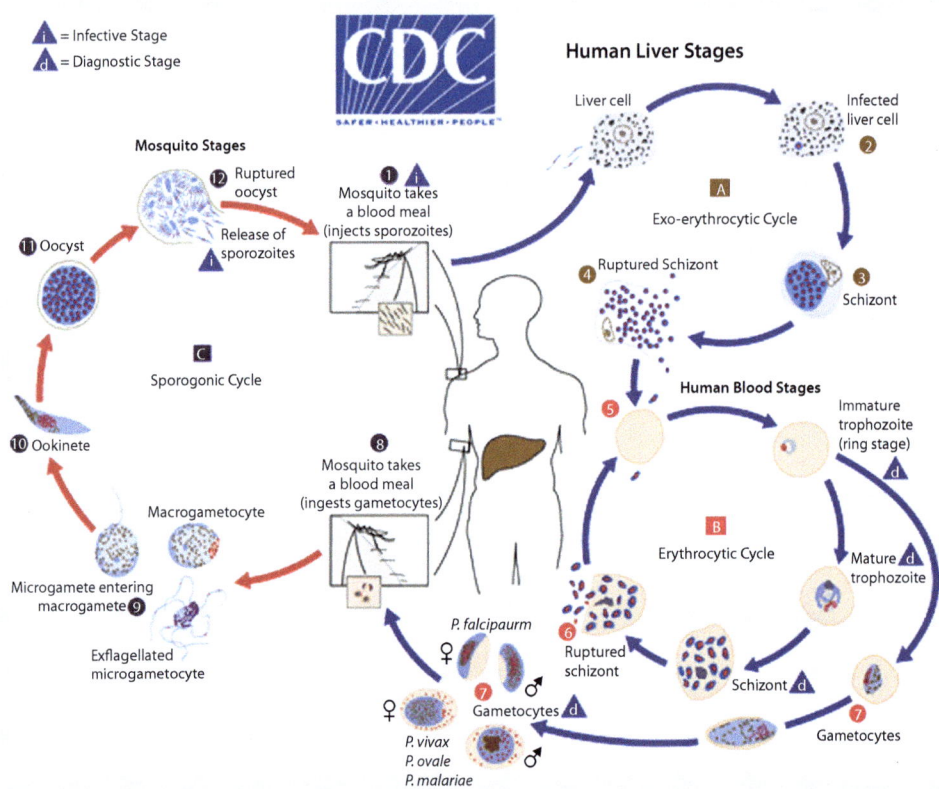

◻ **Fig. 32.1**   Plasmodium life cycle. (CDC)

32.1.3 **Diagnosis**

In case of pyrexia of unknown origin, the patient always should be asked about previous stays overseas. Additionally to the symptoms, a blood test is the most important diagnostic tool. The parasite can be demonstrated using a blood smear and thick drop. A single negative smear does not exclude malaria. A negative smear should be repeated three times within 12–24 h. In the thick drop, existing parasites with a low count can be accumulated and detected. After a positive test, the number of parasites in the erythrocytes should be calculated. A parasite count >2% might be an indication for complicated malaria. A PCR-test for *Plasmodium* DNA is a good diagnostic tool and commonly used. It is slightly more

sensitive than the blood smear. It also allows a discrimination of the malaria species. Another test is the antigen detection. These immunologic tests often use a dipstick or cassette format and provide results within 2–15 min. Hence, they are referred as "Rapid Diagnostic Tests" (RDTs). RDTs should be followed up by microscopy. RDTs and smear microscopy currently provide the best results in testing for malaria. The *Plasmodium* antibody test is not suitable in the initial phase, as antibodies only can be detected after 6–10 days. It is only to retrospectively confirm a previous infection. Regular monitoring of the blood count and renal function and a careful fluid balance is necessary during the treatment of malaria. A CXR may be necessary, if respiratory symptoms are present.

32.1.4 **Treatment**

The treatment depends on the severity and the pathogen. In *complicated malaria*, admission to the intensive care should be considered, if more than one of the following criteria exists:

- Inability of the oral intake of medication
- Parasite load of erythrocytes >2%
- Severe symptoms of malaria (see table above)

The treatment options of complicated malaria are:

- *Artesunate* (allowed only in some countries): 2.4 mg/kg/bw iv; first dose on admission, repeated after 12 and 24 h, minimum duration of therapy 24 h and then once a day, till oral therapy is tolerated.
  or
- Combination of quinine + doxycycline or clindamycin.
  - *Quinine:*
    - First dose: 20 mg/kg/bw iv over 4 h or 7 mg/kg/bw iv over 30 min with subsequent administration of 10 mg/kg/bw iv over 4 h.
    - Maintenance therapy: 10 mg/kg/bw iv over 4 h three times a day, beginning 4 h after the completion of the first dose.
    - Exemption: if the patient received three or more doses of quinine in the last 48 h or had an Mefloquine prophylaxis in the last 24 h or received a Mefloquine treatment in the last 3 days. +
  - *Doxycycline*: 100 mg iv twice daily for 7 days (iv or oral)
    or
  - *Clindamycin*:
    - Initial dose: 10 mg/kg/bw
    - Maintenance dose: 5 mg/bw every 8 h for 7 days (iv or oral)
- After clinical improvement medication can be changed to a complete cycle of the oral therapy of an uncomplicated malaria (Riamet® or quinine with doxycycline or clindamycin).

Uncomplicated malaria can be handled on the normal ward. Outpatient therapy with close supervision can be considered under the following conditions:

- Parasite load of erythrocytes <1%.
- Age > 12 months.
- No co-morbidity.
- Pregnancy is excluded.
- Ability of oral medication intake.
- *P. falciparum* is excluded.
- Clinically stable under medical therapy for the last 24 h.

A daily blood smear is necessary during treatment to follow the process of the disease. The patient can be discharged from the hospital and continue treatment at home; if oral therapy is tolerated, a clinical improvement is achieved and the parasite count decreases. A week and a month after discharge, blood smears should be repeated. Primaquine as eradication therapy is approved in some countries. It is the only drug that can be used to eliminate hypnozoites, which are the dormant forms of the malaria parasites that occur with *P. ovale* and *P. vivax*. Because primaquine causes haemolysis in G-6-PD deficiency, G-6-PD status prior therapy needs to be established. If an eradication with primaquine is required in patients with G-6-PD deficiency, a dose up to 45 mg weekly for 8 weeks, with monitoring for haemolysis, could be considered. In children methaemoglobinaemia can be provoked by giving primaquine. A single dose of primaquine 45 mg for *P. falciparum*, *P malaria* and *P. knowlesi* can be given to sterilise the gametocytes. If malaria caused by *P. vivax* or *P. ovale* or co-infection with these parasites is suspected, a 14-day treatment with 15 mg of primaquine twice a day is recommended.

Treatment of uncomplicated malaria:

- Artemether 20 *mg* + *Lumefantrine 120 mg* (*Riamet®*): four tablets (appropriate dose for children, 5–14 kg; one tablet; 15–24 kg, two tablets; 25–34 kg, three tablets) in following time interval: 0, 8, 24, 36, 48 and 60 h; for *P. falciparum*, site of action: inhibits nucleic acid and protein synthesis

or
- *Atovaquone 250 mg* + Proguanil 100 *mg (Malarone®):* four tablets (appropriate dose for children: 11–20 kg, one tablet; 21–30 kg, two tablets; 31–40 kg, three tablets) with a high-fat meal or milk daily for 3 days; for *P. vivax* (Papua New Guinea and Indonesia) and *P. falciparum*; site of action: inhibits metabolic enzymes and thus the growth of parasite

or
- *Mefloquine (Lariam®):* first dose 750 mg, second dose 500 mg (6–8 h after the first dose), third dose 250 mg (only at bw > 60 kg, 6–8 h after the second dose); for *P. falciparum* and *P. vivax*; site of action: schizoid

or
- *Chloroquine*: Dose first day 10 mg/kg/bw, second day 10 mg/kg/bw, third day 5 mg/kg/bw; for *P. malariae, P. knowlesi* and *P. falciparum* (if there is no chloroquine resistance); site of action: erythrocytic, unknown mechanism

or
- *Chloroquine + primaquine* (with normal G-6-PD)
    - Chloroquine: Dose first day 10 mg/kg/bw, second day 10 mg/kg/bw, third day 5 mg/kg/bw; site of action: erythrocytes
    - Primaquine: 15 mg twice a day for 14 days (adults), 0.25–0.5 mg/kg/bw daily for 14 days (children); *P. Ovale* and *P. vivax* (all countries except Papua New Guinea or Indonesia and no chloroquine resistance); site of action: extra-erythrocytic inhibits plasmodium mitochondria

    or
- *Combination therapy* (except for patients, who had Malarone® as prophylaxis); for *P. Falciparum* and *P. vivax* (Papua New Guinea and Indonesia)
    - *Quininsulfat*: 600 mg (children 10 mg/kg/bw) three times a day for 7 days; site of action: unknown, probably inhibits the *Plasmodium* DNA transcription/replication

+
- *Doxycycline*: 100 mg twice a day *or* clindamycin 300 mg (children 5 mg/kg/bw) three times a day for 7 days; site of action: probably inhibits the dissociation of peptidyl t-RNA at the ribosome, inhibits protein synthesis by binding onto the 50 s ribosome subunit

or
- *Clindamycin* 20 mg/kg/bw three times daily for 7 days; site of action: inhibits protein synthesis by binding onto the 30 s and 50 s ribosome subunit

32.1.5 Prophylaxis

- **Exposure Prophylaxis**

Before commencing holidays overseas, medical advice should be given in order to assess the malaria risk of the particular country. In nearly all tropical areas, there is a risk of getting infected with malaria. In some tourist areas, this risk might be small, but infection is still possible. In particular day trips to more remote areas pose a risk. Some areas have malaria outbreaks and therefore should be avoided. In general, mosquito bites should be avoided to minimise the risk of any mosquito-borne infections. Mosquitoes transmitting malaria are mainly active at night, sunrise and sunset. However, mosquito bites are also possible throughout the day. Long-sleeved shirts, long pants and closed shoes cover the skin and provide protection against insect bites. Insect repellent for the skin and clothes offer additional protection. Higher concentrations offer better and longer protection. The protection period of a normal insect repellent lasts usually only 1–2 h. Slow release products can prolong the effect. Mosquitoes avoid air-conditioned rooms. So staying in air conditioned rooms itself provides certain protection. Spraying insecticides in rooms and surroundings can be helpful to repel and minimise the quantities of mosquitoes. The bed should be covered with a mosquito net (◘ Fig. 32.2).

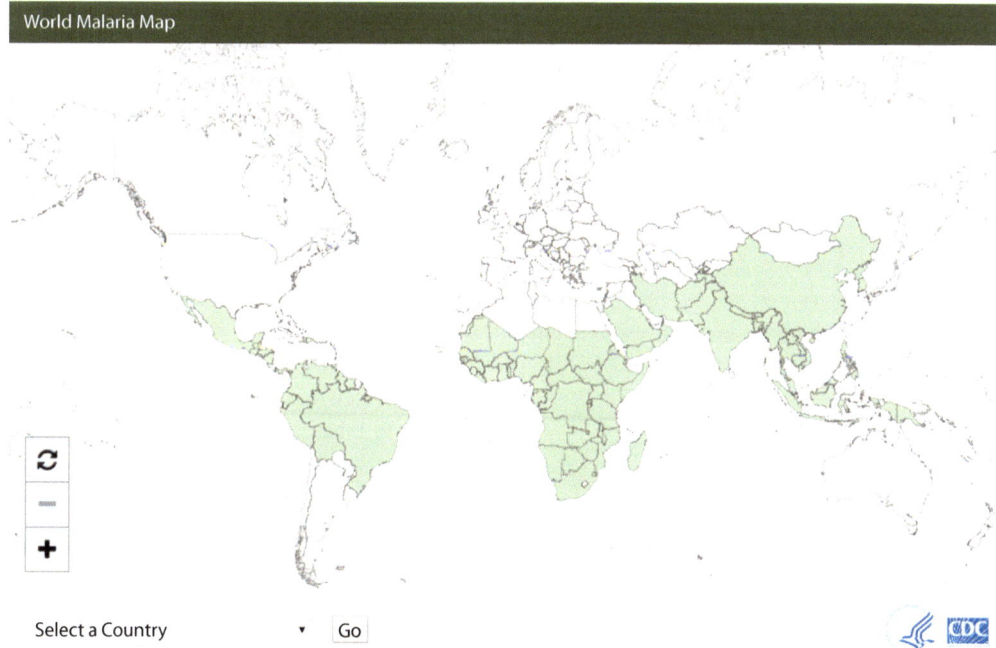

World Malaria Map

Select a Country ▾ Go

◘ **Fig. 32.2** Malaria map. (CDC)

■ **Chemoprophylaxis**

Chemoprophylaxis is important, because the main cause of malaria deaths is still inadequate chemoprophylaxis. There are different drugs for chemoprophylaxis available. They are subject to the travel location and the parasite's resistances to certain drugs. In addition, they differ in side effects, dosage and cost. Except Malarone®, all other drugs for the chemoprophylaxis against malaria have to be taken 4 weeks after leaving the country as they aren't sufficiently effective against the primary liver stages of malaria. Mefloquine (Lariam®) is the only malaria prophylaxis without absolute contraindication in pregnancy.

— *Chloroquine*: schizontocidal; 300 mg (<75 kgbw), 450 mg (>80kgbw)/week; begin 1 week before entering the malaria-endemic country and 4 weeks after return. Adverse reactions: gastrointestinal, photosensitivity, haemolysis (with G-6-PD deficiency), neuropathy (with long-term treatment), cardiomyopathy, eye damage (deposit in the cornea and irreversible retinopathy), narrow therapeutical window

— *Doxycycline*: chemoprophylaxis for *P. falciparum* with Mefloquine resistance, 100 mg/d. Begin 1–2 days before entering the malaria-endemic country and 4 weeks after return. Adverse reactions: gastrointestinal, photosensitivity contraindication, lactation and children <8 years of age

— *Atovaquone + Proguanil* (*Malarone®*): 250/100 mg/d for adults, the dose for children is weight dependent; Begin 1–2 days for entering the malaria-endemic country till 7 days after return; Adverse reactions: gastrointestinal, headaches and vivid dreams

— *Mefloquine* (*Lariam®*): 250 mg/week; long half-life (21 days). Adverse reactions: gastrointestinal, elevation of transaminases, psychiatric (anxiety, agitation, depression, vivid dreams, hallucinations, seizures, suicidal ideations), AV-block, bradycardia, leuco- and thrombocytopenia, rash, alopecia, extrasystoly; contraindication for diving (decrease in vigilance); 2–3 weeks (at least 1 week) before entering the malaria-endemic country and 4 weeks after return; Lariam® is a category B medication and is the only medication against malaria without absolute contraindication in pregnancy. The use in the first trimester should only be considered, if the expected benefits justify the potential risk to the foetus. However, recent studies suggest that even in the first trimester this medication is safe to take.

32.2   Other Mosquito-Borne Diseases

32.2.1   Dengue

■ **Introduction**

The dengue virus is an arbovirus. It has four different serotypes (DENV 1–4). Dengue has a worldwide distribution in the tropics and subtropics, especially in Asia and South America. Approximately 50–100 million cases and about 100,000 with serious complications per year occur. There is a 10% mortality, which can be reduced to 1% with timely diagnosis and appropriate treatment. It has an increased risk for children under 15 years and persons with previous dengue infections. The dengue virus is transmitted by the Aedes aegypti mosquitoes. These mosquitoes mainly bite at day and in twilight (■ Fig. 32.3).

■ **Symptoms**

The incubation period is 2–10 days. There is a wide range in severity of dengue symptoms. The majority of infections cause minor symptoms. But dengue infections can be also quite severe (■ Table 32.3). In particular recurrent infections with dengue are associated with complications and severity of the disease. It is important for the treating doctor to remember that after the initial fever, the critical phase follows. Therefore, the patient must be monitored closely during this time. The disease goes through three stages:

- Fever phase (day 1–3): sudden high fever 40 °C occasional associated with bradycardia; myalgia mainly in the spine, arms and legs ("breakbone fever"), headache; retrobulbar pain; rigors; metallic/bitter taste; vomiting; and dehydration.

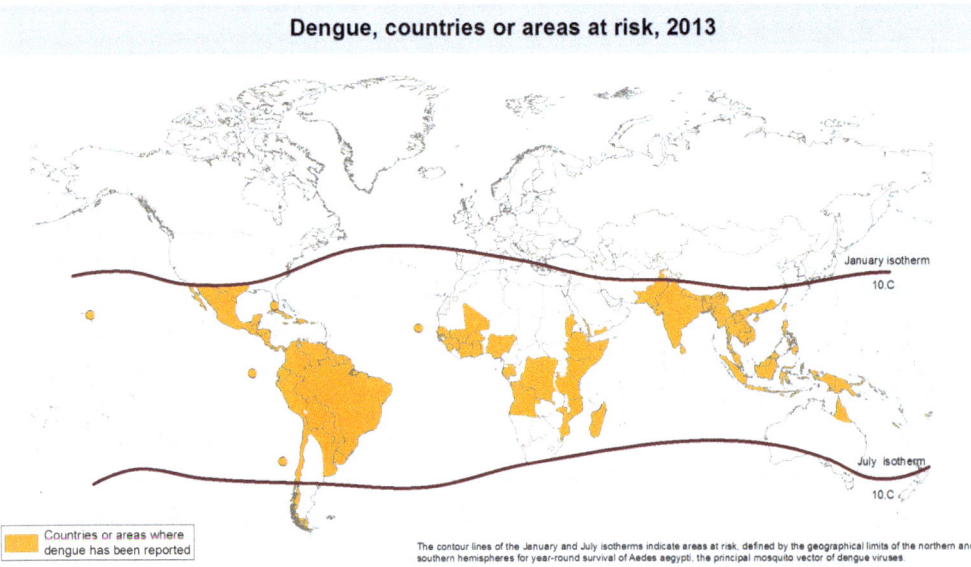

Dengue, countries or areas at risk, 2013

Countries or areas where dengue has been reported

January isotherm 10.C

July isotherm 10.C

The contour lines of the January and July isotherms indicate areas at risk, defined by the geographical limits of the northern and southern hemispheres for year-round survival of Aedes aegypti, the principal mosquito vector of dengue viruses.

■ **Fig. 32.3**   Dengue distribution; 2013 (WHO)

◻ **Table 32.3** Dengue classification

Grade 1	Grade 2	Grade 3	Grade 4
Fever Positive blood pressure cuff test High permeability of the blood vessels Hepatomegaly Thrombocytopenia	Plasma leakage Spontaneous bleeding (skin, epistaxis)	Early shock Disseminated intravascular coagulation (DIC)	Shock Severe bleeding

— Critical phase (day 4–5): normal temperature with possible mild fever later on, leucopenia, exanthema, petechiae and lymphadenopathy. Severe dengue: abdominal pain, spontaneous bleeding, volume shift in to the peritoneal space ("plasma leak"), pleural effusion, hepatomegaly (≥2 cm), rapid increase in haematocrit and decreasing thrombocytes, shock (dengue haemorrhagic shock = DHS or dengue shock syndrome = DSS), increased bleeding (dengue haemorrhagic fever = DHF) and organ failure (particularly liver).

— Remission (after 6 days lasting sometimes for weeks): risk of hyperhydration is given when extravascular fluid is reabsorbed without reducing the intravenous fluid administration. In particular in long remissions, fatigue and depression may be present. Normally there are no long-term damages after a dengue infection, and the vascular changes recover completely.

■ **Treatment**

There is no medication available to treat dengue directly. The diagnosis of dengue can be demonstrated by PCR in the initial phase and using IgM and IgG a few days later. Due to severe complications, the haematocrit, coagulation parameters, leukocytes and platelets have to be tested daily. Thrombocytes <100,000 cells/mm³ can rise the suspicion of DHF. If pleural effusion is suspected, a CXR should be obtained. By tightening a blood pressure cuff petechiae can be provoked (medium pressure of the systolic and diastolic pressure for 5 min). This can be used as a diagnostic tool. An increase of the haematocrit of >20%, pleural effusion, ascites or hypoproteinaemia could be a sign for extravascular fluid loss. The extravascular fluid loss is typically found in the initial phase. Hence, fluid replacement therapy is crucial in this phase. As the extravascular fluid loss can come to an end quite quickly, a complication of the fluid replacement therapy is hyperhydration. Decrease of haematocrit of >20% after fluid administration can represent a fluid excess and hyperhydration. Hence, careful monitoring of the fluid balance and weight are necessary. The therapy is adjusted according to its severity. If necessary, DIC, blood loss or shock require specific treatment.

32.2.2 Chikungunya

Like dengue, Chikungunya is a mosquito-borne disease. The species transmitting the Chikungunya virus (CHIKV) are *Aedes aegypti* in the tropics and subtropics and *Aedes albopictus* in colder regions (◻ Fig. 32.4).

These mosquitoes bite day and night, but mainly in the early morning hours and late afternoon. The incubation period is between 2 and 12 days. The symptoms are similar to that of dengue. Patients suffer from sudden fever with headache, skin rash, fatigue, strong limbs and muscle pain. Affected joints often are swollen. The symptoms generally last for few days but can persist for weeks and years. The disease has no long-term effects. For diagnosis RT-PCR and virological methods can be used in the initial phase. Later, it can be diagnosed by IgM and IgG. IgM peaks after 3–5 weeks and can be detected up to 2 months. The treatment requires analgesia only.

32

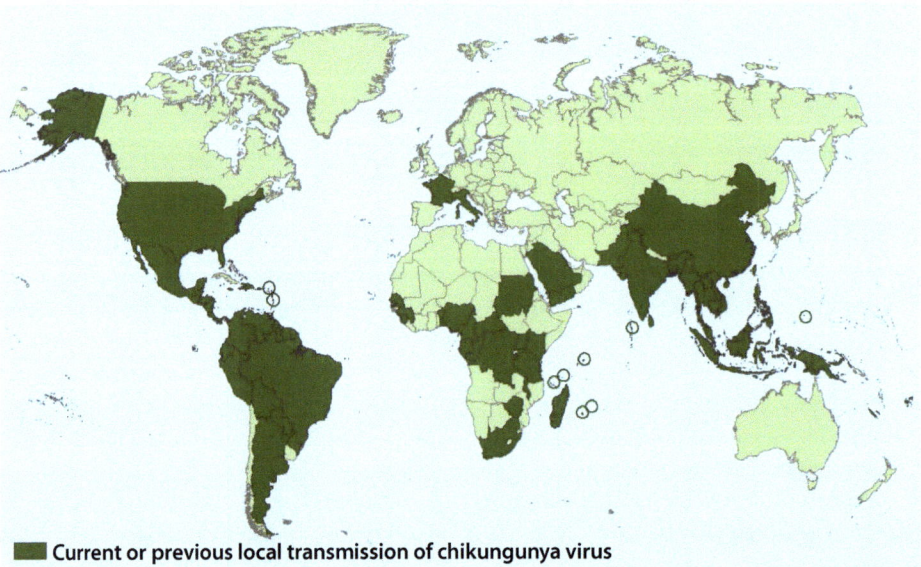

Countries and territories where chikungunya cases have been reported*
(*as of April 22, 2016*)

■ Current or previous local transmission of chikungunya virus

*Does not include countries or territories where only imported cases have been documented. This map is updated weekly if there are new countries or territories that report local chikungunya virus transmission.

Data table: Countries and territories where chikungunya cases have been reported

AFRICA
Benin
Burundi
Cameroon
Central African Republic
Comoros
Dem. Republic of the Congo
Equatorial Guinea
Gabon
Guinea
Kenya
Madagascar
Malawi
Mauritius
Mayotte
Nigeria
Republic of Congo
Reunion
Senegal
Seychelles
Sierra Leone
South Africa
Sudan
Tanzania
Uganda
Zimbabwe

ASIA
Bangladesh
Bhutan
Cambodia
China
India
Indonesia
Laos
Malaysia
Maldives
Myanmar (Burma)
Pakistan
Philippines
Saudi Arabia
Singapore
Sri Lanka
Taiwan
Thailand
Timor
Vietnam
Yemen

EUROPE
France
Italy

AMERICAS
Anguilla
Antigua and Barbuda
Argentina
Aruba
Bahamas
Barbados
Belize
Bolivia
Brazil
British Virgin Islands
Cayman Islands
Colombia
Costa Rica
Curacao
Dominica
Dominican Republic
Ecuador
El Salvador
French Guiana
Grenada
Guadeloupe
Guatemala
Guyana
Haiti
Honduras
Jamaica
Martinique
Mexico
Montserrat

Nicaragua
Panama
Paraguay
Peru
Puerto Rico
Saint Barthelemy
Saint Kitts and Nevis
Saint Lucia
Saint Martin
Saint Vincent & the Grenadines
Sint Maarten
Suriname
Trinidad and Tobago
Turks and Caicos Islands
United States
US Virgin Islands
Venezuela

OCEANIA/PACIFIC ISLANDS
American Samoa
Cook Islands
Federal States of Micronesia
French Polynesia
Kiribati
New Caledonia
Papua New Guinea
Samoa
Tokelau
Tonga

■ **Fig. 32.4**   Distribution of Chikungunya 2015. (CDC)

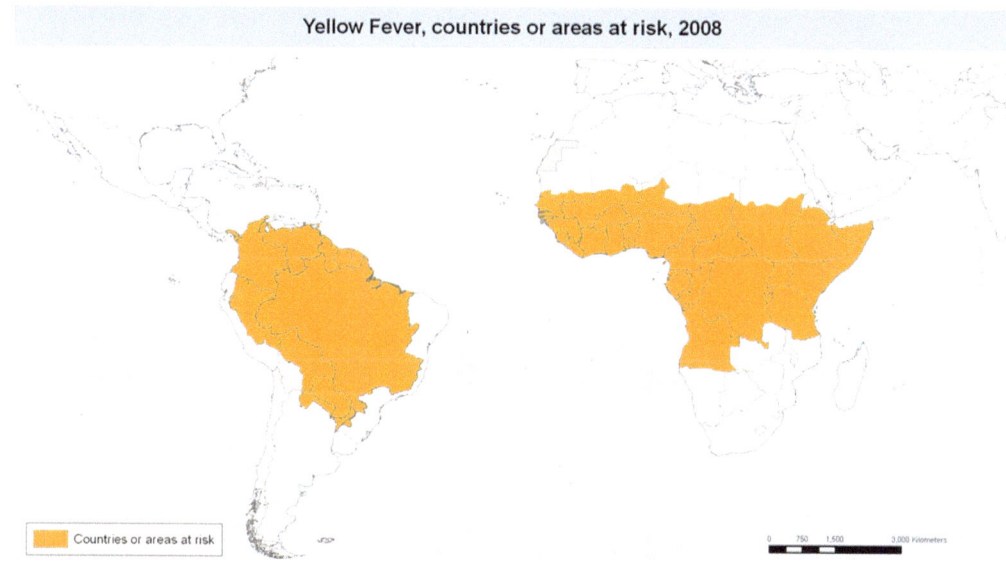

□ **Fig. 32.5**   Yellow fever 2008 (WHO)

32.2.3 **Yellow Fever**

Yellow fever is a disease transmitted mainly by the *Aedes aegypti* mosquito but also by other mosquitoes or ticks. The pathogen is a RNA-containing Flavivirus. It has approximately 200,000 infections with approximately 30,000 deaths annually. 90% of cases occur in Africa and the remaining 10% in South America. The risk of getting infected with yellow fever is with 1:200–2000 in Africa and higher than 1:20000 in South America (□ Fig. 32.5).

The transmission occurs in rainforest areas (jungle or sylvatic cycle), where mosquitoes transfer the virus from monkeys to humans, in endemic areas of the savannah (savannah or intermediate cycle) either transferred from monkeys or human to humans via mosquitoes or in urban areas from human to human via mosquitoes.

The incubation period is 3–6 days. The disease has two phases. The acute phase comes with fever, headache, myalgia, head- and backache, loss of appetite, nausea, vomiting and diarrhoea. The second phase occurs only in approx. 15% of infected humans

within the next 24 h. Jaundice, abdominal pain and vomiting are rapidly developing, followed by diffuse bleeding (epistaxis and GI bleeding) and multi-organ failure (mainly kidneys). If symptoms of the more severe second phase develop, 50% of the patients die within the next 10–15 days. Patients who survive usually recover without significant organ damage.

The diagnosis can be made via a blood or tissue biopsy of the liver. There is no cure for yellow fever and only supportive measures can be taken. However, a very effective life-vaccination (Stamaril®) is available. Only authorised doctors are authorised to prescribe and give the vaccine. Severe side effects of these vaccinations are severe allergic reaction (1:55000), vaccine-associated neurotropic disease/post-vaccinal encephalopathy (1:125000) and vaccine-associated viscerotropic disease/multi-organ failure (1:400000). For travelling into countries where yellow fever is endemic, vaccination is mandatory. The side effects seem to be age-related and occur increasingly with progressive age or in young children. The vaccination is contraindicated in children below 9 month and during pregnancy. Analysis of yellow fever vaccines adverse events demonstrated an increased frequency of serious adverse events in persons age 60 years and older. The risk of viscerotropic side effects in <65 years is 1:400000, in a population of 65–75 years of age 1:40000 and in >75 years of age 1:4000. A failure to be vaccinated or being documented can lead to a refusal of entry into other countries or to a certain time in quarantine when leaving the area where yellow fever occurs. If there is a clinical indication against receiving yellow fever vaccine (e.g. children <9 month or poor immune status), a written medical exemption can be granted, to enable to travel to these countries without vaccination.

Absolute contraindications for a yellow fever vaccination are:

- Allergy against the vaccine or egg protein
- Age < 6 months
- Immunodeficiency
- Neoplasia
- Transplantations
- Immunosuppressive therapies

Relative contraindications for a yellow fever vaccination are:

- Age 6–9 months
- Age > 60
- Asymptomatic HIV infections and CD4+ T lymphocytes 200–499/mm^3 (15–24% of the total in children <6 years of age)
- Pregnancy
- Lactation

32.2.4 Others

Aedes aegypti spreads also the *Zika virus*. However, it is also sexually, intrauterine and perinatal transmitted. Currently the main distribution is countries in South and North America as well as the Caribbean Islands, Singapore and some countries in South Pacific Islands. Symptoms of Zika infection may be fever, rash, arthralgia, myalgia, headache and conjunctivitis. But in most cases, an infection is asymptomatic (~80%). These symptoms are lasting for several days to a week. The incubation period is 3–14 days but is likely to be a few days to a week. The diagnosis can be made via PCR or serology. Blood PCR can be detected only in the first week of the disease. Urine PCR can detect the virus up to 2 weeks. There is no specific treatment available. Deaths are unlikely. There is a potential risk during pregnancy, as microcephaly or other birth defects (~20%) may develop. The Zina virus cane be also transferred via semen and can affect unborn life.

Ross River virus (RRV) is transmitted by the bites of Culex annulirostris, Aedes vigilax, Aedes normanensis and Aedes notoscriptus in Australia, Papua New Guinea, parts of Indonesia and the Western Pacific Islands. The main transmission time is in the humid summer month from December till March. The main symptoms are fever, rash, headache, myalgia, arthralgia and fatigue. The initial symptoms with fever last usually for 1–2 weeks. Myalgia and arthralgia usually last longer. Symptoms of fatigue and depression can be late complications. The incubation time is between 3 days and 3 weeks. The diagnosis is made with IgM. There is only symptomatic treatment available.

Barmah Forest virus (BFV) is transmitted by the same species as the RRV. It mainly can be found in Australia. Many people don't develop any symptoms. The incubation time is 3–11 days. If symptoms appear, they are similar to the one of RRV. The initial symptoms last for 1–2 weeks, and the arthralgia and myalgia may last for 6 months. The diagnosis is made with IgM. There is only symptomatic treatment available.

Sindbis virus (SINV) is related to the Chikungunya virus. It is mainly transmitted via the Culex and Culiseta mosquitoes. It can be found in Europe, Africa, Asia and Oceania. The symptoms and the duration of the symptoms are quite similar to RRV and BFV. The diagnosis is made with IgM. There is only symptomatic treatment available.

The *o'nyong-nyong virus (ONNV)* is related to the Chikungunya virus but is restricted to Africa. It has similar symptoms as the Chikungunya virus but has additionally mainly cervical lymphadenopathy, and the affected joins rarely show signs of an effusion.

32.3 Gastrointestinal Infections

Most of the gastrointestinal tract infections are caused by poor hygienic conditions of the travel destination. Occasionally ingested seawater can cause intestinal infections too. The main transmission routes are either food-borne or by contact. However, the most common cause for gastrointestinal infections is eating contaminated food. Old, warmed up food, salads, unpeeled fruits, poorly cooked food, contaminated water (ice and already opened bottles with refilled water) and ice cream often have substantial quantities of pathogens and pose a risk. Hence, the best protection against GI infections is avoiding contaminated food or drinks. Usually gastrointestinal infections last for a few days and are self-limiting. If diarrhoea contains blood or mucus in combination of high fever for more than 2 days, more thorough assessment is required. Blood and mucus without fever are most likely related to a parasitic disease. If fever is present, it's most likely a bacterial or viral disease. But also climate change by itself or dehydration may be caused by autonomic dysregulation gastrointestinal symptoms such as nausea, weakness, vomiting and diarrhoea.

With dehydration the DCI risk increases. Rehydration and supply of certain electrolytes such as sodium, chloride and potassium are the most important treatments for gastroenteritis. Fatigue is a common associated symptom. Tannins of black tea boiled for more than 10 min might be beneficial for diarrhoea. The consumption of bananas is recommended because of the high content of potassium. But the best options are rehydration preparations in form of drinks, powders or icy poles. Loperamide may slow down the peristaltic and give some relief from diarrhoea. Probiotics may support recovery. A low fibre diet is rec-

ommended in the active phase of diarrhoea. Administration of antibiotics is rarely necessary and indicated. It only is used for serious illnesses or symptoms.

32.3.1 Salmonellosis (Salmonella Typhimurium + Enteritidis)

- Reservoir: poultry or meals prepared with egg
- Incubation: 8–48 h
- Symptoms: fever, vomiting nausea, diarrhoea, occasionally blood and mucous in the stool
- Duration: 4–7 days
- Treatment: symptomatic; azithromycin 1 g OD for 5 days or ciprofloxacin 500 mg BD for 7 days or ceftriaxone 2 g OD

32.3.2 Typhus (Salmonella Typhi + Paratyphi)

- Reservoir: water and food
- Incubation: 1–2 weeks
- Symptoms: headache, myalgia, bradycardia, roseola in the abdominal area, continuous fever 39–40 °C, porridge – like diarrhoea, intestinal bleeding and decrease of the fever after 4 weeks
- Treatment: symptomatic; azithromycin 1 g OD for 5 days or ciprofloxacin 500 mg BD for 7 days or ceftriaxone 2 g OD; vaccination available

32.3.3 Shigellosis

- Reservoir: human, flies, food and faeces
- Incubation: 2–5 days
- Symptoms: fever, diarrhoea, sometimes with blood and mucus in the stool and severe abdominal pain
- Treatment: symptomatic; ciprofloxacin 500 BD for 5 days, norfloxacin 400 mg BD for 5 days or bactrim 160/800 mg BD for 5 days

32.3.4 ETEC (Enterotoxic *E. Coli*)

- Reservoir: food and water
- Incubation: 0–2 days
- Symptoms: mild to severe diarrhoea with fever and blood and mucous in the stool, most common cause for diarrhoea overseas
- Treatment: symptomatic; norfloxacin 400 mg OD and ciprofloxacin 500 mg OD

32.3.5 Amoebiasis (*Entamoeba histolytica*)

- Reservoir: food (particular strawberries) and water
- Incubation: 1–4 weeks
- Symptoms: diarrhoea like raspberry jelly, no fever! Blood and mucous in the stool, risk for developing a liver abscess
- Treatment: symptomatic, asymptomatic carrier, paromomycin 500 mg TDS for 7 days; invasive, tinidazole 2 g OD for 3 days or metronidazole 400 mg TDS for 7 to 10 days

32.3.6 Cholera (*Vibrio cholerae*)

- Reservoir: contaminated food and water
- Incubation: 0–5 days
- Symptoms: often mild GI symptoms, 5–10% develop severe symptom with nausea vomiting, rice water-like diarrhoea and severe dehydration, mortality risk of 25–50%
- Treatment: rehydration, electrolyte substitution; vaccination available; azithromycin 1 g single dose, ciprofloxacin 1 g single dose

32.3.7 Hepatitis A

- Reservoir: food (in particular sea food) and water
- Incubation: 15–50 days
- Symptoms: initial phase (2–7 days) – flulike symptoms, gastrointestinal,

hepatomegaly; hepatic manifestation (4–8 weeks), no jaundice (approx. 70%), jaundice (30%) with dark urine, jaundice, pruritus; hepatitis A has no chronic form, rarely fatal (fatality is age dependent)
- Treatment: symptomatic, bed rest, avoidance of liver toxic substances (alcohol, medication); vaccination available

32.4 Japanese Encephalitis

Japanese encephalitis is caused by a *Flavivirus*, which is transmitted by mosquitoes (*Culex particularly C. tritaeniorhynchus*). The hosts are usually pigs and water birds. In humans there are usually not sufficiently high concentrations of virus to serve as a host. The distribution is the Asia, especially in rural areas. Epidemics occur every 2–15 years (☐ Fig. 32.6).

The transmission can occur throughout the year but frequently peaks in the rainy season. There are about 68,000 cases per year. Only about 1% of the patients are symptomatic. However, if symptoms develop, the mortality rate is 20–30%. Approx. 30–50% of patients who survive have long-term neurological or psychiatric complications. Mild courses of Japanese encephalitis may be accompanied by mild fever and headache. Severe cases show high fever, neck stiffness, photophobia, headache, disorientation, coma, convulsions, spastic paralysis or death. Consequential damages may be behavioural disorders, convulsions, paralysis and speech disorders. The diagnosis can be established with blood tests and lumbar puncture. There is currently no treatment option. The vaccination is usually well tolerated and available for prophylaxis.

32.5 Other Tropical Diseases

There are various tropical diseases, which are present in poorer countries causing more or less severe symptoms. These diseases are termed "neglected tropical diseases" (NTD). The more common NTDs are summarised in this chapter.

Geographic Distribution of Japanese Encephalitis Virus

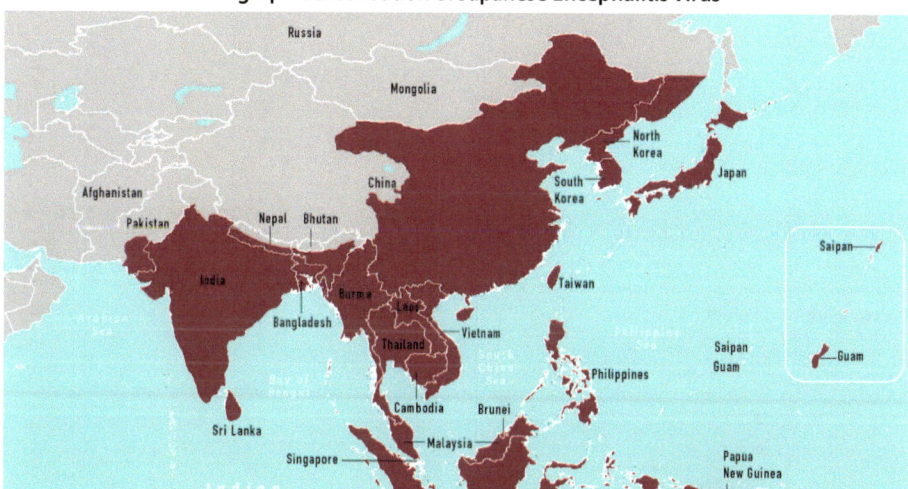

Data Table: Countries in which Japanese encephalitis virus has been identified			
Australia	India	Pakistan	Sri Lanka
Bangladesh	Indonesia	Papua New Guinea	Taiwan
Brunei*	Japan	Philippines	Thailand
Burma	Laos	Russia	Timor-Leste
Cambodia	Malaysia	Saipan	Vietnam
China	Nepal	Singapore	
Guam	North Korea	South Korea	

*No data but presumed to be endemic.

☐ **Fig. 32.6** Japanese encephalitis 2007. (CDC)

32.5.1 Trypanosomiasis

There are three main conditions caused by these pathogens.

The *African trypanosomiasis (sleeping sickness)* is transmitted by the tsetse fly. The distribution is only in some countries of the sub-Saharan Africa. Seventy percent occur in the Democratic Republic of Congo.

Tsetse flies are mainly found in rural areas. There are two forms causing sleeping sickness, *T. brucei rhodesiense* and *T. brucei gambiense*. *T. brucei gambiense* has an incubation period of months to years and *T. brucei rhodesiense* weeks to months. The initial phase is the haemolytic-lymphatic phase, in which pathogens replicate in tissues, blood and lymphatic tissues. Symptoms are intermittent fever, headache, myalgia and pruritus. Additionally, a painless, indurated chancre on the skin 5–15 days after the bite and lymphadenopathy (axillary and inguinal) can be associated. In the second phase, the CNS affected causes continuous headache, behavioural disorders (mood swings and depression), delirium, sensitivity disorders, coordination problems and disruptions of the sleeping cycle (daytime somnolence). The diagnosis is mainly made clinically. Only for the T. b. rhodesiense, a blood test (centrifuged or wet preparation) to

■ **Table 32.4**   Treatment of sleeping sickness

Species	Drug of choice	Adult dosage
T. brucei rhodesiense, haemolymphatic stage	Suramin	1 gm IV on days 1, 3, 5, 14 and 21
T. brucei rhodesiense, CNS involvement	Melarsoprol	2–3.6 mg/kg/day IV × 3 days. After 7 days, 3.6 mg/kg/day × 3 days. Give a third series of 3.6 mg/kg/d after 7 days.
T. brucei gambiense, haemolymphatic stage	Pentamidine	4 mg/kg/day IM or IV × 7–10 days
T. brucei gambiense, CNS involvement	Eflornithine	400 mg/kg/day in 4 doses × 14 days

detect the parasite is available. Examination of buffy coat increases sensitivity. A biopsy of the lymph node to detect the pathogens can be diagnostic for *T. brunei gambiense* or be used for a culture and PCR. The card agglutination test for trypanosomiasis (CATT) is a field test suitable for mass population screening in endemic areas for T. b. gambienses but has a low specificity and is hence only used for identifying suspected cases. All diagnosed patients need to have their cerebrospinal fluid examined for staging, which influences treatment options (■ Table 32.4). The treatment is dependent on the pathogen and the staging. If untreated, infections of both forms lead to coma and death.

Leishmaniasis has three forms: visceral, cutaneous and mucosal (Kala-Azar). There are about 30 different pathogens, from which approx. 20 are held responsible for these diseases. The disease is transmitted by mosquitoes or sandflies (*Phlebotomus* and *Lutzomyia*). The cutaneous form is the most common one, which causes skin ulcerations. Typically this form appears weeks to months after the initial mosquito bite. Initially papules are formed, which later ulcerate. They can be painful or painless. The visceral form affects organs, especially the liver, spleen and bone marrow. Therefore, this form can be quite dangerous. The changes occur within months and years. Hepatosplenomegaly and

pancytopenia develop. The mucus form is rare. Ulcerative changes of the mucous membranes (e.g. nose, mouth and throat) are typical for this. Endemic areas for leishmaniasis are East Africa, some Arabic countries, India, Bangladesh, Brazil and some other South American countries. Historically, the diagnosis was made by taking a biopsy (skin, bone marrow or other tissues) for culture. Now PCR or serological testing with high sensitivity replaced biopsies for making diagnosis. As the visceral disease is fatal without treatment, it needs to be treated in any case. All other forms require normally no treatment. Following medication is available:

- Pentavalent antimonial (Sb^V) compounds (20 mg per day IV or IM for 28 days)
- Liposomal amphotericin B (3 mg OD IV on day 1–5, 14 and 21)
- Miltefosine (in adults > 45 kg 50 mg 3 times daily for 28 days)
- Azoles (fluconazole 200 mg OD for 6 weeks, itraconazole 200 mg BD for 28 days, ketoconazole 600 mg OD for at least 28 days)
- Paromomycin (uncommonly used)
- Pentamidine isethionate (uncommonly used)

The *Chagas' disease* is transmitted via an insect bite ("kissing bug") or by contaminated food. It occurs in Central and South America. It has

Table 32.5	Treatment of Chagas' disease	
Drug	Age group	Dosage and duration
Benznidazole	<12 years	5–7.5 mg/kg per day orally in two divided doses for 60 days
	12 years or older	5–7 mg/kg per day orally in two divided doses (max 300 mg/d) for 60 days
Nifurtimox	≤10 years	15–20 mg/kg per day orally in three or four divided doses for 90 days
	11–16 years	12.5–15 mg/kg per day orally in three or four divided doses for 90 days
	17 years or older	8–10 mg/kg per day orally in three or four divided doses for 90 days

an acute and chronic phase. In the acute phase within 1–2 weeks after the infection, localised swelling of the area of the insect bite (skin or mucous membranes), lymphadenopathy, bilateral orbital oedema, meningoencephalitis and myocarditis can occur. 20–30% of all infections become chronic, causing arrhythmias with risk of "sudden death", cardiomyopathy and enlargement of the oesophagus (megaoesophagus) or of the colon (megacolon) even after years or decades. The cardiomyopathy consists of fibrosing myocarditis, causing arrhythmia (RBBB, left anterior fascicular block, ST changes, premature ventricular beats and bradycardia) and ventricular failure. The diagnosis in the acute phase is made by a blood smear (thick and thin) to visualise the parasite. A serological test is also available.

Treatment is recommended in the acute phase and in patient up to the age of 50 and no advanced cardiomyopathy with chronic Chagas' disease (■ Table 32.5). In age groups above 50, benefits and risk need to be outweighed.

32.5.2 Helmetides

Worm infections are a major problem in underdeveloped countries. They occur mainly in rural areas. These conditions may cause insignificant symptoms but also lead to serious consequences or even cause death. Because

some dive sites are located far away from tourist centres, these infections should be discussed before travelling.

■ **Ascariasis (Roundworm)**

This kind of roundworm is found in the tropical and subtropical regions of Africa and Southeast Asia. The transfer follows on oral intake of eggs by contaminated food. The larvae are entering the bloodstream after hatching in the intestine. They reach the lungs via the blood and penetrate the lung tissue, and the larvae can be coughed up. If the sputum is swallowed again, the larvae reach the intestine, mature there within the next 2–3 months and lay eggs, which are then excreted via the faeces. The adult worms live about 1–2 years. Infection is usually asymptomatic. However, abdominal pain, flulike symptoms, allergic skin manifestations, malnutrition, productive cough and a stridor can occur. The diagnosis can be made by examining the faeces (eggs, worms) or sputum (larvae).

■ **Ancylostomiasis (Hookworm)**

Hookworms are found in tropical and subtropical regions of Africa and Latin America. The transmission is percutaneously or orally by ingestion of contaminated soil. In contaminated soil the larva is able to survive for about 3–4 weeks. Larvae can penetrate the skin and enter the blood and reach the alveoli in the

32

lungs. From there they ascend in the airways, are swallowed again and finally get into the intestines. There larvae mature to adult worms. The worms attach themselves to the wall of the intestine and feed on blood. The eggs are excreted in the faeces and reach again the soil. The eggs can survive up to 2 years. Common symptoms are pruritus and rash at the entry site, abdominal pain, diarrhoea, weight loss, anaemia and extreme fatigue. The diagnosis can be made of the faeces.

■ **Filariasis**

Filariasis has a worldwide distribution in tropical and subtropical regions. It is caused by *Wuchereria bancrofti* and *Brugia malayi*. It is transmitted by mosquitoes. The infective filariform grow inside mosquitoes and enter via its saliva during the bite. They migrate to the lymphatic vessels and lymph nodes where they develop into adults. They can live there for about 6 years. The female worms produce microfila, which are circulating in the blood. Absorbed by mosquitoes they develop within 1–2 weeks to the infective filariform. Initially there are no symptoms. Later lymph oedema in extremities or genitals is a common symptom. In men hydrocele can develop. The skin typically swells and hardens ("elephantiasis"). The diagnosis is made via the blood. Detection in the blood smear has to be performed at night, as larvae only circulate in the blood at night. There is also a serological detection of anti-filaria IgG4 available for diagnosis. The treatment with DEC is the drug of choice. Concurrent disease of Loa Loa or onchocerciasis is a contraindication for DEC, because of the serious side effects (encephalopathy and deaths). Ivermectin is used as a prophylaxis, but not as a therapy.

■ **Schistosomiasis (Bilharziose)**

Schistosomiasis can be found in tropical and subtropical regions worldwide. In addition to malaria, it is the most common parasitic disease. The parasite schistosoma is housed in freshwater snails. By being exposed to freshwater in these regions, infections can occur. The eggs are excreted in urine or faeces of the host. They hatch under optimal conditions and release miracidia. These miracidia infect freshwater snails and develop into sporocysts. These develop into cercariae and get released into the water, where they can penetrate the skin of the host. There, they shed their tail and become schistosomulae and migrate to the liver. In the liver they mature into adults. The paired adult worms migrate to the bowel and bladder, where they lay the eggs. A rash ("swimmers itch") may develop at the entry site on the skin. Suprapubic pain and haematuria, abdominal pain, myalgia, fever, swelling of the lymph nodes, liver and spleen enlargement and eosinophilia can be additional symptoms. The risk of bladder cancer is increased with schistosomiasis. The diagnosis can be made in the stool and urine. The maximum excretion of eggs in the urine is between 12 and 3 pm.

■ **Trichuriasis (Whipworm)**

Whipworms have a worldwide distribution in the humid tropics. The eggs are orally absorbed via soil or unwashed vegetables or fruits. The whipworm grows in the large intestine. The eggs are excreted via the faeces. In the soil the eggs pass through various stages before getting absorbed again. The symptoms are abdominal pain, chronic diarrhoea, nausea, vomiting, inflammation of the intestine, anaemia and eosinophilia. The diagnosis is made with a stool sample. The treatment on the infection is dependent on the parasite (◘ Table 32.6).

32.5.3 **Leptospirosis**

Leptospirae are long, motile spirochetes. They have a worldwide distribution, but infections occur more commonly in tropical and subtropical regions. They spread through infected urine, which enters water or soil. Leptospires can survive for several weeks and

■ **Table 32.6** Overview over the common tropical worm infestations

Drugs	Ascariasis	Ancylostomiasis	Filariasis	Schistosomiasis	Trichuriasis
Albendazole single dose 400 mg	x	x			x
Mebendazole 100 mq/d for 3 days or single dose 500 mg	x	x			x
Ivermectin single dose 200 μg/kg/bw	x				x
Diethylcarbamazine (DEC) 6 mg/kg/bw/d for 1–12 days			x		
Pyrantel 11 mg/kg/bw For 3 days (max. 1 g)		x			
Praziquantel twice daily for one days 4 h apart, 40^a or 60^b mg/kg/bw				x	

[a]For S. Mansoni, S. Haematobium, S. Intercalatum; [b]for S. Japonicum, S. mekongi

months. Infections can be caused by contact with either direct contact with the urine or other body fluids except saliva as well as with contaminated soil and water. The bacteria enter the body through the skin or mucous membranes. A broken skin increases the risk of infection. Increased risk is after heavy rainfall or flooding. The incubation period is usually 5–14 days, but can range from 2–30 days. Symptoms vary greatly. Usually sudden onset of headaches, fever, chills, myalgia, nausea and vomiting, diarrhoea, rash and jaundice are common signs of the first phase for 3–8 days. If the patient doesn't recover the second phase (Weil's disease) develops, with renal failure, ARDS, hepatomegaly, jaundice, haemorrhage and meningitis. This has a fatality rate of 1–5%. Untreated symptoms can persist for several months. Treatment is either doxycyclin 100 mg BD or benzylpenicillin 1.2 g QID or ceftriaxone 1 g OD for 7 days.

32.5.4 Rickettsial (Spotted and Typhus Fever) and Related Infections (Anaplasmosis and Ehrlichiosis)

Infections caused by *Rickettsia*, *Orienta*, *Ehrlichia*, *Neorickettsia*, *Neoehrlichia* and anaplasma are summarised as Rickettsial infections. Rickettsias are divided into the typhus group and the spotted fever group. Orienta make up the typhus group. The reservoir is found in mainly animals, like rodents, but some species are found in fish. The vector is commonly ticks. In scrub typhus the vectors are larval mites. Others have fleas and lice as a vector. Infection occurs either by bites of the vectors or by direct contact, inoculation or inhalation of contaminated fluids or faeces. The clinical presentation varies. Mild symptoms are headache, myalgia, abdominal pain, cough and rash. Some rickettsial infections,

32

like Rocky Mountains and Brazilian spotted fevers, Mediterranean spotted fever, scrub typhus and endemic typhus, have a fatality rate up to 20–60%. Diagnosis is made clinical and by serology. The treatment should be started early by suspicion as serology reports can take quite some time and a delay in treatment may be fatal. Doxycyclin 100 mg BD for 7 days or azithromycin 500 mg OD at the first day 250 mg OD for further 4 days are the antibiotics of choice.

32.5.5 Q-Fever

Q-fever is a zoonosis caused by the protozoa *Coxiella burnetii*. The bacterium is quite resilient due to its sporelike life cycle and remains virulent for months even up to more than a year. The primary reservoir is cattle, goats, sheep and other wildlife like kangaroos, rats and cats. Rarely is it transmitted by tick bites or by ingestion of unpasteurised milk or dairy products. The incubation time is usually 2–3 weeks but can range from 2 days to 6 weeks. The initial acute Q-fever comes with sudden onset of high fever up to 40 °C, headache (retrobulbar), myalgia, chills, non-productive cough and sweats. The symptoms settle within 5–14 days. 50% of all infections are however asymptomatic. Often thrombocytopenia and abnormal LFTs are found. Complications are ARDS, endocarditis and meningoencephalitis. The diagnosis is based on detecting phase II and phase I antibodies (IgG) 4 weeks apart. The initial test (phase II) should be taken at the end of the first week of illness. IgM and IgG rise almost at the same time. A fourfold rise is diagnostic. An initial negative titre doesn't rule out Q-fever. Seroconversion occurs usually between days 7 and 15 but is almost always present by 21 days. PCR testing can be used in the first 2 weeks but before antibiotic administration. However, a negative PCR result doesn't rule out Q-fever. Chronic Q-fever develops in 0.2–4%. It can result in endocarditis, aneurysms, osteomyelitis, hepatitis, neurogic (mononeuritis, optic neuritis), pulmonary (interstitial fibrosis, pseudotu-

mor) and renal (glomerulonephritis) disease. Chronic Q-fever usually develops shortly after the infection. However, chronic endocarditis may not come apparent until 2–4 years or even longer. Chronic fatigue syndrome is described in approx. 10%. Typically in chronic Q-fever, the initial IgG titre is increasing (>1:800). The treatment for acute Q-fever is doxycyclin 100 mg BD for 14 days or for at least 3 days after fever subsides and until clinical improvement. As serological confirmation takes time, treatment should not be delayed. Early treatment is effective at preventing severe complications. For chronic Q-fever, 18 months of doxycyclin 100 mg BD and hydroxychloroquine 200 mg TDS is recommended as standard treatment.

32.6 Rabies

Rabies has an almost worldwide distribution. More than 95% of deaths occur in Africa and Asia. About 40% are children under 15 years of age. Dogs are the main vectors. In Asia, there is also a risk of transmission through monkeys. In addition to other diseases, like the Lyssavirus, bats or flying foxes can transfer rabies. It is transmitted by bites or scratch wounds but also by inoculation of saliva onto mucous membranes or eye of an infected animal. Thorough cleaning of the wound and vaccination within hours can prevent the disease.

The incubation period is usually 1–3 months but can be less than 1 week and more than a year. Initial symptoms include paraesthesia in the wound area. The disease can pass in two forms. The *hyperactive* form (70%) shows up with hyperactivity, manic behaviour, paranoia, hallucinations, delirium, hydrophobicity and occasionally aerophobia (triggered by the extremely painful spasms in the larynx area). The *paralytic form* (30%) is characterised by a slow but steady increasing paralysis. The paralysis begins in the area of the infection. The diagnostics can be established on the animal that has inflicted the wound. The tissue samples of the animal are taken from the brain (brainstem and cerebellum). The diagnosis in humans is difficult and unreliable. Investigation of blood (antibodies), saliva (PCR), spinal fluid (antibodies) and skin biopsies (rabies Antigen) are available. The vaccine and the immune globulin can be given during pregnancy. Typical side effects of the vaccine are headache, myalgia, malaise, fatigue and nausea.

Treatment after potential infection (post-exposure prophylaxis PEP) includes:

- Irrigation of the wound for a minimum of 15 min and washing of the wound with water, soap, iodine or other disinfecting substances
- Rabies vaccine
- Rabies immunoglobulin into the wound area within 7 days after the first vaccination

Following data should be recorded when a rabies vaccine is given overseas:

- Address, email and telephone of the practice or hospital
- Date of vaccinations
- Batch number, name of the vaccine and manufacturer
- How many vaccinations are given
- Application: subcutaneous or intramuscular injection

WHO recommends the following approach with potential rabies after animal contact:

- *Category 1*: Feeding of animals, touching animals or being licked at the intact skin; no PEP
- *Category 2*: Nibble of unprotected skin, minor scratches without bleeding; immediate PEP and rabies vaccination
- *Category 3*: Single or multiple bites (transdermal), scratches, licking of open wounds, mucous membrane contact with saliva, contact with bats or fruit bats; instant PEP, rabies vaccination and rabies immunoglobulin

Vaccination against rabies is recommended for:

- Travellers, who for more than 1 month in areas, in which rabies is present

- Professions that deal with bats or fruit bats
- Professions, in which might get with rabies in contact (e.g., veterinary surgeon or nurse)
- Laboratory workers who handle objects with rabies or Lyssavirus
- After animal contact category 2 + 3

Pre-exposure prophylaxis (PreP) includes three vaccinations on day 0, 7 and 21–28. The dose is 0.1 ml intramuscularly or subcutaneously. The vaccination lasts for 10 years. Follow-up vaccinations (post-exposure prophylaxis = PEP) include four vaccinations on day 0, 3, 7 and 14. The dose is 1.0 ml intramuscularly. Immunocompromised patients should receive five vaccinations with an additional vaccination on the 28th day. With previous vaccinations, two vaccinations are recommended on day 0 and 3 after exposure. It is not recommended to change the brand or the manufacturer during the course of vaccinations. However, it is possible, if that particular vaccine is not available. Immunoglobulin should be administered with the first vaccination. The dose is 20 IU/kgbw. The immunoglobulin preferably should be given in proximity of the wound. The immunoglobulin can be diluted, if the wounds is large, to enable to cover the entire wound area. The immunoglobulin is not recommended, if the first vaccination was given more than 7 days ago, if PreP or PEP was completed or if an adequate serologic detection of VNAb titres (≥ 0.5 IU/ml) is present.

To avoid infection, no animals should be fed. Bringing your own food or carrying items like handbags, water bottles, etc. should be avoided, if you stay in the range of monkeys. Distance should be maintained to stray cats and dogs.

32.7 **MERS**

The Middle East respiratory syndrome (MERS) is caused by a corona virus. Corona viruses can cause mild flulike symptoms but also severe symptoms like the severe acute respiratory syndrome (SARS). The MERS-CoV occurs mainly on the Arabian Peninsula (Iran, Jordan, Kuwait, Lebanon, Oman, Qatar, Saudi Arabia, United Arab Emirates and Yemen). But through international travel, it can spread worldwide. Recently it resulted in some cases in Korea. MERS has 37% mortality. The disease is transmitted through droplets or direct contact. The MERS-CoV also has a wide range of symptoms, from mild common cold symptoms and infections of the upper respiratory tract to a rapidly progressive pneumonitis, respiratory failure, septic shock and multi-organ failure. It seems the MERS-CoV has a low virulence, since the transmission occurs usually only through close contact by human to human, such as the care of a person suffering from MERS. Camels seem to be the original reservoir. Mild forms with fever and mild respiratory symptoms, MERS should be considered, if close contact with infected people existed prior to these symptoms.

MERS can be asymptomatic but also lead to respiratory failure and death. Typical symptoms include fever, cough and shortness of breath. Pneumonia or pneumonitis is often associated with MERS. Sometimes gastrointestinal symptoms such as diarrhoea and vomiting can occur. It has a high mortality of 36%. The treatment depends on the severity of the disease. Caution in contact with camels in affected countries should be taken. Eating insufficient heated camel meat and milk should be avoided.

A suspicion of MERS should be considered in individuals with the following risk profile:

- Fever and pneumonia/pneumonitis and stay in endemic areas or contact with a symptomatic person from an endemic area within 14 days before onset of symptoms
- Fever and pneumonia/pneumonitis and hospitalisation in endemic areas or contact with camels and camel products in an endemic area within 14 days before onset of symptoms
- Fever and pneumonia/pneumonitis and contact with a MERS diseased person within 14 days before onset of symptoms
- Cluster of patient (especially medical personnel) with severe respiratory symptoms with unclear aetiology

32.8 Tuberculosis (TB)

Tuberculosis is caused by an acid-resistant *Mycobacterium*. *M. tuberculosis* is responsible for tuberculosis in more than 95%. It has global distribution but occurs more frequently in countries with low hygienic standards. Tuberculosis spreads around the globe through international travel and immigration. It also shows a rising rate of resistances to conventional therapies. The time between the initial infection and tuberculin conversion takes approx. 8 weeks. The transmission is caused by droplets. Initial infections can be asymptomatic or cause unspecific symptoms such as cough, night sweats, loss of appetite, fatigue or erythema nodosum. People with normal immunity develop symptoms of tuberculosis only to 10%. The initial infection usually turns into latent tuberculosis. Tuberculosis can affect other organs to approximately 20%. The latent tuberculosis can be reactivated at a later stage when the immune system is weakened. The tuberculosis has three stages:

- *Exudative stage:* Caseation with cavern formation or caseous pneumonia
- *Productive stage:* Tubercle formation
- *Secondary changes:* Scarring and calcification

Complications of primary infection are hilum lymph node tuberculosis, pleurisy, miliary tuberculosis, caseous pneumonia and Landouzy sepsis (usually only people with immunodeficiency).

The diagnosis can be made with the tuberculin skin test (TST/Mendel Mantoux). 3 days after the strictly intradermal injection of the substance, the induration at the injection site is measured. An induration of >5 mm may be suggestive of tuberculosis. It is considered a positive test if either the patient has a radiological proof, had close contact with someone with tuberculosis, and has symptoms of tuberculosis, is HIV positive or suffers from immunodeficiency. An induration >10 mm is considered as positive, when the patient who travelled to a country with high TB prevalence is an iv. drug user, homeless and a resident of nursing home or prison and has diabetes mellitus, silicosis, M. Hodgkin's or end-stage renal failure. An induration >15 mm is considered as evidence of tuberculosis without any risk factors or symptoms. The TST can be negative in the first 8 weeks after an infection as well as in patients suffering from miliary tuberculosis, M. Hodgkin, sarcoidosis, viral infections, and lowered immunity, receiving an immunosuppressive therapy or at high age. A false-positive test can occur after multiple TSTs, after vaccination against tuberculosis and infection of other mycobacteria. The interferon-γ test (QuantiFERON® TB gold) offers an alternative testing method. This test has the same sensitivity as the TST but a higher specificity. Moreover, this test is a confirmation test and isn't affected by previous BCG-immunisations. It consists of three parts, the control (to determine the baseline-interferon-γ), mitogen control (determining the ability of an immune response) and antigen detection (detection of prior infections). A CXR may demonstrate caverns or hilar lymph nodes, but is not a diagnostic tool to exclude tuberculosis.

The treatment duration of uncomplicated tuberculosis is 6 months, of complicated tuberculosis 9–12 months (◨ Table 32.7). It's a combination treatment of different drugs.

Medications for the tuberculosis treatment are:

- *Isoniazid*: 5 mg/kgbw, max. 300 mg /d; side effects: elevated serum transaminases, polyneuropathy, prophylaxis to avoid side effects of pyridoxine 40–80 mg/d

- *Rifampicin*: 50 mg/kgbw, max. 600 mg/d; side effects: elevated serum transaminases, cholestasis, anaphylaxis, thrombocytopenia and flu syndrome
- *Pyrazinamide*: 25 mg/kgbw max. 1500–2500 mg/ d; side effects: elevated serum transaminases, hepatitis, nausea, flush, myopathy, arthralgia and hyperurikaemia
- *Ethambutol*: initial 25 mg/kgbw, max. 2500 mg/d; side effects: retrobulbar neuritis

A vaccination BCG vaccine is not recommended due to its side effects and the lack of efficacy.

32.9 Travel Vaccination

All vaccinations should be given 28 days before travelling. Minimum time for a sufficient protection is 2 weeks (◨ Table 32.8).

32.10 Diving Organisations

32.10.1 Description

■ **DAN**

Divers Alert Network (DAN) is a non-profit organisation for divers. They provide medical information and articles, diving insurance, life insurance and travel insurance. They also offer courses, support and research. DAN has an international hotline for support and coordination of diving accidents but also for general medical advice overseas.

■ **EUBS**

European Underwater and Baromedical Society (EUBS) is a European organisation for diving and hyperbaric medicine. They provide guidelines for hyperbaric treatment and training of medical professionals for the hyperbaric medicine.

■ **GETÜM**

The German organisation for diving and hyperbaric medicine is the "Gesellschaft für Tauch- und Überdruckmedizin" (GETÜM).

◨ **Table 32.7** Treatment of uncomplicated and complicated tuberculosis

2 Month	4 Month
Isoniazid	Isoniazid
Rifampicin	Rifampicin
Pyrazinamide	
Ethambutol	

■ **Table 32.8** Travel vaccinations

Vaccine	Combinations	Vaccination schema	Comments
Hepatitis A (e.g. Havrix®)	(Twinrix: Hepatitis A + B, Vivaxim: Hepatitis A + Typhus)	Two vaccinations (0 and 6 month)	
Hepatitis B (e.g. Engerix®)	(Twinrix – hepatitis A + B)	Three vaccinations (0, 2 and 6 month)	
Influenza (e.g. Vaxigrip®)		Annual	Updated influenza A + B
Measles (e.g. MMR-Priorix®)	Measles + mumps + rubella	Two vaccinations (0 and 6 months) no further vaccinations necessary	
Polio (Ipol®)	Boostrix: diphtheria + tetanus + pertussis + polio Infarix: diphtheria + tetanus + pertussis + polio + hepatitis B + *Haemophilus influenzae* Type b	After three vaccination (0, 2 and 6 months) vaccinations every 10 years (only for polio or Boostrix)	
Japanese encephalitis (e.g. Jespect® or Imojev®)		Jespect: two vaccinations 28 days apart, further vaccinations within the two years (between first and second year).	Imojev: Only single dose required (only available in Australia)
Meningococcus (quadrivalent meningococcal conjugate vaccines, e.g. Menveo®, Nimenrix®)		Every 3 or 5 years	Menveo or Nimenrix preferred for protection overseas, Menveo: Meningococcal group A, C, W_{135} and Y conjugate vaccine; Nimenrix Meningococcal group A, C, W_{135} and Y tetanus toxoid conjugate vaccine
Rabies (e.g. Rabipur®)		Three vaccinations (day 0, 7 and 21 or 28) further vaccination with antibody-titre ≥0,5 IE/ml	Post-exposure treatment after vaccination recommended with WHO category II and III; also with I, if it can't be clearly defined: two doses at day 0 and 3
Tuberculosis			Generally not recommended as risk outweighs benefits
Typhus (e.g. Typhim® or Vivaxim®)	Vivaxim: hepatitis A + typhus	Every 3 years	

(continued)

32

▣ Table 32.8 (continued)

Vaccine	Combinations	Vaccination schema	Comments
Cholera (e.g. Dukoral®)		Two doses at least 1 week apart	Commonly not required, protection for approx. 2 years (adults); protection against *Vibrio cholerae* and ETEC
Varicella		2 vaccinations	
Yellow fever (e.g. Stamaril®)		Single dose	Certificate is valid for 10 years, a new vaccination may be required after 10 years to renew the certificate

They provide guidelines for hyperbaric treatment and training of medical professionals for the hyperbaric medicine.

■ **SPUMS**

The South Pacific Underwater Medicine Society (SPUMS) is the organisation for diving and hyperbaric medicine in Australia. They provide guidelines for hyperbaric treatment and training of medical professionals for the hyperbaric medicine.

■ **UHMS**

The Undersea and Hyperbaric Medical Society (UHMS) is the organisation for diving and hyperbaric medicine in the United States. They provide guidelines for hyperbaric treatment and training of medical professionals for the hyperbaric medicine.

■ **VDST**

The organisation for German recreational divers "Verband Deutscher Sporttaucher" (VDST) provides diving curses, information about environmental issues, research, sportive diving activities and an emergency hotline.

32.10.2 Contact Details

— DAN Europe: C/da Padune, 11 – 64026 Roseto – Italy, Tel: +39-085-893-0333, Fax: +39-085-893-0050; Emergency contact: +39-06-4211-8685

— DAN International

America: 6 West Colony Place, Durham, NC 27705 USA, Tel: +1-919-684-2948 or +1-800-446-2671, Fax: +1-919-490-6630, or +1-919-493-3040 (medical); Emergency-Hotline: +1-919-684-9111.

Brazil: 150 – Térreo- Edif. Galleria Plaza, Campinas – SP, CEP: 13091–611, Brazil; Office: Tel: +1-919-684-2948, Emergency-Hotline: +1-919-684-9111.

Japan: Japan Marine Recreation Association, Kowa-Ota-Machi Bldg, 2F, 47 Ota-Machi 4 Chrome Nakaku, Yokohama City, Kagawa 231–0011,Japan; Office: Tel: +81-45-228-3066, F ax: +81-45-228-3063; Emergency-Hotline: +81–3–3812-4999;

Asia-Pacific:PO Box 384, Ashburton, VIC3147, Australia;Office: Tel: +61-3-9886-9166, Fax: +61-3-9886-9155, Emergency-Hotline: 1800-088-200 (inside Australia), +61-8-8212-9242 (outside of Australia).

Southern Africa: Private Bag X197, Halfway House, Midrand 1685, South Africa; Tel: 0860–242-242 (Sharecall in South Africa), +27-11-266-4900 (Int.), Fax: +27-11-312-0054 (Int.); Emergency-Hotline: 0800–020-111 (inside Southern Africa), +27-828-10-60-10 (outside Southern Africa),

- *EUBS*: webmaster@eubs.org
- *GTUEM*: c/o BG-Unfallklinik, Professor-Kuentscher-Str. 8, D-82418 Murnau, Tel: +49-8841-48-2167, Fax +49-8841-48-2166
- *SPUMS*: 630 St Kilda Road, Melbourne, Vic, 3004
- *UHMS*: 631 US Highway 1, Suite 307, North Palm Beach, FL 33408, Tel.: +1-919-490-5140, Fax: +1-919-490-5149
- *VDST*: Berliner Str. 312, 63067 Offenbach, Tel.: +49-699819025, Fax: +496998190298

32.11 Web Links

- *CDC*: ▶ www.cdc.gov
- *DAN*: ▶ www.diversalertnetwork.org
- *DAN Europe*: ▶ www.daneurope.org
- *Emedicine*: ▶ http://emedicine.medscape.com
- *EUBS*: ▶ www.eubs.org
- *GTUEM*: ▶ www.gtuem.org
- *The Rubicon Research Repository*:
  ▶ http://archive.rubicon-foundation.org
- *SPUMS*: ▶ www.spums.org.au
- *UHMS*: ▶ www.uhms.org
- *VDST*: ▶ www.vdst.de
- *WHO*: ▶ www.who.int.

32

Suggested Reading

Ahmed SH. Schisotsomiasis. 2015. At: http://emedicine.medscape.com/article/228392 Accessed 05 July 2015.

Busowski MT. Yellow fever. 2015. At: http://emedicine.medscape.com/article/232244. abgerufen am 30 June 2015.

CDC. Chikungunya virus. 2015. At http://www.cdc.gov/chikungunya/. Accessed 23 June 2015.

CDC. Dengue, unter. 2015. http://www.cdc.gov/Dengue/. Accessed 23 June2015.

CDC. Japanese Encephalitis. 2015. At http://www.cdc.gov/japaneseencephalitis/. Accessed 25 June 2015.

CDC. Malaria, unter. 2015. http://www.cdc.gov/malaria/. Accessed 10 June 2015.

CDC. Middle East Respiratory Syndrome (MERS). 2015. At http://www.cdc.gov/coronavirus/mers/. Accessed 25 Sep 2015.

CDC. Parasites – African Trypamosiasis (also known as Sleeping Sickness). 2015. At http://www.cdc.gov/parasites/sleepingsickness/. Accessed 05 July 2015.

CDC. Parasites – American Trypanosomiasis (also known as Chagas Disease). 2015. At http://www.cdc.gov/parasites/chagas/. Accessed 05 July 2015.

CDC. Parasites – Ascariasis. 2015. At http://www.cdc.gov/parasites/ascariasis/. Accessed 10 July 2015.

CDC. Parasites – Filariasis. 2015. At http://www.cdc.gov/parasites/lymphaticfilariasis/. Accessed 08 July 2015.

CDC. Parasites – Hookworm. 2015. At http://www.cdc.gov/parasites/hookworm/. Accessed 10 July 2015.

CDC. Parasites – Leishmaniasis. 2015. At http://www.cdc.gov/parasites/leishmaniasis/. Accessed 05 July 2015.

CDC. Parasites – Schistosomiasis. 2015. At http://www.cdc.gov/parasites/schistosomiasis/. Accessed 05 July 2015.

CDC. Parasites – Trichuriasis (also known as Whipworm). 2015. At http://www.cdc.gov/parasites/whipworm/. Accessed July 2015.

CDC. Rabies. 2015. http://www.cdc.gov/rabies/. Accessed 15 July 2015.

CDC. Tuberculosis. 2015. http://www.cdc.gov/tb/. Accessed 20 Sep 2015.

CDC.Yellow fever. 2015. http://www.cdc.gov/yellowfever/. Accessed 20 June 2015.

Gompf SG. Rabies. 2015. At: http://emedicine.medscape.com/article/220967. Accessed am 15 July 2015.

Gupta S. Whipworm. 2015. http://emedicine.medscape.com/article/1000631. Accessed 20 June 2015.

Haburchak RD. Hookworm Disease. 2014. http://emedicine.medscape.com/article/218805. Accessed 20 June 2015.

Haburchak RD. Ascariasis. 2015. http://emedicine.medscape.com/article/212510. Accessed 10 June 2015.

Helps SC, Gorman DF. Air embolism of the brain in rabbits pretreated with mechlorethamine. Stroke. 1991;22:351–4.

Hennessy TR, Hempleman HV. An examination of the critical released gas concept in decompression sickness. Proc R Soc London B. 1977;197:299–313.

Herold G, et al. Innere Medizin. 2008.

Jani AA. Japanese Encephalitis. 2015. http://emedicine.medscape.com/article/233802. Accessed 25 June 2015.

MIMS Online (Australia). Accessed 12 Nov 2017.

Natesan SK. Chikungunya Virus. 2015. http://emedicine.medscape.com/article/2225687. Accessed 23 June 2015.

Odero RO. African Trypanosomiasis. 2015. http://emedicine.medscape.com/article/228613. Accessed 05 July 2015.

Salazar DM. Middle East Respiratory Syndrome (MERS). 2015. http://emedicine.medscape.com/article/2218969. Accessed 12 Sep 2015.

Shepherd SM. Dengue. 2015. At: http://emedicine.medscape.com/article/215840. Accessed 23 June 2015.

Stark CG. Leismaniasis. 2014. http://emedicine.medscape.com/article/220298. Accessed 05 June 2015.

Tolan RW. Trypanosomiasis. 2015. http://emedicine.medscape.com/article/1000389. Accessed 05 July 2015.

Wanyangankar S. Filariasis. 2015. http://emedicine.medscape.com/article/217776. Accessed 08 July 2015.

WHO. Malaria. 2015. http://www.who.int/topics/malaria/en/. Accessed 10 June 2015.

WHO. Middle East respiratory syndrome coronavirus (MERS-CoV), unter. 2015. http://www.who.int/emergencies/mers-cov/en/. Accessed 12 Sept 2015.

WHO. Rabies. 2015. http://www.who.int/mediacentre/factsheets/fs099/en/. Accessed 15 July2015.

WHO. Tuberculosis. 2015. http://www.who.int/topics/tuberculosis/en/. Accessed 20 Sept 2015.

Supplementary Information

© Springer International Publishing AG, part of Springer Nature 2018
O. Rusoke-Dierich, *Diving Medicine*, https://doi.org/10.1007/978-3-319-73836-9

Index

A

B